SOCIAL COGNITION

TEXTS IN SOCIAL PSYCHOLOGY

Abraham Tesser, *Editor*

Social Cognition: Understanding Self and Others
Gordon B. Moskowitz

SOCIAL COGNITION

Understanding Self and Others

GORDON B. MOSKOWITZ

THE GUILFORD PRESS
New York   London

© 2005 The Guilford Press
A Division of Guilford Publications, Inc.
72 Spring Street, New York, NY 10012
www.guilford.com

Printed in the United States of America

This book is printed on acid-free paper.

Last digit is print number: 9 8 7 6 5 4 3 2 1

Library of Congress Cataloging-in-Publication Data

Moskowitz, Gordon B.
  Social cognition : understanding self and others / by Gordon B. Moskowitz.
    p. cm.—(Texts in social psychology)
  Includes bibliographical references and index.
  ISBN 1-59385-086-7 (hardcover)—ISBN 1-59385-085-9 (pbk.)
  1. Social perception. I. Title. II. Series.
  BF323.S63M67 2005
  302.'12—dc22
                                                    2004017501

About the Author

Gordon B. Moskowitz, PhD, was drawn to social psychology as an undergraduate at McGill University. He received his PhD from New York University in 1993. While at NYU, he developed interests in impression formation, automaticity, minority influence, accessibility effects, stereotypes, and the effects of goals on each of these processes. Following graduate training, Dr. Moskowitz did a year of postdoctoral study at the Max Planck Institute in Munich. After a year as a faculty member at the University of Konstanz, he then decided to return to the United States and moved to Princeton University, where he was Assistant Professor in the Department of Psychology from 1994 to 2001. In the fall of 2001 Dr. Moskowitz moved to Lehigh University, where he is now Associate Professor in the Department of Psychology. In addition to his research presented in journals such as *Journal of Personality and Social Psychology* and *Journal of Experimental Social Psychology*, Dr. Moskowtiz has edited a book titled *Cognitive Social Psychology*, has served on the editorial boards of several journals, and has been awarded a grant from the National Science Foundation for his research on the control of stereotyping.

Preface

Civilized men have gained notable mastery over energy, matter, and inanimate nature generally, and are rapidly learning to control physical suffering and premature death. But, by contrast, we appear to be living in the Stone Age so far as our handling of human relationships is concerned. Our deficit in social knowledge seems to void at every step our progress in physical knowledge. . . . Gains in medical science are widely negated by the poverty that results from war and from trade barriers erected largely by hatred and fear. At a time when the world as a whole suffers from panic induced by the rival ideologies of east and west, each corner of the earth has its own special burdens of animosity. Moslems distrust non-Moslems. Jews who escaped extermination in Central Europe find themselves in the new State of Israel surrounded by anti-Semitism. Many of the colored people of the world suffer indignities at the hands of whites who invent a fanciful racist doctrine to justify their condescension. . . . Rivalries and hatreds between groups are nothing new. What is new is the fact that technology has brought these groups too close together for comfort. . . . We have not yet learned how to adjust to our new mental and moral proximity.

—ALLPORT (1954, p. xiii)

It has been more than 50 years since Gordon Allport began the preface to his book *The Nature of Prejudice* with the passage above. Although laypersons may still be in what Allport called the "Stone Age" regarding an understanding of "human relationships" and "social knowledge," psychologists have moved a few centuries beyond the Stone Age through the scientific examination of these issues. The advances that have been made are subsumed within the research domain known as *social cognition*.

As I write this, it is August 11, 2004, and I have finished reading the page proofs of this book for the last time. The memorable presidential election of 2000 was just heating up as I started to write this book in the spring of that year. It has been an amazing 4 years, largely spent with my nose buried in my laptop as I wrote and read drafts of chapters. During this time, I have seen my two children, Benjamin and Isaac, born. My wife, Cindy Gooch, and I have moved several times, each changed jobs, purchased our first home, and watched with the rest of the world as our country has tried to find its place among the too many nations who see their borders threatened by horrible violence. I was teaching in the very class that this book will now serve when (unbeknownst to me) my former home, New York City, was under attack. It has been a hectic time, during which this book—and my family—have been my personal constant. Cindy must be thanked at the outset for her amazing patience throughout this process. Few other wives would put up with a husband attempting to add a section on nonverbal behavior to his book while simultaneously timing labor pains. Or reading drafts of chapters on almost every extended car trip or vacation. As might be imagined, both she and I are thrilled that this book is finished. We both are indebted to our parents—Howard and Gerry Moskowitz, and Harold and Joan Gooch—who provided love and lots of support and help with the kids during this time.

What is even more thrilling is to see that, every day, the relevance of the topics discussed in this book continues to be made clear in the media and in our personal lives. Many scientists will claim that their specific area of study is essential to understanding human life. Biologists, chemists, neuroscientists, and physicists will quite appropriately feel that they study the very processes that make life and living possible. But, to me, social psychology (and social cognition in particular) is at the heart of understanding human life, since it explains our social nature—the ways in which we think, act, and feel (and make sense of the world) in relation to each other. And it explains these things not at the level of the neuron, but in the context of the cultures and situations in which we live. It examines the power of others to shape the thoughts, deeds, and feelings of an individual.

Despite my personal fascination with social cognition and its centrality to daily life, why did I write a book about it? In the spring of 1999, I thought my life was going to be slowing down a bit, and against all advice, I decided to occupy myself by writing a book. I had been teaching person perception at Princeton and saw no comprehensive text to accompany the course. The Fiske and Taylor *Social Cognition* book was at that point 8 years old (and I did not know Ziva Kunda had a book about to be released). Thus, with a perceived vacuum in the text market and a great deal of naiveté, I approached Seymour Weingarten at The Guilford Press, and we agreed to do a book.

Prior to deciding to write this book, I had the unusual good fortune of being at two extremely special places—New York University and Princeton University—that together had provided me with a sense of great excitement about the current happenings in social psychology. With that unique perspective, I somehow felt that I had a voice and the experience to take on the task, and felt great enthusiasm about sharing what I had seen and learned from the amazing people who had passed through those institutions during my time there. NYU especially was a place where social cognition grew from being a fringe element at the start of the 1980s to occupying the heart of social psychology by the decade's end, and I was there as the group (both faculty and graduate students) gathered together and bonded to help lead this movement. These mentors at NYU (faculty members such as John Bargh, Shelly Chaiken, Tory Higgins, Yaacov Trope, and Jim Uleman; and older graduate students such as Chuck Stangor, Tim Strauman, Len Newman, Felicia Pratto, and Akiva Liberman), as well as those at Princeton (colleagues such as John Darley, Dale Miller, Joel Cooper, Debbie Prentice, Nancy Cantor, Danny Kahneman, Anne Treisman, and Marcia Johnson) and Peter Gollwitzer at the Max Planck Institute, have provided me with a wonderful experience in the field and given me a dedication and passion for telling the story of social cognition. This book is dedicated to these people who have mentored me and given their energy to inspiring others through great teaching and research.

I want especially to thank those people who have provided critical commentary on this book. Robert Roman, Lee Ross, John Bargh, Serena Chen, Steve Neuberg, Bertram Malle, Doug Krull, Jacquie Vorauer, Neil Macrae, Ap Dijksterhuis, and Jeff Stone each read one chapter and provided fantastic feedback. Jeff Sherman went above and beyond the call of duty and read many of the chapters, providing much-needed encouragement and criticism. Remarkably, Abe Tesser read every chapter, both in first-draft form and in revised form. I am eternally grateful for all the effort he has put into making this book a better product. It was an unusual dedication of time and energy. Finally, two of my Lehigh graduate students, Elizabeth Kirk and Peizhong Li, have read the entire book at various stages. Peizhong, especially, has been my primary collaborator for most of the time I have been working on this book, and has been patient with me and provided excellent feedback. I have been lucky to have had such wonderful students to collaborate with, both at Lehigh and at Princeton. With such luck and good will from others, as well as with the patience of Seymour Weingarten and the folks at The Guilford Press, I attain closure on this project at last.

Contents

Introduction

WHAT DOES IT MEAN
TO "KNOW" SOMETHING?

A fire engine whizzes past your window. You race to the window to see where it is head-ing. Are you concerned for your safety? Perhaps. Worried about the house of the guy down the street? Maybe. Just plain old curious? Most likely. Curiosity regarding strange events and noises is not unique to humans. My cat lifts his head and jumps to react when he hears the same siren. This is an adaptive process essential for survival. We need to detect danger if it is present in order to cope with it, just as we need to approach stimuli that allow us to survive. It is neither our concern with survival nor our concern over the cause of an event that separates us humans from cats. Rather, it is our *ability to reason and to process information about the causes of events* that distinguishes us in this domain. Consider the individuals who escaped from the World Trade Center's sec-ond tower after the first tower had been struck on September 11, 2001. It was only their ability to infer the possible cause of the initial damage (or someone else's inference, which was then conveyed to them through either an order to evacuate the building or a friend's encouragement to evacuate) that allowed them to predict possible danger to their building, thus leading them to flee the (as yet untouched) second tower. This unique ability to reason about causes is one of the defining and most important ele-ments of being human.

As Heider (1944) asserted, each new event that happens in our surroundings is experienced by us as a disruption to our environment. This initiates a process of attempting to figure out the reason for the change in our environment. We attempt to discover *why* the change has occurred—*Why* has the fire engine raced down our street? *Why* has an explosion occurred in Tower 1?—and adjust our actions accordingly. You and I are constantly in pursuit of answers to what we will call *the "why" question*. This is true of the smallest of changes (e.g., a piece of paper falls off your desk) to more complex changes in your environment (e.g., the building next to you is on fire following an explosion). For small changes to your world, the answer to the "why" question may be easily attained (the window was open and a gust of wind has blown the paper). For more complex changes, you may wrestle with finding the answer to the question for quite some time. (There is no rule requiring that complex changes be effortfully analyzed; it is just that when effort does occur, it is usually expended to explain complex changes. However, as we shall see throughout the book, even complex events can be perceived using minimal mental effort.) The point here is that any change to our surroundings initiates what the pragmatist philosopher John Dewey (1929) referred to as "a quest for certainty." The individual moves down a path to find an answer—to attain understanding and knowledge. And this path can either be smooth and easily traveled, or a rocky one fraught with effort.

The goal of this book is to clarify how we, as perceivers of the social world, go about attaining our understanding of self and others, moving beyond our naive lay theories about how we operate. This will be accomplished by examining the processes underlying perhaps the most important element of our mental life, one philosophers have grappled with since people began reflecting on the human condition—the search for knowledge about the causes and reasons for events. Among the most important and interesting types of changes to our environment that initiate the search for knowledge are those produced by people (including ourselves). Social interaction is an essential part of human existence, and we need to understand the characteristics and motives of those around us. The behavior we observe creates a need to understand the behavior, with each new event bringing a new need to understand whatever changes to our environment that behavior has produced. *Why* has the behavior occurred? The person across the room is staring at you. Is it sexual attraction, hatred, or something embarrassing sticking to your face that is the cause of the attention? Members of your gym start avoiding you. Has there been some rumor (false or true) spread about you? A member of a minority group is denied a job at the office where you just started working this summer. Was this person simply not qualified, or was the person the victim of prejudice? You find yourself agreeing with every word your new friend Erik speaks. Are you fascinated and enthralled by Erik, or being ingratiating in hopes of some material gain? These examples all illustrate how simple events involving people (including some people that have nothing to do with you at all) trigger attempts to discern the cause for their actions. Their presence has caused a change in your immediate environment and has set you off on a quest for understanding that change.

Thus understanding other people—from detecting their presence, to focusing attention on them, to labeling them, to making inferences about what they are like and what they are likely to do, to remembering them—is one of the most frequent and important activities we humans engage in. *Person perception* refers to the examination of the processes concerned with how we come to "know" and understand what other people are like. A more familiar term, *epistemology*, is the study of the origin and nature of knowledge, and the concern of this book is with the origin and nature of a specific type of knowledge—that formed about people. The beginnings of this field of study in psychology are typically traced to Fritz Heider, who, in the title of his seminal book from 1958, described this domain of inquiry with the term *interpersonal relations*:

> The term "interpersonal relations" denotes relations between a few, usually between two, people. How one person thinks and feels about another person, how he perceives him and what he does to him, what he expects him to do or think, how he reacts to the actions of the other. (p. 1)

These types of thoughts are ubiquitous, since they occur in circumstances ranging from those in which our judgments of others are highly consequential to the other person (such as when we are witnesses or jurors in a trial), to those that are highly consequential to ourselves (such as when we attempt to figure out why a friend has failed to return a call or why an object of our unrequited affection seems to be acting friendly), to those that seem to have no consequences whatsoever (such as when we try to ascertain why the cashier at the market said hello). We humans engage in an unending pursuit of answers to the "why" question, with each new moment bringing new stimuli to us that we need to examine and comprehend.

The scientific study of this type of social knowledge is relatively young (in comparison to physics and biology, for instance). In its short empirical history, the pursuit of how people understand their social environment has been called *interpersonal relations* (Heider, 1958), *person perception* (Schneider, Hastorf, & Ellsworth, 1979), and the amalgam *interpersonal perception* (Jones, 1990; Kenny, 1994). However, the main concern of this area of investigation has not varied—analyzing processes of attribution. An *attribution* is the end result of a process of classifying and explaining behavior in order to arrive at a decision regarding the reason or cause for the observed behavior. For example, Roger throws a bat at Mike during the course of a baseball game. Whether the cause for Roger's behavior is determined to be something about his personality (he is hostile; he hates people like Mike) or something about the situation he is in (he has failed to see Mike; the situation is promoting extreme anxiety), or some combination (in situations such as these, Roger is hostile to people like Mike; when extremely anxious, Roger can lose his cool), the perceiver is nonetheless trying to understand why the event occurred and uses the information at hand to make an attribution about why the bat was thrown toward Mike. As perceivers, we all continually ask ourselves this question: "To what cause can the event I am now observing be attributed?" The ways in which we go about forming attributions for what we observe—especially attributions about a person's *personality* as the cause for his/her behavior—is the focus of Chapter 6 of this book. Chapters 7 and 8 continue examining this issue, focusing on how our attributions are affected by our taking "cognitive shortcuts" and relying on limited amounts of information, as well as focusing on how attributions can be distorted by our personal biases.

How might the ways in which we interpret others be biased? Despite the obvious importance of the behavior and situation of the person being observed on how we reason about the causes for that person's behavior, equally important to our analysis are the perceptions and conclusions we draw about those behaviors *as observers*. In the example above, is the person observing the bat being thrown prejudiced in favor of Roger or against Roger? For example, the fact that a perceiver identifies with a group to which Roger belongs has no bearing on whether, where, how, and why Roger threw a bat toward Mike. Yet perception of the physical evidence and the type of conclusion drawn—the attribution—are indeed often altered, distorted, and dependent on such seemingly irrelevant factors as the perceiver's readiness to see one type of interpretation over another. The same behavior (throwing a bat) in the same situation (a game), under the same perceptual conditions (seen on TV, from an identical angle, with identical commentary from the announcers), is often attributed to very different (sometimes diametrically opposed) causes/reasons by two people who have different personal biases.

Thus the study of the processes involved in perceiving each other and coming to "know what we know" about the people in our world is essentially a question not only of what behavior we have seen, but of our cognition as individual perceivers—our social cognition. *Social cognition*, therefore, is the study of the mental processes involved in perceiving, attending to, remembering, thinking about, and making sense of the people in our social world. Although the term *social cognition* was used as far back as Heider's

(1944) article titled "Social Perception and Phenomenal Causality," the term did not take on real currency until well after the cognitive revolution in psychology. Perhaps seminal in making this term a common descriptor for the psychological processes that are involved in organizing experience and in the individual's pursuit of making sense of the social world was the use of the term in the title of the first volume of the Ontario Symposium book series (Higgins, Herman, & Zanna, 1981). Several years later, Fiske and Taylor's influential textbook, *Social Cognition* (1984), helped to not only cement the term, but move the study of social cognition to the heart of social psychology, where it still resides.

The current text examines social cognition with an emphasis on the person as perceiver of other persons in a social situation. The contributions that the perceiver makes to the perceptual process is the focus of Chapter 1, where it is discussed how insidious our biases can be, due to their furtive nature. (The word "furtive" is used because we perceivers naively assume that our perception is an unbiased reflection of the facts that have been presented to us, rather then identifying our own distortion of the so-called "facts" while perceiving them.) Chapter 2 focuses on how quickly and unknowingly the mental processes that shape our attributions operate. It is argued that we can be "biased" not in a deliberate attempt to distort and deceive, but because the basic mental processes that determine how and what we see operate outside of our awareness, delivering to us a distorted view of the world before we realize that any thinking has occurred. The world is filtered through a personalized lens.

The theme of how social cognition is shifted beyond what the facts/data that have been observed suggest is one that returns throughout the book. Chapters 9 through 12 examine some of the specific types/sources of personal bias and subjectivity that distort how we see the world. Chapter 9 focuses on individual differences, and Chapter 10 on momentary fluctuations, in what is called *construct accessibility*. The argument in those chapters will be that whatever thoughts are readily accessible in our minds will have an unusually large influence on what we think we see. Chapters 11 and 12 shift the focus to distortions and biases in person perception arising from the expectancies and stereotypes that we, as perceivers, have learned from our own past experience and from our culture. What we expect to see in another person is often what we believe we actually have seen in that person. Throughout the book, it will be emphasized that we the perceivers are active participants in interpreting the behavior we have observed, with our psychology as perceivers often being a larger factor in determining how a behavior is interpreted than the actual behavior that is observed.

WHY ASK THE "WHY" QUESTION?: SOCIAL KNOWLEDGE AS A BASIC HUMAN NEED

> The organism is a biological unit whose internal activities tend toward a relation of equilibrium. To maintain these functions and their equilibrium the organism directs itself in the strongest way to the surroundings, engaging in a constant commerce with them. . . . In the environment the organism seeks first a field of operations, a region in which it can move and act in accordance with its structure. It is sensitive to those aspects of the surroundings that are of prime relevance to its life functions.
>
> —ASCH (1952, pp. 44–45)

In the quote above, Asch (1952) describes humans as biological organisms pursuing a set of specific physical needs that are linked to survival—such as the needs for food, reproduction, and shelter from harm—and that can promote a state of equilibrium. By *equilibrium*, he refers to a state of balance, of a system that is in a state of rest or satiation: All of the organism's needs are met. When a biological need is not met, such as when hunger is felt, an imbalance exists. All organisms, from ants to people, are motivated to attain equilibrium when it has been disrupted. To do so, we humans must engage in what Asch calls a "commerce" with the environment. We look to the environment to return us to a state of equilibrium—in the current example, by providing food that will put an end to the state of hunger.

Psychologically, a similar type of commerce between the individual and the environment exists. When a person's psychological needs are not met, the person is said to lack equilibrium. For example, as long as a killer has not been brought to justice, the family of the murdered victim is in a state of psychological tension—lacking equilibrium. So long as you do not understand the reason your girl-/boyfriend has dumped you, you dwell on the event and suffer the emotional consequences. Just as devouring food restores the equilibrium that hunger shatters, the imbalance experienced from a psychological need can be restored to equilibrium through a commerce with the environment. The family turns to the legal system to bring the killer to justice; you turn to interaction with friends and conversations with your "ex" to help you understand why you have been dumped. When interaction with the environment provides a sufficient explanation for our psychological state, this psychological issue no longer plagues our minds or drives us to seek answers.

What types of psychological needs cause us to constantly pursue the "why" question? That is, why are we so caught up with understanding why every little change in our environment has occurred and why people act the way they do, even when they are not acting in a way that has a direct impact on us? The answers that psychologists provide invoke three basic needs: (1) feeling as if we are approved of/loved and belong to a group of others that is larger than ourselves (affiliation needs); (2) having positive self-regard (self-esteem needs); and (3) understanding and deriving meaning from the actions of others in a manner that is sufficient to allow us to plan our own behavior and interact in an appropriate manner (epistemic needs).

Affiliation Needs

A popular introductory-level textbook in social psychology (Aronson, 1988) reminds us that we humans, by our very nature, are "social animals"—we need each other to survive. This is not merely so because the physical dangers and pleasures of the world are, respectively, best avoided and attained through the help of others (it is impossible for us to reproduce without the help of others; it is more difficult to defend ourselves from harm if we are alone than if we are protected by a group or army; it is easier to get nourishment if some of us are hunting and others are gathering). In addition, we humans have an emotional need to "belong" to something outside ourselves; to commiserate and share experiences with others; and to feel wanted/loved by a group, such as a family, colleagues, or a team (e.g., Baumeister & Leary, 1995). This need to develop, affirm, and protect social relationships affects even basic information processing, since individual thought is a product of social activity, directed by the norms of the culture we are linked to and the social bonds we seek to maintain (see Hardin & Conley, 2001, for a review of this connection between affiliation needs and epistemic needs).

To deny the needs for love, identity, and community would be to remove oneself from human existence, much like the character in the Simon and Garfunkel song who declares, "I am a rock." Objects (like a rock) can exist void of these characteristics, but to be human requires a pursuit of the psychological need to affiliate to deliver a sense of love, community, and identity that can only be attained through being linked to others (and that often deliver the unwanted negative consequences of this pursuit, such as loss of love, ostracism, and negative identity). Perhaps identity seems like a fairly personal issue that is attained simply through knowledge of the self. But identity needs are discussed here as a component of belongingness and needs to affiliate because a significant portion of identity comes from the social groups (religious groups, nation-states, ethnic groups, etc.) to which one belongs (e.g., Brewer, 1991; Tajfel & Turner, 1979). Identity is multitiered, so that it is partly determined by individual qualities such as traits and abilities. However, it is also determined by membership in a variety of groups, and by affiliations with others who share those group memberships. One person can derive identity from all of the following social groups: Yankees fans, New Yorkers, Jews, McGill University graduates, music lovers, Lehigh Valley residents, baseball/softball players, academics, hikers, authors, homeowners, Americans, Beatle devotees, liberals, cat lovers, fathers, summer camp alumni, brothers, Democrats, Ivy Leaguers, social psychologists, and more. Thus, we need to affiliate to have an identity.

The pursuit of this basic need to affiliate gives rise to many types of "why" questions aimed at understanding the actions and reactions of others: Is this individual someone I could love? Does that behavior mean I am accepted and liked? Is that person's assertiveness a sign of hostility? Is this other person's reference to Yom Kippur meant to signal that we share a religious affiliation and cultural heritage? The need to affiliate propels the search for meaning, so that we may know whom to approach and whom to avoid when we are seeking love, identity, and community.

Self-Esteem Needs

Linked to our human need to belong is our need to feel positive about ourselves—to have high self-esteem. These are linked because we feel good about ourselves typically after evaluating our performance, and it is difficult to evaluate ourselves without having a group of important and relevant other people against whom to compare ourselves (Festinger, 1954b). In addition, we derive a substantial portion of our self-esteem from the groups we are associated with (see Tajfel & Turner, 1979). The groups we identify with also serve to set our most important standards that we use when evaluating our abilities (e.g., Higgins, 1989) so that we derive pleasure when we meet those socially defined standards (and experience negative emotions when we don't live up to these self-guides). Thus a good deal of our experience of self-esteem is linked to social comparison and depends on how we perform relative to others. Finally, it is difficult to experience heightened self-esteem without being able to share accomplishments with others. (If you were kissed by the most attractive person in town, how long would you be able to wait before wanting to tell someone?)

The esteem and belongingness needs, though linked, are not redundant, since we do not have to belong to a group or feel accepted by its members to use the group as a reference point. (In fact, we often compare ourselves to groups of disliked others, safe in the knowledge that we will come off positively in the comparison; see Lambert & Klineberg, 1967.) And certainly not all feelings of positive worth need be experiences shared with others or derived from experiences with others. This fact does not deter the human drive to feel positive about the self. Just as with affiliation needs, this drive for positive worth has implications for social cognition, in that it gives rise to a host of "why" questions relating to assessing how we are doing relative to others and understanding our own and others' behavior for the purpose of making social comparisons.

Epistemic Needs

An *epistemic need* is the need to identify/label, understand, and be able to make predictions about the people and objects in our world. It is a need to have meaning. Heider (1944, p. 359) stated that "some authors talk of a general tendency towards causal explanation, a 'causal drive,'" thus likening this psychological need to the physical drives (hunger, reproduction) that allow us to survive.

The Functions of Attaining Knowledge

Why has this cognitive activity been elevated to the status of a basic need? Almost every thought and action we undertake during the course of our waking moments is aimed at either avoiding aversive stimuli or approaching pleasurable ones. (Take a moment to analyze any of your behaviors, asking yourself why you are engaged in it. Eventually you will arrive at the fact that the behavior is serving a basic goal of approach or avoidance.) But how do we know what is dangerous and painful in order to avoid it? What alerts us as to which stimuli will bring us pleasure and should be approached? This information is delivered by our cognitive systems' fulfilling several essential functions.

First, the things in our environment are *categorized*—labeled as being an instance of some type of thing that is known to us and possessing the features of this class of things (e.g., Bruner, Goodnow, & Austin, 1956). For example, when you observe a round object that has a hole in it sitting on the kitchen table in a box, you label it as an instance of the category "donut" (and had it not been in a box, but had a cigarette sitting on it, you might have categorized it instead as an ash tray). Second, having placed the stimulus into a category provides for us an *understanding* of its features and *inferences* about what to expect (e.g., Allport, 1954). Thus labeling the object as a donut leads immediately to the inference that you can eat it, and the knowledge that it will be sweet. Third, possessing such basic understanding of a stimulus (whether we are talking about an object or a person), once attained, allows us to *make predictions* (e.g., Bruner, 1957) about how it will influence us—whether it is likely to pain or pleasure us, based on our inferences. If you are like me, you predict that the donut will give you pleasure. Fourth, these expectancies and predictions prepare us for behavior, so that we are *ready to respond appropriately* (e.g., James, 1890/1950). Thus you respond by approaching the object and sticking it in your mouth—a response that would be inappropriate had this round object been categorized differently (say, as an ash tray).

This sequence of cognitive events delivers an understanding of the elements in our environment and is what allows us to know what to think and how to act from moment to moment. A final function that such understanding provides for us is that it allows us to feel in control of what happens to us. Such feelings of efficacy are essential to attaining well-being and avoiding depression (e.g., Lerner, 1980; Seligman, 1975). These processes of categorization, and their functions for us as individuals, are the focus of Chapter 3. For the time being, let us consider a simple example in the domain of person perception.

If I am lost while walking in Central Park at night, whether or not I approach a stranger depends on how I label that person and the inferences I draw from having categorized that person. Is it a man or a woman? Does the person seem physically imposing and dangerous? Is it likely that the person is armed? Will the person speak my language? Will the person perceive me as a threat? These questions get answered relatively quickly, as my mental apparatus races to provide information about whether a situation poses an opportunity for help or harm. Let us say that the person is categorized as a woman, and that her clothes identify her as a jogger. Her status as a jogger suggests that she knows her way around the park. The revealing nature of her sportswear suggests that she is not carrying a weapon. Our relative physical sizes suggest that she poses no physical threat. All this information is provided in milliseconds, much of it without my consciously intending to ask (or answer) those particular questions. But armed with these answers, I can reduce my fear of being lost in a potentially dangerous place by approaching the woman. And the wise person will take into account that the woman also is engaged in these processes of perception, and will herself be wary of being approached in a dark park by a stranger more physically imposing than she.

An Emphasis on the Ordinary (Not the Extraordinary)

The example just described is not typical. Rarely do we find ourselves in interactions where we *desperately* need information from other people. The need to understand is usually not driven by extraordinary circumstances. What makes this need to understand others amazing is how often we engage in satisfying it, even in mundane circumstances where we would not imagine that any inferences need to be formed. As stated above, any action that occurs in our environment causes a change to that environment and sets these processes of attaining meaning into motion, triggering answers to the "why" question. If you encountered the same jogger running toward you during an afternoon trip to the park with your brother, you would be likely to engage in all of the same inferential steps described above—noticing someone running, detecting her gender, making assumptions about her physical ability. This would occur despite the fact that she is now irrelevant to you in any way other than having entered, and disrupted, your immediate environment. But labeling her as a jogger answers the momentary "why" question (Why is this person running at me?), despite the facts that (1) asking it is irrelevant to you and your brother, and (2) these cognitive processes happen without your even realizing them.

The Invisibility of Attaining Knowledge

The example above illustrates that these processes (categorizing, inferencing, predicting, and preparing appropriate action) that produce answers to our "why" questions are such pervasive parts of life that we do not even need to attend to them consciously. That is, we seek answers to questions about the events that occur around us so routinely/frequently that these very processes come to happen automatically, without our awareness, our conscious intent, or even the knowledge that we are engaged in any mental activity (e.g., Bargh, 1997; Bruner, 1957). Much of the mental activity that allows us to navigate through our social world has essentially become invisible to us. This may seem counterintuitive. Surely, a complex change in our environment will not be handled so recklessly by us as to leave us negotiating the situation without the use of our conscious powers of reason. Perhaps this is true, and consciousness will be used to help us understand the change. But it is also true that much of our understanding of the event, and our eventual conclusions about the event's cause and how to act in return, are determined by psychological processes that occur outside our awareness. Chapter 7 will review the evidence for the notion that inferences, particularly those about the traits of people we observe, occur quite spontaneously and outside conscious awareness.

Bargh (1997) assures us that this is not laziness or stupidity on our part. As we will see in Chapter 2, it is precisely because such activities are important that they have come to operate unconsciously (e.g., James, 1890/1950). Just as you do not need to consciously monitor something as important as every breath you take, important psychological events, like making inferences about the causes of events in your environment, are unconsciously handled, freeing your conscious mind to work on more complex tasks. Almost as often as you inhale, you make some type of inference, judgment, assumption, categorization, rationalization, or conclusion about the people that surround you. Dating back to the time when you can first remember being, your mental life had already developed to such a degree that these important mental activities had come to operate by force of habit, providing the information you need to know to act and survive without your needing to experience that any mental production has taken place (e.g., Helmholtz, 1866/1925). If you doubt this is possible, simply recall the last time you drove your car while daydreaming and seemed to have driven 2 miles without being able to recall any of it. If driving can happen without much conscious control, imagine how many psychological events, such as answering simple "why" questions, you are able to carry out without being aware of them.

THE PROPERTIES OF THE DATA VERSUS THE ACTIVE CONSTRUCTION OF THE DATA

If it is granted that basic psychological processes relating to attention, categorizing, and inferencing deliver meaning, we must still deal with the questions of where attention is focused, how people are categorized, and which inferences seem reasonable. Two themes repeated throughout the book deal explicitly with the manner in which social meaning is achieved. We have touched on these themes already. The first is that what we come to know about the social world is determined by the properties of the people and events that we observe: They have an inherent meaning that experience has taught us and that can be discovered by an analysis of their properties. Thus we attend to features that are most salient in the object/person being perceived; we categorize according to the features that capture attention; and we make inferences based on what the properties of the object/person being perceived dictate. The second is that what we come to know is determined by what we (the perceivers) contribute to the epistemic process via selectively perceiving, attending to, and interpreting the information received. Thus the features that seem salient and capture attention are those we select to attend to; the categories we use are those serving our interests; and so on. Each of these themes is linked to a philosophical perspective: Meaning as something acquired through experience with data is associated with empiricism, while meaning as a constructed product of the perceiver is associated with pragmatism.

Empiricism and Addressing Epistemic Needs

The term *empiricism* is not meant to imply that we perceivers are relying on naturally/naively conducted experiments to discern the truth about a person or object, but to suggest that knowledge originates in experience. It is a philosophical approach beginning with the assumption that there is meaning inherent in the things we experience. If there is meaning inherent in the people and things we interact with, such meaning can be attained if we seek it out through experience with those persons/things. Therefore, "truth" is something to be attained, although it may require a thorough appraisal of the data. But the data are the starting points of the search for knowledge, and they drive and motivate the search for knowledge. Locke (1690/1961) presumed that the mind starts out like a piece of white paper—"void of all characters, without any ideas: How comes it to be furnished?" His one-word answer was through "experience." Knowledge of coldness comes through experiencing the way in which an object labeled as cold to the touch affects the sense of touch. This basic type of knowledge was labeled a "simple idea," and Locke claimed that (1) "the mind is wholly passive in the reception of all its simple ideas" (p. 37), and (2) such ideas serve as the material and foundation for more complex ideas. Hume (1748/1961) described the process through which the "elements" of knowledge—simple ideas gained through sensation—are combined to produce more complex knowledge through a process of association:

> Though our thought seems to possess unbounded liberty, we shall find, upon a nearer examination, that it is really confined within very narrow limits, and that all this creative power of the mind amounts to no more than the faculty of compounding, transposing, augmenting, or diminishing the materials afforded us by the senses and experience. When we think of a golden mountain, we only join two consistent ideas, gold, and mountain, with which we were formerly acquainted. (p. 317)

Thus the philosophical position of the British empiricist school (e.g., Berkeley, Hume, Locke) stressed the role pure sensation plays in shaping perception. Experience is where knowledge is to be gained, and truth is what the pursuit of knowledge seeks to uncover. In relating this approach to person perception, we might say that if we seek to understand a person such as a politician, then we must maintain that there are "truths" about the person that can be revealed through a rigorous examination of his/her behavior. The uncovering of such truths is our goal in attempting to understand the politician.

Most of us would like to believe that we are empiricists—that there are inherent qualities about the people and things we come into contact with, and that through our experience with them, the properties and essential features that make up the "essence" of the observed persons/things are simply revealed to us. We like to believe this for two reasons. First, our knowledge is what we use to guide our behavior, so we feel that obviously it would be ill advised to do anything other than react to what would be considered factual properties and qualities. And since we do typically act successfully (we don't get slapped in the face or run down by cars very often), this suggests to us that we are correctly receiving the signals that the stimuli are sending us, and that the knowledge we possess comes from fact. Second, our psychological experience of the world is typically one of meaning "raining down" upon us, where we simply receive the sensory transmissions provided to us. Thus a donut has certain essential features that tell us, "This object is a donut," and also tell us what we can do with it. We know what it is and what it does, because it tells us. It does not feel as if we are inferring these properties.

This same belief in ourselves as empiricists explains our experience of how knowledge is produced about the people in our social world. When we have the sense that a politician is a liar, or that a grandfather is a respectable man, this knowledge seems to us to be facts dictated to us by the qualities of the people in question. It seems to us as if our role is to observe what they have done, and the essential knowledge about them is revealed to us by their words and deeds. In essence, the pursuit of the "why" question is experienced by us as a pursuit of facts. We gather information to tell us what to expect and how to act, and we presume that the information we gather is factual and is based on accurately assessing the features of the persons/things in question.

Pragmatism and the Pursuit of Knowledge

The pragmatist perspective begins with the assumption that our goal as perceivers is not to obtain absolute truth. Rather, knowledge serves the function of telling us how to act toward and think about the people and objects entering our environment. Until we understand the qualities of those people and objects, we will have uncertainty and doubt about how to act and think. Removing this uncertainty and doubt, attaining "closure," is said to be the goal of seeking knowledge. Thus human understanding is attained by any knowledge that can structure the situation in a *sufficiently meaningful* way that allows for making predictions about what to expect. This approach came to be labeled *pragmatism* by James (1907/1991), since pragmatism's root (from Greek) is the word "practical." From this perspective, since knowledge exists essentially to service action, it is very practical in nature: We need to know simply enough to allow us to act. This is often accomplished without knowledge that is perfectly rooted in experience, or without the complete facts about an object or person we are interacting with. Instead, we are willing to rely on theories about the data, rather than close inspection of the data themselves. If adequate knowledge (that which allows for useful inferences and appropriate action) is capable of being produced without exhaustive effort or extensive experience with the person or thing being perceived, then we perceivers will be satisfied to stop the epistemic process before a thorough appraisal of the person or thing has been conducted. The nature of the theories and information/beliefs/expectancies that we hold about people and use to deliver meaning in lieu of extensive thinking about people will be the concern of Chapter 4. Chapter 4 addresses how we are able to make adequate and pragmatic responses (how we formulate sufficient answers to our various "why" questions) in the absence of a thorough appraisal and by expending relatively little mental energy.

Let us examine an example of how an epistemic need can be satisfied by *producing* a truth rather than *discovering* a truth. If you seek to understand a politician who is addressing you (an epistemic need), this can be satisfied by exhaustively analyzing his/her every word and past stance on issues. However, you can also form an impression that adequately accounts for what is being stated and that allows you to predict what can be expected from this politician by relying on prior beliefs about types of politicians, rather than exhaustively attending to this particular politician. For example, in the 2000 U.S. Presidential election campaign, pundits had predicted that the "professorial" Al Gore would handily defeat the "affable" George W. Bush in the televised debates, thus providing a large advantage for Gore toward winning the Presidency. To examine the common perceiver's reactions toward the candidates, a television network gathered a group of prospective voters to watch the candidates and provide reactions to the candidates' positions on various policies. Following the debate, a reporter asked one of these observers, "Who do you think won the debate and will likely get your vote for President?" The reply was something to the effect of "I really liked George Bush. I thought he had the better positions on the issues." The reporter followed up by asking "Which issues? What was it about Bush's policies that won you over?" The individual thought a bit, and responded with something to the effect of "I thought he was a nice guy; he seemed trustworthy and the kind of guy you could have a beer with."

Invited to a television studio for the explicit purpose of analyzing positions and thinking deeply about issues, this individual nonetheless was happy enough to process the information provided by the candidates only to the level that allowed for the formulation of an opinion. The person was satisfied to ignore the details (he/she was unable to recount any of the specific policy points discussed), and simply to formulate a sufficient impression to allow him/her to make what was believed to be a good enough prediction—"George W. Bush will do just fine as my President." It may be that if the person had analyzed the issues carefully, he/she still would have favored Bush. This is not the point. The point is that a prior theory about what Bush is like (or what affable people similar to Bush are like) determined the conclusions drawn and the amount of effort spent analyzing what Bush had to say. This is how people operate when their goal is not to be accurate and uncover "truth," but simply to form a sufficiently reasonable opinion (to get closure). They analyze only deeply enough to feel comfortable with their opinions and to feel as if the opinion suggests to them a reasonable course of action.

Charles Peirce (1877) referred to this type of knowledge attainment as the struggle to remove doubt—a process he labeled *inquiry*. Peirce believed that "the sole object of inquiry is the settlement of opinion. We may fancy that this is not enough for us, and that we seek not merely an opinion, but a true opinion. But . . . as soon as a firm belief is reached we are entirely satisfied, whether the belief be false or true" (p. 67). Thus, even if we perceivers are charged with forming an accurate impression (as the prospective voter described above was), we may nonetheless settle on the first acceptable opinion and press our mental capacity no further. Imagine how much less "truth seeking" might be found if we did not have an explicit goal of forming an impression or if we did not have the pressure of being on camera in front of millions! If we are not compelled to think as deeply as possible when asked to and when so many are scrutinizing us, how likely is it that we do so when walking around from moment to moment? However, let us conclude by recalling that just because we are not thinking as deeply as possible does not mean that we are thinking badly or coming to conclusions that will lead us astray. The approach is called pragmatism because this strategy is practical—it works the bulk of the time. Finally, the idea that we operate in this fashion does not rule out the possibility that we are capable of thinking more deeply. We should still be able to kick into mental overdrive when it is desired. The principles that govern switching from simple to complex processing, from being pragmatists to empiricists, are the focus of Chapter 5.

HOW DO PSYCHOLOGISTS EXAMINE EPISTEMOLOGY?

Despite the fact that philosophers for centuries have been contemplating questions that we would today label as questions of psychological processes (and we need not begin with the debate between empiricists and pragmatists, as any brief review of philosophical writings from Descartes back to Aquinas back to Socrates and beyond will reveal a concern with the nature and function of human knowledge), the systematic experimental investigation of these matters is relatively new. The methodologies of the science have evolved somewhat in its young existence.

Wundt and Scientific Introspection

Wilhelm Wundt was the first to use the term *experimental psychology* in print (Wundt, 1862, p. vi) and he founded the first formal psychological laboratory in 1879. Wundt and his students (such as Külpe, Cattell, and Titchener) relied on an experimental method called *introspection*. Introspection as a method for examining psychological processes did not refer to casual processes of reflection, as the word might be used in everyday language. Instead, people had to be trained to introspect on their mental sensations, stripped of any higher-order inferences and complex reactions, through a training process that contained thousands of practice introspections in "perception, apperception, discrimination, judgment, and choice" (Boring, 1953, p. 172). Thus, through training in this method, reports about the most elemental sensations and images experienced in the mind were generated by research participants.

Introspection came under attack from theorists who believed that much of mental life proceeds in the unconscious. Within Wundt's own lab, Külpe (1904) concluded that the introspective technique was ineffective when it came to examining higher-order thought processes; he hypothesized that unconscious guides steer conscious processes, and thus that people do not have access through introspection to the processes that direct thinking. Much later, Sigmund Freud similarly argued that introspective reports only scratch the surface of mental life because of the unconscious motives that introspections do not access. In addition (as might seem obvious today), introspection as a scientific approach was somewhat unreliable, with observations regarding exactly the same stimulus varying both within a given person and between different people. As experimental psychology developed as a science, alternative methods emerged and seized upon these shortcomings, generating the first great controversy of the young discipline.

Behaviorism and the Borrowing of Methodologies from the Physical Sciences

The direct examination of one's mental state through introspection was labeled by behaviorists as impervious to and unavailable for scientific study. Instead, behaviorists took as their template the "exact" science of physics, where the emphasis is not on the world of subjective experience, but objective and external observation. This approach was succinctly summarized by Köhler (1930):

> Both the physicist and the chemist are interested in knowing how a system which they are investigating will react when exposed to a certain set of conditions; they also ask how the reaction will change with a variation of those conditions. Both questions are answered by objective observation, registration, and measurement. This is exactly the form of real experimentation in psychology, too: a subject of a certain type (child, adult, man, woman, animal) is the system to be investigated; certain conditions are given and objectively controlled. . . . a reaction occurs which is observed quite objectively . . . behaviour, i.e., the reaction of a living system, is its only subject matter. (p. 12)

This reflects the impact of the British empiricist school. Observable experiences are the domain of inquiry, and the notion of abstract or unobservable "causes" or unobserved entities is rejected. Laws describing human behavior are not predicated on the assumption of some unseen entity or mental state. From this approach, it is simply enough to know that a person seeks food when hungry and to use the term *motivation* to describe this, rather than to believe in the notion of a mentalistic state that the individual experiences as a purpose or intent and that impels the behavior. Unseen entities are nice metaphors, but not the domain of science. Instead, science is founded on measuring and manipulating associations, which have been forged through experience, between stimuli and responses made in the presence of those stimuli (and the aversive and appetitive states addressed by responding to those stimuli).

Gestalt Psychology

Just as introspectionism as a methodology came under attack by the behaviorists, behaviorist tenets came under attack by Gestalt psychology (and later cognitive psychology). This time, it was not the methodology that was questioned—simply the assumptions about what was to be allowed in the domain of examination by this methodology. Gestalt psychology attacked the behaviorist belief that mental activity cannot be studied through the scientific method because, as behaviorists felt, it is unobservable and equivalent to terms like *spirituality* (reflecting a "prescientific mythology," Köhler, 1930). From the Gestalt perspective, psychologists were "throwing the baby out with the bath water." Simply because the methods introspectionists employed were deemed questionable for building the foundation of a science, this need not mean the content area being examined by those methods should also be discarded. In fact, Köhler (1930, pp. 23–24) mocked the behaviorist belief that mentalism should be ignored because one cannot prove the existence of mental states. He pointed out that

> it is a truism in epistemology that I shall never be able to "prove" conclusively the existence of an independent physical world. As an extreme purist I might argue this point exactly as the behaviourist disputes the assumption of direct experience in others. Somehow it does not occur to the behaviourist to apply his epistemological criticism to the assumption of the physical world. He does not say; Thou shalt not work upon a physical world, the existence of which will always remain a mere assumption. On the contrary, he assumes it is a reality with all the healthy naivete which he lacks in psychology.

Köhler's point is that one can study cognitive activity and still follow the scientific method. The methodological criticisms that fit introspection do not level all attempts to examine cognition. Out of this criticism of behaviorism eventually grew a cognitive revolution that took hold in the middle to latter part of the 20th century, and that maintains its grip on psychological science to this day. Cognitive processes—from reasoning, to attention, to memory, to encoding of information, to language comprehension and production, to knowledge structure (the nature of mental representation)—all became dominant themes of psychological inquiry.

Social Psychology and the Pursuit of Knowledge: The Person within the Situation

Thus far we have examined a simplified summary of two philosophical approaches to epistemology and a brief review of the ways in which psychologists have studied epistemology. The social-psychological approach to person perception uses the scientific method espoused by Gestalt psychology, cognitive psychology, and behaviorism, and draws from both the pragmatist and empiricist philosophical traditions. In social psychology, the perception of people is believed to be multiply determined. It is contributed to by the observed behavior (behavior can suggest meaning quite clearly and diagnostically), the situation that this behavior occurs in (behaviors change meaning according to the context in which they are observed), and the biases that the perceivers of the behavior bring into the perceptual process (e.g., their goals, norms, values, and expectancies).

This position was originally articulated in social psychology by Kurt Lewin, who asserted that a person's behavior is best seen as the interaction of the person, who possesses a variety of goals and desires, with a situation. Lewin said that the person and his/her situation form a unit, which he referred to as the *life space*, and that only by focusing at the level of this unit can human behavior be examined. Lewin (1935) claimed that understanding what drives a person to act involves understanding the relationship between the goals/needs of the person and the opportunities to pursue those goals that are afforded by the situation he/she is in. The person acts one way in one situation because the possibility of pursuing goals that are served by that behavior exists in that situation, whereas the possibilities of pursuing other goals are less strongly represented in that situation. Lewin used the term *valence* (more recently the term *affordance* has taken hold) to capture this relationship between situational opportunity and individual desire. Social psychology adopted this position to posit that only in the intricate relationship among what the situation affords, what the person wants, and what behavior can be performed in the service of the person's goals/needs is the person's behavior understood. For example, if I have the goal of finding a place to eat when I meet some friends later in the day, restaurants on the city street become salient to me even at moments when I am not consciously scanning for them (and even though I would have failed to notice them if that goal had not been in place). My view of the city changes to meet my goal. Similarly, with perceiving people, if I have the goal of finding a partner for a project, the traits and qualities that leap out are different from those that I might otherwise observe. As a consequence, the person I am drawn to approach might be different from the person I would approach if I was operating with the goal of finding a tennis partner.

As a means of understanding behavior, the life space approach can get quite complicated. Obviously, each person has many goals in any given situation, and each situation affords, to relative degrees, the opportunity to pursue many goals. As an example, a boy studying for an exam in his room may be enticed by his bed to lie down, by a novel on the bookshelf to procrastinate, or by the Internet to download songs he promised to send to a friend. Each of these goals (sleeping, studying, procrastinating, helping a friend) may be important to this student, and each affords the opportunity to be pursued by stimuli in the environment. This is not meant to imply that the student mechanically responds to stimuli (the bed alone does not trigger sleeping; the Internet, downloading; the exam notes, studying), but that there is an interaction of objects in the environment and the student's intentions/goals. This interaction between one's goals and the ability of various people and objects to afford one the opportunity to attain those goals is what directs thought and behavior. Whether the student in this example sleeps, reads, downloads, or studies depends on his needs and goals within that situation and which of the objects in his life space speaks to those needs most clearly. It is because of this approach that in social psychology (and social cognition particularly), self-esteem, affect, intent, goals, identity, love, attitude, and a host of other unseen mentalistic concepts come under the realm of inquiry, in addition to cognitive processes such as attention, memory, and encoding.

PERSON PERCEPTION VERSUS OBJECT PERCEPTION

Our understanding of the people in our world has been said to be jointly determined by the situations we are in; the qualities of the people we encounter; and our own biases that shape our interests, expectancies, and goals. Though we may cling to the belief that our knowledge of ourselves and others is relatively objective and accurate, many different factors determine what we know about the people that make up our social world. But how does perception of people differ in this regard from perception of objects, such as donuts, chairs, and weather patterns?

Similarities between Object Perception and Person Perception

Understanding people involves psychological processes that in many ways are similar to the processes used in understanding objects. Consider a perceived object. It becomes present in our life space, occupies the focus of our attention, and is immediately (often preconsciously) categorized. The raw material on which the categorization is based consists primarily of the shape, color, and other physical properties of the object that allow it to be classified. And with categorization comes the triggering of an associated set of inferences that provide us as perceivers with expectancies and informs us about how to act. "We assume that there are real, solid objects with properties of shape and color, things placed in particular positions in real space, having functional properties making them fit or interfere with our purposes, and in general defining their place in the space of means–end relations" (Heider, 1958, p. 21). Essentially, an object defines itself, with perception and categorization providing for us a complete description of the function of the object, what it can do for us, and what we can do to it. These relations are specified by the very nature of the thing. An object categorized as a chair is something on which we can sit, and from which we are likely to receive comfort and rest. An apple pie is something we can eat, and from which we are likely to enjoy a sensation of pleasure as well as satisfaction for a feeling of hunger. A lake can provide feelings of both serenity and fun (boating, swimming, etc.). These feelings are caused by the object, and are caused simply by observable physical qualities of the object, as defined by the function of these physical properties.

Now consider a perceived person. Many of the processes in person perception may be the same as those used in object perception. Like nonsocial objects, people are real and solid objects with properties of shape and color that have functional relations to us. Thus, as with object perception, the raw materials that allow a person to be categorized also contain physical properties. In addition, a person, like an object, enters our life space, is attended to, and is categorized (e.g., as a man, a Hispanic, etc.). As we will see in many chapters of this book, people are simplified, structured, and assigned to categories in much the same manner that objects are. Despite the thousands of words in the English language for making sense of (or individuating) people, there is a tendency to assign people to categories that render them similar to other classes of people. This process simplifies the act of perception, structures our environment for us, and provides much-needed closure. Finally, person perception, like object perception, represents a search for meaning. An object (social or not) that enters our life space must be understood, so that we know how to respond and what to anticipate as a response from it. However, we come now to a discussion of the many differences between person and object perception.

Differences between Object Perception and Person Perception

Inferring What Has Been Seen

The raw materials of person perception include behavior: People *perform actions directed toward us*. Just as in object perception, a categorization is made and inferences are drawn from the raw materials in person perception. Furthermore, just as in object perception, these raw materials often go unnoticed when we are reflecting on our inferences. In this case, the raw material may be the behavior of others, and the inferences we make perhaps require a far greater level of complexity and sophistication. In object perception, the nature of the inference process is simply an identification of an object's features (e.g., it is round, has a hole in the middle, is covered with something, it is sweet-tasting, etc.) that allows us to place the object in one category or another (e.g., it is a donut, not a bagel). The inference is a simple one: the object belongs in one category and not another. In person perception, we need to do more than detect features and assign them to one class or another; we must engage in inferential processes that first tell us how to identify and interpret the type of behavior being enacted.

This increased complexity does not mean that we make inferences about people in a more conscious fashion than we make inferences about objects. It is still wholly possible (and frequently the case) that we identify behaviors without conscious awareness. Indeed, figuring out what type of behavior we have seen, and even making further inferences about what type of person is likely to enact such a behavior, can occur in less than a second; we only consciously experience that an inference has been made—a person has been categorized—and not the mediating steps that deliver that inference. For example, we may say that Susan seems unhappy with us without being able to pinpoint what it is about her reaction that makes us feel this way. The raw material consists of her physical features combined with her behavior (both verbal and nonverbal); yet we cannot point to having made inferences about those materials in arriving at our conscious experience of the person. All we experience is the end product, the percept—Susan is displeased.

It is not a requirement that we fail to notice the raw materials that contribute to our perception of others, as there are times when we are well aware of the factors that contribute to our inferences. Heider (1958) suggested that such awareness is most likely to occur when the materials that contribute to our inferences consist of more than direct visual properties (e.g., size and shape), such as behavior. The implication is that while the behaviors and features that lead to our impressions need not become aware to us, and we may simply experience the final percept (e.g., Susan is displeased), person perception presents a heightened possibility for such awareness to emerge. When behavior serves as the raw material for our inferences, which is exclusively the case in person perception, the chance of noticing how those raw materials are contributing to our percept is increased (though not always detected). Thus person perception, especially when it is based solely on detecting physical characteristics and not on behavior, can be as removed from conscious awareness as object perception is. But the fact that it includes features not found in object perception (behaviors) presents a potentially more complex set of inferences that need to be performed, and thus an increased chance of consciously detecting that such processes are occurring.

Stability

According to Kenny (1994), one distinction between object and person perception revolves around the stability of the perceived objects. People as objects of perception are in greater flux and are more likely to change from moment to moment than are physical objects: "An individual's behavior changes when he or she is with different interaction partners" (Kenny, 1994, pp. 1–2). This point is reminiscent of Heider's (1944) earlier observation that because others change from moment to moment, we seek features that are stable to give ourselves coherent knowledge on which to base predictions of their future behavior. Trait inference (assuming that a person's behavior occurs because the person has personality traits causing that act) provides this stability and a sense that we can predict what others are likely to do (Bruner, 1957).

Deducing Internal States

Another way in which perceiving people differs from perceiving objects is pointed to by the analysis of the concepts "try" and "can" (see Chapter 6 and Heider, 1958). We do not have access to the internal states of others—only to their overt acts, from which we must assume that an accurate reflection of their internal states is being provided. Objects, in contrast, have no internal states we must deduce. These internal states deduced in person perception include motives (which dictate a person's effort), as well as aptitude/efficacy at a task (which dictates a person's ability). Thus, while the function of an object and its causal relationship to us are revealed by the physical properties of the object, these properties are not immediately revealed to us upon perceiving the shape, color, behavior, and other properties of a person we perceive. Further inferences need to be made that allow us to understand the cause for the person's action, and to explain why he/she has entered our life space and what effects he/she may have on it. These further inferences involve attempts to glimpse into the internal state of the perceived person.

Motives and Goals

This need to deduce internal states reveals another important property of person perception that distinguishes it from object perception: People *act with purpose* in ways meant to affect or influence us, in either a positive or a negative way. Although it is true that objects have the ability to harm or help us, they do not do so with intent. A chair may provide comfort, but we cannot say that the chair intends to comfort us. This means that person perception, as opposed to object perception, requires inferring the intent of an action, because people, unlike objects, are *causal agents*. That is, in addition to inferring what we have seen, we need to infer why it happened. For example, we may categorize a person's behavior as providing comfort, yet still need to infer the *reason why* that comfort is being provided. Is the person concerned for us, being ingratiating, being nurturing, or being sarcastic? The motive/goal needs to be examined. Heider (1958) made this plain:

> The fact that [we are interacting] with another person and not an object means that the psychological world of the other person must enter into the analysis. Generally, a person needs to react to what he thinks the other person is perceiving, feeling, and thinking, in addition to what the other person may be doing. In other words, the presumed events inside the other person's skin usually enter as essential features of the relation. (p. 1)

Dynamics

Finally, this quote from Heider alerts us to one more difference between object perception and person perception: Person perception is a *dynamic process*, in which the people we are perceiving are simultaneously perceiving us. In object perception, we may cause an object to move (when we push a chair), or that object may cause us to behave in some way (when we step on a tack); however, the object does not respond to this action, nor does it attempt to make sense of our action. But social interaction is a dynamic process of interpersonal adjustment—I act in response to or in anticipation of you, while you simultaneously do the same with me. It is a dance, where our actions are dynamic/coordinated, even if we are not focused on this interpersonal coordination. This interpersonal nature of action will be the focus of Chapter 13.

Differences in Object versus Person Perception in the Brain

Recently, researchers have begun to ask whether this dynamic nature of person perception might lead to quite different processes for object versus person perception in the brain. That is, although the type of processing people engage in when facing social versus nonsocial stimuli may seem quite similar when certain types of measures are used, real functional differences in the purpose of each type of perception may exist. Thus person perception may be more than just an extension of the principles and processes that govern object perception; it may be a unique (though similar) type of processing that has evolved its own specific set of mechanisms served by distinct and observable regions of the brain. Mitchell, Heatherton, and Macrae (2002) have examined this issue by using functional magnetic resonance imaging (fMRI) techniques. Many people are familiar with this technology, from knowledge of how medical doctors use the fMRI scanner to produce data about various parts of the body. Psychologists scan the brain to get images of what sections of the brain are being triggered by various cognitive tasks. More sophisticated fMRI procedures can be used to allow us to get much more information besides what portion of the brain seems to be involved, but these issues are too complex for the current interest. Mitchell and colleagues have simply started to ask whether fMRI data can be used to answer initial questions about social perception, such as "Are similar brain regions involved in person and object perception?" and "Is information about the self processed in different brain regions than information about others?"

Regarding the former question, the initial evidence points to unique brain areas dedicated to processing people as opposed to objects. Consider the following experiment of Mitchell, Heatherton, and Macrae (2002). Research participants are placed in the scanner and are asked to perform a cognitive task while images of the brain are taken. The task is quite simple: People are shown two words simultaneously and are asked to decide whether one can be used to describe the other. Sometimes the first word in the pair is the name of a person, and at other times it is the name of an object. The second word, which is being paired with either a person or an object, can then either be used to describe the first word or not. For example, one might see a pairing of "Adam" and "assertive," and although one does not know Adam, one can conclude that the word "assertive" might be used to describe him; it is appropriate to use traits to describe people. However, one might also see a pairing of "mitten" with "fickle." In this case one would conclude that "fickle" cannot describe mittens. Thus the same type of judgment is being made in each case, but some of the time it concerns a social object (e.g., Adam), and some of the time it concerns a nonsocial object (e.g., mittens). The results show that different brain areas are showing activation for each of these tasks. Using fMRI data in this way provides some suggestive psychobiological evidence that social perception involves specific brain regions that have evolved specifically for this unique function.

CODA

The concern of this book is with our knowledge of the people that inhabit our social world—how we understand their qualities, make inferences about their traits and characteristics, form judgments about the pressures of the situations they are in, predict what they are likely to do, and decide how we are to act in return. All social exchanges begin either with the perception of other people in our immediate presence, or with the contemplation of other people who are not currently present. What we infer about these people will dictate the way in which we choose to behave and the nature of our cognition. For instance, if you are to enter a room full of students, the manner in which you think, act, and speak depends on your having formed inferences about what is expected by the others in the room. Are you the lecturer, a teaching assistant, or a fellow student? What expectancies do others have for you in each of these social roles? This will dictate how you dress, where you sit, how you prepare, and so forth. What expectancies does your mother have for you? Even though she won't be in the room, the standards she holds may have an impact on all the same issues. Knowledge of the characteristics and expected actions of the people in our social world is what drives our own ability to act, think, and navigate through life.

The emphasis throughout the book will, therefore, be placed on how an individual makes sense of the people with whom he/she comes into contact (either physically or mentally). This will involve an interaction of various forces that drive social cognition—the context in which behavior is observed, the features/qualities of the behavior (the actions that are performed, or at least perceived to have been performed) those interactions occur), and the individual perceiver's subjectivity in construing the context and the behavior observed within that context. Chapter 1 emphasizes the role played by first the context, then by the perceiver's subjectivity, and finally by the qualities of the data that are observed (the features of the people and objects observed within the situation).

1 Naive Realism

THE CONSTRUCTION OF REALITY
IN THE PURSUIT OF SOCIAL KNOWLEDGE

When George H. W. Bush, the 41st President of the United States (and father of the 43rd President, George W. Bush), was running for reelection against Bill Clinton in 1992, he made a statement (which I paraphrase) that conveyed the following effort to distinguish himself from his opponent: "I never attended Oxford University." (His reference was to the fact that Clinton, as a student, had won a Rhodes Scholarship and attended Oxford, and later Yale law school.) Bush's motivation for this statement seemed to be to capitalize on an anti-intellectualism/elitism he assumed was dominant in the electorate. Bush realized that perception was what mattered most, and he wanted to create the perception of himself (in others) as a man of the people. Clinton was to be labeled, in this war of person perception, as the Ivy Leaguer, Ivory tower dweller, and leftist intellectual who could not relate to the people. This would explain Bush's appearance at the Country Music Awards during the reelection campaign, armed with the hard-to-swallow declaration that he loves pork rinds! Never mind that Bush himself (and his son George W., another so-called "man of the people") graduated from Yale University, one of the most elite academic institutions in the world, or that the Bush family comes from extreme wealth (while Clinton was a child of a broken home with depressed financial means, who made it to the elite institutions through sheer academic achievement). The handlers for the 41st President probably knew that the way in which we interpret other people is often irrelevant to the facts about those others, and more directly related to *what we are prepared to see in them*. The person who can set the agenda for what perceivers are prepared to see in others has already won half the battle. This is not to say that reality does not matter. People ultimately came to see Bill Clinton as an intellectual, but as a man with the "common touch" as well. But the creation of an expectancy or a stereotype in the mind of a perceiver will go a long way toward directing the outcome of that perceiver's impressions.

However, just because person perception is directed by what we expect to see, what we want to see, and what we hope to see, this does not mean that we recognize in ourselves that the ways in which we see other people are influenced by these expectancies, wants, and wishes. If we have inferred that Carol (a person we have observed) acted violently, we conclude that it must be because her behavior was clearly violent. If we believe that Carlos acted intelligently, it must be because his actions reflect his underlying intelligence. We see ourselves as merely transcribers of the qualities displayed by others, despite the fact that our construal of them is heavily influenced by subjective forces (existing wholly in our own minds as perceivers) that are divorced from the actual qualities of the persons being perceived. We remain naive to our biased perception of others, clinging to the image of ourselves as objective. For example, when a person asserts that "George W. Bush is the President of the United States, so he must be highly intelligent" (a statement recently made to me), the person is ignoring the fact that this perception may not be an accurate transcription of the actual qualities of the President, but an impression constructed in the perceiver's mind to satisfy his/her expectancies of what a President should be. The perceiver may point to selective evidence to support this view (such as the President's delivering a series of coherent speeches), while selectively ignoring other evidence that would argue against it (such as the speeches' being scripted by others and simply being read off a teleprompter). The issue here is not whether the 43rd President is or is not highly intelligent, as I have no way of answering that question. It is that the perception exists in some that he is (and in others that he is certainly not), and this perception seems to the perceiver to be based on fact.

This failure to see how we subjectively arrive at the conclusions we draw about others can be referred to as *naive realism*. This term captures the idea that when trying to make sense of the world, we begin with the perception of the people and objects that enter our visual field. Both objects and people have features that are independent of us. They existed prior to coming into our life space and will continue to exist once they have departed. This enduring character of the people and things we observe gives rise to the belief that our experience of things is one of an objective reality opening itself up to us. Asch (1952, p. 46) has summarized this well: "This insistent character of things, their stubborn independence of us, is a primary mode of our experience. . . . There can be nothing more objective, more real, than this world of things. Their reality character is not a result of inference or belief; it is the source of inferences and beliefs."

Asch (1952) soon warns us, however, that this sense of our basic perception of people and things being driven solely by the events that we observe is an illusion. Rather, our understanding of an object is transformed and "constructed" according to the specifications we bring as perceivers to meet the world of stimuli that bombard our senses. As Bruner (1957, p. 123) put it, our use of prior categories in inferring the identity of a perceived object "is as much a feature of perception as the sensory stuff from which percepts are made." Even the most simple forms of knowing, such as knowing that a thing on a desk is a "pencil," require us to make *inferences* that are not directly revealed by the properties of the thing (pencil). Such inferences represent a leap beyond what is objectively revealed to us by the stimulus, so that a pencil cannot exist for us before the sensory experience has been transformed through an interface with our prior knowledge about writing utensils. Bruner (1957, p. 133) labeled this process, where we go beyond the information given in order to imbue the stimulus with meaning, "the most ubiquitous and primitive cognitive activity." Such inferences occur unconsciously; we are unable to recognize that our minds are manipulating and transforming the information that hits the senses. James (1890/1950) made this quite explicit in his criticism of the empiricists:

These writers are bent on showing how the higher faculties of the mind are pure products of experience; and experience is supposed to be of something simply given. . . . [They] regard the creature as absolutely passive clay upon which experience rains down. The clay will be impressed most deeply where the drops fall thickest, and so the final shape of the mind is moulded. . . . These writers have, then, utterly ignored the glaring fact that subjective interest may, by laying its weighty index finger on particular items of experience, so accent them as to give to the least frequent associations far more power to shape our thought than the most frequent ones possess. . . . [Interest] *makes* experience more than is made by it. (p. 403)

You may be thinking that this tendency toward naive realism is somewhat attenuated when it comes to judging people. After all, objects may seem to have an immutable set of features, because they lack the subjective qualities that characterize humans. But when we are judging people, we know that they possess intentions and inner thoughts that are not known to us, so it might make sense that we take this into account when perceiving them. Because the causes for a person's actions are ambiguous and unknown, the assumption that we have perfect insight into a person's "essence" from observing his/her behavior (i.e., the notion that the person has characteristics that are simply revealed to us) might be deemed inappropriate. However, our willingness to accept that we are sometimes anything less than rational—that we produce impressions that are not tied explicitly to the data provided—seems to be thrown out the window when it comes to social perception as well. Ichheiser (1943, pp. 145–146) captures this point eloquently:

The psychologically naive, unreflective person lives in the belief that he experiences and observes other people in an objective, unbiased way . . . he is not aware of the fact that certain processes [of misinterpretation] are at work within himself, which distort and falsify his experience of other people even on the level of immediate observation. It remains concealed from him that what he considers as "facts" is permeated by—and partly the result of . . . unnoticed and unconscious but nevertheless systematically proceeding misinterpretations.

Despite the fact that people, as targets of perception, are hardly as objective (by definition!) as objects, we rarely recognize the perceptual distortions and inferences that we often make; we maintain a healthy dose of naive realism in the realm of social perception. When a sports fan sees the home team as unfairly penalized, he/she truly perceives the play in a manner totally opposite to that of the opposing team's fans. When a White eyewitness testifies against a Hispanic defendant as having aggressively attacked another person, the eyewitness may believe that he/she saw an unarguable act of aggression, despite the fact that another person may have categorized the same behavior differently. When a negotiator sees an opponent as extreme and unyielding, the negotiator may see the same acts on his/her own team as examples of flexibility and moderation.

This chapter examines general forces that shape social cognition, even though we remain naive to their influence. The first force examined is the context in which a behavior occurs, with the same behavior changing in meaning as the situation changes. Next, the ways in which we perceivers "make" experience—how we construct perception—are examined. The chapter concludes with a reminder that the power of the data in shaping an impression of other people should not be ignored or assumed to be irrelevant. Although what we expect and want to see in others is a powerful force, so too are the actual behaviors and qualities those people possess.

THE CONSTRUCTED NATURE OF PERCEPTION: THE ROLE OF CONTEXT

There is More to Perception than What Meets the Eye

If you are having trouble accepting the fact that much of your experience of the world is a distortion—something less than a replica of the facts provided for you by the stimuli that hit your senses—conduct a brief thought experiment. Think of a time you saw a huge sun setting on the horizon, or observed a giant yellow moon creeping in your window. Now consider the facts. Has the size of the sun or the moon actually varied from one moment of the day to the next? No; your perceptual system has automatically distorted the image. Try another exercise to illustrate to yourself that your perceptual system is constantly manipulating the information it receives to provide for you a coherent and constant perception of objects. Imagine that you are at a town hall meeting held by a nominee for President. When you observe the nominee walking around the room, first he/she is 10 yards away from you, then 5. The pure image on the retina informs you that as the person approaches, the individual grows in size. But you do not perceive an emerging giant. Although the physical object remains constant, the stimulation that strikes the sensory apparatus varies (Köhler, 1930). Yet your experience agrees with the constancy of the object.

These examples illustrate the point that perception is not merely a case of transcribing data, but of making sense of data. And *the way we make sense of data is partly determined by the context in which those data are received*. Our understanding of even simple stimuli is dependent on the background against which objects are seen (e.g., distance of the moon from the horizon):

> Instead of reacting to local stimuli by local and mutually independent events, the organism reacts to an actual constellation of stimuli by a total process which, as a functional whole, is its response to the whole situation. This is the only viewpoint which can explain how to a given local stimulus there may correspond altogether different experiences as soon as surrounding stimulation is changed. (Köhler, 1930, pp. 80–81)

Thus part of our perceptual experience is determined not by the properties of the object or person we have observed, but by *the context in which the observation occurs*. To illustrate to you that perceivers are not aware of the ways that context leads them to twist the data they receive, let us begin by reviewing some perceptual illusions from Gestalt psychology. With these familiar examples, you can clearly see (once they are pointed out) the distortions (due to context) in your perception of the illusions, even though you cannot report how or why they occur.

Gestalt Psychology and the Construction of Perceptual Experience

Holism

A fundamental tenet of Gestalt theorizing is that the parts of a stimulus array interact to make up a structure, and those interacting parts are dynamic in that they influence one another. Understanding is not achieved by examining the individual elements, but by examining the nature of the relationship between the parts and the emerging properties that the dynamic system reveals. The Gestalt perspective introduces us to the notion of *holism*: Perception is not a sum of the parts of a series of stimuli taken individ-

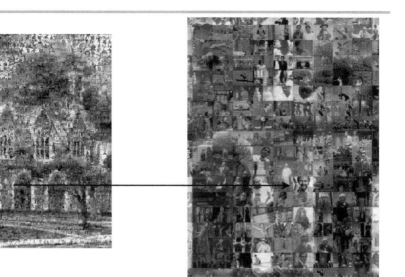

FIGURE 1.1. The emergent meaning from the sum of the parts. Photos courtesy of Robert Silvers of Photomosaic and the McCarter Theatre Center in Princeton, New Jersey.

ually, but the result of the placement of a stimulus in a field from which it derives meaning. An example is provided by the picture on the left-hand side of Figure 1.1. Each individual unit of the picture (McCarter Theatre in Princeton, New Jersey) is itself a picture (of people and things associated with the theater), as can be seen from an enlarged section of the image on the right-hand side of the figure. But the individual units, taken as a whole, have an emergent meaning (similar to a pointillist painting) when organized and pieced together by the visual system: It becomes a picture of a building. The same is true of person perception. A person is more than the sum of his/her traits and behaviors.

Some classic optical illusions make a similar point. In the Mueller–Lyer illusion (Figure 1.2), the perception of the length of a line is altered by the surrounding features in which the line is embedded. The top line, despite being equal in length to the lower one, seems longer because of the context in which it is encountered. In the Ebbinghaus illusion (Figure 1.3), the perceived size of the inner circle of each set is altered by the size of its surrounding circles. Despite the identical size of two inner circles, they look different because of the contrast with the immediate context. Thus the same image (line or circle) is perceived differently by the same person, depending on the context in

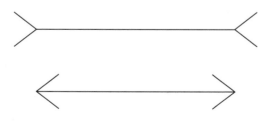

FIGURE 1.2. The Mueller–Lyer illusion.

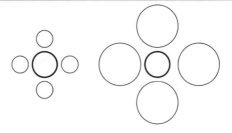

FIGURE 1.3. The Ebbinghaus illusion.

which the image is seen; This occurs despite the fact these are concrete and clear objects. Imagine how much more easily perception can be distorted by context if the thing being perceived is not as clear-cut and seemingly unalterable as a line or circle (such as a person's behavior).

Closure

The notion that the parts must be seen as a functional "whole" leads us directly to a second Gestalt principle of how our perceptual system works. The pieces of information that are observed are put together by the perceptual system so they make sense as a unit. The system strives toward a structured and coherent organization, and when this is not achieved—when our perceptual experience lacks a sense of structure and meaning—there is a drive toward producing it and reducing ambiguity. The perceptual system can supply information to our experience to complete that experience and give it meaning (the figural components are observed, understood, and separated from the background). Consider the image in Figure 1.4. Rather than seeing a set of discrete lines that have no meaning, our perceptual system strives for closure by filling in the gaps in the diagram and producing for us a percept that has meaning; we see a triangle. In person perception, we make inferences or seek input from others to fill in the gaps and give meaning to a person's behavior. For instance, if we ask ourselves, "Why was I dumped by my ex?", we do not leave this question open; we seek to get closure, by any means necessary. We need the tidiness of an explanation.

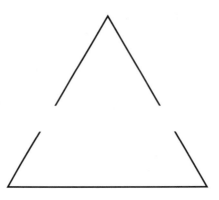

FIGURE 1.4. Closure provided by the perceptual system.

Prägnanz

A related principle of Gestalt psychology addresses the *manner* in which our perceptual system seeks to provide closure. Do we analyze all of our faults in coming to understand why we were dumped, or do we accept simple (and clearer/cleaner) solutions? The principle of *Prägnanz* (the German word for "terseness" or "precision") asserts that we tend to perceive and structure information in the clearest, least ambiguous way. In addition, there is a tendency toward perceptual rigidity, intolerance of ambiguity, and viewing new experiences from the standpoint of an existing set (Heider, 1944). If a simple and tidy explanation accounts for being dumped (e.g., "I am too selfish"), we may reach closure and seek no further complexities. Thus, in Figure 1.5, it is difficult to see the image of a young woman if one has already seen the image as that of an old woman (and vice versa). One view, not multiple views, of the image is seen.

Figure and Ground

In perception, some aspects of the entire field are the focus of attention, jumping out and capturing the eye—they are figural. The rest of the situation fades into the background. Figures 1.2 and 1.3 illustrate the relationship between the background context (*ground*) and the object of perception within that context (*figure*) as providing an emergent meaning when considered as a whole unit. We can take this principle one step further. Figure and ground do more than form a structure with emergent meaning; the perception of the figure is actually determined by its ground, such that changes in ground alter the interpretation of what is figural (see Figure 1.6, where the shading of

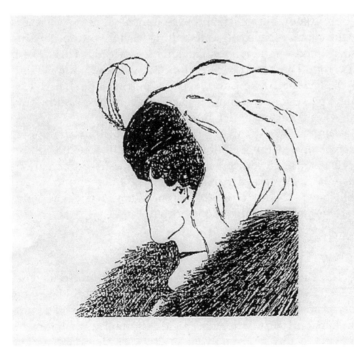

FIGURE 1.5. What is seen as figural can vary.

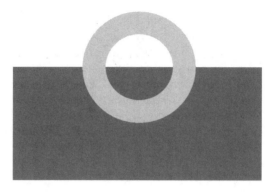

FIGURE 1.6. Change in ground alters figure.

the circle seems to change as we move around it). The same act, such as telling a joke with the punch line "A pig like that you don't eat all at once," can be perceived entirely differently if told at a party or during a presentation to a group of animal rights activists. The meaning shifts from funny to insensitive and stupid as the context shifts.

In addition to the meaning assigned to a figural item changing when the ground changes, what is actually seen as figural can alter from person to person, depending on where we choose to focus our attention. As an example, consider the illustration in Figure 1.5 again. Whether we see an old or a young woman depends on what is seen as figural. But what is seen as figural is not absolute, it is dependent on where we happen to focus our attention. This is partly determined for us by the context we are in. Situations specify appropriate ways to act, and what jumps out at us—what is figural—will be determined by the context specifying and limiting what is appropriate. Imagine that you walk into a funeral and one person is laughing hysterically. This person will leap out against the background and capture attention. But take the same person and the same behavior, and change the background, such as putting him/her dockside (at a boat party) rather than graveside (at a funeral), and perhaps the person would no longer be seen as figural; you might not notice him/her at all.

Ideally, this foray into Gestalt psychology and illusions has convinced you that although our senses provide information that seems real, the data we consciously experience are already distorted by our perceptual apparatus. Yet we remain naive to the distortions. Let us now begin to apply this idea to social perception and discuss how we may remain oblivious to the forces at work in the situation (such as context) that determine how we act toward and think about people.

Field Theory

In the early part of the 20th century, Kurt Lewin worked in Berlin, the center of the Gestalt movement. Lewin applied Gestalt principles to what could be labeled as the earliest of social-psychological theories—field theory. Lewin endorsed a view that behavior could only be understood within the entire field of stimuli, as an interaction of a person with a situation. Lewin emphasized a dynamic approach that reflected the Gestalt principle of holism, in that action could only be understood within the context of the entire "field" or against a background:

Every action one performs has some specific "background," and is determined by that background. A statement or a gesture which may be quite appropriate between companions in a swimming pool may be quite out of place, even insulting, at a dinner party. Judgment, understanding, perception are impossible without a related background, and the meaning of every event depends directly upon the nature of its background . . . the background itself is not often perceived, but only the "figure." (1935, p. 175)

Many classic experiments in social psychology have illustrated this fundamental point regarding how social behavior is determined by context. The way in which a perceiver construes his/her environment can change dramatically (and produce in response drastically different behavior) when a person is observed in one context versus another. Early theorists influenced by Kurt Lewin made this point explicit, such as when Sherif (1936) declared that behavior is determined in large part by one's culture and its norms, and when Festinger and Carlsmith (1959) illustrated that a person's attitude toward a boring task will depend on whether the context rewarded them with $1 or $20. The way in which people respond, despite the fact that they often fail to recognize its influence on them, lies in the power of the social situation.

For example, Milgram (1963) famously illustrated the important role that context plays in shaping behavior. Few people would admit to being capable of willingly delivering dangerous, even lethal, levels of electric shock to other people, all because they believed it was part of an experiment and the experimenter said they must. When asked independently of the experiment, most people vehemently denied that they would even approach giving dangerous levels of shock to others. After all, this would be inhuman. But the power of the situation is far more overwhelming than many of us would like to believe. Shockingly (no pun intended), it is far too human to follow orders, even if it means presenting danger to others. When people were brought into a lab at Yale University and instructed to shock a person who was sitting in an adjacent room whenever the person answered a question in the experiment incorrectly, people were willing to do this. However, the willingness to do so was not limited to low levels of shock. Even when the person in the next room screamed in pain, begged for it to stop, and seemingly was in extreme peril, people persisted in moving to extreme levels of shock (in reality, there were no shocks administered and no person in the other room—just a tape-recorded voice to provide the illusion). Not everyone, but far more people than we would have expected, gave far greater levels of shock than we might have predicted. Why?

One answer to this question allows us to drift away from the "knee-jerk" response that some people are just cruel. These were not "some people" who believed they were administering dangerous shocks, but most people. There was something about the power of this situation that got people to act in ways they would never have intended, despite the fact that they were clearly free not to do it (and just to walk out of the experiment). They yielded to the power of the situation and followed the "script" of what one is supposed to do in an experiment—one does what one is told and asks questions later. In this case, the research participants allowed the routine associated with being in an experiment and the authority associated with an experimenter and the prestige of the institution ("Yale University would never condone harmful behavior," they opined) to guide how they thought and acted.

However, Milgram's experiments, while illustrating the power of the situation, are not exactly an illustration of naive realism. Naive realism is the steadfast belief that one's actions and perceptions are based on the qualities of the stimulus alone, unaltered by the context it appears in (or by one's own personal biases). Participants in the

Milgram experiment, however, typically pointed out that it was the situation that caused their behavior. They were all too aware of the power of the context and asserted that they acted this way only because the experimenter said they must. Although they may not have anticipated that they would have followed orders before doing the experiment, it was clear that they attributed their behavior to the power of the situation, thus detecting the role of context in shaping their judgment and action. We will next examine a clearer case of participants' failing to detect the impact of the situation, despite there being a clear and powerful contextual component to their perception and action.

Latane and Darley (1968, 1970) conducted a famous set of experiments showing that people would fail to do things they always assumed they would do. These authors found that people did not act altruistically and help others who appeared to be in dire need. Research participants were placed in a situation where they observed what seemed to be an emergency for another person, and the researchers observed just how helpful people were (i.e., whether they intervened to offer aid). As in the real-life event that triggered the research (a murder in New York City observed by many people who watched from the comfort of their apartment windows, without one person helping or even calling for help from the police), bystander intervention often did not occur. In fact, they found that the more bystanders present at the time of the emergency, the less likely the person experiencing the emergency was to receive help.

Rather than concluding that people are callous and lacking in concern for one another, the researchers tried to explain these findings by assuming that the context in which the behavior is observed plays a significant role in defining the construal of the behavior. A behavior seen when alone seems altogether different from the same behavior seen along with other bystanders who fail to offer aid. First of all, a context in which one is alone offers a quite clear set of social norms: If a person is potentially in need, and no one else is present, norms dictate that a bystander should offer the person help (or at least inquire whether he/she needs help). However, let us consider what occurs when other people are also present to observe the event. If a person is potentially in need of aid, presumably others will detect this and either look alarmed or offer assistance (or both). What happens if others do not offer aid or look alarmed? The individual perceiver, having turned to the other people in the context to help define and understand the behavior unfolding in that context, is now likely not to construe the event as an emergency or one where the individual needs to intervene. This is the opposite construal from that formed when the perceiver is alone, without the benefit of a social context to shed meaning on the event. Of course, this still leaves unaddressed the question of why people in a group context are less likely to look fazed or offer assistance than when they are alone. Latane and Darley asserted that the more people present in a context, the less personal responsibility any one individual feels, and thus the less likely it is that one will act (safe in the assumption that someone else will act). They referred to this as *diffusion of responsibility*. As just mentioned, the failure to act that arises from diffusion of responsibility has a damaging social component, because when people fail to act, they also *look at each other not acting*. This leads them to assume that there is no need to act. This nonaction causes each individual perceiver to alter the way he/she defines the situation.

Asch (1952) provided a similar illustration of people remaining naive to the influence of powerful contextual forces on how they construe the world. Research participants were presented with lines of varying lengths and asked to make perceptual judgments regarding which was longer. This task was performed in groups, with judgments made aloud in front of the group. To manipulate the context, and examine its force, the other group members were actually confederates working with the experimenter who were told to provide undeniably incorrect responses (e.g., labeling an obviously short line as "tall"). The manipulation of context was the degree of unanimity in the group members' reports. Did the entire group see the obviously tall line as short? Did the entire group, with the exception of one person (who could thus validate the participant's own perceptual experience), report an obviously false judgment? Did more than one person report correctly, but still present those responses in a context where the majority of people reported incorrectly? Asch expected to find the context playing a small role in this situation of judging lines. Given the clarity of the perceptual data, it was assumed that features of the stimulus would dictate what was reported as having been seen and what was experienced as having been seen.

Surprisingly, context played a larger role. The participants came to see the lines in the (incorrect) fashion reported by the group, despite the physical, verifiable evidence provided by their own perceptual experience. An objectively short line was labeled as "tall" by an individual when seen in the context of a group whose members called the line "tall." One might be tempted to conclude that this merely reflected superficial conformity, with people not wanting to deviate publicly from what the group reported for fear of standing out or causing trouble. However, the written responses of participants made it evident that many came to doubt their own perceptual ability rather than doubting the group. They began to question themselves and used the opinion of others to undermine what they should know to be true. Importantly, people were oblivious to the power that the social force held over them. They contended that even if the majority had not been present, their responses would have been unchanged. And they were expected to be unchanged even if they were to confront (alone, without the group) the person who dissented with the group (and who in reality was providing an accurate judgment). This is a fine example of naive realism, because this is not how people perform when asked to give a judgment without a majority present. They do not incorrectly call a short line "tall": "the members lacked awareness that they drew their strength from the majority, and that their reactions would change drastically if they faced the dissenter individually" (Asch, 1952, p. 182).

The Inherent Meaning of the Data Seems to Change with a Change in Context

We have been examining how the context can alter what a person attends to and what one ultimately sees. The features of the data may suggest specific meanings, but which features are attended to (and have their associated meaning forced on a perceiver) can shift from situation to situation. However, context can play an even more subversive role in determining how people see the world. Context can alter the very meaning they ascribe to the behavior/data they observe and can determine what they think they see. We have already noted that a laugh at a funeral is interpreted differently from the same laugh on a boat or at a party. Let us review another example before reviewing research findings illustrating the subtle force of context on our interpretation.

Imagine that you were involved (but not hurt) in a car crash. A police officer at the scene determines that the other person is to blame. A 1-year-old television that is no longer under warranty was in your trunk and was destroyed. It will cost you $1,500 to replace. This damage to the TV was not covered by your or the other driver's insurance, so you have sued the other driver for $1,500 to cover your damages. Now imagine your attorney has arranged a settlement that the other driver will accept for sure (100%

chance). In this settlement, you will get only $900 of the $1,500 you had to spend to replace your equipment, but you will definitely get this $900. If you go to court, there is a 40% chance that the judge will decide against you and you will get nothing, and there is a 60% chance that the judge will decide in your favor and you will get the full $1,500. Based on this information, which of the two options would you choose (see Figure 1.7A)?

Now let's imagine the settlement again. This time, imagine that your attorney has arranged an out-of-court settlement that the other driver will accept for sure (100% chance). In this settlement, you will lose $600 of the $1,500 you had to spend to replace your equipment, but you will definitely not lose the full amount. If you go to court, there is a 40% chance that the judge will decide against you and you will lose the full $1,500, and there is a 60% chance that the judge will decide in your favor and you will lose nothing (see Figure 1.7B). Based on this information, which of the two options would you choose?

If you are astute, these settlements should sound pretty similar. In fact, they are exactly the same in terms of outcomes. In each case, you can accept a 100% sure thing in which you end up with having spent $600 (and getting $900 from the other driver). In each case, you can accept a gamble or risk—going to court—and each scenario presents you with a 60% chance of ending up with $1,500 and a 40% chance of ending up with nothing. Therefore, these are the same outcomes for you, just described in two different ways (e.g., "six of one, a half-dozen of the other"). In fact, each situation describes the same utility of taking the risk versus taking the sure thing. The sure thing

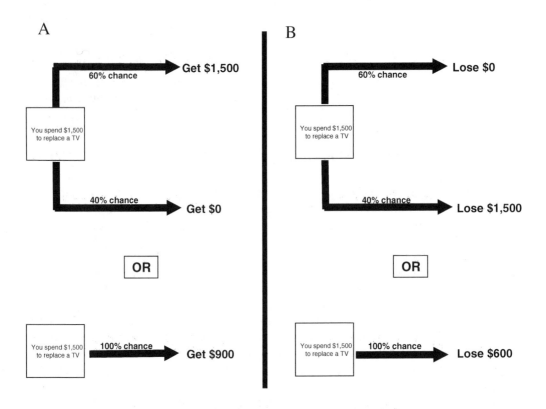

FIGURE 1.7. Framing the same outcomes as gain versus loss.

gets you $900; the risk presents you with a 60% chance of having $1,500 (and 60% of $1,500 is $900). Remarkably, the decision people make and the behavior they choose to pursue are determined by how the question is framed. Even though the two outcomes relating to going to court are the same, people are less likely to go to court when the context is described one way versus another (Tversky & Kahneman, 1981). That is, you will make an important decision one way if I tell you it will make you lose $X, but you will decide totally differently if I tell you it will allow you to recoup $Y, even if the amount you end up with is the same and all that changed was how I framed it (as a gain or loss).

The Framing Effect

The court scenario (and others similar to it) have been used in research to examine how the context in which a decision is made alters the very nature of the decision-making process. Tversky and Kahneman (1981) presented research participants with scenarios similar to the one described above, and then gave them the corresponding options (as represented in either Figure 1.7A or Figure 1.7B). In some conditions of these experiments, people were asked to make a decision that was framed in terms of loss; that is, they were asked to choose between two options that both involved losing money (a sure thing where they lost vs. a risk where they lost, as in Figure 1.7B). In other conditions of these experiments, people were asked to make a decision that was framed in terms of a gain; that is, they were asked to choose between two options that involved saving money (a sure thing where they gained vs. a risk where they gained, as in Figure 1.7A). In both the gain and loss conditions, the risk associated with the risky choice (going to court, in our example) resulted in the same outcomes. Despite the outcomes' being the same, the way in which they were framed altered the participants' willingness to take a risk. The data show that people are much more likely to take the sure thing when the options are framed in terms of gains. Thus, in our example, when people are asked what they would choose when the car accident and the lost TV are described in terms of a gain, most people say they would settle out of court and take the $900. However, when people see the situation framed in terms of loss (losing $600 of the $1,500, which is the same thing as getting $900), most people do the very opposite and decide to take their chances and go to court. This impact on one's decision to pursue an outcome as determined by whether the outcome is framed as a loss or a gain is known as the *framing effect*.

In Tversky and Kahneman's research, people were willing to choose the riskier option when the choices presented to them were framed in terms of what they stood to lose. In contrast, people were more cautious in their choices (more likely to choose the sure thing) when the options were framed in terms of what they had to gain. Why? When a situation is described to people in terms of what they have to gain from it, people are placed in a state that has been called *risk-aversive*—they try to keep what they have for sure. When the same situation is described to people in terms of what they stand to lose, people are placed in a state that has been called *risk-seeking*—they are willing to take chances in hopes of preventing loss. The point is that a subtle aspect in how information is presented, a change in context, influences how people respond by altering the way in which the data are interpreted. They come to see the choices as more or less risky in one or the other context.

The framing effect has obvious implications for person perception. The way in which we interpret a person's behavior and qualities can depend on a shift in context as subtle as altering how the behavior and qualities of the person are framed. Framing can determine whether we choose to attend to the positive or the negative features that are present in a person. With a change in the framing of a person's features can come a total reversal in how we react when evaluating that person. Shafir (1993) demonstrated that the same person (in this case, a child's parent) could be seen both as more desirable than an alternative (a child's other parent) *and* less desirable than that same alternative! To shift whether a parent is seen as more or less desirable requires merely altering the way in which the information describing the parent is framed. Research participants were asked to assume the role of a judge deciding to which of a child's two parents to award custody following a divorce. One parent was described with fairly average features, such as having decent working hours and having a good rapport with the child. The other parent was described in a much more "enriched" way that contained both more extreme positive information (such as having an extremely close relationship with the child) and more extreme negative information (such as having a job that required being away from home often).

When the custody case was framed in terms of awarding custody, the participants were likely to award custody to the "enriched" parent with the extremely positive (and negative) features. However, when the opposite question was asked—that is, the decision was framed in terms of loss—participants chose the same parent. That is, when asked which parent should be denied the opportunity to get custody, the participants were likely to respond by denying custody to the "enriched" parent! This same parent was both more likely to be rejected and more likely to be accepted as the parent receiving custody, depending on the framing of the question (even though in content it was the same question). Presumably, the decision to award custody made the positive features of the "enriched" parent more strongly salient than the negative features. In contrast, the decision to reject custody made salient the negative features of the "enriched" parent. Similar reversals in people's preferences as a function of how questions were framed were shown by Ganzach and Schul (1995) for making decisions regarding whether to cancel a trip, postpone taking a course, and vote for a political candidate.

Seemingly Useless Information

It is bad enough that how a question is framed can alter how we evaluate important information and make life-altering decisions. Unfortunately, even the addition of useless information to our context can change what we see as salient and what types of evaluations we make, so that the very same data change their meaning and have their impact on us shifted and reversed. For example, Redelmeier and Shafir (1995) examined how decisions made by doctors, in domains involving life and death, change when extra information is added to the context—information that should not, if doctors make decisions based on the data alone, alter the decision. A group of over 400 neurologists and neurosurgeons were experiment participants. They were asked to evaluate descriptions of several patients who were awaiting to have surgery on the carotid artery. Their task was to prioritize the patients to determine whose symptoms warranted getting surgery first. Some of the physicians read about two patients, and 62% selected Patient 1 as receiving top priority, while 38% selected Patient 2. A second group of physicians read the same two descriptions of Patients 1 and 2, but also received a description of a third patient with symptoms similar to those of Patient 1. Because there were now three choices instead of two, we might expect that the percentage of doctors selecting Patients 1 and 2 would now decrease as some of the doctors would have their decisions siphoned off to Patient 3. In addition, because Patient 3 was similar to Patient 1, and

Patient 1 was earlier deemed to be the one to receive higher priority, a rational out-come would have doctors experiencing conflict over Patients 1 and 3, with the majority selecting one of these two patients (and still only a minority of them should have selected Patient 2).

However, this was not what happened. Patient 2 who, in the two-patient scenario, received only 38% of the doctors endorsing him for top priority, suddenly jumped to receiving a commanding majority of top-priority endorsements (58% of the doctors in this scenario chose Patient 2). It thus seems that a doctor's decision regarding whom to operate on could be altered by something as trivial as whether a third person is also in the waiting room. The context alters the way in which a doctor attaches meaning to and evaluates the data, so that a person who was a low priority in one context suddenly becomes a high priority, when all that changes in the context is the addition of another person. You might think that the doctors in this research were just not trying too hard or thinking too deeply, and that in real emergencies they would be more rational. Redelmeier and Shafir stress, however, that thinking harder would no more help than it would in trying to avoid seeing the moon illusion or Ebbinghaus illusion. The context has an impact people do not see, and naive realism prevents overcoming the bias simply by thinking harder.

When Questions Determine Answers

We have already seen that the manner in which a question is framed influences the manner in which people respond, altering drastically what people think and do with changes in the context of the question. Such a finding should certainly raise speculation that many other factors relating to the context in which a question is asked can alter the types of answers people give. This would present a serious problem for survey results, seemingly suggesting that researchers could get just about any answer they desired from a respondent if they were clever enough to set up a context for the question that would promote the answer they were looking for. Schwarz (1999) provides some excellent examples of how contextual forces—ranging from the phrasing of the questions asked, to the order in which the questions are asked, to the types of scales provided to respond to those questions—can influence person perception:

> When asked what they consider "the most important thing for children to prepare them for life," 61.5% of a representative sample chose the alternative "To think for themselves" when this alternative was offered on a list. Yet, only 4.6% volunteered an answer that could be assigned to this category when no list was presented (Schuman & Presser, 1981). (p. 93)

> When asked how successful they have been in life, 34% of a representative sample reported high success when the numeric values of the rating scale ranged from –5 to 5, whereas only 13% did so when the numeric values ranged from 0 to 10 (Schwarz, Knäuper, Hippler, Noelle-Neumann, & Clark, 1991). (p. 93)

> Whether we conclude that marital satisfaction is a major or a minor contributor to general life-satisfaction depends on the order in which both questions are asked, with correlations ranging from .18 to .67 as a function of question order and introduction (Schwarz, Strack, & Mai, 1991). (p. 93)

These examples illustrate dramatic changes in what people presumably think about themselves and others, due to minor alterations in the context in which the questions assessing those thoughts are placed. When people are answering questions, the first step is to understand the question being asked, and the context in which the question is asked—including detailed features of the context—can change that interpretation. For example, Schwarz, Strack, Müller, and Chassein (1988) wanted to illustrate how the types of options listed for respondents to select from could alter the question the respondents thought they were being asked. The respondents were asked, "How frequently have you felt really irritated?" To answer this question required deciphering what was meant by "really irritated." They found that the way in which people interpreted the meaning of this phrase, and therefore the way in which they perceived themselves, were both determined by the types of responses offered. When the choices offered focused on infrequent occurrences of irritations (such as a response scale ranging from "less than once a year" to "more than once a month"), then participants assumed that the question was asking about severe cases of irritation. However, when the choices included larger frequencies as options (such as "once a day" being the lowest amount, rather than "more than once a month"), participants answered the same question differently, now inferring that the data (the question being posed) meant something different (much more minor types of annoyances), due to the context in which it was encountered.

It is not just the rating scale used that can alter how people interpret questions (and hence cause the context in which the questions occur to dictate the types of answers provided). The surrounding questions, particularly those answered immediately prior to a particular question, can have an impact on what one believes a given question is asking and the way in which one describes the self. A very nice illustration of this context effect was provided by Strack, Schwarz, and Wänke (1991). Research participants were asked their attitudes about a fictitious issue. Thus they essentially had no basis for an answer from their own prior experience, and one would assume that differences in responses between participants would simply have been random. However, the differences were not random, but were influenced by the context in which questions about the fictitious issue were embedded. The participants were all German students asked to give their evaluation of an educational program that was not well defined and purely fictitious. The question about the fictitious issue was preceded for some participants by a question asking about estimated tuition costs at American universities, and for other participants by a question concerning the Swedish government's financial support for students. The ratings of the fictitious German program changed as a function of the context, presumably because one context led participants to infer that the question referred to some plan to charge students, and the other context led them to infer that it was a plan to provide financial aid to students. This impact of context takes us back to the discussion of the Ebbinghaus illusion at the start of this chapter (see Figure 1.3): The context in which a circle is embedded alters the perception of the circle. Here, the context in which a question is embedded alters the perception of the question, due to the standard, or frame of reference, one uses in evaluating the question. As the standard or point of comparison shifts, perception shifts.

This same principle can be used to describe perception of people. To illustrate, examine Figure 1.8 and imagine what your impression of former President Ronald Reagan would be if the first image you had seen of him was the "Presidential"-looking first image as compared to the other two images. This same person would be perceived differently in the three contexts, despite the almost uniform facial expression in each picture. The context determines the meaning the data seem to possess.

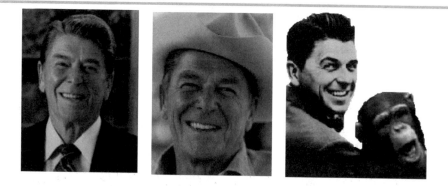

FIGURE 1.8. Impressions of the same individual vary with the context. Reprinted by permission of the Ronald Reagan Library.

THE CONSTRUCTED NATURE OF PERCEPTION: THE ROLE OF THE PERCEIVER

Thus far, we have examined one form of the tendency to place almost perfect trust in the information our senses provide, by reviewing evidence that subtle changes in context will alter what we think we see. Even when the same objective features/qualities are presented, a change in context changes our perception. Our trust in the accuracy of our senses is so strong that we do not stop to think that our judgment, inference, and perception are biased by the situation in which that information is encountered. In this section, we examine another powerful force that directs our perception of people: our subjectivity as perceivers. Our norms, goals, stereotypes, expectancies, culture, prior knowledge, mood, affect, needs, and other characteristics can all direct what we think we see. While classic social psychology experiments have focused on illustrating the power of the context to subtly alter people's perceptions of each other (and thus their decisions about how to act appropriately), we must keep in mind that the concept of *life space* that has forcefully guided this focus on context also includes the person who is within the context. Thus differences between people (such as coming from different cultures, or having different expectancies/stereotypes, or being in different moods) should alter the way in which the context is experienced, and the way in which the behavior that is observed within that context is construed.

Sherif (1936) argued that whenever we perceive, we rely on *reference points*. That is, we use other elements in the environment as standards (such as when the outer circles in the Ebbinghaus illusion are used as a reference for evaluating the size of the inner circle). In object perception, the standards are typically other objects with which the target shares physical space. In person perception, when we are attempting to understand people, the norms of our cultures often serve as an internal frame of reference that we lean on in perception. For example, our internal representations of our cultures instill values and norms in us that emphasize some aspects of the visual field over others. Thus people from different cultures can perceive the same stimulus differently:

> In the course of the life history of the individual and as a consequence of his contact with the social world around him, the social norms, customs, values, etc., become interiorized in

him. These interiorized social norms enter as frames of reference among other factors in situations to which they are related, and thus dominate or modify the person's experience and subsequent behavior in concrete situations. (Sherif, 1936, pp. 43–44)

In this way, the norms we have internalized from our cultures are important elements of the field, capable of exerting an influence over our perception, judgment, and behavior. In fact, Sherif (1936) held that all our experiences are filtered through culture: "We do not face stimulus situations involving other people or even the world of nature around us in an indifferent way; we are charged with certain modes of readiness, certain established norms, which enter to modify our reactions" (p. 99). Even our perceptions of beauty and art pass through this filter: "To a person brought up on oriental music, which is built chiefly upon rhythm and melody, the harmony of a musical work coming from a great European orchestra is almost sheer noise" (p. 62). It is this fact that allows Sherif to posit that different individuals perceive exactly the same information in different ways: "Different persons may notice different characteristics of the same stimulus field . . . so that the field may take on altogether different modes of organization" (p. 31).

Subjectivity in Object Perception

Let us begin with a review of three experiments that illustrate the impact of forces emanating from within the perceiver—such as norms, expectancies, and preferences—on object perception. Then let us shift to examining how such forces affect person perception.

Sherif (1935) performed an experiment that made use of the autokinetic effect and the assumption that group membership establishes in the individual member of the group an internalized frame of reference. The *autokinetic effect* is a perceptual illusion whereby a small point of light, though stationary, is perceived as moving if the individual is in a dark room where there is no frame of reference against which to see the light. Sherif took advantage of this ambiguous situation by placing participants in a dark room and asking them to estimate how far a point of light traveled. This was an ambiguous situation, because an estimate could not be accurately made, given that the light was not really moving; it only appeared to be moving. Sherif examined the effects of norms established within a group on perception of the light's apparent movement. Participants were asked to judge the light's movement in a group, and it was found that the group gradually converged on a shared norm for how much the light "moved." Later research showed that this socially developed norm continued to persist in directing how people responded as individual members of the group were removed and replaced with new members. The frame of reference was transmitted among members of the group. In addition, the norm established in the group setting continued to influence perception when participants later made the same judgments when alone. Sherif (1966, p. xii) summarized his findings as follows: "Caught in the uncertain situation, the individuals grope toward perceiving their surroundings in an orderly and stabilized way, even though the surroundings lack stable anchorages. Since secure gauges for perceiving the situation are lacking, they grope together toward establishing boundaries, influencing each other."

The norms of society, therefore, do more than lead us humans to conform with each other for fear of becoming outcasts. The influence of norms as seen in Sherif's (1935) research is more subtle. Norms become internalized so that we use them without knowing, without consciously conforming. They become our frame of reference and lead us to experience reality in the way the norms dictate, shaping what is perceived and the type of meaning derived. We actually come to see a stimulus differently through the filter of one set of cultural norms versus another, despite our being oblivious to the fact that we are using such norms to filter perception.

Next we turn to a tradition of research called the "New Look" because at the time it presented a novel empirical approach to perception, attention, and judgment—a focus on the selective/subjective nature of information processing. Rather than describing humans as organisms who transcribe physical stimuli directly into mental representations under the sole direction of what Bruner and Goodman (1947, p. 34) called the "autochthonous determinants of perception" ("the electrochemical properties of sensory end organs and nervous tissue"), the New Look described people as manipulating the data (unknowingly) according to their expectancies, prior knowledge, needs, motives, and values (Bruner, 1957). People see what they expect to see, and are adept at seeing things they value, desire, and like.

Let's start with an example of research from this tradition focused on how expectancies influence perception of something as concrete as an object. Bruner, Busiek, and Mintrum (1952) manipulated what people expected to see. Research participants were presented with line-drawn images flashed extremely briefly on a screen. Some were led to expect that the image was of a particular object by being told that this object would be flashed ("You will see an image of a pine tree"). Other participants were given no specific instructions, and therefore had no expectancies. When attempting to reproduce the image, participants distorted their drawings so that what they described as having been perceived looked like the typical object in the category label that was activated in the instructions. When they had an expectancy, their perception was distorted to fit it. If the expectancy of a pine tree was provided, the drawings looked like typical pine trees. This influence was exerted on attention and judgment, despite the participants' being perfectly unaware of this influence.

Bruner and Postman (1948) shifted their focus from expectancies as a guiding force in perception to affect. Research participants were shown a series of discs with symbols on them, and their task was simply to draw the size of each disc. This was to be accomplished by varying the size of a circular patch of light until it was the same size the person perceived the disc to be. The symbols on the discs were the main variables of interest in the experiment. For half of the research participants, the set of discs contained symbols that were negative (e.g., a swastika) or neutral, whereas for the other half of the participants the discs contained symbols that were positive (e.g., a dollar sign) or neutral. The subjective size of each disc was reliably affected by the type of symbol inscribed on the disc; that is, the discs with positive symbols and the discs with negative symbols were each perceived to be larger than the discs with neutral symbols. Bruner and Postman concluded that the value associated with the thing being perceived leads to accentuation in perception: "Apparently, that which is 'important' to the subject looms larger in perception" (p. 206). Their reasoning as to why a negative stimulus would be seen as larger was that negative stimuli warn people about danger and threat, and thus the accentuated perception of such stimuli would help people prepare to defend against the coming threat. Thus the positive or negative affective tone attached to a stimulus has an impact on the basic perception of the stimulus—in this case, on subjective judgments of size. (We will return to discussing the New Look in Chapter 9, where our focus is on how a person's chronic states affect how the person interprets the social world. There we will shift to considering another dominant guiding force emanating from the perceiver—the perceiver's needs and goals.)

In the research presented above, variations in perception between different individuals were said to occur whether the external information was well defined or not. Thus even cases of perceiving well-defined objects still leave the perceiver open to the influence of elements in the field of stimuli other than the characteristics of the thing being perceived. The influence of these forces is only magnified in ambiguous situations, where the physical stimuli do not impel an obvious meaning. This is the case in judging people. Think of the O. J. Simpson trial and verdict. The same information was viewed in drastically different ways as a function of the social groups to which people belonged. This is obvious to any person who has heard members of opposing political parties discussing a Presidential address, or sports fans from different teams debating a controversial play. They see or hear the same information, but somehow come to opposite conclusions.

Exactly the Same Person/People Perceived Differently by Two Sets of Observers

A classic illustration of this point was provided in an experiment by Hastorf and Cantril (1954). The experiment involved the events surrounding a Princeton–Dartmouth football game of the early 1950s. At that time (though it seems hard to believe today), Princeton had perhaps the greatest player in the nation—Dick Kazmaier. The Princeton star suffered a severe injury during the extremely rough game (as did, subsequently, several Dartmouth players), and tempers were running hot after the game. Each side screamed accusations toward the other concerning illegal and "dirty" play, and the affair was written up in newspapers outside the two universities' towns (because the nation's premier player, Kazmaier, had been hurt). Hastorf and Cantril took advantage of this naturally occurring set of biases to examine the active and constructed nature of perception. A movie of the game was played to both Princeton students and Dartmouth students who came to the labs at their respective universities. Their task was to watch the film of the game and to check off the number of plays that could potentially be categorized as "dirty." The important point is that while the identical movie was shown to two separate groups of students, this identical information was seen differently by the two groups. Dartmouth students saw the same number of infractions being committed by Dartmouth players as by Princeton players. Princeton students saw more than twice as many penalties committed by Dartmouth players as by Princeton players. One (or both) of these groups is being heavily biased in their interpretation. It could be that Dartmouth students saw the game correctly and Princeton students exaggerated the offensiveness of their adversaries. Or it could be that the Princeton students saw it accurately, there *were* twice as many infractions by Dartmouth, and Dartmouth students distorted the information so that their team did not look so "dirty." Perhaps both groups distorted the reality slightly.

Similarly, even the same person can, at two different points in time, hear the same speech or watch the same event and walk away with totally opposing views of (1) what was said/seen and (2) why the person making the speech said what he/she did or why the events observed occurred. Thus, perhaps after having been out of Princeton for 50 years, one of the participants from the original experiment, if asked to watch the original film of the game again, may no longer see the Dartmouth team as so vicious. This can occur because even though the stimulus is perfectly unaltered (we could show him the same film of the game), the goals, affect, expectancies, and mood of the perceiver have changed. We need not *necessarily* wait 50 years for such changes to occur. For example, the same political speech heard 1 hour later may be reacted to differently by the same person as his/her mood and expectancies have altered.

The Mechanisms of Naive Realism

Changing the Judgment of an Object

Why would students from different universities come to such different conclusions when watching exactly the same football game? One explanation is that we all tend to evaluate information in line with our values and attitudes. If something is similar to those things we like, we judge this new thing favorably. If people display traits or behaviors that oppose our attitudes and values, we judge them negatively. In this perspective, naive realism exacts its influence by *influencing how we judge an object*. There is a change in the judgment of the object as a function of the differences (or changes) in the point of view and attitudes between the two sets of perceivers. Our affective or evaluative response to a person or object is applied to things associated with that person or object. If I like Princeton University, I will see the behaviors of Princeton students in a similarly favorable way, because I apply the favorable judgment of the university to other things associated with it (such as the behavior of the members of the school's football team). This is a case of *spreading* of affect or valence.

As an example, contemplate your reaction to this statement by Thomas Jefferson: "I hold it that a little rebellion, now and then, is a good thing, and as necessary in the political world as storms are in the physical." Now imagine what your reaction would be, were you to learn that it was actually said by Lenin. Actually, instead of imagining your reaction, let us examine this point empirically and have you assume you would respond identically to participants in the following experiment by Lorge (1936). Participants were given lists of statements such as these and were told who the author was. Their task was to read each statement and indicate their degree of agreement with the statement—how much they liked it. The number of statements provided was large enough so that some were listed twice. When a statement did happen to appear a second time, the person to whom the statement was attributed was changed. This would provide two ratings for the same statement, with the only difference being who the speaker linked to the statement was. The interest was in whether attitudes toward the statement would change as a function of the view of the messenger (whether the messenger was judged positively or negatively). Lorge found that changes in the ratings of the quotes corresponded with participants' liking for the people to whom the remarks had been attributed. The conclusion was that when a statement is read, a perceiver attaches to it the same evaluative reaction held toward its author. If the author is liked, the quote is liked. If the author is disliked, the quote is disagreed with.

This spreading of evaluation can also be seen in how we form impressions. Rather than spreading from a person we are observing to that person's positions and statements, the evaluation can spread from the traits we have attributed to a person to how we interpret and evaluate other traits of the person. If we are told that a person is intelligent, this might affect how we label other traits he/she exhibits, making us more likely to see these traits as positive than negative (e.g., seeing a sarcastic remark as funny rather than cruel). Also, we might assume that other positive traits, not yet seen, are also likely to be characteristic of the person. This spreading of evaluation from one trait to others is referred to as a *halo effect*: The evaluation attached to one trait known to be possessed by a person imposes itself on how we evaluate other behavior and traits that are also attributed to that person. The judgment (the positivity or negativity) of some subset of traits or behaviors leads to the formation of a general impression, that, like a halo, surrounds the individual and illuminates the entire person with the evaluation associated with the general impression. Asch (1946, p. 260) described halo effects as occurring when this general impression operates as a force (labeled "G") that shifts the evaluation of each individual trait in the direction of the general impression: "the general impression 'colors' the particular characteristics . . . this is the doctrine of the halo effect" (see Figure 1.9). The emerging impression is thus a combination of the set of observed and imagined traits, now biased by the evaluation associated with the general impression and the impact of the valence associated with the general impression on each individual characteristic (represented by the arrows in Figure 1.9).

For example, Nisbett and Wilson (1977) found that people's evaluations of others extend far beyond the behavior actually observed. Once positive or negative impressions have been formed by having observed behavior in one domain, it leads ratings/evaluations of the person in that domain to spread to other domains/dimensions for which there is no reason to like or dislike the person. These researchers conducted a study where students watched an interview with a teacher who spoke with an unspecified European accent. Half of the participants saw the teacher answering the interview questions in a pleasant and agreeable fashion, while the other half saw the same teacher, speaking with the same accent, answering the questions in an autocratic and rigid fashion. Next they asked research participants to provide ratings of the teacher—not only answering questions about performance in the interview and how much they liked him, but also answering a series of questions assessing evaluations of the teacher along other dimensions that really were somewhat irrelevant to the behavioral evidence that was provided (how attractive he was, how participants liked his accent, etc.). These latter questions should have been answered identically by all students; after all, they saw the same teacher with the same accent. His warmth or coldness during an interview should not have had an impact on how attractive the students found him to be or how "cool" his accent was. However, the degree to which they liked the teacher exerted an influence over these irrelevant characteristics, so that the more likable teacher was also seen as more attractive. In other words, halo effects were found to occur: Evaluation

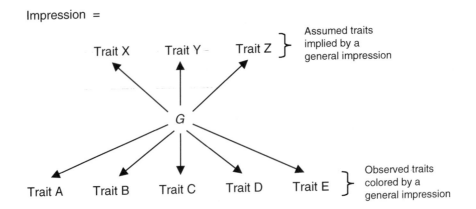

FIGURE 1.9. A general impression (G) combines with new characteristics to produce an impression.

spread from some characteristics to others, even to characteristics that were irrelevant to the behavior observed.

Another illustration of halo effects, or the changing of the judgment of an object, is potentially revealed in a famous study by Asch (1946). Asch gave people lists of traits and asked them to form an impression of the person they described (by writing a description of the person). Asch found that changing one trait in the list changed the evaluation associated with all the traits. People reading a list of a person's traits ("intelligent," "skillful," "industrious," "determined," "practical," "cautious") formed very different evaluations of that person, depending on the addition of one other trait to that list. If that list also included the trait "warm," the evaluation of the person differed sharply (i.e., it was far more positive) from the evaluation formed when the word "cold" was added. In fact, a whole set of positive traits was assigned to the "warm" person that was not assigned to the "cold" person, and this shifted the affect assigned to the other traits provided in the list.

Changing the Object of Judgment

Why should we say that illustrations of halo effects are only "potentially revealed" by these studies? Because, although it is perfectly adequate to describe the findings in terms of halo effects, it was not the way Asch (1946) described his findings. Asch did not believe that adding a trait such as "warm" simply served to make the other traits in the list seem more positive. He argued that there was a new meaning being attached to the "warm" person that made the constellation of traits entirely different, not just in valence, but in interpretation. The set of traits seemed to be an entirely different object when "warm" versus "cold" was included. This is the Gestalt principle of holism coming into play: A set of traits can only be understood not as a series of individual traits that somehow are summed together, but as a meaningful constellation, a unit with emerging meaning. When part of the constellation changes, the emergent meaning changes as well. When the word "warm" was included in the Asch (1946) list, the traits ascribed to the person seemed to suggest this to be a very different person, not just a slightly more positive person. Asch suggested that the arrows in Figure 1.9 do not represent the evaluation that spreads from a general impression to the other features/traits composing the impression, but represent an organizational force that combines the features in a way that produces a coherent meaning. If the general impression shifts, it is not simply evaluation that shifts, but the meaning of the entire impression and the individual traits of which it is composed.

Asch believed that some traits have greater power than others in a constellation of traits and behaviors involved in determining the emergent meaning linked to the set of traits. He called these *central traits*, and contrasted them with what he called *peripheral traits*, whose ultimate evaluation and meaning can be dependent on the central traits. Asch reasoned that "warm" and "cold" were, in the context of the other traits provided to his research participants, seen as central traits, and therefore had the power to alter the way in which the traits that surround them were interpreted. The entire unit of information shifted when a central trait was altered. Altering peripheral traits does not have this severe of an impact on how information is interpreted. However, Asch also illustrated that the meaning of individual traits varies as a function of the context in which those traits are observed. A trait that is central when imbedded in one set of traits can take on a different meaning, and even be peripheral, if it is encountered among a different set of traits.

This review offers a radically different twist on the answer to the question "Why are 'identical' pieces of information evaluated differently by different people?" It is not that each person forces his/her positive or negative views on the information. It is that each believes he/she has seen a different piece of information. In accord with this, Hastorf and Cantril (1954) did not believe that changes in the judgment of the object were what caused the differences in judgment between students in the experiment described earlier. Rather, they believed that the two groups of students, despite being shown the same movie, *saw* different games. This is why they cleverly called the title of their published article "They Saw a Game," highlighting the postmodernist view that people see different realities. Rather than changing their *judgments of an identical object* (their liking), naive realism was believed to exert its influence by changing what people saw as the *object of judgment*! Hastorf and Cantril (1954, pp. 132–133) stated: "It seems clear that the 'game' actually was many different games and each version of the events that transpired was just as 'real' . . . it is inaccurate and misleading to say that different people have different 'attitudes' concerning the same 'thing.' For the 'thing' simply is *not* the same for different people" (emphasis in original).

Asch (1948) made this same point by returning us to the example of a quote that can be assigned to two different authors—Jefferson versus Lenin. The difference in judgment may not be due to the fact that Americans like Jefferson more, but to the fact that the quote changes meaning when ascribed to one man versus the other. The same information, placed in one context, is perceived as a totally different entity than when it is placed in a different context. Different authors lead to the generation of different expectancies, and these expectancies change what one thinks one reads. Asch concluded that changes in ratings as a function of changes in author are due to "*a change in the object of judgment, rather than in the judgment of the object*" (p. 458). The meaning of the word "rebellion," when linked to Jefferson, suggests honest colonial farmers throwing off the yoke of corrupt authoritarian rule. When attributed to Lenin, it suggests streets running red with blood and a new authoritarian regime sweeping into power.

Asch's (1946) seminal article on how people organize characteristics, features, and behaviors into a meaningful and coherent impression provides many excellent illustrations of this point in the domain of person perception. As discussed above, in one of Asch's experiments, the judgment formed about a person altered when a central trait was altered. Changes to a single word in a set of words changed the meaning of the set. For example, when preceded by the word "warm," the word "determined" might be interpreted to mean that the person is *persistent*. However, if preceded by the word "cold," the word "determined" might be interpreted to mean that the person is *stubborn*. In fact, even the very same set of words, traits, and behaviors presented in two different orders could lead to drastically different impressions of the person being described. Although people actually were responding to the same words, they were treated as different stimuli; they meant something different.

For example, in another experiment, Asch (1946) gave participants a list of traits and asked them to form an impression. This list is provided here, and perhaps you too should perform the experiment and form an impression of a person who possesses the following traits: "intelligent–industrious–impulsive–critical–stubborn–envious." Other participants were presented with the same traits and the same instructions. The difference was that the list was presented in reverse order. Continue performing the experiment and now form an impression of a person who possesses the following traits: "envious–stubborn–critical–impulsive–industrious–intelligent." If you are like most people, your impression of these two people will be drastically different, despite getting the same information. This is referred to as a *primacy effect,* because the impression formed is not a summation of the individual elements but a function of the relationship between the items, with the strength of the earlier items in the list exaggerated over those presented later. The meaning of the set is altered as a function of the information that comes earlier.

The Consequences of Naive Realism

Forces emanating from within the perceiver, the impact of which the perceiver would vehemently deny, alter the way in which people are seen. Let us turn now to investigating some consequences relating to this form of naive realism. Lee Ross and his colleagues from Stanford University have demonstrated five consequences relating to perceivers' naively believing that their perceptions of people are accurate transcriptions of the "reality" in the data.

1. Believing That Everyone Thinks Like Us

If we believe that our interpretations of the world are objective, and therefore are not aware of our biases, this should lead to the false assumption that most people see things as we do. After all, other people receive the same information as we do and should respond to that information in the same way we would. We all believe we are simply seeing what is obviously there. The *false-consensus effect* is the name Ross, Greene, and House (1977) gave to the belief that we will all see events and people identically—the tendency to have a self-centered bias in consensus estimates and fail to recognize the likelihood that others will construe things differently.

In an experiment illustrating this effect, Ross, Greene, and House (1977) asked undergraduates whether they would be willing to walk around campus wearing a sign that said "REPENT." They then asked them what percentage of their classmates would be willing to act the same. The students who said they would wear the embarrassing sign believed that 64% of other students would do the same. The students who refused to wear the embarrassing sign estimated that 77% of other students would also refuse. Obviously, it would be impossible for more than 50% of the people to wear the sign and more than 50% of the people to refuse to wear the sign. Participants were revealing their belief that most other people would think and act as they would. The cause of such miscalculations in estimates of what our peers will do is supposedly that we fail to realize that our choices are subjective. Instead, we believe that we are merely responding to the objective realities of the situation. If this is really the cause of this effect, then the false-consensus effect should be less pronounced when people believe that their choices are based on idiosyncratic oddities of their own personality. Gilovich, Jennings, and Jennings (1983) found this to be true: When people listed a dispositional explanation (an explanation linked to their own personality or disposition) for a choice they had made, there was no evidence for false consensus (the assumption that others would make the same choice). When they recognized explicitly that their view was a unique one, they no longer exhibited the bias that others would see the world as they did.

2. Seeing Information in the Opposite Way from a Competitor's View

People who are seeing the same information, but who have different expectancies and goals related to that information, will interpret the information in diametrically opposing ways. They use the same information to support opposing conclusions (e.g., Hastorf & Cantril, 1954). Consider the example of people from opposing political, social, or ethnic groups that have a history of conflict. The members of each group might see the same data as evidence that their own group is righteous and good, whereas their opponents are immoral and bad—never realizing that their opponents are seeing the event in exactly the opposite way, or that the information being observed could be interpreted in any other way.

Lord, Ross, and Lepper (1979) demonstrated this effect of naive realism in action by examining how members of opposing ideological camps reacted to the same information. Their participants were both advocates and opponents of capital punishment who were asked to read a research article on the topic of capital punishment. The article had mixed conclusions about the effectiveness of capital punishment. Rather than the two sides' coming closer together in their judgment based on the inconclusive data, they instead polarized their views further. Each group easily accepted the data in support of their own position, seeing those pieces of evidence as indisputable fact, while evidence opposing them was seen as open to alternative explanations and suffering from methodological problems. The same set of data was used to bolster the beliefs people on both sides of the debate already had (and to shatter the beliefs of their opponents).

3. Believing That Neutral Others are Biased against Us

Given that we expect others to agree with us (the false-consensus effect), when we find out that others actually disagree with us, the conclusion we typically draw is that these "disagreeing" other people are biased. Of course, it is possible that our own position is so extreme that no other persons could possibly agree with us, even if they were totally neutral and unopinionated! But rather than concluding that our own position is somewhat extreme, we instead tend to see other people as the ones who are biased. This is not paranoia; it is a logical consequence of naive realism. If we truly believe we see things as they are, then those who disagree with us would have to be, by definition, biased. For instance, in the political climate of today, there is much talk of a "liberal media bias" put forth by members of the conservative right. It is wholly possible that these accusations are a product of naive realism—that the conservatives who fear a liberal media are simply extreme in their views, yet fail to recognize this extremity in themselves, believing instead that their views are accurate (and that most others agree with them). Thus the media, presenting a more even-handed view, seem somehow opposed to them (and must, they conclude, be biased in favor of their liberal opponents).

Evidence for this consequence of naive realism was provided in an experiment by Vallone, Ross, and Lepper (1985). Members of opposing groups, with fairly extreme opinions, were exposed to identical pieces of information. The research used pro-Arab and pro-Israeli perceivers who were exposed to news reports (from network television nightly news aired in September 1982) relating to a massacre of civilians in refugee camps in Lebanon. The measure of interest was the perception of media fairness. Perhaps somewhat shockingly, given prior evidence showing that people see ambiguous information as favoring their group, perceivers saw the media as *biased against* their group. Despite the fact that network news coverage of international affairs attempts to be neutral, and despite the fact that impartial observers would not have seen any strong bias in the way the news was reported, partisans from either side saw a bias, and saw it as levied against them. Vallone and colleagues labeled this effect of naive realism on judging the even-handedness of the media the *hostile-media effect*. At first glance, this may seem to contradict the point (made above) that we see new information as consistent with our positions. Vallone and colleagues found that, rather than seeing new information (a news report) as consistent with their views, focusing on points of agreement, and ignoring points of disagreement, participants instead saw the information as damaging to them. But these two sets of findings are not contradictory. It simply is the case that sometimes our positions are so extreme that it is difficult to find supportive evidence in the remarks of others whose positions are not as extreme.

What is the psychological mechanism responsible for the hostile-media effect? It has been argued above that people are twisting and distorting their perception in line with their subjective views, and that they do not realize they are doing it. But what is the nature of the distortion and twisting of the data? Two possible forms of naive realism have been discussed earlier: the changing of the judgment of the object, and the changing of the object of judgment. A case can be made for the hostile-media effect's being an instance of people changing the judgment of the object. The logic would be that in the course of their experiences in life, proponents of a particular issue are selectively exposed to evidence in support of their views and develop the belief that the majority of the existing data support their view. Along with this belief that their opinion is consensual comes an overwhelmingly positive evaluation of their position. If new information is then received that does not support their view, it seems unrepresentative of the "real" situation to the perceivers (with their perception of what is real derived from their own knowledge base). The conclusion drawn by the perceivers is then that the information being provided is biased and unrepresentative, since it does not match their own: If their position is accurate and positive, then that which mismatches it must be inaccurate and negative. They evaluate it as bad information, and it is seen as more opposed to them than it really is. They seem to push their evaluation of it in the direction opposite to their own, not see it as consistent with their own (see Figure 1.10).

However, a case can also be made for seeing this phenomenon as arising from a change in the object of judgment. From this perspective, the partisans would be described as coming to see, essentially, totally different news reports (despite the reality that the reports are identical). It is not that they just evaluate the news negatively because it fails to agree with them, but that they come to interpret the information being reported in a wholly different way from someone who has opposing views. Thus, even if the information presented is fairly neutral or factual, they hear it as distorted

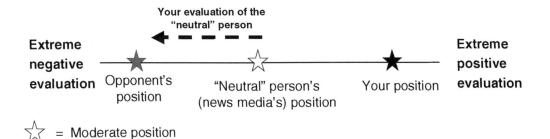

FIGURE 1.10. The hostile-media effect, extreme positions, and changing of the judgment of an object.

against them. In fact, the data from Vallone and colleagues (1985) suggest that despite seeing the same news reports, these two groups "saw" very different information. For example, pro-Arab participants felt that 42% of the references to Israel were favorable, but pro-Israel participants thought that only 16% of the references to Israel were favorable. Each group seemed to see a media presentation that had information heavily stacked against them, and to fear that any persons observing the report (even persons who were neutral on the issue) would see the report as sympathetic to their opponents, swaying them to sympathize with the opponents.

In each of these explanations, people's positions are used as a *standard* against which the media reports are evaluated. If their own positions are extreme, there will be a wide discrepancy between their feelings on the issue and how the media (if actually nonpartisan) present it. This perception of a distance between a media presentation and the "supposedly factual" standard people are using to evaluate the information leads to the perception the media is biased. If, however, people's positions are not extreme, the distance between the media presentation and their own characterization of the events will be small. This would allow new information to be seen as similar to their own and judged to be favorable rather than hostile.

4. The Perceptual Divide (the Negotiator's Naivete)

A fourth consequence of naive realism comes into play when people are not judging neutral reporters, but members of an opposing group. When perceivers are judging others who may be seen as motivated to disagree with them, such as Arabs judging Israelis and right-to-lifers judging pro-choice advocates, these others will be seen as not only being biased, but deliberately biased, or even stubborn or hostile in their bias. Thus naive realism can give rise to perceptions of motivated antagonism. The consequence of this is that perceivers tend to *overestimate the divide or gap that separates them and their opposition.* The opposition is seen as extreme and unyielding, more so than reality warrants.

Robinson, Keltner, Ward, and Ross (1995) investigated the idea that naive realism gives rise to an assumption about group differences that leads opposing groups to overestimate how different they actually are. Robinson and colleagues asked liberals and conservatives to read a story about an actual racially charged incident that took place in the Howard Beach section of Queens in New York City. A young African American (Michael Griffith) was chased by a group of White youths intending to beat him. In an attempt to escape their assault, he ran across a busy highway, where he was tragically killed by the oncoming traffic. The information contained in the story was factual information about the case (e.g., the White kids deliberately chased Michael into oncoming traffic; Michael had been using cocaine that night). The participants (e.g., conservatives) were then asked to make ratings indicating their evaluations of this scenario. However, they were also asked to make ratings of how a typical member of their ingroup (conservatives) and a typical member of their outgroup (liberals) would respond.

The prediction was not only that conservatives would be more anti-victim (and liberals pro-victim), but that people would expect much larger differences between the groups than actually existed. Such an exaggerated gap perceived to be separating groups is called a *perceptual divide* (see Figure 1.11). This was examined in this study by looking at people's ratings of how they thought their own group members would respond and how they thought members of the other group would respond, and then

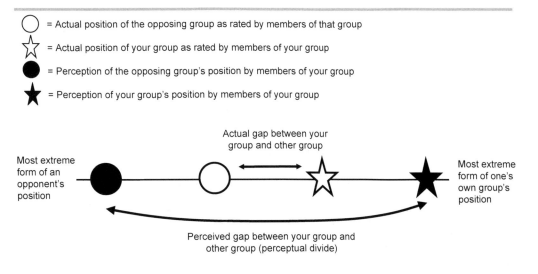

= Actual position of the opposing group as rated by members of that group

= Actual position of your group as rated by members of your group

= Perception of the opposing group's position by members of your group

= Perception of your group's position by members of your group

Actual gap between your
group and other group

Most extreme
form of an
opponent's
position

Most extreme
form of one's
own group's
position

Perceived gap between your group and
other group (perceptual divide)

FIGURE 1.11. The perceptual divide (the negotiator's dilemma).

by comparing these ratings against how people from those groups actually did respond. Robinson and colleagues found that the conservative participants did blame the victim more than the liberal participants did. However, the actual gap between liberals and conservatives was smaller than the imagined gap. Conservatives thought other members of their group would be slightly more anti-victim than those people actually were, and liberals thought conservatives would be *even more* anti-victim than that, painting them as far more extreme than they actually were (as expected, the reverse biases were seen in judgments of liberals).

Thus members of one group see members of an opposing group as far more extreme than they really are (and, interestingly, people see members of their own group as a little more extreme than they really are, with each individual assuming he/she is the moderate one in the group). The conclusion is that people have a tendency to overestimate the gap between their group's positions and those of an ideologically opposed group. This will make it more difficult to resolve differences between the groups, as the inflated perceived gap makes it seem harder to find common ground. This problem is especially dramatic at the negotiating table in cases where perceived differences are large, thus hindering the attainment of a successful resolution. We may refer to this specific application of naive realism to negotiations as *negotiator naivete*.

The perceptual divide does not only affect negotiations. Miller and Prentice (1999) have applied this logic to explain why stereotypes are hard to break. They assert that when differences of opinion arise between a person from one group and members of a different group, the person assumes that the cause for those differences is the difference in the groups. Miller and Prentice posit that once differences are attributed to someone's group, there is the belief that this opinion cannot be changed. Why? Because people feel that members of other groups have more extreme opinions than they actually do. These authors have labeled this the *cultural divide*. Thus, if a Black person and a White person disagree, the perceiver first assumes that group differences are what caused the rift in opinion. This then makes the difference seem greater than it otherwise would have (e.g., if the rift was between White people). According to the cultural-divide hypothesis, perceived differences get even greater when the opposing groups are ones for which the culture has clearly defined stereotypes. In this case, the estimate of how difficult it is to change the opponents' beliefs gets greater as the perceived divide between the two groups widens (since it is hard to imagine people wanting to turn their back on their own group to embrace the other group's opinion).

5. The Bias Blind Spot

One final consequence of naive realism is that although people are naive about the subjective nature of their own perceptions, they are all too aware of, and ready to believe in, these sorts of subjective biases in others. Rather than seeing the reality (that differences in perspective influence everyone), people see themselves as reasonably, and others often as unreasonably, responding to the same set of circumstances. Pronin, Lin, and Ross (2002) argue that people make an invidious distinction between their own susceptibility to bias (which is small) and the susceptibility of other people (which is large). In support of this, they collected survey data from Stanford University students asking them about a series of biases in social judgment. After reading a description of each bias, they were asked in one survey to rate how susceptible the "average American" was to this bias, as well as to rate how susceptible they themselves were to this bias. A second survey asked participants to rate themselves and their fellow students (people in the same class as them). In each case, the results revealed that participants saw themselves as less likely to fall prey to these biases in judgment than other people.

Proof that a blind spot is a consequence of naive realism relies on establishing that people do not recognize that their assumption regarding the accuracy of their self-judgments is a false one. Pronin and colleagues (2002) illustrated this point. Participants were asked to perform a task where they made ratings of their ability on various attributes in relation to other people. For example, they had to rate how considerate of others they were, relative to other Stanford students. Their findings replicated a known bias—that most people see themselves as above average when asked to rate themselves in relation to others (obviously, not everyone is above average). This bias, discussed further in Chapter 8, was not of central concern. The central issue was whether people were aware of this bias. To examine this, people were next told that the bias exists, and that research has shown that 70–80% of people see themselves as above average. Participants then estimated whether they in fact had been influenced by this bias in their prior ratings. The vast majority (63%) of the people claimed that their prior ratings were accurate, and an additional 13% claimed that if anything, they had underestimated their ability in an attempt to be modest. People do not see their own bias, and this leads to a division in their perceptions of susceptibility to bias between self and others—a self-bias blind spot.

THE UNCONSTRUCTED NATURE OF PERCEPTION: THE POWER OF THE DATA

Thus far, the goal has been to convince you that what we "think" we "know" about a person is subjectively determined, actively built by our readiness to see the world in prescribed ways. We all construct reality. What has not been meant by this review is to attempt to convince you that there is no external reality! If we get too lost in subjective distortions, we will soon find out that reality bites. The world "out there" does present meaningful data to the senses that determine what we feel, see, and think, and ignoring these data can have harmful consequences. The prior discussion has focused on our subjective biases as perceivers and on the power of the context, because naive realism renders us unlikely to notice or admit that biasing forces exist. The properties of the person being perceived—the physical data on which perceptions are partially built—are easier to detect and admit as influences on us. The fact that we are influenced by the physical properties of the world is probably not surprising to us. When a man acts like a jerk, he is perceived as a jerk. We are less likely to know that our expectancies make us ready to see him as a jerk, or that the context is what has defined his behavior as "jerky" behavior. Let us now give equal time to discussing the more obvious influences on our perceptions of people—the actual features and behavior we observe in those with whom we interact. The key question will be what properties grab our attention.

Affordances in the Data and the Ecological Approach to Perception

McArthur and Baron (1983) point out that because of psychology's fixation (as a field) on the questions concerning naive realism and subjectivism, many psychologists have almost ignored the analysis of "the structured stimulation that exists in our social environment" (p. 215). They remind us that "to fully understand impression formation or causal attribution or other aspects of social perception we must ultimately identify the nature of the stimulus information that reveals industry, hostility, and the other attributes that we perceive in people" (p. 215). Instead of a focus on our biases as perceivers, McArthur and Baron propose what they call an *ecological approach* to social perception that, like subjectivism, assumes that perception is an adaptive process. By this, they mean that perception tells us how to behave—it serves a practical (pragmatic) or functional role for us, telling us which behavior is appropriate in a given situation. Whereas the subjectivists' focus is on how our norms, perceptual readiness, expectancies, and goals allow us to make sense of a highly interpretable stimulus world, the ecological approach focuses on how the features of the stimuli we encounter specify clear and diagnostic meanings that suggest (in and of themselves) appropriate ways to act, without need for subjective twisting. The behavior and stimuli we encounter in the world "provide information to guide biologically and socially functional behaviors . . . [and] this information is typically revealed in objective physical events" (McArthur & Baron, 1983, p. 215).

However, because the features of the people and things we are perceiving are believed to serve a biological function for us, it must be made clear that even when we focus on the features of the person/thing being perceived, we must speak of those features in terms of how they relate to our needs as perceivers. We may discuss a bear as a "threat" and having features that reveal threat, or a sycophant as a "bother" and having behavior that is bothersome. But these features acquire meaning only because they are relevant to our needs as perceivers—we do not wish to be mauled by a bear or forced to endure the insincerity of a sycophant. This is consistent with the approach of Kurt Lewin, described in the Introduction to this book: The needs of an individual develop links with elements in the situation that are able to address those needs. Proponents of the ecological approach use the term *affordance* to describe this relationship between the meaning of features/behavior and the needs of the person. In McArthur and Baron's (1983, pp. 215–216) words, "information available in events specifies, among other things, environmental affordances, which are the opportunities for acting or being acted upon that are provided by environmental entities." The meaning of a feature/behavior is tangled up with what type of response afforded to the person who observes that feature/behavior. The bear claw says "eat me" when it is a pastry in a bakery and "fear me" when it is hanging at the end of a large, furry mammal. In each case, the meaning of the object, and a reasonable way to respond, is inherent in the feature/behavior itself—but only as it affords a person an opportunity to know how to act. And that meaning can differ between two people, with different goals, observing the same stimulus. A lion on the plains of the Serengeti affords the opportunity to run for your life, but not to the big-game hunter. This does not lessen the ferocity inherent in the stimulus.

What is being described here is an evolutionary "two-way" street: Features have meaning, but only in association with the qualities of the organisms that interact with those features. Birds and flowers may have the colors they do because of what those colors afford the conspecifics or non-conspecifics that respond to them, and in so doing serve the needs of the latter. It is probably not an accident that for us as humans, other people are the most attention-grabbing objects, and that the things about people that we cannot help noticing (gender, age, beauty/health) are all properties with obvious evolutionary significance. In essence, the ecological approach assumes that we humans preferentially pay attention to things/features that have adaptive or evolutionary value. That is, we are attuned to detect information in others that reveals an inherent threat or that, alternatively, affords the opportunity to approach a desirable state. Features that signal a potential pleasant interaction will be at an advantage, just as will be features that signal negativity and threat. As Bruner and Postman (1948) showed, these stimuli loom larger. Like the subjectivist approach, the ecological approach maintains that attention, judgment, and evaluation are selective processes not determined wholly by the features being observed. However, unlike the subjectivist approach, the ecological approach holds that this selectivity is derived from the adaptive value of the behavior being observed—its ability to specify an opportunity to approach a state that will promote the pleasure and satiation of the organism, and to avoid a state that will hinder/hurt it.

The argument here is that the stimuli we observe (whether these are behaviors or some static features) are associated with specific types of evaluative responses, because these stimuli reveal to us that they are either appetitive or aversive to us. Even if a particular person or object has no immediate adaptive value for us, the process of having the affect or attitude associated with that person/object triggered is said to occur regardless, for all objects and people we encounter, in the service of the primary need for survival. This occurs so that we can immediately have information about its potential value/threat to us available (e.g., Bargh, Chaiken, Govender, & Pratto, 1992; Cacioppo, Berntson, & Crites, 1996; Fazio, Sanbonmatsu, Powell, & Kardes, 1986). Researchers refer to this as *automatic affect activation* or the *automaticity of attitudes*. When we say that affect is triggered by a person/object, we are saying that we have learned over the course of our lives that the features and behaviors it exhibits are linked to our approach or avoidance motivation, and that positive or negative affect is therefore associated with the mere perception of the object/person/feature/behavior.

We can now start to formulate some expectations about how the features and behavior of the people we interact with shape what we notice and think. Stimuli that have links to our adaptive and functional responses as perceivers should acquire power to speak directly to us, unimpeded by the subjective twists reviewed earlier. For example, negative and threatening behavior should have adaptive value and should be detected easily in person perception. Features that are linked to powerful appetitive drives should attract attention. Behaviors and features that signal clear emotions and intentions on the part of the other person (thus specifying what we can expect to transpire during our interaction with them) should be perceived quite readily. Unexpected and novel events represent a potential threat and would be expected to have the power to direct social perception. Essentially, any diagnostic feature/behavior exhibited by another person that can specify some inference about how that person can help us to approach some desired state, or avoid some undesired state, should have perceptual weight.

What Grabs Us?: The Salient Features of Data That Pull Attention

Some information is prominent in the perceptual field and seems to leap out from the background/context, making it figural and attention-grabbing. Its prominence in the context renders it able to capture attention and have a greater impact on our cognitive processing than stimuli (or features of stimuli) that are less prominent. Such information is said to be *salient*, or to have increased *salience*. Salience, as Higgins (1996) put it, "refers to something about the stimulus event that does not occur until exposure to the stimulus, and that occurs without a prior set for a particular kind of stimulus" (p. 135). The concept of salience informs us that there are features of the things we observe, the "data" in our social world, that are more powerful at directing our attention and influencing our responses than others. Not all stimuli and features are created equal. Postman, Bruner, and McGinnies (1948) tell us that the properties of objects that make them attention-grabbing are well known in the study of object perception, and include such properties as intensity, novelty, suddenness, repetition, movement, complexity, and unit formation. Snowden (2002, p. 180) provides an evolutionary argument for the attention-grabbing properties of luminous and brightly colored objects, and the visual system that directs attention to detect such stimulus features:

> What is the purpose of color vision? Experiments with individuals who lack color vision (Heywood, Cowey, & Newcomb, 1994; Mollon, 1989; Steward & Cole, 1989) suggest one of its major roles may be to highlight targets for further inspection and thus guide visual attention to locations of interest. Recent theories of primate color vision emphasize the role color information plays in tasks such as gathering fruit hidden within a dappled background (B. C. Regan et al., 1998). Thus, it might be expected that color would be a good cue for grabbing attention, and governing visual behaviors such as moving the eyes so as to foveate a target.

Starting with the assumption that the qualities of objects that make them salient are well known in cognitive psychology, Postman and colleagues shifted their focus to factors in perceivers that determine how they interpret the world. Let us take the time now to shift back to examine the so-called "well-known" factors inherent in objects/people, as they are now less documented than the perceiver-driven factors Postman and colleagues directed psychologists' concern to (so effectively that they never looked back!).

McArthur (1981) began a continuing quest to update the understanding of these factors, focusing on the features and behavior of people that "grab" us, rather than taking the "data" for granted. Specifically, McArthur claims that "in the realm of person perception, as in object perception, perceivers selectively attend to intense, changing, complex, novel, and unit-forming stimuli" (p. 202). These features of a stimulus are said to capture attention because, as discussed in the review of Gestalt psychology, the perceptual system is geared to produce holism and closure; to see units being formed between objects, if possible; and to detect change in the environment and render it meaningful and constant. Thus complex, novel, and sudden/changing behaviors are figural (stand out) in our environment and capture/grab attention.

In summary, salience is the featural prominence inherent in (or momentarily achieved in) an event/person. Independent of our expectancies and goals, the stimulus world already is pulling us in specific directions, with the features or properties of the people/objects we encounter in our environment rendering some more salient than others. Salience is capable of determining what we see and hear within a given situation or interpersonal interaction, thus making it fundamental to person perception. As Taylor and Fiske (1978, pp. 253, 256) asserted, "causal perception is substantially determined by where one's attention is directed within the environment and that attention itself is a function of what information is salient . . . perceptually salient information is then overrepresented in subsequent causal explanations."

Salience and Causal Weight

Why is causal perception so much a function of what is salient to the person? The causal explanation we produce, the meaning that we arrive at when answering the "why" question, begins with a cognitive process of *selective attention*. In this process, features of our social world are detected, and from the multitude of features that hit our senses at any moment, a select few are allowed further processing. That to which we selectively attend will have a greater opportunity to influence the final perceptions and judgments at which we arrive. According to Heider (1944, 1958), a perceptual unit that captures attention will focus us on information associated with that unit, at the expense of attending to information linked to other elements of the environment. If we are focused on a person and his/her behavior, we are less likely to notice other forces in the situation that may have been responsible for the behavior other than the person. Thus what is salient will have extra causal weight in determining explanations for how and why a behavior occurred. Salient information acquires this power by directing attention, allowing us to select from among the myriad of stimuli that bombard our senses those subset of stimuli that will be considered when making sense of our environment. Although a variety of perceiver-driven forces serve to filter the stimuli in our world, so too can the salient properties of the stimuli themselves that pull attention and that force their way through the filter of selective attention. With salience comes attention, and with attention comes causal weight. This discussion introduces a logical question: "What makes something salient?"

Salience and the Natural Prominence of the Data

When there is something fairly absolute that would make an object, feature, or behavior salient regardless of what context it occurred in, it is said to have *natural prominence* (Higgins, 1996). What features of people make them naturally prominent? Social psychologists have attempted to apply the list of salient properties described in research on object perception (intensity, repetition, complexity, novelty, suddenness, movement, and unit formation) to the features of people. To do so introduces a methodological problem: how to measure or detect whether in fact a given feature of a stimulus is perceived as more salient than other features of that stimulus. A solution to this problem is to examine our reactions to the stimulus and see whether it is overly influenced by the feature that is thought to be salient. If a feature is salient, we should have focused on it to a greater extent, thus making it more likely to (1) be the focus of our attention, (2) make an impact on our impressions, (3) be remembered, and (4) be seen as the cause of whatever events we have observed.

Using such measures, McArthur and Post (1977) manipulated the salience of one person relative to other people in the stimulus field. This was done by placing the person under either a bright light or a dim light. They reasoned that being well illuminated in a context would be a form of natural prominence, similar to that found for vivid and intense objects. A person with features making him/her more vivid than others should be salient and be more likely to capture attention than others. McArthur and Post found that when a person had featural prominence by virtue of being more brightly illuminated than other people, this did indeed make the person more salient, as measured by the degree to which the stimulus person made an impression on others. The person who was better illuminated was seen as a central cause for the events that transpired, despite the fact that the same behavior, when not well lit, was not seen as causal.

In the real world, a famous example of this type of salience was seen in the Presidential debate between Richard Nixon and John F. Kennedy in 1960. The typical description of this debate is that listeners on the radio heard no advantage for Kennedy over Nixon in terms of how well he handled the questions asked. However, those who watched the debate on television perceived a different debate. These individuals observed a strong performance by Kennedy, perhaps one that won him the Presidency of the United States. It may have been that Kennedy, being the more attractive (handsome) of the two, won the support of TV viewers by virtue of his good looks. But a more compelling explanation, given that most people were already well aware of what the two men looked like and how attractive they were, is that the more salient of the two men was perceived as having won the debate because he was interpreted to be more prominent, more causally relevant. Kennedy and Nixon were equally well lit on the stage, but Nixon famously wore a suit that blended into the background, whereas Kennedy's suit contrasted with the background and made him more salient. The result: An analysis of the text of what they said provided no advantage to Kennedy, but the same text combined with each man's prominence altered what people heard, and shaped the outcome of the election and the future of the country.

Novelty is another feature that should, according to research in object perception, make a person salient. McArthur and Ginsberg (1981) illustrated this by picking a feature that is relatively novel in a person—having red hair. In this research, two men were videotaped talking to each other; one man had red hair, while the other had (much more common) brown hair. Behind each of these two strangers was a black-and-white photograph that was unrelated to the conversation the men were having. The researchers predicted that if one of the two men were salient, people would be attending to him more closely and would be more likely to detect and analyze the other elements in that man's surroundings. In other words, the picture behind the red-headed stranger should be better remembered than the picture behind the brown-haired man. How do we know that it was not the picture itself that was more salient, rather than the hair color? McArthur and Ginsberg deliberately varied whether the videotape was shown in black and white or in color. They predicted that when the tape was in black and white, the two men should be equally salient (because the red hair would not be detected), and no differences should be found in attention to (and memory for) the images placed next to them. However, when the tape was in color, the red-haired man would be novel and therefore salient. The salience would capture attention, and this increased attention would be evidenced by better recall for the picture placed next to the man. This is precisely what was found: The recognition of the objects in the picture behind the red-haired man was greater than that found for the brown-haired man, but only when the video was in color.

Novel or unexpected (unusual) behavior has also been shown to have particular weight in blaming a person for some outcome. A behavior can be novel or unexpected for a variety of reasons: (1) One could know the person well, and thus know that a particular behavior is unusual for that given person; (2) one could have expectancies about the groups to which the person belongs and for the social roles the person enacts, and determine that a behavior is novel in relation to what is prescribed by those expectancies; or (3) a behavior can be more objectively novel, in that it is so extreme or rare that without any such expectancies, the perceiver still recognizes the behavior as highly non-normative and unlike anything another person would do. Why would such novel behavior have causal weight? Performing a behavior that most people would perform indicates little about what is responsible for the observed behavior (if everyone acts as this person does, then something in the situation must be causing the person and others to behave in this manner). However, when the person's behavior is novel and unusual, then the behavior is unique to him/her. In this case, the individual's personality is most likely to be seen as the cause for the action. Jones and Davis (1965) asserted this as a fundamental rule of thinking about people: The more a person's behavior departs from what the average person would do, the more causal weight it has.

As reviewed above, one way to determine whether a behavior or feature is salient is to examine whether it plays a significant role in shaping the perceiver's impressions. Given that novel behavior is central to shaping impressions, we can deduce that novel and unexpected behavior is salient to the perceiver and captures attention. Neuberg and Fiske (1987) provided support for this deduced hypothesis. Research participants were asked to interact with someone they were told had schizophrenia. When having their interaction partner described to them through a written report, some participants read about behavior that was typical of people with schizophrenia; others read about behavior that made it clear the person acted in ways known to be unexpected and novel for people with schizophrenia. How did the novel behavior affect the perceivers? It led them to dedicate approximately 30% more time to reading the description of people with schizophrenia. As Neuberg and Fiske concluded, the novelty of the behavior increased the attention that perceivers gave to the person. This is a sign that the person was more salient than the typical person with schizophrenia.

Negative information, just like information that is inconsistent with and disconfirms prior beliefs, also seems more unusual because it violates expectancies and therefore captures attention. Norms dictate that people act positively and in a civil manner, and when negative behavior is observed, it is fairly novel. In addition, base rates from our experience in the world suggest to us that negative events are infrequent. Finally, given the need to identify hazards, dangers, and life-threatening stimuli in the environment, the detection of negative information is essential from an evolutionary perspective. Once again, the faster we are able to identify such information, the more likely we will be to react in a functional manner. If negative events capture attention more easily because they are salient and informative, they should be weighted more heavily in how we form impressions as a function of this increased focus.

To illustrate this, Fiske (1980) asked research participants to examine photographs of people performing behavior that was relevant to the interpersonal domain of sociability and behavior relevant to the domain of social activism. The "sociable" person was observed interacting with friends in a park in a manner that varied in how negative it was (from extremely negative, to moderately negative, to moderately positive, to extremely positive); the "activist" was observed reacting to a petition regarding child pornography, also varying in how negative the reaction was (from extremely negative to extremely positive). Because there were two dimensions with four possible behaviors in each, participants were asked to judge 16 people who were performing behaviors that captured every combination of these two dimensions (e.g., an extremely negative sociability act, an extremely negative activism act, a moderately negative sociability act, a moderately negative activism act, etc.). The participants were asked to make likability ratings of these people. Analyses were conducted to determine what factors were carrying the most weight in determining people's likability ratings. The extent to which the behavior was negative and the extent to which it was extreme were both found to be significant forces in shaping impressions. In addition, attention and salience can be assessed not merely by looking to see what forces have a strong impact on impressions, but by examining more direct types of evidence, such as the amount of time spent attending to and looking at a given photograph. Once again, negative information received greater attention than did positive information; extreme information also received more attention than nonextreme information (such that both extreme positive and extreme negative information received greater attention). This makes sense from the model described above, as extreme information has many of the same properties that make negative information salient—it is unexpected and nonmodal. Thus both extremity and negativity in one's behavior make one salient. Why? "Perceivers must ration social attention or be overwhelmed. In this instance, people seem to allocate processing time in an adaptive manner. Rather than equally weighting whatever comes along, social perceivers apparently attend to the most unusual cues—the nonmodal ones" (Fiske, 1980, p. 904).

Objects are also likely to be salient when they can form a perceptual unit with other elements of the perceptual field. Heider (1944) imported these ideas from Gestalt psychology and object perception to person perception by asserting that people ascribe greater causal weight to perceptual units, with the "units" usually consisting of people and their behavior. Heider assumed that each time another person enters our life space, a change to our environment has been produced by the actions we have observed. The unexplained action triggers a state of doubt, and a pursuit of meaning is initiated. How do we pursue meaning? Through making an attribution for the event in which the action and the actor are linked together as a perceptual unit. Perhaps Heider's most influential assertion was that the origin of the behavior (the person) and the change introduced by that origin (the person's behavior and its effects) form a perceptual unit, such that the two are seen as belonging together. With this salience comes extra causal weight to the perceptual unit, with the person seen as the cause for the behavior:

> The origin and the change which is attributed to the origin form a unit; that is to say, the change "belongs" to the origin. . . . Through causal integration changes or passing experiences are related to the framework of the invariant environment which gives the change its meaning. . . . animate beings, especially persons, are the prototype of origins. (Heider, 1944, pp. 358–359).

In other words, the search for meaning requires a stable and coherent cause to be ascribed to some event. In this case, some interpersonal behavior is the event, and the cause is assigned to what is most salient in the interaction. For us as perceivers, this salience will be determined by what units are most easily formed between the stimuli we observe during the course of the interaction. Such units are most easily formed between the behavior we are attempting to understand and the person who performed the behavior. Thus the underlying personality of the person—his/her invariant and stable disposition and intent—is seen as the origin or cause of the behavior, even if other forces in the situation may have caused the behavior.

An illustration of this notion of unit formation promoting salience is provided in the research of Macrae, Bodenhausen, and Milne (1995). Macrae and colleagues point out that people typically can be described by multiple categories, depending on which features of the person are salient. For example, a Chinese woman might be best described as Chinese if her nationality is salient, but as a woman if her gender is salient. A Black policeman might be categorized as a Black man if race is salient, or as a cop if occupation is salient. According to Heider's logic, the extent to which a particular feature is salient (and would be used in describing a person) would depend on its ability to form a unit with other features of the relevant situation. Macrae and colleagues illustrated this by showing research participants a videotape of a Chinese woman, but varied the features of the social environment that could be used to form a unit along with the woman. Some participants witnessed a Chinese woman eating noodles with chopsticks, thus allowing the woman's nationality to form a unit with the behavior and seem salient. Other participants saw a Chinese woman putting on makeup in front of a mirror, thus allowing her gender to form a unit with the behavior and seem salient. When the same woman was seen putting on makeup or using chopsticks, the concept that formed a unit with the set of data provided shifted, and what became salient was altered. In each case, a natural feature of the person had the potential to be salient, but unit formation determined which would eventually gain prominence.

One way to examine the natural prominence of features is to examine whether the brain has evolved special processes for dealing with them (to illustrate their biological relevance by their association with specific brain functions). Let us begin with an example: Someone is staring at you, and you want to ascertain why. A more fundamental question is this: Why have you even bothered to notice that someone is staring at you? Why does this capture attention? Langton, Watt, and Bruce (2000, pp. 51–52) explain: "Humans and many other species tend to look at things in their environment that are of immediate interest to them. You might be the recipient of another's gaze, for instance, because you are a potential meal, a mate or simply because you are someone with whom they would like to interact." The gaze of another person captures your attention, because, as we have been discussing, it makes good evolutionary sense to know why you have become the focus of attention. Macrae, Hood, Milne, Rowe, and Mason (2002) have argued that the gaze of another captures attention because it is a cue signaling that another person is potentially important to what will transpire in your immediate context. Evidence for the importance of detecting gaze—its natural prominence in capturing attention—can be evidenced by biological adaptiveness, with specific brain systems having evolved for the purpose of detecting eye gaze: "Electrophysiological research has suggested that such a system may be localized in the superior temporal sulcus (STS). . . . Perret and his colleagues located specific cells in the STS that responded selectively to the direction of gaze" (Macrae et al., 2002, p. 460). Macrae and colleagues further posit that the amygdala may be a localized center in the brain for detecting eye gaze, citing neuroimaging research by Kawashima and colleagues (1999) investigating the neural mechanisms involved in detecting gaze. Macrae and colleagues do not present neuropsychological evidence for linking gaze to specific brain systems, but they do provide indirect evidence that gaze is a feature with the ability to capture attention and affect basic processes of person perception. They reasoned that if gaze serves an evolutionary function that gives it natural prominence, you should be able to detect gaze quickly and be faster to identify, categorize, and make inferences about a person who has directed his/her gaze at you. In one experiment, they asked participants to look at faces presented on a computer monitor and to respond by indicating the gender of the person depicted—a simple categorization task. They manipulated whether the people depicted were directly gazing at the participants, or whether gaze was averted. They found that people were able to identify gender more quickly when gaze was direct. The best explanation for such a finding is that the gaze of another captures your attention and facilitates processing of the target upon which attention has been focused.

The suggested role of the amygdala in directing attention to people's features is perhaps derived from LeDoux's (1995) evidence that the amygdala plays a central role in emotional responses. Given that attention-grabbing features of stimuli are proposed to have an adaptive nature, such features are likely to be ones with emotional significance, particularly those associated with emotions such as fear and threat. The need to detect stimuli relevant to fear and threat (in order to avoid danger and survive) suggests that a specific relationship would have evolved between stimuli linked to these emotions and specific regions of the brain. What types of stimuli should acquire the ability to capture attention because of their relationship to specific brain centers dealing with fear and threat? Images that look threatening and dangerous, such as a fierce-looking animal or an angry-looking person. In essence, evidence that the features of a stimulus implying threat and danger have specific brain regions dedicated to their detection would provide good evidence that such features not only capture attention, but do so because they have natural prominence. This is precisely the argument put forth by Öhman (1993), who has argued that specific neural mechanisms are in place for the purpose of scanning the environment to detect such features in a stimulus and to prepare the individual to respond to threat. This includes directing attention to the threatening stimulus, as well as triggering autonomic arousal.

Do threatening stimuli receive preferential attention? If gaze can be conceived of as a potential threat, then we have already reviewed evidence suggesting that the answer to this question is yes. However, is there other evidence, and to what extent does this evidence reveal involvement of specific brain systems in detecting threat and focusing attention on it? Mogg and Bradley (1999) provide one such illustration. They modified a technique in which words relating to threat and neutral words were shown to people simultaneously, with one word appearing above the other. One of the words was quickly followed on the screen by a dot, and people had to respond to the dot by indicating where it had appeared. The logic was that people would respond faster if they had already been attending to the spot where the dot was soon to be located. Thus there should be faster responses to the dot if it occupied the spot where the threatening stimulus had been if, and only if, that stimulus had already captured attention (e.g., Mogg, Bradley, & Williams, 1995). Mogg and Bradley's modification to this technique was to include more realistic stimuli—threatening versus nonthreatening faces. They predicted that threatening faces would capture attention and facilitate responding to the dots (relative to happy faces and neutral faces). Furthermore, to drive home the point that this is an adaptive process that has evolved efficient systems to execute this direction of attention, they posited that this effect would be found even if the faces being present were never consciously detected by the individual! Subliminally presented, threatening faces should capture attention, thus illustrating the natural prominence of these types of stimuli.

What did Mogg and Bradley (1999) find? When threatening faces appeared on the left-hand side of the screen (and neutral faces on the right-hand side), participants were faster at detecting the location of the dot when the dot appeared on the left (in the spot where the threatening face had formerly been). The complementary pattern was not found when threatening stimuli appeared on the right side of the screen; people did not respond faster to dots that also appeared on the right. Thus it seems that attention was directed to threatening stimuli, even when the stimuli could not be consciously seen, but only when the stimuli appeared on the left side of the visual field. This finding, replicated in subsequent research, suggests that the right hemisphere of the brain is responsible for detecting threatening stimuli. This is consistent with other research suggesting that the right hemisphere exerts dominance in the perception of faces expressing emotion, and in emotional processing more generally. Such a difference provides the type of evidence for brain localization needed to support the idea that attention is being directed because of the natural prominence of threatening stimuli.

Salience and the Relative Distinctiveness of the Data

Not all salient information is something inherent to a person, or a quality that is salient (or even physically present) in every situation. One can display features that are salient and attention-grabbing only in certain contexts. Thus an important aspect of the salience of a person's behaviors and features is the fact that they are often relative: A laugh at a funeral is more salient than a laugh at a party; a loud yell heard while you are walking on a quiet street is more salient than the same scream at a football game. When a person's features and behaviors are salient or prominent because they stand out in relationship to other things, but do not grab attention in different contexts is known as salience due to *comparative distinctiveness* (Higgins, 1996).

For example, when a White person sees a Black police officer, the fact that this is a Black person may seem more salient if the encounter takes place in a restaurant, in a gas station, or on a date. However, race may not seem salient if the White person is the victim of a crime and is awaiting assistance (see Taylor, 1981). In that case, the fact that the Black person is an officer of the law will be what grabs the White person's attention and dictates the assignment of a category. Let's take a different example, where the context does more than select one feature to be salient from among other competing, potentially salient features (such as Black and police officer, Chinese and woman, skinny and blonde, etc.), but an example where a feature typically not salient is made salient by the context in which it occurs. A Chinese colleague recently told me a story about how when he was a boy, in his village a Westerner was so rarely seen (either in person or on television) that children would swarm around and stare whenever a White person happened to visit the village. However, one must imagine that the same White person, if moved to downtown New York, Sydney, or Munich, would never be salient. The color of one's skin, the presence of a hat on one's head, the pattern on one's dress, the loudness of one's voice, and the length of one's hair are all features that are comparatively distinct, with their salience dependent on the context.

One factor that determines whether a person will be salient within a situation is his/her physical position within the context. Position in a context can make people momentarily salient because they are suddenly well lit, or because they are located in a position where all eyes happen to be focused. Taylor and Fiske (1975) examined the impact of where a perceiver's physical gaze is focused by manipulating the seating arrangements in a group of research participants. Two confederates working for the experimenter were asked to engage in a scripted dialogue while six research participants watched. Among the six, two were seated so that their gaze was focused on one of the confederates, and two were seated so their attention was directed toward the other confederate. The final two participants were seated so that both confederates were equally visible, and gaze was not directed more strongly toward either one (see Figure 1.12). The participants were asked to watch the interaction and make judgments about which person was more responsible for directing the tone and topics of the conversation. The findings revealed that focus of attention had an impact on judgments. The person who was more salient by virtue of being momentarily the recipient of visual focus was seen as playing a greater causal role in shaping the interaction. Similar results were found when a second experiment presented two targets on a split screen, and participants were asked to focus attention on one of the two sides of the screen. The salient person was seen as more responsible for the shape of the discussion.

Being the focus of the direct gaze of others is not the only contextual force that makes a person salient. Taylor, Fiske, Etcoff, and Ruderman (1978) examined several hypotheses concerning what features get attended to and direct attention to a person. They state that

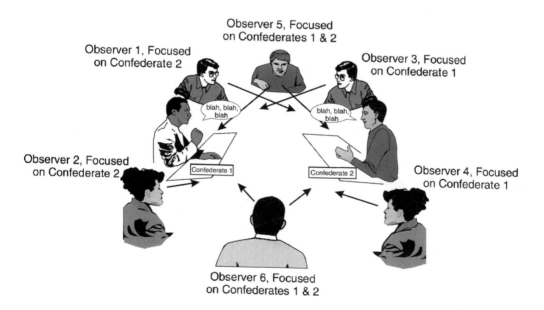

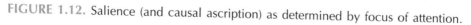

FIGURE 1.12. Salience (and causal ascription) as determined by focus of attention.

instead of perceiving a group of persons as a set of unique individuals, the perceiver may . . . select salient social or physical dimensions to use as discriminating variables for grouping and managing person information. If this is true, certain variables such as race or sex would be likely candidates for such categories, since they are physically salient as well as useful social discriminators. (p. 779)

Physical features such as gender and race, however, are only salient if the context places such a feature in isolation. We would not argue that women are salient by virtue of their gender alone, because approximately half of the population is female. Similarly, Blacks may be a minority in the United States, but they are hardly surprising to encounter. But contexts can make members of these groups surprising and salient. Blacks certainly are rare on the campuses of the last three universities at which I worked (Konstanz, Princeton, and Lehigh), and this might make their race something that is attention-grabbing in those settings. Women were certainly rare at the last three technology jobs at which my wife worked as a programmer, or in the engineering departments in which her closest female friends were receiving their PhDs. Once again, because of the relative "solo" status of women in these contexts, gender might be particularly attention-grabbing. Attributes such as race and gender (as well as others) attain heightened salience when the context places people with these attributes alone instead of among others of their group.

Taylor and colleagues (1978) illustrated this importance of "solo" status for grabbing attention by manipulating whether people were novel in a particular context by virtue of either their gender or their race. For example, in one experiment participants listened to a dialogue among six group members with the aid of a visual display; each time a person was heard to speak, his/her picture appeared on a screen. Participants were to make ratings of how influential, talkative, and prominent a given person was over the course of the group discussion. What was important about this research was that participants in the different conditions of the experiment did not hear different things; the person they were evaluating spoke exactly the same number of times and said exactly the same things. What differed between participants was whether the person was novel in this context or not. They arranged the materials so that people in the different conditions of the experiment believed they were watching groups of different compositions. Some participants saw and heard a group that had one woman and five men; others saw and heard a group with three women and three men; finally, others saw and heard a group with one man and five women. The findings were impressive: Despite the same words' being spoken, evaluations of the person's contributions to the group differed as a function of whether the person was salient, novel, within the context. The solo man was perceived as disproportionately more influential and prominent than in the condition when there were three men and three women. Identically, the solo (novel) woman was disproportionately more influential and prominent than in the condition in which she said the same words but in a group that contained two other women. Novelty within a context leads to salience and attention, with the attention-grabbing powers of one's novelty being evidenced by an overemphasis on one's contributions and importance to a situation.

A person belongs to many categories—a gender (male or female), a generation (baby boomer, Gen X, etc.), an occupational group (academic, medical professional, etc.), an ethnicity (African American, Hispanic, etc.), a religious group (Jew, Muslim, etc.), a nationality (American, Canadian, etc.), and a social subculture (Goth, punk, etc.). How other people categorize us seems to be determined partly by which of these many categories is temporarily made salient and captures the attention of the perceiver. Novelty within a context is one such factor, even with self-categorization. My own identity as a Jew was never more salient than when I moved to Munich, Germany, where my religious affiliation was a fairly novel one. Does this overemphasis on a person because of his/her solo status lead that factor to be seen as responsible for the person's actions? For instance, if a person is novel because of his/her race, and thus race is what grabs attention and shapes how others categorize this person, does this mean that race is overemphasized as what causes the person to act and speak as he/she does? The possibility exists for a perceptual and interpretive overemphasis on whatever factor makes one novel. The only female in a workforce of 20 computer programmers will perhaps be defined and reacted to according to gender. The Blacks on a college campus that is mostly White may be attention-grabbing because of their race; this may lead people to react to them in terms of race and to ascribe race as the cause for why they speak, don't speak, act, or fail to act in a given situation. Taylor and colleagues (1978) found support for this, in that the solo woman in a group was presumed to have more stereotypic features and play a more stereotype-prescribed role in the group than the same woman in a gender-mixed group. For example, the solo woman was more likely to be described as "motherly" and the solo man more likely to be described as "macho" than the same individuals saying the same things, but in a gender-mixed group.

Stangor, Lynch, Duan, and Glass (1992) propose that what makes a particular feature salient to perceivers depends not only on the novelty of that feature within the context, but on the utility the feature has for the perceivers within that context. Stangor and colleagues believe that the feature that has the most information value for perceivers provides them with a useful basis for making inferences that are relevant to them within that context. If the goal is ultimately to predict what others are like so that the perceivers can act and react, then they should choose to attend to those features that will provide the type of information that suits those contextual goals. Hair color is usually not very informative—there are few useful stereotypes about hair color that would allow perceivers to make inferences and plan appropriate behavior. However, gender is a fairly useful and inference-laden social category. The utility of this category will make it the more likely one to capture attention and become salient (thus making perceivers more likely to pigeonhole the person according to that feature and the stereotypes/inferences prescribed by it).

To examine what grabs attention, Stangor and colleagues (1992) showed research participants a series of photographs of people and an accompanying text of statements made by each one. The people in the photographs varied on several dimensions or features that could potentially have captured attention. After the participants had examined a stack of such items, a surprise memory test was given in which the participants had to try to recall which people had made which statements. One way to assess what types of features were capturing attention would be to look at the types of errors people made: Did they routinely confuse people with particular types of features, so that women (if gender was used as the potential attention-grabbing feature) were routinely believed to have made statements made by other women (but rarely to have made statements made by men)? Such a pattern would suggest that gender, and not some other feature (such as shirt color or race), was what grabbed attention. These researchers predicted that the more utilitarian types of categories—those that carried much meaning for the perceivers (such as race and gender)—would capture attention.

To test this hypothesis, Stangor and colleagues (1992, Experiment 5) pitted a utilitarian category against one that was not particularly informative to see whether errors in memory were more likely to align along the utilitarian dimension. The photographs contained pictures of people who differed from each other in terms of race (the utilitarian category) and clothing color (a noninformative and not very useful category). However, one could predict that differences in clothing color would make a person salient and would capture attention. Stangor and colleagues proposed that, given the presence of a more utilitarian feature, the attention-grabbing power of clothing color might fade. The photographs were of four White women and four Black women. Two of the White and two of the Black women wore white shirts, while two of the White and two of the Black women wore black shirts; this creating two features, each presented an equal number of times. The number of within-race errors and the number of between-race errors were computed, as were the number of within-clothing errors and the number of between-clothing errors. Although there was no difference between how many errors were made within one clothing color (mistaking a white-shirted person for a different white-shirted person) as there were between clothing colors (mistaking a white-shirted person for a black-shirted person), such differences were in fact found for race pairings. People were more likely to make errors that confused something said by a person of one race with something said by a person of the same race than they were to confuse something said by a person of one race with something said by a person of a different race. Stangor and colleagues concluded that salience is not determined by novelty alone, but by the value that a feature holds for the person within the context. Some features, such as race and gender, have natural informational value because of a rich history of stereotypes and beliefs and inferences that perceivers feel they can lean on.

CODA

Perception is a construction. And what we see is built not solely from features of the data being observed, but from the context the data appear in and from the meaning we impose as perceivers on the data. Despite this constructive nature of perception, our experience of the perceptual process is that we are objective, acting on fact, responding solely to the data. Asch (1952) stated:

> Although phenomenally we see objects directly, with no process intervening, objectively the process is mediated. [We cannot maintain] that the perceived object is a photographic reflection of the real object. We have to say that the object in the environment and our experience of it are two distinct, though related, events. (p. 47)

Although our experience is that we are empiricists, the reality seems to be that we are instrumentalists, seeing that which suits our goals. We see what we want to see—that which we already believe to be true. Shakespeare (1602/1974) reminds us of this when Hamlet likens Denmark to a prison. When his friend Rosencrantz disagrees, Hamlet retorts, "Why then 'tis none to you; for there is nothing either good or bad, but thinking makes it so. To me it is a prison" (p. 1155). Kant (1781/1990) stated this more formally: "Without the sensuous faculty no object would be given to us, and without the understanding no object would be thought" (p. 45).

One source of this subjective twisting of the data we receive is the context in which those data are embedded. Ichheiser (1943, p. 151) tells us:

> The behavior of the individual is always determined by two groups of factors: by personal factors (attitudes, dispositions, etc.) and by situational factors. The situation plays its part in determining behavior in two ways: as a system of stimuli which provokes reactions, and as a system of opportunities for action (or obstacles to action). We cannot understand the underlying motivation of behavior without taking into account the dynamics of the situation involved . . . the importance of situational factors is often greater than the importance of personal factors: individuals endowed with different traits (attitudes), nevertheless, behave in the same way in identical social situations.

Ichheiser's (1943) point in the quote above is that even when the situation is relegated to the role of ground or context, it can still play a part in shaping perception. It does so in two ways: (1) as a system of stimuli with specific features that we react to, and (2) as a system of opportunities for taking action. What we notice is determined by what is "out there" to be noticed. A second source of subjectivity in perception arises from our state as individual perceivers, the persons within the situation (what Ichheiser called the "personal factors"). Our goals, expectancies, stereotypes, needs, affect, attitudes, mood, and other qualities will all dictate what is attended to, how it is interpreted once attention is focused on it, how it is organized in and retrieved from memory, and ultimately the type of judgment we form of the observed person and his/her behavior.

This chapter's analysis of the constructed nature of perception has highlighted the fact that the processes that determine our social judgment often occur outside of conscious awareness and without intent. These processes are often difficult to control even if we have been forewarned about their occurrence. This is a very different type of analysis from that focused on by Heider in his classic 1958 analysis of interpersonal perception. Heider's interest was in everyday psychology, analyzing what each of us is capable of finding out about our own social cognition. Heider compared each person to a "naive scientist" who reflects on what might be the causes for events the person has observed and inferences he/she has formed. This was said to be accomplished by engaging in reflection and carefully considering the potential causes that could have compelled another person to act. As Heider (1958) stated explicitly at the outset of his book, "Our concern will be with 'surface' matters, the events that occur in everyday life on a conscious level, rather than with the unconscious" (p. 1). Heider's rationale was that despite the fact his approach was essentially mapping out lay psychological processes—specifying what each of us could observe in ourselves, had we taken the time to introspect carefully enough—the act of carefully scrutinizing these conscious processes would yield important insights into how we function, providing a set of principles that describe how we operate as naive scientists. The main contribution of this analysis was the important revelation that the study of common sense does not always reveal common or obvious findings.

But the approach in the current analysis is to combine Heider's interest in surface matters that are under our conscious control as perceivers with those matters lurking beneath the surface. Those processes that occur automatically and preconsciously have been incorporated into this analysis of interpersonal perception. But this raises another question: What are automatic and controlled processes? To this question we turn in Chapter 2.

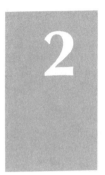

2 Automaticity and Control

We automatically interpret manifestations of other persons in specific ways without being aware of our doing so and without noticing that our observations are based on, and guided by, those unconscious interpretations. What we consider to be "objective facts" are actually products of our unnoticed interpretative manipulations.

—ICHHEISER (1943, p. 146)

Evaluation of other persons, important as it is in our existence, is largely automatic, one of the things we do without knowing very much about the "principles" in terms of which we operate. Regardless of the degree of skill which an adult may have in appraising others, he engages in the process most of the time without paying much attention to how he does it.

—TAGIURI (1958, p. ix)

When Paula Jones accused President Clinton of sexual harassment, it led most of us to question her motives and to try to form an impression of her in order to ascertain whether her claims were real or not. It also led us to consciously question and reevaluate our opinion of the President. When the pregnant Laci Peterson was found dead, and we then learned that she was allegedly murdered by her own husband (who had been having an adulterous affair), most Americans exerted considerable effort thinking about the motives and behavior of Scott Peterson in order to figure out whether he was responsible for his wife's death. And if we didn't exert the effort ourselves, we turned to the media, consumed with these stories, to do it for us.

This exercise of our volition for the purpose of understanding a person is a case of our exerting *control*: We have the goal of forming an impression, and we regulate our thoughts and behavior to allow us to pursue that end. Often the impressions we form of others are made in order to help us attain some goal other than simply forming the best possible impression of the person. Examples of such control in person perception include the following: We want to impress someone, so we form an impression of him/her focused on what that person would find impressive; we want to suck up to the boss, and we need to know what his/her expectancies are, so we can act in an ingratiating way; we want to see a defendant we dislike convicted, so we attend most closely to the damaging parts of the case and ignore parts that would speak to an acquittal; we want someone to be attracted to us, so we smile pleasantly and sit close to that person when the opportunity arises; we want another person to detect that we are displeased with him/her, so we give that person the silent treatment, complete with stern glances and a furrowing of the brow. In all these cases, our impressions are controlled—they are the results of thought processes performed to help us attain some goal we have selected. The thoughts we have about others are often controlled in this sense of the word; that is, our thinking is said to serve some end state. The types of goals that relate to person perception and that dictate the types of impressions we form are discussed at the end of this chapter.

While it is obvious that we exercise control to willfully examine the people in our world, it is also true that we infer motives, form impressions, detect and send communicative signals, and make attributions without a great deal of conscious effort. We engage in these activities somewhat incidentally and outside of awareness, so that rather than being explicit and obvious, they are *implicit processes*. As Ichheiser (1943) and Tagiuri (1958) have asserted in the quotes above, inferences about the qualities of others occur without conscious intent or awareness. Consider the two examples given above. Even if you were not aware you were trying to form an impression of Paula Jones, Bill Clinton, or Scott Peterson as you read/heard about them in the press, you still were likely to have formed such impressions. And you would not argue that someone else forced you to form impressions, or these impressions were not made of your own free will! Rather, your thought processes were under your direct control, even if you were not consciously attending to these thoughts, attempting to form impressions, or even aware of having formed impressions.

THE UNCONSCIOUS NATURE OF NAIVE REALISM

Chapter 1 has asserted that one reason we are not aware of the many influences on and biases in our judgment is that such influences occur outside of conscious awareness. Naive realism occurs because at the very primary stages of information processing (such as determining where our attention is focused and how we identify a stimulus), selectivity of stimuli has already started to direct what we see and hear, prior to the involvement of our conscious will or conscious awareness of what we have done. The current chapter begins with two examples of this to help convince you that this is plausible, and the rest of the chapter is spent fleshing out these intriguing ideas in the realm of person perception. First, imagine that you come across a photograph of (or are lucky enough to meet) Rosa Parks. Rosa Parks falls into multiple identity categories: elderly, African American, female, activist, heroine, and others. How will she be identified, given the many possibilities? Smith, Fazio, and Cejka (1996) demonstrated that the identification of a stimulus person is influenced by the subjectivity of the perceiver, such that the way in which a person is categorized and identified (e.g., Bruner, 1957) is directed by the perceiver's attitudes. Thus what you believe you have seen (how you categorize Rosa Parks—as a heroine, an elderly lady, etc.) can be determined by your preferences without your even realizing there may have been several perfectly acceptable alternative ways to label her.

With a similar focus on the unconscious impact of attitudes on the early stages of information processing, Roskos-Ewoldsen and Fazio (1992) posited that the selective focus of attention would be directed toward objects associated with one's attitudes. To test this, research participants performed two tasks. In the first one, a visual display of six objects (e.g., frog, books, bread, music; see Figure 2.1) arranged in a circle was briefly flashed. Attention to these items was measured by a recall test that occurred later, with the researchers' hypothesis being that items better recalled would be the ones that had been attended to. They found that the objects on which participants were more likely to focus attention, and therefore were more likely to remember later on, were the ones they liked best (preferences were assessed in a separate part of the experiment). People who liked books best would be more likely to remember books from the circle of items, whereas a person enamored of food would be more likely to recall the bread. Even when items were briefly flashed at participants so that they did not have time to detect all the items in the array, they still had time to direct attention to some items more than others. Therefore, preferences unknowingly guide where to focus attention.

What we see, and how we identify and label what we see, has already been twisted according to the subjective forces within us as perceivers; yet we remain unaware that such forces have been at work. Given this fact, naive realism in judging people seems an almost foregone conclusion. If the perceptual products that we use to build our impressions are biased, the final outcome of the judgment process must, it seems, be biased as well. The focus in this chapter is on the perceptual/cognitive processes serving as the building blocks of impression formation. We have already noted how these processes may be biased. What is even more intriguing is the idea that we lack awareness of far more than an influence on these cognitive processes contributing to person perception. In addition, *we often even lack the awareness that any cognitive processes have occurred at all*—we are unaware that we have attended to something, or engaged in a process of categorizing that which we have attended to. These processes are implicit.

An implicit process can be defined as *automatic* if it has the following features: being (1) unintended (it is initiated without conscious intent); (2) impossible to control (the decision not to engage in the process does not stop the process from occurring); (3) extremely efficient (it occurs despite our working on other activities at the same time); and (4) able to proceed without our awareness. In sum, the processes producing

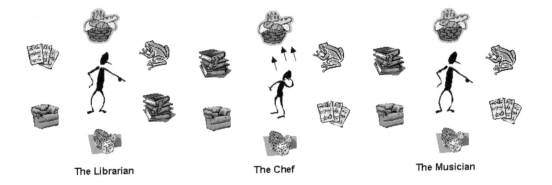

The Librarian   The Chef   The Musician

FIGURE 2.1. Preferences guide attention.

our impressions can be automatic, and though they are automatic, they can still be biased.

Phenomenal Immediacy

We concern ourselves in this chapter with the automatic processing of information relating to other people, for two very important reasons. The first is that such processes are ubiquitous and contribute a much greater component to our moment-to-moment thoughts than many of us would have guessed or believed. We like to believe that we are in conscious control of most of what we think and do, when the reality is that we are far more efficient creatures than that. Habit, routine, and evolution have given us the ability to relegate much of our mental life to the preconscious. The second reason is that we *fail to recognize* just how much mental activity we are constantly engaged in (such as forming inferences about people and making judgments about what others are like), and therefore do not recognize its impact on how interpersonal perception and social interaction unfolds. Chapter 1 has made it clear that our phenomenological experience is simply to feel as if the qualities of the people we observe are inherent—embedded in them, not inferred by us through our own undetected mental activity. Why assume the qualities we observe in others are indicators of some objective essence, when we know all too well that we have no insight into the true motives in another person's mind?

One explanation is the simple ease with which inferences about them come to mind. If our goal to form impressions of others operates outside of our conscious awareness and without conscious intent, then we are likely to have formed impressions without consciously realizing that we had done so, and without realizing that these impressions are controlled by our intentions/goals to have formed them. In essence, if we do not experience our own subjective manipulation of the data in producing these impressions, then we probably do not even think that either an impression or any manipulation of the data has occurred. When knowledge is arrived at easily, and we do not even experience it as being "arrived at" by us through perceptual or impression formation processes, then it is likely to be interpreted as a perceptual given, a "true quality" of the person. In such instances, the characteristics of the person being perceived have *phenomenal immediacy*. Just as gazing at the sky we perceive the color blue, and the appearance of this thought is held as an indisputable fact, the appearance of an impression about another person can be experienced as if (its phenomenology is as if) it effortlessly popped into the head, and therefore it has the character of "feeling true" (or being an immediately recognizable, inherent quality of the person). The reason we don't feel we need to answer the question "Why is the sky blue?" is because most of us never stop to ask that question. Our experience of it simply is that the sky just *is* blue. This quality exists independently of our perception and simply presents itself to us upon our merely being exposed to the sky. In social perception, our experience is similar: We simply feel we know what others are like, because we do not experience the machinations of the brain that give rise to such impressions. They occur automatically.

Implicit Communication and Perception via Nonverbal Cues

Perhaps the simplest way to illustrate the automatic nature of social cognition is to examine a domain where this seems obvious and intuitive—nonverbal communication. Imagine you are lost and need directions, and you bump into a man who looks like a "punk." You might consciously decide to form impressions of this man based on nonverbal cues he sends you before you have even interacted with him. You decide to attend to the expression on the face to detect whether he is friendly; you plan on avoiding him if his actions seem erratic and potentially threatening; and you use his manner of dress as a cue as to how informative the person might be. In addition to the conscious choice to attend to these cues, you are likely also to notice and distill information from a host of other bodily movements he makes that you are not aware of having noticed or intended to use in forming your impressions. For example, the extent to which eye contact is made may affect whether you approach or avoid this man, without your realizing this factor has even been something you noticed. The types of hand gestures exhibited could also play a role in shaping how communicative he seems and how helpful and trustworthy the information is. Kenny (1994) calls situations such as this, where we form impressions of people we have never met, *zero acquaintance*. Despite having never met, the perceiver (in this example, you) observes the target (in this case, the "punk") and is able to imagine what type of person this is.

The next section of this chapter reviews the importance of nonverbal behavior in social interaction, as a way of introducing the concept of automaticity in an important domain of person perception. This is followed by a review of the idea that much of human behavior and cognition can be characterized by a distinction between that which occurs automatically and outside of conscious awareness, and that which is controlled and driven by conscious intent. Social cognition is complex and involves the coordination of many mental and physical activities, some of which we have relegated to the domain of the preconscious and have become so skilled at pursuing that these activities require no conscious monitoring on our part, even to initiate them. The domain of nonverbal behavior is but one interesting area for illustrating this idea.

BODY LANGUAGE, FACIAL EXPRESSION, AND NONVERBAL COMMUNICATION

Most of us are familiar with the expression "body language." It is probably not surprising to learn that we send signals and conduct a good deal of the communication we have with others through a nonverbal language—our own personal sign language. We all readily recognize that our bodies, our faces, and the tone of our voice all communicate tremendous amounts of information to others, and that we receive signals from others in these domains that we use as an important source of information for determining what they are like and what they want. The wave of the hand that means "hello," the lean forward, the wink of the eye, the furrowed brow, the middle finger, an uncertain smile, a push away, a pull toward, the outstretched thumb, a hug, a tear, and a look of fear are all part of the silent exchange directing the course of our social interactions. What we may not recognize is just *how* silent these exchanges can be. Not only do we fail to utter any noise in initiating many of these responses, but we often do not initiate any conscious intention to display a particular nonverbal behavior. In other words, these processes are not only quiet, but not conscious to us. Can it be said that we always consciously intend to lean forward slightly when interacting with a person we like, or to lean away slightly when interacting with a person we dislike? Do we always mean to reveal our emotions in our facial expressions so that our hearts are "on our sleeves," open to inspection? It is true that many nonverbal behaviors are initiated with the conscious intent of communicating a particular feeling or piece of information. When we wave hello, we have intended to signal our friendliness, and when we use our middle finger, we are intending to express anger and hostility. However, these same emotions can "leak out" unintentionally in our nonverbal behavior, in addition to being consciously controlled.

For example, Ekman (1992) described one nonverbal sign—a smile of true joy—that has features associated with it that are difficult to control and are produced quite spontaneously. A joyous smile involves the movement of muscles surrounding the eye that are difficult to control, and a person cannot adequately duplicate this movement if trying to fake a smile. This one component of nonverbal behavior communicates something meaningful, and it happens without the awareness or conscious intent of the person sending the message. Another example may have helped shape the 2000 U.S. presidential election. Al Gore famously rolled his eyes and looked visibly annoyed when George W. Bush was providing answers to questions during their first debate. The ability to control one's facial expressions is extremely difficult, especially when one hears something that truly generates a strong emotion, such as outrage, joy, and fear. It is certainly possible to control such expressions once one recognizes them in oneself, but the micromanagement of these *microexpressions* is extremely difficult in the short run, when for a fleeting moment one's true emotions may be betrayed by the rolling of one's eyes upon hearing something one considers outlandish. Perhaps Gore's inability first to control these expressions, and then to recognize they were occurring and rein them in, led him to appear arrogant and superior—which hurt his public image. Of course, perhaps Gore was using these expressions deliberately to attempt to communicate nonverbally to viewers that Bush was not too bright. If that was his intent, it backfired, because people did detect his nonverbal cues and saw them as a sign of Gore's arrogance, not Bush's lack of intelligence. In either case, the signals were being sent and received, and it is possible to imagine these signals operating either through automatic processes (which Gore was unable to control) or controlled processes (which Gore was using strategically). Finally, it is easy to imagine nonverbal behavior operating outside of conscious control by considering how you behave when speaking with someone on the telephone. You are likely to use your hands and arms as expressive aids, or to express emotions in your face (even though no one will see them). Yet you are probably not aware of, and have no control over, the sending of these nonverbal signals.

Lack of Awareness that a Nonverbal Communicative Exchange Is Occurring

It has been suggested that people detect and send information via nonverbal channels—through what has been called *nonverbal communication*—that help to drive the engine of interpersonal perception. A defining feature of an automatic process is the person's lack of awareness of the process. We next review evidence for the implicit sending and detecting of nonverbal cues. Let us begin with a common form of nonverbal communication that we may usually think of as consciously controlled—the hand gesture. We all know people who speak with their hands. They may gesticulate quite robustly, waving their arms about while they speak. Even the most nonexpressive person you know must animate his/her speech somewhat through hand gestures. Much of this form of communication is consciously intended and deliberately used to accompany and exaggerate speech. However, people may not be aware of the extent to which they are doing so or the precise way they use gestures to accompany their speech, just as the recipients of those signals may not be aware of the nonverbal signals that are being sent to them or the subtleties of interpretation and decoding that are going on. Therefore, this description of people who "speak with their hands" introduces two important questions: First, to what extent are people even aware of the fact that they are using hand gestures to accompany their speech (if they are the messengers) or reacting to and detecting hand gestures in others (if they are the perceivers)? Second, do hand gestures actually help people communicate (nonverbally), allowing perceivers to understand the motives and feelings of those with whom they are interacting?

Gestures as Nonverbal Cues: Nonsemantic Information

One experiment illustrating the ability of people to detect and use nonverbal cues without being aware of their reliance on these skills comes from Chawla and Krauss (1994). Research participants were asked to distinguish between whether another person was speaking to them spontaneously and extemporaneously, or whether the person was delivering a rehearsed speech. First, people were taped having a conversation, and portions of this tape were used to present to research participants an unrehearsed, spontaneous narrative. Several such narratives were created. In addition to the spontaneous narratives, rehearsed narratives were created. These were made by having a trained actor rehearse the spontaneous narratives and recreate them on tape as a monologue. Thus two versions of the very same words were created—one that was spontaneous, one rehearsed. These narratives were then played for research participants to see whether they could distinguish between them, but the manner in which they were presented was also manipulated. Some participants only heard the narratives on audiotape without an accompanying video; others saw a video without sound; and finally, some people watched the narratives under normal videotape conditions (with sound and vision).

The findings revealed that having audio alone and having video alone were fairly comparable. Participants in each of these conditions were able to perform at better than chance levels in guessing which narrative was rehearsed and which was spontaneous. However, people who received both audio and video were far superior at making this distinction, attaining accuracy 80% of the time. This group of people also provided evidence that they were making better use of nonverbal cues in the narratives. Each person was asked to rate how real and spontaneous each narrative seemed; these ratings were then correlated with the use of nonverbal cues, such as hand gestures and pauses in speech, in the actual videotapes. The spontaneity ratings of the perceivers were significantly correlated with hand gestures and pauses in speech used by the speakers. However, this was only true for certain types of gestures and pauses. What types of hand gestures and pauses were seemingly related to people's ability to tell the difference between spontaneous and rehearsed speech? They were those gestures and pauses that were known (from previous research) to be related to problems with lexical access. For example, when people have trouble pulling thoughts and words out of memory (trouble with lexical access), they use particular types of hand gestures, as well as pauses in speaking as they search for the right thing to say. Participants in the condition of the Chawla and Krauss experiment where they heard the audio and saw the video seemed to be detecting these gestures and pauses, because their ratings of spontaneity of the speech were correlated with the occurrence of these types of hand gestures and pauses. Their ratings did not correlate with hand gestures more generally or with pauses in speech more generally, just with these specific type of gestures and pauses known to be associated with trouble accessing words from the lexicon.

Troubles with lexical access are more likely in spontaneous than in rehearsed speech. Did you know that? Probably not. We would be hard pressed to argue that the research participants were aware of this and were therefore deliberately searching for signs of trouble with lexical access in order to do the task better. We would also be hard pressed to argue, even if the participants were deliberately looking for signs that the speech was spontaneous, that they were consciously aware of the fact that certain hand gestures indicate problems with lexical access, and that they deliberately tried to make themselves aware of the fact that others were or were not revealing these cues to them. Thus, here is an instance where perceivers seemed to be clearly attending to nonverbal cues without being aware that they were doing so. They were using cues suggesting trouble with lexical access, despite probably not being aware that such cues have anything to do with lexical access or that lexical access has anything to do with how spontaneous speech seems. A clever speaker can make use of this information to deliver a speech that seems fresh and spontaneous, despite being rehearsed, by using the proper hand gestures and pauses (such as when pretending to be trying to think of just the right word) that will implciitly signal to perceivers the speech is "off the cuff."

Using the Chawla and Krauss (1994) research to answer our first question (are people aware of their use and detection of nonverbal cues?) also provides a partial answer to the second question (are nonverbal cues useful at helping the communication process along?). Nonverbal cues helped the participants to detect whether others were being spontaneous or not, so they certainly were communicating information from speakers to perceivers. However, this is only a partial answer to a complex question whose answer is best derived from reading Krauss, Chen, and Chawla (1996). To summarize their view, nonverbal behavior is only useful at communicating specific types of information between persons in a social interaction. The usefulness of nonverbal behavior (hand gestures) in identifying spontaneous speech is not dependent on specific semantic meaning being associated with a given behavior. That is, the nonverbal behaviors being detected are not symbolic representations of specific words that are being uttered, such as when a person waves one hand to signal hello or shakes his/her head in disagreement. They refer to more abstract states, such as the person's attitude. The extent to which a person is leaning away from you while talking may not tell you about the specific meanings of the words being uttered by the person, but it may tell you about that person's evaluation of you. Krauss and colleagues propose that gestures communicate *nonsemantic information*, such as a feeling that a speaker is having trouble producing speech—a syndrome usually associated with spontaneity. They argue that while gestures can silently signal nonsemantic information, they do not automatically communicate specific semantic meaning.

Thin Slices of Behavior

People detect features of others as revealed by their looks, posture, and gestures, and they make inferences and form impressions about those others based on those features, even in the absence of any interaction with such others (what Kenny, 1994, calls *zero acquaintance*). Yet they often deny that they use nonverbal cues, even when the effects are clear. One convincing example is the extent to which people are influenced by the physical attractiveness of others. They may deny that they use such nonverbal information for any purpose other than evaluating whether another person is attractive or not, but what they really mean to say is that they are not aware of the influence that such information has over their evaluation and judgment. This is what is illustrated by halo effects as discussed in Chapter 1. A halo effect occurs when one variable unknowingly influences people's impressions of a person along a different variable, because it shades the manner in which the person's overall character is interpreted. You probably would accept the idea, without an empirical illustration, that evaluations of physically attractive people on dimensions that have nothing to do with attractiveness are unknowingly influenced by the nonverbal communication of their good looks and sexy bodies. But let's review a classic social-psychological study that makes this point quite clearly.

Dion, Berscheid, and Walster (1972) described an effect on person perception that has been highly replicated over the years (see a meta-analysis by Eagly, Ashmore, Makhijani, & Longo, 1991); it has been dubbed the *"what is beautiful is good" stereotype*. The basic idea is that when people detect the physical attractiveness of others through examining their features, these nonverbal signals influence the impressions of these people along a wide variety of traits and behaviors. The physical attractiveness of a set of photographs (male and female faces) was determined by having 100 judges rate the faces for attractiveness. Once these ratings were made, different research participants were shown the faces and were asked to make a variety of judgments about each person's personality and his/her likely behaviors and expected outcomes in life. The results revealed that being physically attractive led to the perception that a person was kind, sociable, poised, interesting, warm, outgoing, and modest; had a fulfilling life, prestige, good moral character, and professional success; and was socially adept. In other words, a positive halo shone around such people, all emanating from the detection of a few features in the face.

Ambady and Rosenthal (1993) illustrated that while physical attractiveness does influence perceivers' ratings of a person they are observing in an interaction, so too does a host of specific nonverbal behaviors, such as head shakes, smiles, nods, yawns, frowns, emphatic gestures, and biting the lip (or my own personal vices of fiddling with an object while I teach, touching my face while I speak in public, and moving about the room when I am talking to a group). Ambady and Rosenthal took videotapes of teachers, which had been made for the purpose of receiving feedback from a teaching laboratory, from the library of the teaching lab. These were edited into short clips (10 seconds from the start of class, followed by a segment of 10 seconds from the middle of class, and ending with 10 seconds taken from the end of class) to show to research participants. The clips were rated by participants to detect how frequently each of the nonverbal behaviors mentioned above was performed, as well as to provide more molar evaluations of each teacher's attractiveness and nonverbal behavior relating to personality dimensions (such as confidence, competence, attentiveness, enthusiasm, professionalism, etc.). Finally, the ability of perceivers to quickly detect these nonverbal cues in teachers was assessed by correlating the evaluations made by the participants with the actual teaching evaluations of students who had taken the class with the teachers in question. First, the findings revealed that the ratings of the teachers were correlated with physical attractiveness: The more attractive the teacher, the better the student evaluation of the quality of that teacher's performance as a teacher. However, other nonverbal cues that perceivers were detecting quite quickly from the videotape were also correlated with the ratings of the actual students who took the class. Teachers who received positive evaluations from actual students received more favorable ratings on the molar nonverbal behaviors from the participants watching the short video clips. In addition, the specific nonverbal behaviors judged to be present by participants only briefly exposed to a teacher were also shown to predict how skilled at his/her profession the teacher was perceived to be by the actual students in the class. It seems that perceivers, even those in different contexts at different points in time, make similar inferences about a target person. In this research, people with extended contacts with the teachers made inferences compatible with the nonverbal cues that seemed to be detected by people who were in zero-acquaintance contexts (seeing only 10-second clips).

Ambady, Hallahan, and Conner (1999) have referred to these very brief observations of nonverbal behavior ranging from 1 to 30 seconds in length as *thin slices of behavior*. As is obvious in the example above from Ambady and Rosenthal (1993), in many cases the people whose behavior is being judged are not aware that they are being judged and not aware that they are generating any nonverbal behaviors to be used by others in judging them. Whether the perceivers are aware that they use nonverbal behavior in making their judgments is often less clear. If people are asked to make a judgment of another person based on a short, silent video clip, the perceivers are probably aware of the fact that they are using nonverbal behavior in forming an impression. They may not realize the extent to which they do this, the exact influence it has on them, or which dimensions/types of nonverbal behavior they are using or find influential (e.g., Nisbett & Wilson, 1977), but they must surely be aware of the use of such behavior in forming a judgment. A further illustration that people use nonverbal cues in thin slices of behavior, communicated without the communicator's awareness, to make important evaluations of the other person (e.g., whether a teacher is effective or not; whether a person is homosexual or heterosexual) was provided by Ambady and colleagues, who asked participants to make judgments concerning the sexual orientation of the communicator (gay or straight).

Ambady and colleagues (1999) recruited gay and lesbian students and male and female heterosexual students from campus social groups to play the role of the communicator. These individuals did not know they were being selected because of their sexual orientation, but believed they were helping the researchers in a study on how students balance academic activities with extracurricular involvement in social groups. Videotapes were made of these students discussing how they managed to maintain such balance, and were then edited into silent films. The films were shown to research participants, who were asked to decide whether each person depicted was gay or straight. Some of the participants saw a 10-second film; some saw a 1-second film; and some saw a still picture (the still picture was included to allow the researchers to detect whether the use of nonverbal cues was carried by static elements such as hair style or color, and manner of dress, or whether it was captured in more dynamic elements such as gestures and body movements). Could sexual orientation be perceived accurately from brief observations of video clips, and did such clips promote more accurate assessments of sexual orientation than photographs? Participants rated the clips on a 7-point scale, where 1 meant the person was clearly heterosexual and 7 clearly homosexual. The results showed that the gay men and lesbian women serving as targets were perceived to be "more gay" than the heterosexual targets. Accuracy was significantly greater in the 10-second videos than in the 1-second clips or the photographs.

Albright, Kenny, and Malloy (1988) similarly found that under such conditions of zero acquaintance, different perceivers have fairly similar reactions to a target person (there is a consensus in impression formation). This suggests that, as discussed in Chapter 1, much of the information communicated in person perception is implied by the features of the target and is not necessarily a subjective inference of the perceivers. It also suggests that these features of the target are being detected in a similar fashion by perceivers, despite the fact that these perceivers have not had any interaction with the target, but have merely observed him/her behaving. Kenny, Horner, Kashy, and Chu

(1992) concluded that consensus in impressions between different perceivers is determined by the fact that these perceivers each attend to and detect the same set of nonverbal cues and behaviors, which they may not even know they are using (or which the target may not even know he/she is sending). Why would people develop an ability to detect cues so subtle that the person sending them is ostensibly not even aware of doing so? One possible answer is the same answer provided in Chapter 1's discussion of the factors that determine where perceivers selectively focus attention. Gibson (1979) and McArthur and Baron (1983) have proposed an *ecological approach* to person perception, in which certain elements of the environment are said to attain power to grab attention because they have adaptive value for an individual. Thus being able to attend to and quickly identify features in others that reveal important properties related to the perceiver's needs would be extremely adaptive, especially if much of this detection could be automated so that it proceeded without awareness or conscious intent. It would be functional to identify nonverbal signals that a threat is present. "Similarly, the ability to perceive variables related to sexuality, such as gender and sexual orientation, may also facilitate adaptive behavior; accurately perceiving such attributes could be helpful for identifying available and receptive romantic partners" (Ambady et al., 1999, p. 539).

Unintentionally Detecting and Expressing Information from the Face

If we continue this line of reasoning—in which the features of a target that have adaptive value for a perceiver are believed to develop such strong associations with the needs of the perceiver that they can grab attention even without the perceiver's being aware of this or intending to focus on those features (e.g., McArthur & Baron, 1983)—then we should be able to identify variables other than threat and sexuality that fit this ecological approach to person perception. Often the cues/features associated with such ecologically important variables are provided in the faces of the target persons. Thus a quick glance at the facial expression and facial features of others can often provide enough information for impression formation to occur (e.g., Asch, 1946), and for physical reactions/responses to these others to be planned and enacted. This can occur even though perceivers do not consciously intend to examine the faces of others; or, if perceivers do consciously intend to look at the face to examine facial expressions, they may unintentionally attend to and detect specific types of features associated with evolution-relevant responses. Let us examine some of the research on the power of the information expressed in the face for automatically communicating specific meanings to perceivers (as lack of intent is another hallmark of automaticity).

The Baby Face

One important candidate was identified by McArthur and Apatow (1983–1984), who wrote that "it is essential to species survival that we be able to recognize infants, and that their distinguishing features elicit caregiving, nurturant responses and suppress aggressive ones" (p. 317). It is essential that babies trigger paternal and maternal instincts in others. However, adults whose facial features resemble the structure of an infant's face should unintentionally trigger these same impulses. It is possible that our instincts to protect infants have led us to become so skilled at detecting babyish features that we will have the instinctive responses triggered merely by observing these features in people, even if they are not infants! Lorenz (1971) used this to explain why people show strong preferences for certain types of pets and dolls: "The products of the doll industry . . . and also the various types of animals (e.g., pug-dogs and Pekinese) which are taken over . . . as substitute objects for their parental care drive, permit a clear-cut abstraction of these babyish characters" (p. 154). The ecological approach offers an evolutionary perspective on why my mother-in-law collects dolls and has had a series of Pekinese dogs—they trigger nurturing feelings by virtue of their babyish features.

McArthur and Apatow (1983) predicted that having a facial appearance with features characteristic of infants would trigger specific types of impressions, despite the fact that perceivers were not aware of the influence of, or intending to focus on, those particular features in forming their impressions. Having a baby face was posited to be a cue that would be associated with personality traits such as being kind, lovable, flexible, nonthreatening, weak, and naive. The procedure of their study was to identify what the features of a baby-faced adult would be, manipulate those features in pictures shown to research participants, and ask the participants to form impressions of the individuals from the pictures. The features of the baby-faced adult included large eyes relative to the rest of the face; a high forehead and a short chin (with vertical placement of the eyes being more toward the center of the face rather than higher up, giving the illusion of a higher forehead); and a short nose and ears (see Figure 2.2). These features were manipulated in drawings that research participants were asked to evaluate by rating each picture on several scales—strength, dominance, naivete, warmth, and honesty. They were also asked to rate the likelihood that the person in the picture would perform certain behaviors, such as "Does she look like the kind of roommate who would comply with all your wishes about the furniture arrangement, quiet hours, radio station, etc.?" and "Does she look like the kind of person who would turn a cold shoulder to your attempts at friendly conversation?"

The results showed that as babyishness of the face increased, there was a decrease in the perceptions of the physical strength of the target. It had a similar effect on perceptions of social strength: The more baby-faced the targets, the less dominant they were seen to be, and the more likely they were rated to submit to a roommate's

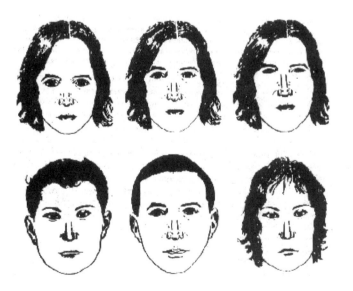

FIGURE 2.2. Baby-faced versus mature-faced adults (decreasing babyishness from left to right). From McArthur and Apatow (1983–1984). Copyright 1983–1984 by The Guilford Press. Reprinted by permission.

requests. Similarly, the baby-faced targets were seen as more naive and more likely to fall for a far-fetched story. On the more positive side, they were seen as warmer and more honest. The findings provide support for the position that the physical features of, and cues given off by, the person being perceived exert a strong impact on the manner in which the person is perceived. The effects showed very little variation across participants, suggesting that some cues have extremely strong powers to communicate associated attributes, even if the people perceiving them are not aware of the nature of the features guiding their perceptions.

What is the impact of constantly sending nonverbal signals that a person does not consciously intend to send? Collins and Zebrowitz (1995) reported the remarkable fact that American soldiers serving in World War II and the Korean conflict who had baby faces were more likely to receive awards for their military service. There are two possible explanations for this. First, it could be that the expectancies held by perceivers that baby-faced people would be weak and dependent led them to see these people as more heroic and brave than they really were, because their mildly brave behavior seemed extraordinarily brave in the context of the expectancy of these people as weak and dependent. In this case, the impact of having babyish features would be felt in how others evaluated these persons, establishing a context with which their current behavior could be contrasted (see the discussion of contrast effects in Chapter 10). Alternatively, it could well be that baby-faced people actually behaved in a more courageous fashion and deserved to receive recognition from their country to honor their heroism. Here, the impact would be felt in the very behavior of the baby-faced adults.

People with baby faces may be treated by others as weak, dependent, submissive, and intellectually inferior. They may be liked and treated warmly, but others may constrain their opportunities by constantly trying to care for and nurture them. One possibility is that through a self-fulfilling prophecy, baby-faced adults will come to develop the qualities others expect them to possess (see Chapter 13; e.g., Darley & Fazio, 1980; Snyder, Tanke, & Berscheid, 1977). However, another possibility is that these adults will rebel against these expectancies and become the opposite of what other people expect. Zebrowitz, Andreoletti, Collins, Lee, and Blumenthal (1998) provided evidence that baby-faced adults come to act in ways that rebuke the stereotype. It is proposed that this behavior arises as a way of compensating for the continuous stream of expectancies and inferred qualities that result from other people's unintentional reactions to the nonverbal cues in the faces of the baby-faced adults. Zebrowitz and colleagues found that baby-faced adolescent boys had better academic performance than boys of the same age and socioeconomic status (SES) with more mature faces. They presume that in order to compensate for the expectation of others that babyishness is associated with intellectual inferiority, these individuals developed better academic skills that led to intellectual achievement.

Furthermore, Zebrowitz and colleagues (1998) examined delinquent boys to see whether baby-faced boys were more delinquent than their mature-faced peers (presumably as a compensation for other people's expectancies and behavior). Two measures of delinquency were used—first, whether a boy was a delinquent or not; and second, if a boy was delinquent, how delinquent he was. To assess the latter, the frequency of delinquent acts was measured by looking at the number of criminal acts committed by boys labeled as delinquent. The participants were delinquent and nondelinquent White men who were adolescents in the 1930s and 1940s, and whose behavior had been culled from archival records at correctional schools and public schools. The two samples were matched for variables such as intelligence, ethnicity, and age. The results were a little more complicated than predicted. The first finding was that baby-faced boys were only more likely to be delinquent than mature-faced boys if they came from low-SES backgrounds. Middle-SES boys did not show this tendency. The second finding was that baby-faced delinquents were indeed charged with more crimes between the ages of 17 and 25 than delinquent boys who had more mature faces. However, these results were qualified by an interaction of babyishness and height, such that baby-faced delinquents were only more likely to be charged with crimes when they also happened to be short. The results, despite showing that babyish features interact with other variables, reveal that having features that are associated with infants sends signals to others that are detected and trigger expectancies, and that these expectancies in turn have an impact on the behavior of the baby-faced persons.

Detecting and Expressing Emotions

Babyishness in the face is only one feature of the face that sends signals to others. Perhaps a more common and intuitively obvious facial characteristic that sends such signals is the expressiveness of the face. Facial expressions are how we communicate emotions to one another even before words have had the chance to leap from our mouths (and when words cannot adequately capture what we are experiencing). Charles Darwin (1872/1998) proposed that many of our emotional expressions that leak into the face are biological remnants of once-needed behaviors. For example, we humans bare our teeth when we are enraged. Why? It is plausible that this behavior was required in the evolutionary past of our species, when we used biting as a far more common tactic of expressing rage and hostility than we do today. Baring our teeth is seen as a *vestige of an evolutionary adaptive behavior*. It persists because while it may no longer have adaptive value (we do not need to prepare to bite others), it has communicative value. Our goal here is not to review behavioral ethology or the theory of evolution, so don't worry. It simply is to highlight the point that many of our facial expressions are perhaps biologically derived, and because of this fact, it is quite likely that we do not consciously prepare such expressions—or are even aware of the fact that we are revealing these expressions and sending them to others as nonverbal forms of communication. If emotional expressiveness in the face is biologically based, it stands to reason that it can be triggered by the appropriate stimuli in the environment, rather than consciously willed or something we intend to use as a means of communication. Instead, such expressions simply appear when we experience the emotion. Thus, while the communicative value of your facial expressions is something intuitively obvious to you, the biological basis of these expressions, the cross-cultural consistency in these expressions, and the unintended nature of these expressions may be more surprising to you and reveal an implicit communication network that you were not aware of.

Universal Expressions of Emotions

A biological basis for emotional expressiveness was proposed by Darwin (1872/1998), who argued that emotions such as anger, happiness, and sadness are innate, not learned. We are born with these responses to stimuli already in place, allowing the response to be elicited in the absence of conscious intent. Darwin, in the first line of his 1872 book, referred to these expressions as "involuntarily used by man." The type of evidence that would support this position would show cross-species similarity in emotional expressiveness as well as cross-cultural exactness in expressiveness. If a dog looks similar to me when threatened, and a Mongolian has exactly the same expression as I do when experiencing joy, these similarities are suggestive of an evolutionary component to these reactions, and would imply that we do not merely learn how to respond and then intend to respond in that way in the appropriate conditions. Rather, we are wired to respond, and conditions trigger responding with or without our conscious intent, regardless of the culture in which we have been raised. Darwin eloquently expressed this view in the first of his three principles of expression:

> *The principle of serviceable associated habits.* Certain complex actions are of direct or indirect service under certain states of the mind, in order to relieve or gratify certain sensations, desires, etc.; and whenever the same state of mind is induced, however feebly, there is a tendency through the force of habit and association for the same movements to be performed, though they may not be of the least use . . . it is notorious how powerful is the force of habit. The most complex and difficult movements can in time be performed without the least effort or consciousness. (pp. 34–35)

To examine the universal nature of emotional expressiveness, Ekman and Friesen (1971) used an inventive approach. They traveled to visit a culture that was totally isolated and had had no previous contact with other cultures. This approach nicely illustrates the controversy behind the scenes in much scientific work. Paul Ekman reports in his afterword to Darwin's (1872/1998) book that his work on the universal nature of emotional expression raised the ire of Margaret Mead and many of her colleagues, who had argued for the better part of 50 years (see e.g., Mead, 1935) against such a possibility and for the cultural basis of behavior. Some of Ekman's earlier research had already found evidence that strongly suggested a universal component to emotional expressiveness. Photographs of faces that each clearly depicted a single emotion (such as a woman whose face had a happy expression or a man whose facial expression depicted sadness) were shown to research participants in 23 countries. Each face had to be labeled with an emotion, with participants choosing from a list containing anger, disgust, fear, happiness, sadness, and surprise. The results revealed unusual agreement, with the majority of people in every country agreeing on the same labels. Members of the Mead camp, however, challenged the results as being due to cultural transmission of emotional expressiveness through the media.

To illustrate the universality of emotional expressiveness, Ekman (1971; Ekman & Friesen, 1971) needed to find a culture where there was no contact with the modern world. To do so, Ekman and Friesen (1971) traveled to visit the South Fore culture in Papua New Guinea—a culture still using stone utensils and tools; without a written language; and without exposure to television, movies, or pictures of any kind. The researchers read an emotional story to residents and then presented them with a series of faces similar to those used in the cross-cultural study involving 23 countries (in that they depicted single, unambiguous emotions). The participants were to point to the picture that best captured the emotions of the person described in the story. The results were strikingly similar to those found in the earlier study, but eliminated the possibility that the results could be due to mimicking emotions learned through the media. In an additional experiment, Ekman (1971) asked the New Guinea participants themselves to display, through facial expressions, the reactions they would have in a variety of scenarios. The expressions, examples of which are provided in Figure 2.3, look very similar to the expressions created by the actors whose faces were used in the stimulus photographs of the earlier, cross-cultural study. New Guinea residents showed happiness and sadness in their faces in the same way as people from cultures with which they have had no contact.

It seems that people all over the world reveal the same emotional expressions and communicate these to others, regardless of whether they intend to do so. Although

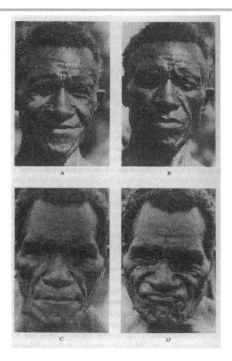

FIGURE 2.3. Expressions of a Papua New Guinea resident not exposed to other cultures or the media: (A) when depicting happiness over a friend's visit; (B) when contemplating the death of a child; (C) when depicting anger and readiness to fight; (D) when imagining a dead pig lying around a while. From Ekman (1998). Copyright 1998 by Oxford University Press. Reprinted by permission.

Ekman and Friesen (1971) and Izard (1971) provided illustrations of this, the range of emotions they examined was limited. More recent research has broadened the spectrum of emotions that seem to have universally distinct patterns of facial expression. For example, shame, embarrassment, and guilt have unique nonverbal displays (e.g., Keltner, 1997). Indeed, as Darwin suggested, it seems that much of emotional expressiveness is reflexive and induced through the force of habit and association, with minimal effort and without the intervention of consciousness.

Just because emotions are often expressed without intent and have a biological basis that makes certain expressions somewhat universal, this does not mean that we have no control over our facial emotional expressiveness, or lack awareness that we are revealing our emotions in our faces. Once we become aware of this expressiveness, we can try to conceal it and control it. Success at controlling emotional expressiveness (essentially, being a good liar) requires a good understanding of what nonverbal cues are sent that have the power to communicate specific emotions. For nonverbal cues to be controlled, we must know what cues have the power to betray our emotions. Because we so often use the face as a means of distilling that information from others, we may have developed quite good theories about how emotion is expressed in the face, even when it is not intended. Thus, because of our experience with using the face to send signals and read others' signals, we are likely to have developed fairly good (though not perfect) skills at controlling the face. But there are more subtle forms of nonverbal communication that are more difficult to control. The next section reviews just how easy (or hard) it is to control nonverbal communication once we become aware it is happening. Recall that inability to control a process is another feature of automaticity.

Nonverbal Leaking of What We Wish to Conceal: Failures to Control Emotional Responsiveness

If we want to ascertain whether someone is being sincere with us, what better way to do so than to have an accurate window into their true emotions and opinions? Because nonverbal behavior is often not consciously intended, it comes to have great value for us as perceivers. Why? What other people say, we may feel, is likely to be tainted by whatever goals those other persons have. They can easily, we deduce, control what they tell us. However, if the body and face are harder to control and unintentionally leak information, these cues from the nonverbal channels should be especially useful to us perceivers, as they would be a pipeline to the truth (e.g., Mehrabian & Wiener, 1967). If the verbal and the nonverbal messages being sent are in contradiction, we might be better served to heed the messages sent to us from the less controlled nonverbal channel (e.g., Ekman & Friesen, 1969). Darwin (1872/1998) argued that because of the principle of serviceable associated habits (emotional expressiveness is triggered by stimuli related to the emotion, no matter how feeble the stimulus), emotional expressiveness is hard, if not impossible, to control when an emotion is experienced or an emotionally charged stimulus is encountered:

> Some actions ordinarily associated through habit with certain states of the mind may be partially repressed through the will, and in such cases the muscles which are least under the separate control of the will are the most liable still to act, causing movements which we recognize as expressive. In certain other cases the checking of one habitual movement requires other slight movements; and these are likewise expressive. (p. 34)

Is there evidence that nonverbal behaviors are hard to control, and therefore provide this type of window to the truth (or what Zebrowitz, 1997, has called a "window to the soul")?

Lying is explicitly an attempt to control what one expresses to others. The word has negative connotation, but in some instances lying—even the most subtle and seemingly difficult type, such as concealing one's nonverbal facial and body responses—is not bad. Cultural norms often force people to "lie" by this definition, requiring that they hide their true feelings. It is inappropriate to cry in a meeting with one's boss just because one gets negative feedback and feels like crying. It is inappropriate to offer unsolicited, horribly negative commentary on a person's physical appearance (e.g., "Say, Connie, you have awfully ugly, hairy arms; I never noticed before you wore that short-sleeved shirt"), even if refraining from doing so is a concealment of the truth. Deception is a prominent component of social life and required in many instances by the rules of society. Aptly summarizing the position of Goffman (1959), DePaulo, Kashy, Kirkendol, Wyer, and Epstein (1996) have stated that "many of the lies of everyday life are told to avoid tension and conflict and to minimize hurt feelings and ill will" (p. 980). DePaulo and Kashy (1998) report that, including small "white" lies, people lie to approximately 30% of the people they know each week (with Mom being the number one recipient of lies). However, lying is also a pervasive and true social problem that can cause great trauma to interpersonal relationships. For instance, the husband who deceives his wife about an adulterous affair is placing that relationship in peril (in more ways than one).

Thus people should acquire skill at deceiving and detecting deception. And there is reason to believe that they do acquire this skill to varying degrees. A good amount of research has been focused on the nature of the ability to detect deception coming from different channels, such as speech, facial expression, body posture, etc (e.g., O'Sullivan, Ekman, Friesen, & Scherer, 1985). We will not delve deeply into this literature, but instead will focus just briefly on one example to illustrate how deception can be revealed by nonverbal communication, in specific channels, of which one is not aware and that one is trying (but unable) to control.

Ekman and Friesen (1969) proposed that while it may be possible to verbally suppress certain ideas or emotions, the body and face are not always willing accomplices to attempts at deceit and evasiveness. Ekman and Friesen (1974) have offered the following proposition: "When an individual is engaged in deception, his body, more than his face, is a source of *leakage* (i.e., the nonverbal act reveals a message otherwise being concealed" (p. 288). Thus leakage is more likely to be evidenced in the body than the face, presumably because people have more experience in learning to monitor their facial expressions and greater awareness of the way in which their expressions might communicate with others. Although the body can be similarly controlled and disguised, people are simply less aware of the communicative signals sent through this channel. Thus, when a person is engaged in deception, the body should be better than the face at revealing the true and hidden emotion—or, if not the actual emotion, should at least reveal to the observer that something is amiss (what Ekman & Friesen, 1974, call *deception clues*).

An experimental situation was arranged where an interview was to take place and the interviewer was led to believe that in any one of four interviews that would transpire, he/she would be deceived. The interviewer's goal was to try to ascertain when he/she were being lied to. The deception involved concealing one's negative emotions and replacing it with a false expression of affect (thus creating two deceptions in one—concealment and false expression). The negative emotions were created by having the person being interviewed watch a distressing film (e.g., a movie documenting an amputation) and then tell the interviewer that he/she had watched a pleasant film that led the person to experience positive emotions. Thus four films were watched, and the instructions as to whether to lie or not were provided for each film, with the case of most central interest to our discussion being the one where the viewer had to lie about having seen the negative film. Observers watched a sample of nonverbal behavior pulled from the interview sessions and had to try to ascertain in which cases the person being interviewed was being honest or deceitful (after first having been provided with a sample of behavior from the same person that they were told was representative of how the person acted when not concealing anything). The findings revealed that observers were more accurate at detecting deception when they used nonverbal behaviors focused on the body than when relying on facial feedback. In addition, when the people being interviewed were asked at the end of the experiment what they needed to do to be a successful deceiver, more of them mentioned controlling leakage through the face than through the body, supporting the idea that people are less aware of the body as a source of information that is being communicated to others and "revealing their hand."

Interestingly, the more important a lie becomes, the less expert people seem to be at controlling the nonverbal sources of communication that stand to undermine the successful execution of the deception. DePaulo, Lanier, and Davis (1983) found that when the motivation to lie was increased, the nonverbal signs that revealed the deception were less successfully controlled and more likely to be detected by perceivers. The motivation to lie was manipulated by telling some of the research participants that lying is an essential interpersonal skill that is predictive of success in life, and that to see how skilled they were in this important domain, they would be asked to lie on videotape and then have their performance repeatedly evaluated by others. The remaining participants were told that they were simply performing a game that involved telling some lies, and that lying itself is not a particularly relevant skill for success in life. All the participants then told lies on videotape and were actually evaluated by others, who were asked to try to detect when each person on tape was lying. The lies told in the high-motivation condition were especially easy to detect. This was not true when the text of what the person had said was all that was provided—the lies were not being detected in the words that they said, but in the cues provided in the voice and body that accompanied the words. It is not that people cannot create good lies; they just cannot deliver them well without revealing their deceit, because they have difficulty controlling the nonverbal cues they send.

It may well be the case that anxiety is what causes people to lose their ability to control their cues to deception. Schlenker and Leary (1982, 1985) have found that when people are anxious they are less skilled at communicating, and some of the conditions that cause social anxiety are high expectations (or fear) of being discovered as fraudulent, low expectations for success at an interpersonal task (such as expecting not to succeed at lying well), and high motivation to do well on an interpersonal task. Some, if not all, of these conditions may well have been present in the research of DePaulo and colleagues (1983). To examine this more closely, DePaulo, LeMay, and Epstein (1991) explicitly manipulated both the expectations for success associated with a lie and the person's motivation to engage in the deception. They illustrated that detecting the cues of deceit in the nonverbal behavior of another person was increased (lies were more detectable) when the person asked to lie believed that the recipient of the lie was especially likely to be able to detect that he/she was lying (i.e., the person had low expectations for success at the lying task), and when the liar was fairly motivated to lie (i.e., it was more important for him/her to lie).

The ability to control nonverbal behaviors was limited, and it seems that conditions that make people want to control nonverbal leakage seem only to increase the likelihood that the unwanted signals will be communicated. It is for this reason that perceivers are believed to rely on nonverbal behavior as information that will betray a target person's true feelings. As perceivers, we know to trust the reactions of others that they have difficulty controlling, as these are more likely to be a reflection of these other persons' true reactions. If they cannot stop themselves from revealing cues in nonverbal communication despite wanting to, the cues must be betraying something real. As we shall soon see, this inability to control a process (such as repressing unwanted nonverbal cues), despite explicit attempts to do so, is one of the "calling cards" of an automatic process.

AUTOMATIC PROCESSING OF INFORMATION

What does it mean to say that someone has responded in an *automatic* fashion? In everyday language, we take it to mean that something happens immediately and without conscious reflection. These qualities that spring to mind from our everyday use of the term are actually components of automaticity in the way psychologists define the term, but there is more. An automatic process is one that is triggered directly and immediately from stimuli in the environment, rather than initiated by a conscious choice. Once cues in the environment unconsciously trigger a response, if it is automatic that response will then run to completion without disruption, all the while providing benefits to the perceiver in terms of mental efficiency. These steps will all occur without one's awareness, such that *consciousness is not involved at any stage of processing* (Bargh, 1984, 1989, 1994, 1997).

How does a process become automatic? Through practice, repetition, and habit. Bargh (1990) proposed that a response that is routinely paired with a specific set of environmental features can eventually, with time and practice, lead to the activation of the response in the presence of the stimulus. Thus the root of the concept of an automatic process can be traced to William James's (1890/1950) definition of *habit*: "A strictly voluntary act has to be guided by idea, perception, and volition, throughout its whole course. In an habitual action, mere sensation is a sufficient guide, and the upper regions of the brain and mind are set comparatively free" (pp. 115–116). Echoing James, Wegner and Bargh (1998, p. 459) have defined automatic processes as mental habits, "patterns [that] become the deep grooves into which behavior falls when not consciously attended." However, certainly these notions were lingering before James's discussion of habit. For example, Darwin (1872/1998, p. 45) presented the basics of the idea in describing how complex behavior is routinized: "It seems probable that some actions, which were at first performed consciously, have become through habit and association converted into reflex actions, and are now so firmly fixed and inherited, that they are performed, even when not of the least use, as often as the same causes arise, which originally excited them in us through the volition."

The use of the term *automatic processing* in person perception can be traced to 1970s social psychology research embracing the methodologies of cognitive psychology. Researchers in this era equated automaticity with one's lack of conscious control over a process (e.g., Hasher & Zacks, 1979; Posner & Snyder, 1975; Schneider & Shiffrin, 1977). They maintained that even if a person deliberately wills a process to occur, the process is still automatic if it is capable of running to completion without the intervention of conscious monitoring (i.e., the process is autonomous). For example, as mentioned in Chapter 1, it is possible for you to drive your car, sometimes for miles, without consciously attending to each movement you make. In fact, it is often possible for you to drive between two places so lost in thought that you later have no recollection of what you were doing while you were in transit or how you decided what route to take. You were not consciously attending to driving the car while you were in transit. The process was initiated by a conscious intent to drive your car, but was completed without conscious awareness.

The Elements of Automaticity

Bargh (1984) took issue with the notion that a process could be called automatic even if the instigation for the process comes from a conscious choice. Since most cognitive processes contain some components that occur outside of awareness, practically all processes should be called automatic if automaticity is defined by a lack of conscious awareness at any point in the process. For example, Chapter 1 has reviewed how naive realism permeates many of the social judgments we make. If we equate an automatic process with lacking awareness of how our responses are being produced, then almost every social judgment we make should be called an automatic one (since naive realism means that we are not aware of our biased processing). Similarly, if complex behaviors such as driving, which are consciously willed and consciously terminated, are called automatic just because we may lack awareness of our responses at a particular moment, then almost any behavior should be called automatic, since most actions involve some component that is routinized and performed without conscious attention. Therefore, driving your car is not an automatic process, because the mere presence of a car does not cause you to mindlessly jump in and begin racing down the highway. Driving, once initiated, might proceed with your consciousness having deserted you, but consciousness must have been there to trigger the action, and most likely will return at some point during your travels. Thus automaticity is not merely a cognitive process or behavior that lacks the devotion of conscious monitoring and attention. Such a definition would render the term so vague as to be useless. Bargh (1994) has described four elements necessary for identifying an automatic process: lack of conscious intent, efficiency, lack of awareness, and lack of control.

Lack of Conscious Intent

An automatic process is one that is not consciously initiated, but determined by the stimuli to which we are exposed. As stated earlier, when we look up at the sky, we do not consciously intend to perceive its color. The color is simply perceived. In our perception of the people we encounter, there is likewise a good deal of processing that proceeds without our conscious intent. We have already examined this possibility in the domain of expressing and detecting emotions nonverbally. However, the possibility that nonverbal communication via facial expressions is unintended and not consciously initiated was not explicitly demonstrated by the research reviewed. The evidence was convincing, but indirect, relying mostly on two points: (1) People use cues that it seems highly unlikely they would consciously be able to report; and (2) the biological and universal nature of emotional expression suggests that it is somewhat innate and not consciously willed. One manner in which researchers have more directly illustrated that facial features can be detected without conscious intent has been to present a stimulus subliminally—below the participants' threshold for conscious recognition. If the participants never consciously detect the presence of a stimulus, yet that stimulus is able to trigger responses associated with it, then the processes associated with detecting it and responding to it must not have been consciously intended. People cannot consciously intend to react to something that they have never even consciously perceived.

For example, Murphy and Zajonc (1993) subliminally showed faces to their research participants, manipulating whether the facial expressions depicted positive or negative emotions. Participants did not consciously see the faces, so they could not intend to detect the expressions or intend to have a mood triggered in them by virtue of being exposed to these faces. Furthermore, they could not intend to be influenced in their judgments of some new and unrelated picture by having seen these faces. Nonetheless, the valence associated with the faces was shown to influence the judgment of an ambiguous (neutral) stimulus. The stimulus, a Chinese ideograph, was liked more when it was preceded by the subliminal presentation of a face with positive (as opposed to negative) valence. Detecting the mood associated with facial expressions, and the subsequent impact of those mood states, met the automaticity criterion of being unintended.

Another powerful illustration of the fact that components of perception of other people occur largely without the need for conscious will or conscious intent is provided by showing that perceivers often engage in thoughts and actions relating to other people that are exactly the opposite of what the perceivers had consciously intended. That is, if the lack of intention refers to the initiation of a response without a conscious act of willing that response, with the response proceeding immediately upon exposure to a triggering stimulus, then a good way to prove that a response is unintended is to prove that people explicitly intend to do something else. If the response occurs despite a lack of conscious intent to initiate it, then it relies on an unintended process. For example, concealing emotions when we engage in deception may be what we intend, but as reviewed earlier, we unintentionally continue to send signals that reveal the emotion we wish to conceal. The experience of the emotion is a stimulus that unintentionally initiates the sending of relevant nonverbal cues. As another example, if I ask you to ignore the meaning of the words written in this sentence, and focus only on whether the shapes of the particular letters are curved or angled, you are still likely to extract the meaning of the words despite being explicitly asked to intend to do otherwise. Extracting word meaning is automatic and occurs even when we have no conscious intent to comprehend word meaning.

Stroop (1935) provided a classic experimental illustration of the fact that people initiate cognitive processes without conscious intent. Research participants were shown either words that named a host of different colors ("red," "blue," "green," etc) or patches of the colors. The words were always printed in colored ink, but in each case, the color of the ink never matched the word. For example, the word "red" might be printed in blue ink, while "blue" might be printed in yellow. The task was extremely simple: "Name the ink color." This was facilitated by *not* reading the words. Stroop's participants found that naming the ink color was difficult when it was presented in a word as opposed to a rectangular patch, and they tended to name the printed word rather than the ink in which it is printed. Why? Because the task called for them to ignore word meaning and focus on ink color, but processing of word meaning occurred immediately upon their perceiving the letter string (the word). This phenomenon—the interference that is found in attempts to name the ink color of a word, where the word is the name of a color that is different from the color of the ink—has come to be called the *Stroop effect*. The effect essentially shows us that detecting word meaning happens without intent, and once it happens, it interferes with other processes that are consciously intended (if the tasks are incompatible). In the Stroop effect, indicating that we have seen the color red when we encounter the word "blue" in red ink is in conflict with the more automatic response of reading the word (which is what we usually do with words). This is what causes errors and slows responses.

Researchers have used this same (or a similar) methodology to illustrate that processes in person perception are unintended. For example, Geller and Shaver (1976) presented words to people and asked them to name the color of the ink for each word. This time, however, instead of being color names, the words were either self-relevant to the people who were reading them or neutral words that were not relevant to the research participants. The logic was that stimuli that were relevant to participants would be automatically detected and processed, even if they had no conscious intent to read the words (such as when a task was facilitated by word meaning's being ignored). People cannot help reading words that are presented to them, and when those words are self-relevant, they find themselves distracted by them and wanting to linger on them. This increased attention to the word meaning will be in conflict with the task. Rather than saying the color of the ink as fast as they can, people are momentarily sidetracked by the processing of information in the environment that is relevant to them. Thus, if the processing of self-relevant information occurs without conscious intent, it should be found to slow down the response time for naming the ink color relative to words that are not self-relevant and that do not initiate any unintended processing. This was precisely what Geller and Shaver found: Their participants took longer to name the color of the ink of a self-relevant word relative to a neutral word. Bargh and Pratto (1986) replicated this finding. People should ignore word meaning, yet unintentionally attend to it.

Efficiency

Rather than being constrained by limits on people's ability to attend to a stimulus, *efficient* processes are able to operate even in the face of such limits (e.g., being rushed, working on many tasks simultaneously, having divided attention). An efficient process requires relatively little mental energy and effort. Indeed, it requires so little cognitive effort that it occurs despite other ongoing mental activity; it will run to completion without being disturbed. You can strain your memory for the year Mark McGwire and Sammy Sosa chased (and broke) Roger Maris's home run record (it was 1998), or the year that Barry Bonds broke the home run record again (it was 2001), while at the same time you detect that the color of a passing car is red. Color detection is an efficient process: It can occur despite straining mental capacity on the more difficult task of retrieving trivia from long-term memory. If performance on a task is disrupted by a secondary task, this suggests that the process in question is not automatic; it lacks efficiency. In social cognition research, many of the processes used to characterize other people (and the self) proceed with such efficiency. Being lost in deliberation, or straining to retrieve information from memory, or trying to remember the grocery list does not incapacitate the ability to form impressions of other people. These impressions might not be as accurate or as detailed as the ones you might otherwise draw, but person perception persists despite the mind's being engaged in multiple mental tasks.

Bargh and Thein (1985) provided evidence for efficiency in social cognition by predicting that the processing of information about the self is efficient. They argued that detecting information relevant to the self is something people are skilled at. But, more than this, people will recognize these traits in others more easily, form inferences about these qualities from the behavior of others fairly easily, and use these inferences as organizing principles for structuring their emerging impression of these others. All these seemingly complex processes of person perception should be carried out by perceivers efficiently and effortlessly, and should persist even in the face of drains on their mental capacity. For example, Bargh and Thein selected some research participants for whom traits related to honesty were highly self-relevant; honesty was a trait that truly mattered to these people. Other participants had no particular affinity for the trait of being honest. Participants then read a series of behavioral description about other people. One of the series of descriptions provided information about a person performing either honest, dishonest, or neutral behavior. Descriptions were presented one at a time on a computer. Some people were asked to read the sentences in only 1.5 seconds, making the task highly demanding of their mental energy. Such people were described as being under *cognitive load*. Other participants performed the task while they were not under cognitive load. A given list of behaviors had 24 sentences—12 implying a self-relevant trait (such as honesty), 6 implying an inconsistent trait (dishonesty), and 6 being neutral. After reading the information, participants completed an impression rating form. In summary, people who either did or did not value honesty received information about another person that was either relevant to honesty or not, and they received this information while either under or not under cognitive load.

If inference formation and organizing the information being presented according to the traits implied by the behavior are efficient processes, they should have occurred in this research, regardless of whether participants were under cognitive load. If they are not efficient, the extra effort from working on the task quickly should have disrupted participants' ability to process the information and form an impression that drew accurately on the information provided. The data showed that people who did not value honesty had no trouble processing the information when there was no load—their impressions reflected the proportion of honest behaviors that actually were presented. However, when such participants were doing the same task under cognitive load, the behavioral information that was actually provided no longer predicted the type of impression they formed. Organizing lists of information about other people was assumed to be an inefficient process, since the ability to do so appeared to be impaired once mental resources were taxed. Thus people under cognitive load cannot engage in the process of producing a coherent impression, as participants in the Asch (1946) experiments did. That is, if people are presented with a set of traits, they should be able to integrate them so that an initial impression is formed around some central traits, and subsequent information should be evaluated based on whether it is inconsistent or consistent with the impression. But to integrate information requires some exertion of mental effort. If people are asked to perform another task simultaneously, this interferes with their ability to form a coherent impression.

However, participants in the Bargh and Thein study for whom honesty was a self-relevant trait did not have such an impairment. For these people, the proportion of self-relevant traits presented could be detected and was used to guide their impressions. This was true both when cognitive load was absent and when it was present. This suggests that processing information about the self, even when it is being observed in others, is efficient; it can proceed despite performing a taxing mental task.

Lack of Awareness

Phenomenal immediacy is said to exist because perceivers lack awareness that any mental production exists. The feeling that gears are churning is absent. People may be aware of the output of an automatic process (they experience the sky as blue), but remain unaware of the occurrence of some process they have actively performed that has caused that output to be experienced. The inability to consciously recognize that any mental activity is taking place is another mark of an automatic process. Once again, social cognition often involves a lack of awareness that the processes of impression formation, attribution, inference, and so forth are taking place. We have already examined this issue in the domain of nonverbal communication, where perceivers were detecting nonverbal signals from thin slices of behavior without realizing that such cues were being sent and received. Nisbett and Wilson (1977; see also Wilson & Brekke, 1994) provided social psychology with yet another citation classic, this time focused on illustrating just how much people lack awareness of the processes contributing to their perception of one another. Nisbett and Wilson performed a clever experiment in which participants were asked to memorize a series of word pairs. For some of the people, the pairs of words included the pair "ocean–moon." Shortly after finishing this task, the participants were asked to answer some mundane questions, and this included among them a question that asked them to name a laundry detergent. Remarkably, the number of people who responded with the brand "Tide" was double for people who had previously seen the word pair "ocean–moon," yet these people saw no way in which the word association task could have influenced their responses to the mundane questions.

Let's bring this type of lacking awareness of influence on judgments back to the domain of person perception tasks. Nisbett and Wilson (1977) found that people not only lack awareness that something might be influencing their impressions of other people; they are even unable to accurately report what the nature of that influence is when they do correctly suspect that something is influencing them. For example, Chapter 1 has reported an experiment by Nisbett and Wilson that provided evidence of halo effects. Students watched an interview with a teacher who spoke with a foreign accent, and some people saw the teacher respond in a "warm" and positive fashion, while others saw him respond in a "cold" and negative way. The degree to which they liked the teacher was shown to influence other ratings formed of the teacher, even ratings on dimensions that should not have been influenced—how attractive they found him to be, how much they liked his accent. The important point for the current discussion is not the fact that such halo effects were found. It is that participants could not accurately guess the direction of the influence! They seemed to know that their ratings of the teacher might be biased, but they believed that the attractiveness of the teacher was what influenced how much they liked him, rather than the other way around. This is an excellent example of people trying to monitor their mental processes, even suspecting that they might be biased, yet having no clue as to what really determines how they come to their conclusions and judgments (how they "know what they know," or why they have behaved the way they have). If people are asked to explain how they came to know something, they get it completely wrong; when asked to reflect about what they do when forming impressions, they do not have very good access to what it is they are doing and cannot even reproduce it when asked. Thus another way to establish that people lack awareness of an influence is to see whether their predictions of how they are being influenced fail to match the actual influence.

Another illustration of how people lack awareness of the factors that bias their impressions of other people can be provided by presenting perceivers with information that will bias their impression, but presenting it in such a subtle way that the perceivers do not realize the bias exists, and therefore have no reason to suspect that they are being biased. For example, in the earlier-reported experiment by Murphy and Zajonc (1993), people were influenced by facial expressions in photographs that were presented subliminally. If the influencing force (the facial expression) was never consciously seen, obviously the participants would not have been aware of its influence. Yet an influence was evidenced all the same. Thus a cleverly designed experiment can create situations where people clearly are being influenced—a fact that becomes obvious to anyone who is aware of the experimental manipulations. But the participants in the experiment (who are naive to these manipulations) may be unable to report any influence on their behavior and cognition, even though that influence is apparent to the clued-in observer. Thus, in the Murphy and Zajonc research, perceivers were not aware of the processes through which a subliminally presented picture of a face influenced their evaluation of an object. Indeed, they were not aware of the existence of the influencing force, of the fact that their evaluation had been influenced, or the processes that led the influencing force to exert its influence.

Lack of Control

A final mark of an automatic process is the inability to stop the process from happening. Once the stimulus that triggers the process is present, the process will start—and, once started, it cannot be stopped. Even if a person consciously decides not to perform the process prior to seeing the triggering stimulus, knowing full well that the stimulus is about to be presented, the person still cannot stop its occurrence in the face of this preparation. To stick with the running example of color perception, if I asked you to look at the sky and not perceive its color, you could not do it. The mere presence of the stimulus (the sky) triggers the response (color perception), regardless of any goals that you have to prevent this response from happening. We have already discussed a similar type of inability to control body movements that nonverbally leak cues to people's true attitudes and emotions. Indeed, DePaulo and colleagues (1991) found that the more their participants tried to control such cues to deceit, the more they displayed them.

This inability to control a process despite the conscious intent to do so is the last feature of an automatic process. We have already seen some evidence of this in discussing how lack of intent is a characteristic of an automatic process. One illustration of this particular feature of automaticity has been that if people are intending to do one thing (such as to name the color of the ink in which a word is written), yet a different process that is incompatible with the intention is initiated (such as reading the word), then we have evidence that they could not have intended the response, since they were explicitly intending to do something else. We can take this logic one step further. In addition to asking people to intend to do one task, we can explicitly ask people to make sure they only do the task asked of them and explicitly tell them not to initiate any other response. We can even be specific and tell them, "Do not do x." If the response that they were explicitly told to avoid is initiated anyway, then we have evidence that they cannot control it. Despite deliberate goals to control the process, it is initiated in the mere presence of its triggering stimulus. As Shiffrin (1988, p. 765) stated, "If a process produces interference with attentive processes despite the subject's attempts to eliminate the interference, then the process in question is surely automatic." In person perception there are many instances of failures at control, and we will review them in various chapters of the book. For example, people may have the explicit goal not to think of others in stereotypic ways, yet it seems that for most people the very opposite occurs when they encounter a member of a stereotyped group (e.g., Devine, 1989). Chapter 11 reviews such failures at controlling.

Let us review one example in detail here, to make the case that the explicit attempt to control a particular response can fail because of the automatic processes triggered by person perception. One technique researchers have used to diagnose whether people can control a response is to explicitly ask participants not to perform the response, and then observe whether the presence of a stimulus associated with the response triggers the response, even though the participants were explicitly asked not to respond (i.e., will it occur despite the attempt to control it?). Gollwitzer (1996) has reported an experiment using a paradigm developed by cognitive psychologists working in the area of attention, called a *dichotic listening task*. In this task, people wear headphones and have separate streams of information presented to each ear. They are asked to ignore the information presented in one ear and to attend to the information in the other (by repeating these words aloud—a task referred to as *shadowing*). However, if information in the ear people are asked to ignore is not ignored, but grabs attention, this suggests that people are unable to control the processing of this information despite being explicitly told to do so (and despite the fact that it interferes with performing the task they have been asked to perform). What type of information will be processed despite attempts to control it? Gollwitzer reports that information related to people's current goals has this power. How can this failure at control be detected? Two methods have been used. First, researchers can examine performance on the shadowing task. Participant's speed at pronouncing the words aloud, and their accuracy at performing this task, should each be impaired if they are uncontrollably directing attention to the words in the ear they should be ignoring. Second, researchers can present the participants with a secondary task, such as turning off a light whenever it comes on. If the timing of the light is arranged so it appears whenever a word related to participants' important goals is being presented in the to-be-ignored ear, then this synchronicity should result in an impairment of their ability to turn off the light quickly. They should be able to do it faster when relevant words are not coinciding with the appearance of the light. The uncontrollable attraction of attention to the ear participants should be ignoring usurps just enough of their capacity for expending mental and attentional effort that there is less capacity remaining to respond to the light (Kahneman, 1973).

Gollwitzer (1996) describes an experiment using both these methods of assessing people's ability to exert control. First, the experiment required creating a goal state in research participants that would uncontrollably lead them to seek out information in their environment related to that goal. The participants were asked to name a project that they wanted to complete in the near future, and to plan how they would attain this goal by dividing the pursuit of the goal into five steps. They were then asked to commit themselves to exactly when, where, and how they would implement each of the five steps. From these descriptions, the researchers selected words that were related to participants' current goals, and then used these words in the dichotic listening task by placing them in the audio presentation presented in the ear that participants were supposed to be ignoring. Thus participants were to ignore the material in one ear (material that would occasionally contain words relevant to their personal goals) and attend to the information presented in the other ear, pronouncing that series of words aloud, all the while awaiting the appearance of a probe light that they needed to turn off as fast as possible. If participants were uncontrollably drawn to the goal-relevant information, unable to pursue the goal of ignoring the information presented in that ear, the presence of those goal-relevant words should have been a momentary distraction and disrupted their ability to turn off the light quickly. This was precisely what Gollwitzer reported: Attention to goal-relevant information could not be controlled, as participants took longer to shut off the light when these words (as compared to non-goal-relevant words) were presented in the ear they were instructed to ignore. In addition, shadowing performance was deteriorated in these instances. There were slower reading speeds reported, as well as increased errors.

Varieties of Automaticity

The concept of automaticity has evolved since the 1970s—largely due to the fact that most information processing contains some subset of these four criteria for automaticity, but not all of them. For example, driving a car does not meet all these features. Driving can be controlled (one does not begin driving in the mere presence of a car, and one can stop oneself from driving, given the goal to do so). Yet driving does not always occur with full consciousness and one's awareness focused on the task. To call this activity fully under control would seem to misrepresent the process. But so too would calling it automatic. To capture the full complexity of most processes, especially those involved in perceiving other people, Bargh (1989) proposed that there are varieties of automaticity. This allows for the possibility that the four features of automaticity can be treated independently and appear in various combinations. If a process (such as the perception of color) possesses all four features, it is said to be a particular variety of automatic processing—*preconscious automaticity*.

If one does not intend to initiate a response, and even lacks awareness that the response has occurred, but its occurrence requires some type of conscious processing, then a second variety of automaticity is said to exist—*postconscious automaticity*. For example, you may unintentionally and unknowingly find yourself sending nonverbal cues to someone you are interacting with. These cues could signal to that person that you are uncomfortable around him/her (e.g., you lean away from the person, fail to make eye contact, etc.). However, this unintended response would not have occurred had you not consciously decided to interact with that person. As another example, consider again the experiment described earlier involving learning word pairs such as "ocean–moon," and then being more likely to name "Tide" as a brand of laundry detergent (e.g., Nisbett & Wilson, 1977). This study showed an unintended and unknown influence on the later task (naming a detergent) resulting from prior conscious and intentional processing (focusing on and learning the word pairs). Finally, some processes occur without conscious awareness and with great efficiency, but require that a conscious goal be in place for the response to be initiated. This third variety of automatic processing is labeled *goal-dependent automaticity*. A perfect example has already been discussed at length—driving a car. You must first have the goal to drive.

Automaticity Is Irrationality (Not)

Identifying the various features of automaticity and incorporating them into the definition are important in distinguishing an automatic process from other responses people make in the absence of conscious awareness. Why is it essential to make this distinction? Because equating the term *automaticity* with a lack of awareness can give rise to the conclusion that automatic processing is irrational processing. There are many times when unconscious processing reflects an almost irrational and nonefficient type of processing, and it is important to distinguish automatic processing from unconscious processes that reflect this irrationality. Automatic processing is not a shortcut people use to avoid thinking deeply. It is a routine set of responses associated with a stimulus that allow people to develop increased efficiency at the task, rather than increased irrationality. Bargh (1984) has made this point by contrasting automatic processing with *mindlessness*—a type of thinking about other people in which mental energy and effort seems to have been eliminated, and people instead operate on automatic pilot. Langer, Blank, and Chanowitz (1978) have posited that mindlessness exists when people act and think without much conscious involvement and end up not making use of (or paying attention to) all the relevant details or actual information in their environment. Langer (1978) assumed that mindlessness results in automatic behavioral responses (behavior produced without the benefit of conscious consideration of the cues in the situation), even arguing that "by the time a person reaches adulthood, (s)he has achieved a state of 'ignorance' whereby virtually all behavior may be performed without awareness . . . unless forced to engage in conscious thought" (p. 40).

For example, our conscious expectations can lead us as perceivers to preclude attention to the environment. Langer and colleagues (1978) assumed that because we have detailed and "scripted" knowledge of specific situations, and how to act in those situations (such as how to behave in a restaurant), we allow the well-learned script to take the control over behavior away from conscious consideration of how to act. We do not exert mental energy to think about how to act; the effortless use of the script dictates the appropriate response. Mindlessness is evidenced in such situations. Each time we enter a restaurant, we do not strain to think what will happen, but know that we will be seated, given a menu, asked for our order, and (at some point after we have been brought our meal and have eaten it) asked to pay the bill. Langer and colleagues suggest that if it can be shown that people fail to consider all available evidence and instead rely on "scripts" to direct behavior, then behavior will have been shown to be produced without conscious processing and to be automatic.

To demonstrate that people operate mindlessly, failing to use relevant information because their expectancies allow them to not even consciously process that information, Langer and colleagues (1978) conducted what is now considered a classic social psychology experiment. They used as (unwitting) participants in the experiment people in the university library who were about to use a photocopy machine. Just as a person was about to start copying, an experimenter approached and requested to make a copy ahead of that person. Langer and colleagues reasoned that asking for a favor of this sort follows a script: If the job is small enough, and if the person making the request provides a sufficiently polite and rational-*sounding* reason for cutting in front, the favor is granted. They then manipulated whether the person asking to cut in front had an explanation to offer for wanting to cut into the line. The logic was that if a reason was provided, it would trigger the script for such requests in the people perceiving the request, thus allowing the script to be followed. If no reason was provided, the script would not be triggered, and people would be less likely to comply because they had no mindless rule to follow. Most important to the study was the type of reason being provided by the person asking to cut in front. One group of participants heard the person offer a reason that seemed legitimate upon close inspection (e.g., "Can I use the machine because I am pressed for time?") However, another group of participants heard what close inspection would reveal to be a totally meaningless and vacuous reason for the person wanting to cut the line (e.g., "Can I use the machine ahead of you because I have to make copies?").

If participants were exerting effort to evaluate the request for a favor, the ridiculous reason should have been no more persuasive than when no reason was provided. Only the good reason should have persuaded them to allow the person to cut in front. If, however, they were simply following the script, any reason, even if totally vacuous, would have been as persuasive as a good reason. Simply hearing the person offer a reason would trigger the scripted response, and people would follow the script regardless of the quality or validity of the reason being offered. The findings revealed that people acted mindlessly in this situation and efficiently followed a script. A perfectly empty and meaningless reason ("Can I use the copy machine because I have to make copies?") was just as effective at getting access to the machine as a perfectly good reason ("Can I use the machine because I have an urgent need to get this done quickly?"). And both of these cases where reasons were offered were more persuasive than when no reason at all was offered (e.g., "Can I use the machine ahead of you?").

Although mindlessness has some elements that seem automatic—the triggering of a social-behavioral script, given a stimulus (e.g., a request to use the photocopy machine)—it is ultimately a process that requires conscious processing and conscious awareness at some stage. According to Bargh (1984), "the features of the situation auto-matically activate the relevant script, which then directs the *conscious* processes of searching for further cues to verify the script as an adequate model of the situation . . . the result is that certain pieces of information are selected by the script over others that may actually be more relevant and useful in the current situation"(p. 35; emphasis in original). Mindless behavior is ultimately the product of a conscious process of search-ing for cues, even though consciousness is abandoned during other stages of the pro-cesses that produce the behavior. And from this quote, we can also see that this uncon-scious aspect of mindlessness is what leads people to act in an irrational manner. A mindless process is one where people are simply not thinking deeply, using expectations to guide how they scan the environment, often at the expense of detecting germane information. They avoid using information they should use, and focus on information they should not use (if they were operating in a rational manner). The failure to detect the relevant information (the irrational response) is then interpreted as a sign that peo-ple have abandoned the conscious evaluation of their environment.

Bargh (1984) points out that such logic equates unconscious responding with irra-tional responding. That is, the evidence that people are acting mindlessly, and hence automatically, is the fact they are operating irrationally, ignoring information that a conscious and thoughtful scan of the environment would not have neglected. This con-clusion is unwarranted. Not all processes that lack conscious awareness are irrational, just as consciousness does not guarantee that people will think rationally. Although some degree of consciousness being removed from a process may produce irrational responding, automatic processing is far more than the removal of some degree of con-sciousness from a process, and hence is not to be equated with such processing and the irrational outcomes associated with such processing. When an automatic process leads people to retreat into the unconscious, it does so in the service of the ability to detect relevant information in the environment, rather than leading them to ignore relevant information. They become so skilled at detection it happens invisibly.

CONTROLLED PROCESSING OF INFORMATION

Control has earlier been specified as one of the four components that must be lacking for automaticity to exist. This might imply that control is the opposite of an automatic process. According to *Webster's New World Dictionary* (1986), *control* is defined as the power to direct or regulate, while *will* is defined as the power of controlling one's own actions. In psychology, the term *control* is essentially equivalent to these lay conceptions; it refers to the ability of the individual to direct and regulate behavior and cognition. Wegner and Bargh (1998, p. 450; emphasis in original) state that "to control something is just to influence it in a certain direction. . . . [Formal] analyses typically begin by dis-tinguishing two features of control—a *control action* (the influence) and a *control criterion* (the direction). Control involves acting upon something until a certain criterion is reached." Control, therefore, is essentially the ability to select, implement, and regulate a goal. Although this might imply that the properties of a controlled process should be the opposite of those seen in an automatic process, this section ends with a suggestion that this need not be true.

The Elements of Control

In discussing control, it is important to keep in mind the distinctions among terms we often use interchangeably in everyday language: *needs*, *motives*, *incentives*, and *goals*. A *need* is a drive state, usually conceived of as arising from a physical (tissue) deficit of some sort. For example, hunger is a drive state that results from the body's requiring sustenance, and it results in the need to reduce that feeling of hunger or else the physical being will suffer (if not perish). A *motive* may be conceived of as a quasi-need, in that while there may be no tissue deficit, a similar process of being driven to reduce some perceived discrepancy between the current state of the organism and some desired state of the organism exists. In this case, it is a psychological deficit that impels people to reduce the discrepancy. The Introduction to this book has reviewed several motives that are seen as powerful forces in directing social cognition, and has referred to them as psychological needs—affiliation, self-esteem, and epistemic needs. *Incentives* are those people/things in the environment that will reduce the drive (the tension state) associated with a need/motive. Finally, *goals* are the end states people seek to attain by having pursued an incentive and addressed a need/motive. For example, the motive to affiliate with others points to various classes of incentives denoting a variety of goals, such as being popular or being admitted to a fraternity/sorority. One's goals permit for successful pursuit of the incentives, such as the goal of being funny at a party or drinking as much as norms dictate. As can be seen, incentives can denote broadly defined goals that can subsume a wide variety of lower-order goals (Geen, 1995).

The role of needs in determining the nature of control is central. Goals will affect a person's behavior differently, depending on what kind of need is the source of that goal (Deci & Ryan, 1991). If, for instance, two people in a music class are asked to create a composition, they each have the same goal. The motive they are seeking to satisfy will alter the nature of the goal that is selected and pursued. The first person (Britney) may set the goal of pleasing others, whereas the second person (Missy) may focus on creating an interesting piece of work. Missy's goal is in the service of a motive to derive intrinsic joy in an artistic process, whereas Britney's is in the service of a motive to be liked. Goals in the service of autonomy, competence, and social integration needs lead to greater creativity, higher cognitive flexibility, greater depth of information processing, and more effective coping with failure (Deci, 1992). When one's goals are not marked by autonomy of choice, such as when one is given a discrete task to perform by an authority or when a goal is selected based on an obligation, performance suffers.

Selecting Goals

A person's motives and needs produce more wishes and desires than can possibly be realized. Therefore, the individual is forced to make a choice between the variety of goals they could pursue at any given moment. For example, one's needs for social contact and affiliation will likely produce more wishes, desires, and goals than one could possibly pursue and attain at any given point in time. These could include goals like attending a party, talking on the phone, visiting a chat room, going to a bar, watching a play with friends, going to the park, and so forth. Only one goal can be selected at any point in time to satisfy the need for social contact. The choice as to which goal to pursue involves deliberating over the *feasibility* (i.e., thoughts about whether and how the goal can be realized) and *desirability* (i.e., the value of the goal) of one's wishes and desires (see Atkinson, 1964; Gollwitzer, 1990, 1993). Selecting a goal, such as deciding to go to a bar as opposed to any of the other options for having social contact, not only depends on the desirability ("How much would I enjoy a bar?") and feasibility ("Is it possible to get to a bar and meet people there?") of the multiple goals one entertains, but on the ability of the current situation (and consideration of future situations) to address those goals ("Are there good bars?").

Implementing Goals

Similar to selecting among goals, attaining the goal that has been selected requires choosing among multiple paths. Thus, once having deliberated among goals and selected one to pursue (such as deciding to go to a bar), the next task for the individual is the successful implementation of a particular goal-directed action. This task may be simple when the necessary goal-directed actions are well practiced or routine. But it may be complex when one is undecided about where and how to act ("What bar?", "Who should I go with?", "How do I get there?", "How do I get home if I am drunk?"). In complex cases, the implementation of goal-directed action needs to be prepared through the individual's reflecting on when, where, how, and how long to act, thus creating a plan for implementing action (e.g., Gollwitzer, 1993, 1999).

Regulating the Pursuit of Goals

When obstacles are placed in the way of goal attainment, or when failure is encountered, people do not simply quit. Rather, they often step up their efforts to pursue the goal. *Persistence* is one of the features that marks the regulation of goal pursuit. Such regulation is also marked by *flexibility*; that is, the way in which people act in pursuing a goal is determined by the appropriateness of a given goal-directed behavior in a given context. When one route to goal attainment is blocked, another course of action is taken. If a certain attempt to achieve a goal gets disrupted or fails, the individual does not need to give up on the goal. For many goals, multiple alternative pathways to approach them exist. For example, a goal such as being popular can be approached via many alternative paths (having parties, giving compliments, helping others, etc.), all of which can be deemed appropriate.

Of course, not all goal pursuits are successful; sometimes they fail. We may try having parties, giving compliments, and helping others, and still never attain the popularity we desire. Although we may persist at first, eventually we may revise our commitment and desire to pursue this goal—eventually lowering its importance, if not giving up on the goal altogether (this is known as *disengagement*). The roles of commitment to a goal, of evaluating and reevaluating the feasibility and desirability of a goal, and of self-efficacy (perceived personal ability) as it relates to whether we persist in or disengage from pursuing a goal are beyond the scope of this book to review, and would be the topics of an entire independent volume on motivation and goal pursuit (e.g., Carver & Scheier, 1981; Heckhausen, 1991; Kuhl & Beckmann, 1985). These issues are raised here simply to highlight the types of elements that determine how we control our behavior and thoughts in interpersonal interaction and person perception. One famous example will illustrate the operation of these various elements (selection, implementation, and regulation) of control.

The Zeigarnik Effect

Kurt Lewin and his students were reported to have started a line of research based on a lunchtime observation. In many German restaurants, the waiters and waitresses do not write down the orders; they keep them in memory. When it comes time to pay, they are able to recall what was eaten by each person at the table in order to collect the money (rather than keeping a bill that gets paid at a register). What Lewin noticed was that although a server's recall for the orders could last a substantial period of time (the duration of the meal), if the server was questioned soon after the meal had been paid for, it was evident that he/she had terrible recall for what each person had eaten. Why would memory for small facts about other people be sustained for an hour, and then purged in an instant? Lewin suggested that the goal of carrying out the task of being a waiter or waitress required holding information in memory, and until the task was completed there would be sustained cognitive activity for remembering the order. But once the goal had been attained, which only occurred when the meal had been paid for, activity related to it could be released. The term *release* is used because the memory that had been so perfect in one instance did not slowly evaporate, but was seemingly discharged when it was no longer relevant.

Pursuing any goal involves each of the elements of control: selecting a specific goal to pursue in a given context from among one's various goals, deciding how to implement that goal, monitoring one's pursuit of the goal to determine whether one has successfully completed the goal (or is at least making satisfactory progress toward goal attainment). The results of this monitoring process will determine whether increased commitment, a new plan for how to implement the goal, a new goal to pursue for the moment (leaving the selected goal for another time), or disengagement from this goal altogether is needed. To extend the Lewin example, waiters and waitresses have various motives they bring to work with them—to survive (pay rent, eat); to raise money to support some other interest (writing, acting, travel); to affiliate with other people; and/or to achieve (i.e., to be the best possible workers). Each interpersonal motive could lead them to select the goal of being good servers. They must next decide how to go about being good waiters/waitresses. The more specific and well-defined goals are, the more likely they are to be attained (Locke & Latham, 1991). To be a good waiter/waitress, a person would do best to set a more specific, lower-order goal, such as "I will remember all details about each individual I am serving so long as they are my customers." Wegner and Bargh (1998) refer to this setting of the specific goal as the *control criterion*—the particular end state that one seeks to attain. Once one has selected a broad goal or incentive to pursue, how does one go about setting the specific lower-order goal? By relying on information from prior experience and knowledge about the self. Wegner and Bargh call the information that allows one to set the criterion the *input* to the control system. Past experience teaches a waiter/waitress that recalling the information will result in smooth transactions without conflict at payment time (and perhaps larger tips). Such types of prior knowledge and experience shape the manner in which the specific goal is set.

Accompanying the specific goal with a plan for how to implement the goal will be the surest way to ensure success (a server's plan might be "So long as they are at my table, I will constantly remind myself who ordered what, and be mindful of what condiments and special needs their food choices present"). Once a plan is formed, one implements the plan and starts to act. A response made to attempt to attain a goal is referred to as the *control action*. However, how does a person know whether the plan is working and the goal is being successfully pursued (or if it has been achieved)? The next step involves *monitoring* the goal pursuit to know how one is doing. Wegner and Bargh (1998) describe two elements of control essential at this stage. The first is the *output*—the results produced by the control action. The second is the *comparator (monitor)*—the checking of the output against the control criterion to see whether the goal is met. If the goal is met (the meal has been paid for and the server has successfully recalled all the items associated with each person), the action can be ended (the server stops trying to remember the details regarding each individual). If the goal is not met (the meal is in progress), the action continues. Together, these regulatory processes constitute a *negative feedback loop* (Carver & Scheier, 1981). This term refers to the fact that the regulation of the control action (whether the waiter/waitress continues to ruminate about the orders of each individual) is dependent on the relationship between the output and the control criterion (as reported by the monitor). The control action is performed so long as there is a *discrepancy* between the criterion and the output. This produces a psychological discomfort or tension that one seeks to reduce (e.g., Wicklund & Gollwitzer, 1982). This negative state of goal attainment is relayed back through the control system via the comparator, and the behavior continues. This loop of action–comparing–action repeats until the criterion is attained and the goal is achieved (see Figure 2.4).

Zeigarnik (1927) undertook a doctoral dissertation, under Lewin's supervision, to illustrate the power of an unmet goal to direct cognitive activity. Zeigarnik designed a series of tasks for her research participants to work on (puzzles, problems). Participants

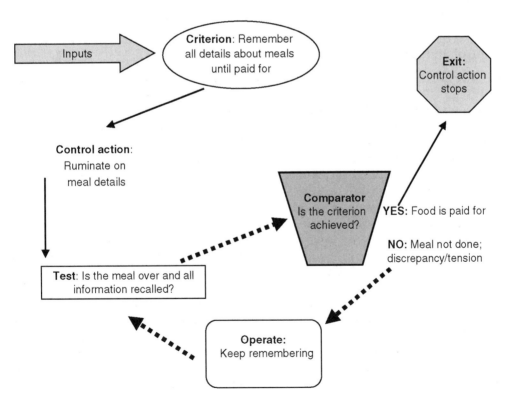

FIGURE 2.4. Regulation/control through a negative feedback loop.

were allowed to work on some of the tasks until they were clearly completed. But some of the activities were interrupted before they were completed. The tasks were then removed from sight so that participants could no longer work on them. What impact would the blocking of a simple, unimportant goal criterion have? Zeigarnik hypothesized that once a goal had been set, and goal-relevant activity had been initiated, participants should continue to focus on attaining the goal and taking actions aimed at attaining the goal until there was no longer a discrepancy between the current state and the desired goal. In this example, if working on a problem had been interrupted, and the materials were even removed from sight, there would be a discrepancy. Participants should perform activities to attempt to attain the goal, even though the task was not very important. Importance and commitment might determine how long they persisted before deciding, in the long run, to disengage. But in the short run, they should persist. To examine whether her participants persisted and continued to work toward unmet goals, Zeigarnik later asked the participants to try to recall the tasks that they had worked on. She found that the unfinished tasks were recalled twice as much as the finished ones; people ruminated on unfinished tasks. According to the Lewinian model, this occurred because the goal of completing the task was left unfulfilled, and being blocked from completing a goal (a discrepancy between the current state and the goal criterion) led to the continuation of goal-directed activity. In this case, with the inability to work on the actual tasks (they were removed), the only possible goal activity was to ruminate over the tasks. People continued to attempt to reduce the discrepancy by devoting mental energy to the task. Just like a waiter or waitress at lunch, participants used memory as a means to work toward an unmet goal (for a review of rumination based on the Zeigarnik effect, see Martin & Tesser, 1996).

Control and Interaction Goals

We have just done a very fast review of the elements that constitute how people regulate and control their thought and action. In discussing control as it is related to person perception, it is also useful to analyze the varieties of goals that people can regulate and pursue when forming impressions of others. What sort of control criteria are commonly in place in person perception? Jones and Thibaut (1958) provided a taxonomy of *interaction goals*—goals that shape the manner in which we perceive information about ourselves and others in a social interaction. Jones and Thibaut specified three general types of interaction goals.

Let's use an evaluation of President Clinton's impeachment process from 1998 as a running example to illustrate the interaction goals common to person perception. The impeachment process arose from an investigation to ascertain whether the President had been involved with a real estate scandal (Whitewater) prior to having become President. A special prosecutor (Kenneth Starr) was assigned to investigate this possibility. While under investigation for this scandal, the President had simultaneously started an adulterous affair with a young woman named Monica Lewinsky. When being questioned about the real estate scandal, the investigators also asked the President about his relationship with the young woman (an issue totally irrelevant to the alleged real estate scandal). The President did not reveal his sexual relationship with this woman, and lied about it to the investigators. Lying while under oath is a crime that carries with it the possibility of impeachment, and the President's opponents pushed for him to be impeached for the act of lying, even though the lie had nothing to do with the scandal in question (in which, as it turned out, the President was found to have no involvement).

Causal-Genetic Goals

Causal-genetic goals are those that we pursue in order to understand others and accurately assess their motives, values, and personalities. They are the goals of simply trying to understand the true causes for events. In attempting to be accurate in assessing causality, we are playing the role of investigators, attempting to be objective in gathering facts. As Jones and Thibaut (1958, p. 166) state, "in one sense, the purely causal-genetic perceiver, A, has no intrinsic concern with the stimulus person, B." We are not motivated to draw any particular type of conclusion, but merely to ascertain the objective facts that govern their behavior and draw the most accurate conclusion. Presumably, prosecutor Kenneth Starr's team was concerned (or at least its charge was to be concerned) with gathering information that is accurate and unbiased in order to draw a conclusion regarding whether impeachment proceedings need occur. The team members were to be impartial gatherers of facts with causal-genetic goals.

Social Sanction Goals

Rather than attempts to draw an accurate conclusion, *social sanction goals* include those that we adopt for the purpose of evaluating other persons to see whether their behavior meets some designated standard or norm. To turn once again to Jones and Thibaut (1958, p. 167), "[a social sanction goal] is to establish whether or not the other person is behaving appropriately, whether the person's behavior 'matches' the norms which apply in the situation." With a social sanction goal we are vested in another person because we are charged with evaluating him/her. Being charged with the goal of gathering accurate data about President Clinton might have led to very different conclusions about him than being charged with the goal of evaluating whether his behavior met appropriate social and legal standards. The latter was the role of (and goal for) the members of Congress who needed to evaluate the President's behavior (lying while under oath about an adulterous affair) against existing legal and moral standards to determine whether the data about the President provided by the prosecutor warranted impeachment, censure, or no particular action at all.

Value Maintenance Goals

Value maintenance goals are goals that we pursue in order to attain something we value for our personal fulfillment. Rather than being accurate, or being judgmental, we are being self-serving. In our running example, this was also a goal adopted by the members of Congress, because their opinions of the President and their ability to support their political party would partially determine their own political future. A problem with the impeachment process was that the people who should have had purely social sanction goals (evaluating the President against some objective standard) also had value maintenance goals (protecting and promoting their own political future). That is, their evaluations of what was appropriate may have been biased by what they valued. The members of Congress trying to ascertain what constituted a "high crime" were the same members of Congress who had to answer to their constituencies come election time, rely on the President should he stay in office, seek political gain, and so forth.

Given the breadth of the notion of "attaining personal fulfillment," Jones and Thibaut (1958) spoke of four subtypes of value maintenance goals, or four domains in which our personal biases can direct our interpersonal interactions.

Accomplishing an Outcome External to the Interaction. With the first subclass of value maintenance goals, the main concern is interacting with others in order to have them help us achieve success on some task that is not itself directly attained through the interaction. Other people can either help or hinder us in achieving a goal because (1) they have some sort of authority that can either promote or prevent us from achieving a goal (e.g., we slow down when driving past a police car, because the police have the authority to prevent us from having a clean driving record); (2) we are partners with these others and need their help to get what we want (e.g., we are working on a joint project that no single individual could finish); (3) the others have something we want, and we need to interact with them in order to make them want to give it to us (e.g., we are interested in attending a sold-out concert, and a friend has one extra ticket that we want). Thus the interaction is focused on getting others to yield to and support our goals. In the running example of the impeachment, the President had the goal of not being impeached, and he relied on the members of Congress to deliver this to him. Thus, when the President was interacting with a particular member of Congress in the weeks before the vote, he could have been reasonably expected to act in a warm and flexible manner toward this person. The outcome desired by the President was external to this interaction, but it could have been promoted by the interaction. We interact with others in a manner that might yield some later outcome.

Maximizing Positive Reactions from Others. With the second subclass of value maintenance goals, our main concern is entering into an interaction with the goal of perceiving that others like us and positively evaluate us. There are two general subclasses of this goal—impression management and belongingness. With belongingness as our goal, we want others to like us so that we can feel loved and experience a sense of belonging and being affiliative with others. With impression management, we want others to like us so that we can control them and be able to get them to do things for us. This will affect the interaction in at least two ways. First, we will structure our perceptions of them around what they can do for us. Second, we will attempt to manipulate what they think about us. For example, a given member of Congress may have wanted to impeach the President, but thought it better to have the President as an ally. Such a person could have used impression management to vote in a manner opposite to his/her true feelings. The vote would then perhaps have given him/her power with the President for being a seeming ally.

Gaining Cognitive Clarity about the Environment. With the third subclass of value maintenance goals, the value to us is provided by others in that they remove ambiguity for us. They help us to gain sufficient information to clarify an aspect of our environment that was previously unclear. We turn to others in an interaction so that they can serve as sources of information to help us achieve closure. Some classic experiments in social psychology demonstrate people following this goal. For example, in Latane and Darley's (1968) famous helping studies (described in Chapter 1), participants failed to help others in a potential emergency situation because other people in their environment defined the situation as not being an emergency (others did not help, or even looked distressed and as if an emergency was being observed). The lack of concern on the part of others provided clarity for the research participants, informing them that the situation was probably not one that called for help or presented danger. In our running example, a conservative talk show host such as Rush Limbaugh would have provided such clarity for people who were opposed to the President. Such people sought information that would explain events to them in a way affirming their values and preferences. Conservative citizens who disliked the Democratic President could receive such information from like-minded people in the media.

A difference should be noted between arriving at a sufficient explanation as described here, and the causal-genetic goals described earlier, which require making an accurate assessment of the behavior of others. When trying to make a sufficient judgment, we try to evaluate others so that we have a sense of simple understanding—their behavior makes sense and is coherent. With a causal-genetic goal, we want to determine causality while maintaining accuracy. This is the same distinction between closure seeking and truth seeking that has been discussed in the Introduction to this book. A person concerned with accuracy would not have turned to a clearly partisan media outlet or talk show host for all his/her information about President Clinton.

Securing Motivational and Value Support. With the fourth subclass of value maintenance goals, we are not concerned with reducing uncertainty, getting positive reactions from others, or attaining some external item. Instead, we enter a social interaction with the goal of getting support for our views or values. If our concern is getting ahead in the world, then we will be attentive to issues of power and cues in others that signal they can help us achieve what we want. If we value the groups to which we belong, then we may enter a social interaction with the goal of promoting a sense of positive group identity or seeing evidence promoting ideologies we value. For example, a Republican member of Congress may have been so concerned with preserving the image of the Republican Party that he/she would have desired to see President Clinton impeached just so the Republicans could seem more righteous and moral. This might have been true even if this member of Congress had also had adulterous affairs and lied under oath. The desire to garner support for the group the member was motivated to promote may have determined his/her behavior when evaluating the President.

Determinism and Free Will

What negative feedback loop models suggest is that we are engaged in constant "tests" of our progress along our goal pursuits. Control involves monitoring ourselves to attain knowledge about where we stand. Although monitoring need not be conscious to us, it suggests that to the extent we are self-reflective, we will have greater success at monitoring our progress. In short, if such testing is indeed as central to regulating goals and controlling responses, heightened states of self-focused attention (self-awareness) should promote goal regulation (Carver & Scheier, 1981). Increasing attention to the self, from something as simple as placing a mirror in front of research participants, is capable of getting them to be more likely to note the discrepancy between their actual behavior and the criterion that serves as their standard. Self-focused awareness can arise from many types of everyday occurrences, such as when we glance into a store window and see a reflection of ourselves, or when we are simply in a social situation where others are looking at us (e.g., Duval & Wicklund, 1972). Such a look into the mirror, whether literal or figurative, gives us greater insight into our shortcomings and motivates us to reduce the discrepancy between how we actually behave and how we desire to behave.

However, this description of control makes it sound as if control is the opposite of an automatic process. With an automatic process, an individual's response is determined by the stimulus; with a controlled response, the criterion is selected by the individual's act of conscious will, and the regulation of the goal pursuit results from actively evaluating how well one is doing in one's pursuit of the goal. The controlled processor sounds like one in possession of free will, while the automatic processor is preprogrammed, almost like an automaton.

The Ghost in the Machine

Some have argued that free will is an illusion. They contend that the feeling of conscious control we have over our responses is nothing more than that—a feeling, an illusion, a ghost. From this perspective, situational forces and prior experience so strongly determine what we do that control is nothing more than an epiphenomenon. We may feel that we choose to act as we do, to select the goals that we do, and to behave the way that we do, but in reality our behavior is mostly triggered by the stimuli we encounter. The feeling of having decided to act, from this perspective, is actually something that occurs after we have already started acting. Consider the following experiment by Libet (1985). Libet relied on the knowledge that prior to a voluntary action there is a brain response—an electrical potential—that can be measured with electrophysiological equipment. Libet measured these electrical potentials during a task in which people were asked to move their fingers whenever a certain event occurred. The resulting data showed that the brain response (electrical activity) occurred about a half second before the physical response. Thus it appears as if brain activity caused the response (finger movement), and the logical conclusion might be that free will, conscious control, was what triggered this electrical activity in the brain. But, if so, there should have been a consciousness of the goal to elicit a response, and it must have occurred *before* the electrical activity in the brain. But Libet found that consciousness of the decision to move one's fingers occurred *after* the brain activity that supposedly caused the action to occur.

Given that consciously "willing" an act such as this seems to occur after the brain response has already initiated the behavior, does this not suggest that our conscious sense of controlling the action is false? The action has already begun before we have the conscious experience of willing it to happen. This raises the possibility that we don't cause things to happen, but the stimuli in the environment do. This returns us to the notion of automaticity as determinism. If the mere presence of a stimulus is what triggers a response, this suggests that the will is not involved. We simply develop a sense of control quickly after the response has occurred, almost simultaneously with it, to allow us to feel as if we have free will. Conscious control, in this scenario, is a ghost in a stimulus–response machine (Ryle, 1949)—a myth we have created to allow us to feel as if we have control. But we are already acting before we experience the decision to act.

Must a finding such as that reported by Libet (1985) suggest that control is epiphenomenal? This is still an issue of philosophical and empirical debate. But we can say this: In the Libet experiment, people were instructed to move their fingers at some point in the experiment. The measures of brain potentials and of conscious willing were then collected at those moments when the finger movements actually occurred. So, while it may be true that a conscious goal was not directing the responding when it actually happened (when the fingers were being moved), it is also true that a conscious goal was required at some point in the process—people would not have moved their fingers at all unless they had been instructed to do so and had adopted this goal consciously. Thus conscious control on our part may be required to select our goals, although it may not be required at the time we pursue and regulate our goals.

Preconscious Control

This may still seem like a shaky attempt to salvage the notion of free will. So let us consider another argument that salvages the notion of free will. Perhaps we should not take the fact that a conscious experience of willing occurs after brain activity has already initiated responding as evidence that our goals are not involved in causing the response. Perhaps it simply means that the conscious experience of our goals operating follows the behavior, but that the goal itself is operating *preconsciously*—prior to our awareness of a goal being pursued, with all the efficiency and lack of awareness that marks automatic processes. Is it possible to pursue goals without consciousness? Does it make sense to say we are "willing" something to happen without being aware that we are making it happen or consciously intending it to happen at the time the response is made? This notion seems impossible, given that everyday use of the notion of control equates it with consciousness. As Wegner and Bargh (1998, p. 453), have stated, "most people think of control in humans as conscious control, so much so that the term 'unconscious control' doesn't seem right at all." But earlier in this chapter, we have already discussed several examples consistent with the notion that control occurs in the preconscious. Think back to the experiments by Gollwitzer (1996) using the dichotic listening task, and by Roskos-Ewoldsen and Fazio (1992) using brief flashes of objects. Attention was automatically directed toward what was important. The Zeigarnik effect offers a similar illustration: People ruminate on tasks that are no longer present without realizing that they are directing mental processes toward the pursuit of the disrupted goal. Let us explore two forms of preconscious control more closely.

Compensatory Cognition. Consider a common experience: When trying to retrieve some information from memory (e.g., who was the most valuable player in the 2000 World Series?), you may experience a *tip-of-the-tongue effect* (Brown & McNeill, 1966). The desired information feels as if it is knowledge you possess and is about to leap out of your mouth. Yet you cannot produce the response. After struggling for some time to access the information, you eventually disengage from the task. Interestingly, the desired information often comes rushing into consciousness at some later time ("It was Derek Jeter!") in an unrelated context, when you are not attempting to retrieve it. This is an example of consciously disengaging from a goal, yet preconsciously pursuing the goal without intending to or being aware that the goal is being regulated. You solve a problem without trying—but you *were* actually trying; you simply were preconsciously trying. And thus the solution to the task, the attainment of the goal, is delivered to your conscious mind as if by magic—it pops into consciousness as if from nowhere. Elsewhere, this type of preconscious cognitive processing aimed at helping one attain an unresolved goal state has been labeled as *compensatory cognition* (Moskowitz, 2001). Compensatory cognition can be said to occur when a discrepancy exists between the desired level and the actual level of goal attainment, thus triggering cognitive activity aimed at reducing this discrepancy and focusing the cognitive system toward goal-relevant stimuli in the environment. People are preparing for goal-relevant behavior by preconsciously directing attention and scanning the environment for information relevant to their goals (Moskowitz, 2002).

Goal regulation can occur without a person's (1) deliberately selecting the goal at the time it is being pursued, (2) knowing that goal-relevant stimuli are present, or (3) knowing that he/she is implementing responses aimed at attaining the goal. A study

was conducted to illustrate this (Moskowitz, 2002): Goals were manipulated in one context and were shown to exert preconscious effects in a totally unrelated context where
participants did not realize the goal was relevant (selected) or being pursued. Research
participants were asked to write about a time in which they acted in an unfair manner,
or failed to live up to the principles that would be exhibited by an egalitarian person.
This task was posited to trigger the goal to be egalitarian. As discussed above, when
people's goal states are not met, compensatory responses are initiated. They desire to
remove the aversive state associated with not attaining a goal.

Once goals were triggered in this fashion, participants were next asked to join a
separate experiment in a different room and perform a task assessing perceptual ability.
In this task, two objects moved on the screen—one vertically, the other horizontally. The
task was to detect which object moved vertically, and to report whether the direction of
movement was up or down. Participants did not know it, but these moving objects were
actually words that moved so quickly that participants could not consciously detect the
content. But the content of the words was essential. On some of the trials, words relating to the goal of egalitarianism were presented as the words that were moving horizontally. If participants were to do the task successfully, they had to ignore the words moving horizontally and focus on the words moving vertically. It was found that on the trials
of the experiment where the goal words appeared, participants were slower at performing the task (naming the direction of the words moving vertically). If the words relevant
to their goal appeared in the to-be-ignored spot (they moved horizontally), participants'
goals led their attention to be diverted away from the task they were supposed to be
focused on (detecting the direction of the words moving vertically) and slowed their
performance on the task at hand. This occurred despite participants' not knowing that
words relevant to their goals were being presented (or that any words were presented!),
or that basic processes of attention were being assessed. People clearly acted in a willful
manner, pursuing goals they selected. Thus there simply is no need for consciousness to
be invoked for goal regulation to occur. In this sense, control is not the opposite of
determinism.

Goal Priming. Bargh (1990) proposed that goals are mental representations that are
stored in memory and capable of being activated. Because links between stimuli and
mental representations lead to the automatic triggering of such representations, given
the presence of the appropriate stimuli, goals should similarly be triggered automatically by stimuli in the environment that are relevant to those goals. Bargh hypothesized
that conscious deliberation regarding the pursuit of a goal, given a specific set of circumstances, leads these two events to be paired. The consistent choice to pair a goal
and a situation leads to the development of an associative link between these two
events. Over time, this link develops enough strength that conscious deliberation is no
longer needed for the goal to be activated, given the appropriate circumstances (Bargh,
1990). For example, if the goal of being egalitarian is adopted whenever one encounters
a homeless person, then eventually merely seeing a homeless person could trigger the
goal to be egalitarian and start one behaving in egalitarian ways, without one's consciously willing these acts. These ideas are discussed more fully in Chapters 9 and 10;
the focus here is on two illustrative examples (for a more complete review, see
Moskowitz, Li, & Kirk, 2004).

Bargh, Gollwitzer, Lee-Chai, Barndollar, and Trötschel (2001) gave research participants a word search puzzle intended to trigger their goal of being achievement-oriented
to varying degrees. Some of the participants had words relevant to the concept of high

performance (e.g., "win," "compete," "succeed") embedded in the puzzle; others had neutral words. Participants then completed three more puzzles, and the experimenters examined how hard they tried to achieve while performing this task. The results revealed that the group with the high-performance goal triggered found significantly more words than the no-goal group. This experiment suggests that performance goals can be triggered outside of awareness and then have an impact on how people achieve, without their realizing that their goal-directed behavior is being influenced or that a goal has even been triggered and achieved without conscious awareness.

Shah (2003) explored how significant others, because they are linked to people's goals, can unknowingly trigger those goals. It was posited not only that cues associated with significant others would lead people to pursue the goals defined by their relationships with those others, but that they might prevent them from pursuing goals deemed unworthy by significant others. A first experiment involved asking each research participant to provide the first name of his/her mother and the first (different) name of a close friend. Participants were then asked to provide attributes that represented separate goals that their mothers and friends had for them. Each participant later performed a separate experiment where he/she was presented with either the mother's name, the friend's name, or a control word. Finally, participants indicated how committed they were in the upcoming week to attaining the attributes they had listed previously and how frequently they would try to fulfill the goals. When participants were provided with the names of their friends, the intention to pursue the goal associated with the friends was heightened. Similarly, when they were thinking about their mothers, participants' commitment to a goal was significantly greater (apparently because mothers have higher standards, or are perceived to have higher standards). In short, relationship partners appeared to be triggering goals associated with the partners and influencing participants' expressed commitment to the specific goals and the intention to pursue those goals, all outside of the individuals' intent and awareness (see also Fitzsimons & Bargh, 2003). Our will is not always operating in conscious ways.

CODA

This foray into the examination of automatic and controlled processing has been undertaken to highlight the point that our interactions are goal-directed. When we examine ourselves and others, we do so for a reason, whether or not that reason is explicit to us at the time. The feeling that we control our cognition and behavior to serve our goals is an insistent one, but the review of automatic processing suggests that much of our responding is guided by processes of which we are unaware, and that we perhaps cannot even intend to stop. Our thought and behavior are determined by cues/stimuli/people in the social environemnt.

Several of the classic experiments in social psychology reviewed in Chapter 1 are perfect exemplars of a central theme of social psychology—that human behavior and cognition are often determined in large part by the powerful social forces that are encountered upon exposure to, or contemplation of being exposed to, other people. But one often-overlooked result of this theme is the fact that if behavior is being determined by the situation, conscious volition on our part is not always a central player in determining how we think and act, with responses instead triggered by the social forces that push and pull us. Wegner and Bargh (1998) stated:

These classic studies share a focus on what the individual does when he or she has to decide or respond in difficult circumstances, under extreme duress, unusually quickly, or in an otherwise stressful, uncomfortable position. As a rule, people in these powerful situations don't acquit themselves very well, as they succumb to pressures that make them do things ranging from merely uncharitable to frighteningly robotic. Classic social psychology, in other words, makes people appear to be automatons. (p. 447)

These experiments share more than the ability to illustrate how some social force is capable of dictating how people behave (indicating the power of the situation and the malleability of human behavior). These famous experiments all involve the processing of information from the environment outside of awareness or without conscious intent, and they all involve the silent detection or communication of internal thoughts and feelings through nonverbal communication. These experiments illustrate how processes of social cognition infiltrate in nonobvious ways into the phenomena examined in each case via the silent exchange of information and nonverbal communication outside of people's awareness and intent. Rather than retrace these steps already taken by Wegner and Bargh (1998), let us just review one example.

Latane and Darley (1968, 1970) found that people did not help others who were in need, despite their best intentions. The researchers explained these findings by assuming that people simply are not aware of their responsibility to help. The more people who are present, the less responsibility any one individual feels, and the less likely it is that one will act. As mentioned in Chapter 1, the failure to act is a socially shared event. People see each other not acting and arrive at an inference that this is not a situation that calls for help. Thus the unconscious inference about the situation's not being an emergency (based on interpreting actions of others) and diffusion of responsibility lead people not to help others in need. This experiment reveals just how dangerous it can be to lack awareness of our own thought processes. Surely if we knew that we are failing to help others because we have incorrectly inferred that someone else has already taken action, or because we have used the inaction of others as a faulty source of information about the nonthreatening nature of the situation, we would help immediately. However, our lack of awareness of these cognitive processes leaves us frozen in inaction, as nonhelpful bystanders. Indeed, Latane and Darley (1968) asked their research participants whether they thought that the number of other people present would influence how they would act. Participants did not think that this would matter at all, whereas the data revealed it to be a quite powerful determinant of whether the participants helped or not. When alone and witnessing an emergency situation, we are far more likely to help than in the presence of a small group, and in a small group we are more likely to help than in a crowd. The ability to recognize the impact of this factor on our behavior has tremendous consequences for an important social behavior. This element of automaticity, lacking awareness, underlies the powerful case of when bystander intervention fails to occur.

This notion of automatic processing as fairly ubiquitous in everyday life may leave us feeling a bit conflicted. It seems to suggest an incompatibility with the supposed goal-directedness of all human behavior and interaction, and we like to feel as if our everyday actions are mostly guided by our own acts of volition (not triggered by external sources, stimuli in the environment). If there is control, how can so much be automatic? If free will dictates our responding, how can it be that we lack awareness of so much of what contributes to our responding? Do we truly have control over our action, or is much of it automatically triggered by the peculiarities of the situiation we are in and the relevant cues that present themselves?

These question presume a dichotomy between determinism and free will—an inherent inconsistency between control and the ability to process information in the preconscious. This dichotomy is uncalled for. Controlled responses can also be determined by stimuli in the environment, so that the mere presence of a goal-relevant stimulus triggers movement toward the criterion—goal pursuit. Control may be more than an epiphenomenon, but may still occur without conscious awareness (for reviews, see Bargh, 1990; Moskowitz, 2001; Moskowitz et al., 2004). Having the will and our goals automated does not make us automata. It simply means that we relegate as much processing as we can to the preconscious, even processing relevant to the pursuit of our most important goals. This makes us more efficient creatures. Thinking less is not the same as irrationality. Thinking less can result in irrational responding, but this does not mean that we must equate all unconscious processing with being irrational. Instead, automatic processing can be a quite pragmatic and rational response to the unique challenges that person perception presents. Chapter 3 examines these issues more closely, asking why so much of our processing of other people occurs outside of our awareness, without intent, beyond control, and rather efficiently.

3 Categories and Category Structure

HOW PERSON MEMORY ILLUMINATES IMPRESSION FORMATION PROCESSES

Our experience in life tends to form itself into clusters, and while we may call on the right cluster at the wrong time, or the wrong cluster at the right time, still the process in question dominates our entire mental life. . . . Open-mindedness is considered to be a virtue. But, strictly speaking, it cannot occur. A new experience *must* be redacted into old categories. We cannot handle each event freshly in its own right. If we did so, of what use would past experience be? Bertrand Russell, the philosopher, has summed up the matter in a phrase, "a mind perpetually open will be a mind perpetually vacant."

—ALLPORT (1954, p. 20; emphasis in original)

My 2-year-old son recently saw an unmarked police car and remarked, "Look, Daddy, a police car with no lights." This ability to understand his environment was dependent first on his having knowledge of the category "police cars"—of the essential features that make something a member of this category. His remark was also dependent on having the ability to include something in the category, despite its lacking one feature one would typically consider to be central for categorization (the lights on top of the car). When he was a year younger, he saw a Hasidic Jewish man in a store and said, "Look, Daddy, cowboy." This statement illustrates two additional points. First, we have categories for groups of people (cowboys, firefighters, lawyers, women, Arabs, Jews, etc.), as well as for groups of objects. Second, our categories are not always appropriately matched to the data that we observe. In this case, the category "cowboys" (one of my son's very first person categories to develop) was defined by very few features, with the feature "wearing a hat with a brim" being the defining one—and, in this case, probably inappropriately applied to the man (who was most likely not a cowboy, but that is an inference on my part).

Chapter 1 has examined the fact that our perception of other people is biased. That is, the data we gather—even data as basic as those allowing us to perceive that an object is a pencil, or that a person is a police officer—are filtered through our existing knowledge and goals. The concern of the current chapter is more basic; it is with the categories that exist in our minds and that allow us to make sense of the new information received by our senses. We cannot filter the external world through the lens of our prior knowledge unless such prior knowledge is stored in long-term memory and organized in a way that makes it meaningful and easily retrieved. Mental representations of the classes or groups of events/things/people that help us to structure our knowledge are called *categories*. (In actuality, cognitive psychologists call a mental representation a *concept*, and the set of examples picked out by the concept a *category*. Thus police cars are a category, and my internal representation of this category in memory is a concept. However, let us use *category* to refer to both the class and its mental representation, for ease of discussion.) A category is a grouping of similar objects/people in memory—a grouping based on the important or essential features that define the class of things constituting the category. Markman and Ross (2003) define categories as "groups of distinct abstract or concrete items that the cognitive system treats as equivalent for some purpose. Maintaining and using equivalence classes involves mental representations that encode key aspects about category members" (p. 592–593). As might be expected, many of our categories overlap. As Allport (1954, p. 171) stated, "We have one category for dogs, another for wolves. . . . A category, in short, is whatever organizational unit underlies cognitive operations . . . related ideas in our minds tend to cohere and form categories."

Imagining life without such prior knowledge is easy if you have ever witnessed a child learning words for the first time. The child is not merely learning to speak, but learning about the world, developing categories. Although the recognition of something as an instance of a category and the naming/speaking of the category are separate processes (Malt, Sloman, Gennari, Shi, & Wang, 1999), they both reflect the emergence of a category system in the developing mind. The child learns to distinguish a cat from a dog, a truck from a car, a fire truck from a dump truck. These categories are forming in the mind in a simplistic way. The child cannot yet clump the dog and cat together into a larger category of "animals" or "mammals," or the Pekinese and the Labrador retriever into the same category of "dogs." We begin with simplistic and concrete knowledge, but through our life history this evolves into a complex and interconnected web of associations. Pekinese and Labrador retriever are soon linked to the same category. "Cats" and "dogs" are seen as distinct categories, but linked together through an association to a higher-order category. Once armed with these associations, we can make sense of most of the information that comes our way and know how to react to it by virtue of that experience and the knowledge stored in our minds (Barsalou & Medin, 1986). My 2-year-old was thus able to appropriately detect police cars, marked or unmarked. In 14 years, this knowledge will tell him how he should act if he is behind the wheel.

In the Allport (1954) quote that has started this chapter, we see that knowledge (experiences) is said to be clustered; we fit our new experiences into one of our existing categories. Although the idea of reacting in a novel way to each and every person may seem like a pleasant thought (i.e., each person would be judged according to his/her merits and the information derived only from experience with that specific person), in the end such an approach would surely leave us unable to interact appropriately. We need categories to make sense of each event/person, leaning on prior knowledge to absorb what currently confronts our senses. Our mental representations of the external world are the building blocks of all knowledge and lay the groundwork to guide social interaction. Allport believed that, as in object perception, person perception simply provides too much information. We perceivers cannot make sense of other people without some internal system for sorting through all this information, organizing it, and making inferences from it. Categories about types of people help us do this, and we have a wide variety of person categories to help us: Americans, Blacks, doctors, extraverts, landscapers, lawyers, Communists, Catholics, Texans, red-necks, liars, Japanese, women, Jews, punks, journalists. The list is endless, but each immediately conjures up a picture of the category and the type of person we might expect to meet if we were told someone belonged to one of these categories. Taylor, Fiske, Etcoff, and Ruderman (1978) put this well: "Instead of perceiving a group of persons as a set of unique individuals, the perceiver may well structure perceptions of the human environment much as perceptions of the object world are structured. He or she may select salient social or physical dimensions to use as discriminating variables for grouping and managing person information" (p. 779).

In a sense, the work reviewed in this chapter is responsible for the active construction of reality reviewed in the preceding chapters of this book. One cannot discuss how people are biased by prior beliefs and goals, or how information about people is processed automatically, unless one first assumes that there are structures in the mind providing the knowledge that allows such psychological events to occur. The discovery that perceivers are involved in the process of shaping their impressions, rather than detecting them, eventually set researchers off on the path to determine what these latent variables were that were guiding what people thought they were seeing and the meanings they ascribed to what they thought they were seeing. In the 1970s and 1980s, social psychology saw a boom in research examining the ways behaviors and traits are represented in the mind, and the relationship that exists between them when stored in memory. Piaget (1970, p. 59) eloquently summarized the subjectivist view: "Even perception calls for a subject who is more than just the theatre on whose stage various plays independent of him and regulated in advance by physical laws of automatic equilibration are performed; the subject performs in, sometimes even composes, these plays." Thus mental representations must be structured in a way that can account for the fact that people fail to perceive a perfectly literal transcription of the world outside, but are involved in the production of what is experienced. Piaget called this *structuralism*, and helped popularize the term *schema* (a term discussed in detail in Chapter 4) in explaining how a child produces his/her experience of the world.

CATEGORIES AND CATEGORIZATION

When we place some new experience into an existing cluster in our minds, labeling and identifying this new experience as an instance of something we are familiar with, we are said to have categorized the experience. The act of *categorization* is the placement of an object, person, or event into some class of familiar things. This is the manner in which we come to identify the people and things in our environment. Despite the fact that we categorize often without needing to consciously attend to or control the process, it is still the case that categorization does not happen in one step. Rather, several processes operate on the new information in order to fit it into one of our existing clusters. It should be noted, however, that before we can categorize a person, he/she must first be perceived. Thus some preliminary cognitive activity has already occurred that allows us to focus attention on a specific person once we start to categorize. Let's begin the analysis here, after attention has allowed us to perceive the person's presence.

The Stages of Categorization

Bruner (1957) describes several stages we must pass through in order to achieve categorization, once having attended to a stimulus. The first is called *primitive categorization*. "Before any more elaborate inferential activity can occur, there must be a first, 'silent,' process that results in the perceptual isolation of an object or an event with certain characteristic qualities. . . . what is required simply is that an environmental event has been perceptually isolated and that the event is marked by certain spatio-temporal-qualitative characteristics" (pp. 130–131). This simply means that the information to which we have attended gets focused on for an analysis of its features. Next we have to determine what these features are representative of. This proceeds through a process called *cue search*. Here we analyze the features (or cues) and check them against categories that contain similar features; we attempt to match the features of the cue to one of our existing categories to which there is sufficient feature overlap. The next step involves concluding that we have encountered an instance of a particular category if there is enough of a feature match between the category and the stimulus. At this stage, we make an *inference* that the new experience is actually just another instance of something we are already familiar with; we place the new experience into one class of things rather than another, assuming that the features it possesses means that it belongs in this class or category. Upon completing these stages, we have gone from encountering an unknown stimulus to having an identity for that stimulus—one that places it within one of our existing categories.

Thus, in an attempt to identify a person, we search for a closeness of match between the features of the perceived person and the features in potential categories to which the perceived person might belong. In this sense, a category is called to mind whenever we encounter stimuli in the environment that possess characteristics of the category. *Category activation* is the end product of an interaction between some stimulus in the environment and the human perceptual system, in which the category attains a heightened state of accessibility and readiness by virtue of being retrieved from memory in this process. A person, therefore, does not directly activate or awaken a category from its dormancy in memory. This responsibility is left partly to cues (e,.g., Higgins, 1996). Cues are information residing outside the mind, such as the features of the person encountered in the environment that have inherent or acquired associations with the concept to be activated. (But cues can also include operations occurring wholly within the mind, such as when concepts already activated in memory trigger associated concepts.)

A given cue may not trigger or activate a category immediately, even if placed within that category. Instead, the activation level of the category will build, like a battery accumulating a charge. Once the activation level reaches a specified *threshold*, the category is activated. The implication is that even if a given stimulus does not sufficiently trigger the category, a weak stimulus that comes along soon after may add just enough charge to push the accumulated charge above threshold and activate the category. Think of a man who acts in a mildly hostile way. This may not have been enough of a cue to trigger the category "hostile" in your mind. If soon afterward another, totally different man also acts in a moderately hostile way, this weak behavior may be perceived by you as hostile because it was enough to trigger the "already warmed up" category. The charge has accumulated above threshold. You may respond by punching the guy in the nose, even though the behavior of the first man may have been more egregious and deserving (or even though neither man deserved to be reacted to as if he was hostile). Obviously, any given instance of categorization can provide a sufficient charge to push the category activation above threshold, without further accumulation being necessary.

Allport (1954) summarized the categorization process well: "Every event has certain marks that serve as a cue. . . . When we see a red-breasted bird, we say to ourselves 'robin.' . . . A person with dark brown skin will activate whatever concept of Negro is dominant in our mind" (p. 21). The perceived person is attended to, identified, and categorized as an instance of a concept we have previously encountered, our knowledge of which is stored in memory and retrieved from memory to allow us to understand the person who currently faces us. Thus our understanding of people and the world around us is dependent on associating each new event with what we have already learned and stored in memory. The past is used to make sense of the present, and our knowledge of the past, though we may not be cognizant of it, drives each and every reaction, starting at the basic level of identifying and categorizing a person's features.

The Qualities of Categories and Categorization

Categories Are Fuzzy Sets

Cognitive psychologists often speak of a "classical view" of categories (Smith & Medin, 1981). In this view, categories are said to be composed of *defining attributes* that are singly necessary and jointly sufficient for category membership (Barsalou & Medin, 1986). This essentially means that categories contain a set of features that *define*, or are equally *central*, to category membership, and an attribute that is not found in all members of the category would not be considered such a defining attribute. Any person (or object) having all of the defining attributes is a member of the category, while any person who (or object that) lacks even one of the attributes is not a member of the category (Lingle, Altom, & Medin, 1994, p. 75). For example, the category of "African Americans" would contain, from this view, only those features that are found in all people who are African Americans. It might include attributes such as these: having a biological connection to a person born on the continent of Africa, being an American citizen, having what might be labeled "dark" skin, and having ancestors in the United States who have been the target of centuries of legalized discrimination (ranging from slavery to "Jim Crow" laws). The categorization of a person as an African American would necessarily entail believing that all of these features are true of the person. The consequence of this type of thinking about categories, as Lingle and colleagues (1994) note, is that because all members of the category have the very same features, each is an equally good representative of the category.

However, not all people (or objects) appear to be equally good representatives of a category. Even if perceivers act as if one person in the category is exchangeable for the next, people are quick to recognize that not all birds are equally representative of the category "birds" (Malt & Smith, 1984), just as not all African Americans are equally representative of the category "African Americans." Tiger Woods is classified by most people as a member of the category "African Americans," but he is not perhaps as representative of the group as other famous members of the category one could imagine, such as Jesse Jackson. Malt and Smith illustrated that the degree of fit to a category leads to variability among perceivers' assessments of how well a given member repre-sents the category. Research participants were provided with a list of birds and were asked to rate how typical of the category each type of bird was, using a 7-point scale. Robins received extremely high ratings (6.89), while owls received moderate ratings (5.0), and chickens (3.95) and penguins (2.63) received very low ratings. Each type is clearly a member of the category, but they vary in how typical they are.

Rosch (1973, 1975) provided a seminal illustration that categories do not seem to possess required/necessary features. If categories consist of a set of attributes that are true of each and every member of the category, then people should respond equally fast when attempting to identify whether any given instance of the category is a mem-ber of the category. Thus trying to answer the question "Is a robin a bird?" would be no easier than responding to the question "Is a penguin a bird?" However, Rosch found that research participants differed in the speed with which they could identify different category members as belonging to a category. In one experiment, participants were asked to judge whether a given stimulus was a member of a particular category. They were presented with a series of statements, all in the same form—stimulus followed by category (e.g., "A robin is a bird," "A penguin is a bird"). They merely had to indicate whether each statement was true or false, and their reaction times were recorded. The critical manipulation in the experiment was the degree to which the stimulus was a typi-cal member of the category in which membership was being judged. Thus some trials of the experiments had stimuli that were very typical of the category (robin), while others had less typical stimuli (penguin). The results showed that it took people longer to say "true" to a real instance of a category when it was less typical (or a poor representative of the category). People did not make mistakes of saying "false" to these poor represen-tatives. They knew they were category members; they were just slower to detect this fact in their minds.

This observation suggests to us that categories have a set of features that are per-haps indicative of category membership (or essential to its definition), and some criti-cal subset of these features must be present for a person to be categorized as a member of the group. These features that are essential to the meaning of the item are still called *defining features* (Smith, Shoben, & Rips, 1974), but each defining feature is no longer seen as necessary or required to be present. Other features may be descriptive of the category, but are less essential, not defining. Rosch and Mervis (1975) described this type of structure—with a set of defining and less essential features being used to catego-rize an object/person—as categorization based on a *family resemblance*. For example, a given type of person shares some proportion of features with other members of the cat-egory, and shares some features with members of other categories. If the proportion is greater (if there is a family resemblance) with members of one category, than the per-son is seen as an instance of that category. Thus an African American may have skin that is not what one would call "dark" at all, yet still be categorized as an African Ameri-can because of a large proportion of shared features with the category (other than this one attribute).

In addition, some features are central to category membership, while others are more peripheral. The feature "able to fly" is more central to the category "birds" than the feature "may eat human flesh." The latter feature, residing at the periphery of the category (since some birds may eat a human carcass), is shared by many other categories (such as lions, tigers, and some space aliens). When you are asked to think of the cate-gory "chairs," a mental image probably comes to mind, accompanied by a set of features that define for you what a chair looks like and does. But what features of this image of a chair are central and give it its essence, and which are more peripheral features that are likely to be found in chairs, but not so important for defining the object as such?

Even the more central features are not always necessary for categorization to occur. Your mental image of a chair is likely to have a back. But if you were to take away the back, the object would still retain its category membership. If you were to remove the arms, once again, the object would remain a chair. However, even though not all the central features need be present for categorization to occur, the more central the features that an object/person possesses, the more easily it/he/she is categorized. Although the feature "primary means of transport is flight" may be considered essential for the category "birds," a few birds, such as the ostrich, are not capable of soaring through the sky. Yet the ostrich is still categorized as a bird because of the sufficient degree of overlap between the other features it possesses and the features that define the category. However, because it has fewer central features of the category, it may take longer to identify and categorize an ostrich as a bird. This is true of people as well. A person with many of the features that constitute a category, and for whom many of the features are more central than peripheral (more defining of the category), will be seen as more representative of the category than someone who has fewer of the essential features and a good percentage of features that reside at the periphery of the category. In this conception, both of these people described would be members of the same category; one would just be more representative of the category.

If each category contains some features that reside at the periphery, it is reasonable to assume that overlap of different categories is likely to occur, and that this will be especially likely to occur at the border between the categories, where the two peripheries meet and the less central features are shared. That is, each category has its boundaries, since it is defined by a set of properties that are more or less central. The qualities that define a category and the boundaries that limit membership in a category are "fuzzy," in that they lack discrete and clear demarcations. For example, if we imagine the armless and backless chair described above, and then alter it slightly so that it is rectangular in shape and perhaps its surface is less comfortable, it may start to shift from one category ("chairs") to another ("end tables" or "coffee tables"). These categories share many features along their respective peripheries where the borders are fuzzy. However, some features of your category "chairs" are more defining or central (e.g., a back, a cushion sized to fit one person, etc.) and can differentiate it from other categories it might share a fuzzy boundary with (such as "coffee tables"). As asserted above, there is often a greater degree of overlap between categories among features that are at the edges of a category. But just because a feature is not at the boundary, but rather is central to a category, this does not mean it cannot be listed among the features that define another category. The ability to fly is a central feature of both the categories "birds" and "airplanes." Thus feature overlap between categories is not restricted to features that reside along the boundaries of the category.

Finally, just because a feature is central to defining a category, this does not mean that this feature is central to defining how we think about the members of the category. Sloman and Ahn (1999) provide a good example. A central feature of a polar bear is that it has white fur, but its white fur is essentially irrelevant when we think about the essence of a polar bear or what it would be like to interact with one: "Naming and thinking about objects impose systematically different demands on the importance we assign to the objects' various aspects" (Sloman & Ahn, 1999, p. 526).

The discussion above informs us that a category need not possess a set of necessary and sufficient features. Rather, categories are marked by a collection of features that vary in how essential they are to the category. Let us examine the issue of categories' lacking defining features that are necessary and sufficient through one more example. Fiske and Taylor (1991) use the example of the category "games" to illustrate this point. What makes baseball, Monopoly, jacks, hide and seek, poker, spin the bottle, Ms. Pac-Man, flag football, peek-a-boo, and twenty questions all members of the category "games"? Are there necessary features that are sufficient to include an activity in this category? Games are typically thought of as enjoyable activities that are engaged in by more than one person, are governed by rules, and have no external purpose other than generating a feeling of pleasure. But does this mean that eating and sex, which sometimes have all of these features, are games? And does this mean that activities that are boring (such as baseball for many people, or Monopoly for people who are running out of cash), are engaged in by one person (such as pinball or Ms. Pac-Man), are not governed by rules (such as playing in the snow and jumping rope), or have an external purpose (such as getting paid millions of dollars to play basketball, or promoting international good will with the Olympics) are not games? Activities that possess some of the features of games (such as eating and sex) are not categorized as such, and activities that lack some of the features of games (such as Ms. Pac-Man and playing in the snow) are categorized as such. This occurs because categorization is not dependent on a perfect fit between the features of a stimulus and all the features denoted by the mental representation. Rather, categorization depends on a sufficient degree of overlap between the representation and the set of features in the stimulus. So long as some subset of a category's features are present in a stimulus, that category may be used to "capture" the stimulus.

Categories Are Socially Shared

Categories are shared among people in a culture. There are at least two good reasons why such a state of affairs should develop. First, it is possible that the origin of people's categories is linked somewhat to the physical realities/features of the objects and people that are being internally represented in the mind. As an internalization of external realities, presumably most individuals' categories will have detected (and represented mentally) the same set of features. However, the socially shared nature of categories is not dependent on assuming that the physical reality of the stimuli is what determines the categories people hold. It is possible that categories are shared because they represent various theories that people hold about the world, and these theories are taught to them by their culture. If they all hold the same theories, they hold the same internal representations of the stimuli explained by those theories (e.g., Murphy & Medin, 1985). This approach would lead us to expect that different members of the same culture would have similar categories, and could lead us to expect cross-cultural differences in categorization. As one example, the *Whorfian hypothesis* (Whorf, 1956) asserts that language influences not just how people communicate, but the structure of their thought. Language causes habitual and obligatory changes in the categories people develop. Whorf (1956) put this best: "Users of markedly different grammars are pointed by their grammars toward different types of observations and different evaluations of externally similar acts of observation, and hence are not equivalent as observers but must arrive at somewhat different views of the world" (p. 221). The Whorfian hypothesis is used here not because it is universally accepted, but because it is a well-known example of how theories might influence cognitive structure.

As a further example, Morris and Peng (1994) describe culture as a powerful force that determines cognitive styles for thinking about behavior. They argue that Western cultures (e.g., Canada, England, Germany, the United States) place a strong emphasis on individuals as autonomous beings, responsible for their own actions and for the effort they commit to attaining their various goals. Such cultures have been labeled *individualist* cultures. This culturally produced cognitive style leads perceivers within the culture to focus on dispositions as causes for behavior. People act in particular ways because they are perceived to have traits that cause them to act in those ways. A culture replete with religious doctrine, folk tales, laws, music, and art (film, books, etc.) that scream of the rights of individuals will develop an implicit theory that individuals are the first and foremost causes of events that transpire. This belief in traits as an enduring characteristic that is primarily responsible for behavior is a mind-set, a cognitive orientation, based on a theory about the meaning of behavior that is linked to the culture's definitions of behavior. Different, non-Western cultures place less of an emphasis on individuals as autonomous beings and more of an emphasis on interconnectedness, social ties, and persons as part of a collective. These types of cultures (e.g., Chinese, Indian, Korean, Japanese) are less likely to lead their citizens to develop cognitive styles that demand the use of enduring traits to describe the character of a person, and that assume this character to be responsible for guiding the person's actions. Instead, social roles, social pressures, and obligations to others are more viable explanations for behavior. The cultural theory about the meaning of behavior alters the very ways in which behavior is categorized and understood, relative to the same behavior as perceived by members of a Western culture. It is not just that they describe the events differently; it is that culture has altered the cognitive styles for framing the world.

As an example of how theories learned through the culture can permeate the manner in which people interpret and categorize the world, Morris and Peng (1994) performed an archival study. They examined how two murders (one committed by a Chinese man and one committed by an American man) were being reported in newspapers. Both papers were based in New York City and served their respective communities worldwide. The findings supported the researchers' predictions, drawn from their notion of culturally derived implicit theories that permeate how the world is seen and described. American and Chinese reporters reported the same event (a murder) in strikingly different ways, categorizing the event differently. American reporters made more attributions to the personal dispositions of the murderer, focusing on the traits and personal characteristics of the type of person who would kill. Chinese reporters, however, made more attributions to situational forces that pushed the killer toward his act. The environment, and the pressures located within the situation, were evaluated and discussed in more detail. In Chinese culture, murder is not simply the act of a crazed or evil person, but of a society that plays a role in how people act. In an experiment meant to supplement this archival finding, Morris and Peng gave American and Chinese students descriptions of a murder case and asked them to describe the reasons why it had occurred. The participants were provided with a list of potential causes, and were asked to weigh each cause for its potential impact. The causes were designed so that some of them were best described as blaming the person and the disposition/traits of the person, whereas others were best described as situational causes. Consistent with the archival results, the Chinese students rated the situational explanations as more prevalent than the Americans did (the Americans, in turn, focused on dispositions as causes). This experiment, rather than looking at how murder was explained by two different cultural groups to its constituent members, examined individual members of each group to see how they categorized the very same event. Theories learned from one's culture altered the way in which the event was categorized.

Categorization Is an Act of Inference

Because no single object or person is likely to have 100% of the features we associate with a category, we must often, in order to categorize, "go beyond the information given" (Bruner, 1957). That is, categorizing requires testing and approximating how some new information fits with our existing knowledge, despite there not being an exact match. This ultimately requires an assumption/inference that those features of the object match closest with a particular category that exists in the mind. An object that has four legs, a back, and arms, and is stable enough to support weight is categorized as the same object as one that has no legs, a base, no back, and a large beanbag curved into its rounded frame. Each object has enough of the features of the category "chairs" to allow us to categorize it. Thus feature matching leads to a degree of probability that each object is a chair, but the final categorization still involves this probabilistic inference that the features match the category. According to Bruner (harkening back to Helmholtz, 1866/1925), even the well-practiced act of categorization, such as identifying an object as a "chair," involves an inference; it is simply an unconscious, automatic one. In the final analysis, each time we see something, we have made an inference about it; we are inferring it is yet another instance of some category of things/people that we already have knowledge about (pens, chairs, Italians, women, etc.).

Categorization Typically Proceeds Automatically

Bruner (1957) believed that the act of categorizing is the most ubiquitous and primitive cognitive activity, so much so that the inference process that accompanies categorizing can occur without conscious awareness; it is often a "silent or unconscious process . . . we do not experience a going-from-no-identity to an-arrival-at-identity" (p. 125). If an object or event or person we encounter is one we are highly familiar with, or one that has a high *cue–category linkage* (meaning that the links between the attributes and the category are clear, well learned, familiar, and well practiced), then we can categorize it without the conscious experience that any acts of inference have occurred. We do not expend conscious effort trying to figure out what it is or to match its features against existing categories. The percept appears in consciousness ready-made for us. An object is encountered, and we state, "That is a chair." This ease of categorization occurs despite the fact that no chair is exactly like another. Yet we infer from degree of overlap that each instance is a representative of the group.

However, if the linkage between cue and category is low—if this is an object or event or person that is not familiar, that we are not well practiced with—then we do not simply experience it, and the feature matching and the attempt at placement do not occur so silently. We consciously attempt a cue search. For example, the first time one encounters a chestnut on a tree, it may be hard to infer quickly and unconsciously that it is actually a nut. One might instead first assume that it is a bizarre fruit (due to the round shape, fuzzy texture, and green color) or wonder if one has stumbled upon a tennis ball tree. For the inexperienced person with an underdeveloped category, the inference that the green, fuzzy objects are chestnuts is difficult and requires conscious effort; it is probably only arrived at after the tree has been categorized as a chestnut tree (hence allowing one to deduce that the things growing on it are chestnuts, not tennis balls).

Categorization Can Be Incorrect

At the end of the section on the "fuzziness" of categories, we have noted that this fuzziness can give rise to incorrect categorizations—to errors. Anyone who saw the movie *The Crying Game* knows that sometimes the inferences we draw based on categorizing according to observable features are wrong. The features we think we see lead us to a category that does not adequately describe the person, and to behavior that is not appropriate. As Allport (1954, p. 20) says, "Sometimes we are mistaken: the event does not fit the category. . . . Yet our behavior was rational. It was based on high probability. Though we used the wrong category, we did the best we could." Because finding an exact match between a stimulus and a mental representation is limited by the fuzzy nature of our categories, we may call on the wrong category; the inference we make about what category best captures the stimulus may be incorrect.

A dramatically tragic example of miscategorization was evidenced among the passengers of the airplanes that were strategically used as terrorists' weapons to attack the World Trade Center on September 11, 2001, in New York City. Passengers on these planes probably knew that their planes had gone off course and were not being flown by the pilots. However, they probably categorized the events that were transpiring as a hijacking. This inference would have been accompanied by a set of expectancies appropriate for that category, including the belief that the plane would be landed in some foreign territory and a set of demands issued. Sadly, this categorization was incorrect, and the events transpiring did not represent a hijacking. But these passengers acted rationally in making the inference and could not have known to make any other type of categorization. Passengers on the flight downed in western Pennsylvania an hour later were able to categorize the event differently, due to their knowledge (through cellular phone contact with loved ones on the ground) of what had transpired on the other planes. And because of the new categorization, they were able to act in a strikingly heroic (yet equally tragic) fashion, according to a quite different way of categorizing their situation. Rather than categorizing the event as a hijacking, they categorized it as a suicide mission, which had a totally separate set of expectancies and inferences and led the individuals on board to act in a totally different fashion from passengers on the earlier planes. The earlier passengers, not knowing that they were part of a suicide mission, sat frozen in their seats while the World Trade Center was struck by their planes. The latter passengers, knowing their country was under attack, chose to attack their "hijackers" before the plane could be used to do similar damage, perhaps saving thousands of lives on the ground and preventing the destruction of either the White House or the U.S. Capitol.

Categories Need Not Be Accurate

It is possible for us to correctly place some new information/event/person into one of our categories, but the category itself may contain objectively false information. There is no necessity that our categories correspond to fact. They can be more or less rational. Allport (1954), once again, informs us that "nature unfortunately has given us no sure means of making certain that our categories are composed, exclusively or even primarily, of the defining attributes" (p. 171). Each culture teaches those of us raised within it the various stereotypes that it has defined, and these become culturally shared. Whether these stereotypes are accurate or not, the category exists because the culture has taught it to us. We may later learn to reject these stereotypes as inaccurate, but we do not lose the category. Even those of us who reject stereotypes of women can report what that stereotype is. The category remains even if it is no longer endorsed. Similarly, any category we have can range from containing a set of features that are between 0% and 100% accurate in describing the reality of the class of things/people it is meant to describe. Most categories have a degree of accuracy that falls somewhere in between these extremes, meaning that most categories are not 100% accurate.

Categories Need Not Correspond to Outer Reality

Finally, the mind can contain categories that do not even correspond to any outer reality. For example, there is no such thing as an elf, Superman, or Santa Claus, but we have categories for them. Having a real physical existence is not necessary for categorization. Fictional or not, only being known to us and having identifiable attributes/features are required for an entity to be categorized. We even have categories for things we reject: An atheist has knowledge of religions; egalitarian people have knowledge of various cultural stereotypes; Red Sox fans know (all too well) Yankees' victories.

The Functions of Categorization

Identifying new information in terms of old information that we are already familiar with serves several important functions. First, it saves us from needing to figure out what a stimulus with a particular pattern of features is (and from calculating what we can expect from it) each time we encounter it. The category provides a means for organizing the incoming information that allows it to make sense to us. Bransford and Johnson (1972) provide an excellent illustration of how categories ease identification and classification of information by asking us to try to learn the following description of a task:

> The procedure is actually quite simple. First, you arrange things into different groups. Of course, one pile may be sufficient depending on how much there is to do. . . . It is important not to overdo things. That is, it is better to do too few things at once than too many. In the short run this may not seem important, but complications can easily arise. A mistake can be expensive as well. At first the whole procedure will seem complicated. Soon, however, it will become just another facet of life. (p. 722)

If we had been told before reading this that there was a category that could explain the entire passage, and the category was called "doing laundry," the complexity of this task would have been greatly reduced for us by virtue of having a frame on which to hang the information. Bruner, Goodnow, and Austin (1956, p. 12; emphasis in original) summarize this function of categorization well: "By categorizing as equivalent discriminably different events, the organism *reduces the complexity of the environment*. . . . we do not have to be taught *de novo* at each encounter that the object before us is or is not a tree. If it exhibits the appropriate defining properties, it 'is' a tree." Thus a first function of categorization is that it allows us to classify and label a stimulus quickly and easily.

Second, every person and object we categorize receives its meaning from the class of things to which it has been assigned. That is, the category tells us what features we can expect that have not yet been exhibited, and it allows us to know things about the stimulus that we have not yet derived from personal experience with this particular instance. For example, when you encounter a strange dog, the knowledge you attain from categorization informs you that you may be hurt by the dog, even though the dog has not shown any signs of hostility. Even though there is a distinctiveness to each new person and object we encounter (e.g., the dog may be a rare breed), this occurs within a reasonable range of deviation from the tendencies that are defined by its membership in a particular category. If it is a member of that category, there are certain features that are certainly exhibited, regardless of how distinctive this case is.

Bruner (1957) informs us that attaining this meaning leads naturally to a third function of categorization. Categorization allows us to make predictions about what to expect:

> The meaning of a thing, thus, is the placement of an object in a network of hypothetical inference concerning its other observable properties, its effects, and so on. . . . In learning to perceive we are learning the relations that exist between the properties of objects and events . . . *learning to predict and to check what goes with what.*" (p. 126; emphasis in original)

If given a piece of knowledge about a category, we can predict features and attributes that are not yet witnessed by virtue of the commonality among those objects that, or people who, occupy the same category (e.g., Gelman & Markman, 1986). For example, Sherman, Lee, Bessenoff, and Frost (1998) found that people make predictions about the behavior of a stranger based on the social categories to which the stranger belongs (categories such as race, age, gender, profession). Indeed, stereotyping is nothing more than the triggering of features and beliefs associated with a social category by a person who may or may not actually possess the features assumed to describe the category more generally. It is a prediction about an individual from the category. These predictions may lead us to systematic errors, as we rely on the predictions suggested by the category rather than what we actually have seen!

For example, Sherman and Bessenoff (1999) showed their research participants lists of friendly and unfriendly behaviors that had been performed by either a skinhead or a priest. The category "skinheads" is inhabited by mostly unfriendly behaviors, while the category "priests" is inhabited by mostly friendly ones. Crucially, however, the lists that were shown to the participants did not support these categorical representations. Instead, the very same number of friendly and unfriendly behaviors were performed by the skinhead and the priest. Subsequently participants were shown each of the behaviors from the lists (both skinhead and priest behaviors), but this time without specifying who performed which behavior. The participants' task was to try to remember who performed each behavior. Despite the fact that there was no association between the person (priest or skinhead) and friendliness in the studied materials, participants tended to misremember unfriendly, but not friendly, behaviors as having been performed by the skinhead, and also to misremember friendly, but not unfriendly, behaviors as having been performed by the priest. Mather, Johnson, and DeLeonardis (1999) found parallel results in memory for whether statements were made by Democrats or Republicans. In the absence of being able to recall who performed what behavior, people were using their categories to allow them to make predictions. These predictions were, in this case, inaccurate, but they were based on rational processes in which people relied on whatever information they could; the stored representation of the category led people to predict that the observed behaviors were ones associated with the category.

The predictions people make from their categories are *veridical* (truthful, accurate, precise) to varying degrees. This is not only because people have trouble remembering the real events that have transpired and are doomed to making guesses that will not accurately capture the actual data. It is also because the categories they have representing those data, as noted earlier, are not necessarily accurate. Categories can be incorrect. Categories can range in how accurately they represent the external reality, and the veridicality of the predictions provided by the categories will vary along with the veridicality of the categories themselves. Once again, Bruner (1957) summarizes this function eloquently:

> The results of categorization are representational in nature: they represent with varying degrees of predictive veridicality the nature of the physical world in which the organism operates. By predictive veridicality I mean simply that perceptual categorization of an object or event permits one to "go beyond" the properties of the object or event perceived to a prediction of other properties of the object not yet tested. (p. 129)

Once armed with expectancies and predictions concerning the people and things that cross our path, the next function of categorization should be obvious: The act of categorization allows us, given our predictions and expectancies, to plan our behavior—to engage in what we feel are appropriate behaviors that will bring about an expected consequence. As Allport (1954) stated,

> [Categorization] forms large classes and clusters for guiding our daily adjustments. We spend most of our waking life calling upon preformed categories for this purpose. When the sky darkens and the barometer falls we prejudge that rain will fall. We adjust to this cluster of happenings by taking along an umbrella . . . when we see a crazily swaying automobile we think, "drunken driver," and act accordingly. (pp. 20–21)

Bruner and colleagues (1956, p. 12) referred to this function of categorization as categories providing "the direction for instrumental activity."

This reference to instrumentalism links this perspective directly to the pragmatist writings of William James:

> Let me begin by reminding you of the fact that the possession of true thoughts means everywhere the possession of invaluable instruments of action; and that our duty to gain truth, so far from being a blank command from out of the blue, or a "stunt" self imposed by our intellect, can account for itself by excellent practical reasons. . . . The possession of truth, so far from being here an end in itself, is only a preliminary means towards other vital satisfactions. (James, 1907/1991, p. 89)

Indeed, Allport (1954, p. 167) essentially summarized James's position in stating that "thinking is basically an endeavor to anticipate reality. By thinking we try to foresee consequences and plan actions that will avoid whatever threatens us and will bring our hopes and dreams to pass." Thus categorization allows us to plan behavior and serves the function of facilitating communication and social interaction.

Categorization and Control

In addition to this pragmatic function of categories, the ability to predict what can be expected from others also provides us with a sense of control over our outcomes. Rather than feeling as if we are subjected to the random effects of the social world, we can instead experience a sense of control over the interactions and situations we enter into, determining what happens to us. As Heider (1958, p. 71) stated, in Lewin's (1936) terms, an unstructured region, that is, a region whose properties are not known to the person, can be considered a barrier which makes action and therefore control difficult if not impossible. Perception helps to structure the region and to remove this barrier.

Thus the predictive abilities that categorization delivers gives us an illusion of control over our environment. Chapter 8 will discuss this illusion of control at greater length.

Categorization and Communication

Categorization is essential for communication. Utterances from someone we are speaking with must be interpreted in ways that involve far more than identifying the actual words that are being spoken. We need to make all sorts of inferences about *qualities* of the communication being received, in addition to its content: for instance, "Is it trustworthy? Is it meant to be ignored? Is it relevant, or is the other person prattling on endlessly? Is it meant for me?" Communication is a complex exchange, and we are perhaps not aware of the extent to which we are constantly categorizing the speech of others according to a host of variables. In fact, Grice (1975) provided an extremely influential analysis of the sorts of factors that govern communication and that we presumably are detecting and categorizing with each exchange. These factors constitute a set of principles or maxims that provide the norms or rules governing how we speak to one another. For example, in everyday life, we do not expect that 50% of the information we encounter each day in newspapers, books, and conversations will be false; we treat most of it as if it is true. We follow a rule suggesting that (1) we should try to be truthful when speaking to others, and (2) we should assume that others are being truthful when speaking to us. This is why compulsive liars seem so pathological, and why journalists who betray this trust (and make up stories or facts in stories) are seen as almost villainous (as evidenced by the uproar in May 2003 over Jayson Blair, a reporter at *The New York Times* who admitted to fabricating facts in interviews reported in published articles). The overarching principle that unites these maxims is that communication is meant to be a cooperative exchange between two people, and we develop rules for maximizing the extent to which we can facilitate and ease our partner's understanding of what we say (cooperating with each other as best as possible).

The first of Grice's (1975) maxims of communication deals with this issue of trust and truth. Grice suggested that when people converse with others, either as communicators or as audience, they try to tailor communication for optimum understanding. The *maxim of quality* asserts that speakers should "say only that which they believe and have adequate evidence for" (Clark & Haviland, 1977, p. 1). This implicit assumption governs the communication. The maxim operates not only for currently active communications, but for previous communications as well: Unless otherwise noted, past communications will be assumed to conform to the majority of past communications in being true. This maxim is so essential to communication that violations of the rule are almost always marked in such a way as to make the violation known and to convey it as being intentional (such as when we display sarcasm and say, "Nice job," to our friend who has just failed miserably). The second maxim in Grice's analysis is the *maxim of relation*, which urges speakers to include only information that is relevant to the current communication goal. This maxim has some relationship to the maxim of quality, especially as it relates to how research participants perform in experiments (e.g., Schwarz, 1999). For example, when participants are given information by a researcher as part of an experimental session, the maxim of relation leads the participants to assume that they should use the information, even if it seems illogical to do so. Experimenters think they are revealing irrational behavior on the part of their participants, when in fact all the researchers are doing is leading the participants to use information that the participants otherwise might not have used. The participants end up thinking, "The experimenter would not have provided me with this information if it was irrelevant, and I was not supposed to try to use it." Thus people may use some trait information when categorizing a person not because they think the trait adequately categorizes the person, but because they think the person they are speaking with would not have mentioned the trait to them if it was not true or relevant. In most cases, if information is assumed to be relevant to communication, it is also assumed to be true.

The *maxim of quantity* is the third of the Gricean norms of communication, and essentially informs communicators not to be windbags or to stray too far from the point. It enjoins people to be informative in their communication, but not to provide too much information or unnecessary amounts of information. For those familiar with the 1970s television show *All in the Family*, the character Edith Bunker would violate this maxim each time she told a story, thus creating hilarity for the viewers. Finally, the *maxim of manner* details a stylistic component of the communicative exchange: Speakers are to be clear and unambiguous. Cooperative communication is that which does not equivocate. The maxim requires people to state meaning and intention clearly, rather than to be obscure and duplicitous. It is the violation of this maxim that makes students get so mad at "trick questions" on exams: If only the meaning had been clear, they could have displayed their true knowledge and responded appropriately.

PERSON MEMORY: CLEVER WAYS TO STUDY THE STRUCTURE OF PERSON IMPRESSIONS AND SOCIAL PERCEPTION

The previous discussion informs us that when forming impressions of people, we rely on prior knowledge. The features of the person with whom we are interacting trigger the relevant categories, and these categories consist of sets of attributes (traits), behaviors, and examples that are known to define the category. For example, the category "lawyers" has features and behaviors such as these: being intelligent, being argumentative, making good money, thinking well under pressure, knowing the laws of the state and country, having a JD degree, and so forth. It also includes examples of lawyers we are familiar with (Johnnie Cochran, Hillary Clinton, F. Lee Bailey, Stephen Bilkis, etc.). We then can use those attributes and examples as information about this specific instance of the category—the person who currently confronts us. Our emerging impression will be informed not only by the behaviors we observe and the words communicated to us by the person, but by the inferred attributes and behaviors supplied to us by the category. Social psychologists' interest in categories arises from this functional component of categories. Social cognition concerns itself with categories largely because the categories help tell us how and what to think about the people we see (and in turn to make decisions about how to behave).

However, a large body of literature has concerned itself not only with the *function* of categories, but with the *structure* of categories. The way in which concepts/categories are structured in the mind may in turn have a strong impact on how and when the categories are used. In fact, Hamilton, Katz, and Leirer (1980a) defined an impression of a person as "*a perceiver's organized cognitive representation of another person*" (p. 123; emphasis in original). Person perception is seen as a process of acquiring information about a person, organizing that information according to some structure in a mental representation, and later retrieving that information from storage. Thus the existing mental representations held by the perceiver are used as an aid for structuring the new information. For this reason, the various ways social knowledge can be structured is an important topic in its own right, and one that has received a good deal of attention.

The goal to study the structure of our mental representations of people presents us with a rather large dilemma. How do we go about assessing the structure of a hypothetical and latent construct, such as our information about a particular category of people? If we want to know how we store knowledge about the people in our world inside our minds, we run into the obvious problem of not being able to physically measure the structure of a mental representation. We run into the same problem if we step back and ask a more superordinate question: How do we study impression formation? (This is a superordinate question because, as just discussed, organization of person information is one component of impression formation.) Hamilton (1981) reminds us that this question was already answered in one way by the work of Asch (1946). Studying impression formation can be done by presenting people with sets of traits and examining the ways they are integrated and made to cohere together in the final impressions people form. However, there is a potential problem in Asch's methodology, because it *asks* people to form impressions that connect a set of traits, then records their impressions. The finding that people form coherent impressions may be an artifact of this methodology. It is perhaps misleading to say that we are studying ways people spontaneously form impressions, organize traits and behaviors about a person, and develop coherent and integrated knowledge, by explicitly telling people to form impressions and explicitly measuring their impressions. If we want to know whether information is organized in a coherent way, if we want to know how impressions are structured, if we want to know whether perceivers even form impressions about others without being asked to—then we need methods that are not so explicit about this, but provide a more subtle window to the operations of the cognitive apparatus.

Thus let us review the methods researchers have used to discover what these structures look like. Various techniques have emerged that rely on *looking at what people remember as an index of how information is structured in memory*. The ubiquity of such methodologies in the early days of research on categories and their relation to impression formation led to the development of a subdiscipline called *person memory*. In essence, this area of research examines how recall (memory) can be used to help us better understand person perception processes. (The seminal volume relating to this topic is a 1980 book called *Person Memory: The Cognitive Basis of Social Perception*, edited by Hastie et al.) Given this central role of memory at the foundation of understanding people (what Newman, 2001, called the cornerstone on which a science of interpersonal behavior will rest), we must take a brief foray into understanding the structure and functions of memory.

Memory Systems and Category Activation

In cognitive psychology (and most social-cognitive theories), it is assumed that memory consists of multiple functional components (Pinker, 1997). The functions of these components are the storing and manipulating of information, both perceptual and conceptual (and behavioral as well). Each component stores and/or manipulates data in a different way. *Long-term memory* is for storing a large amount of concepts over a long period of time (Jonides, 1995; think about your computer's hard drive as a metaphor). The entire dictionary of one's acquired language, all knowledge of categories and concepts, and one's autobiographical memory may be stored there. There is theoretically no limit to how much information can be stored there (in keeping with the metaphor, it is hard drive with an unlimited storage capacity). Moreover, once registered in long-term memory, the information is recorded permanently (barring brain damage). Social-cognitive psychologists do not talk much about the capacity of the long-term memory system, probably because its capacity is virtually (and perhaps literally) unlimited, and therefore the issue is moot. On the other hand, social-cognitive psychologists are keenly interested in the formats (the types of clusters and mental representations) in which information is held in long-term memory. We will discuss these formats later in this chapter. Tulving (1972) proposed that there are two subtypes of long-term memory—*episodic memory* and *semantic memory*. Episodic memory consists of memory for experiences, events, people, and situations (such as associating a song with a particular event or remembering one's first date). Semantic memory consists of memory for facts and definitions—the declarative knowledge we possess (such as knowing what a car is, or the meaning of the word "ironic"). In regard to social cognition, this suggests that information about a specific person and that person's behavior is stored in episodic memory, while information about traits is stored in semantic memory (Carlston & Smith, 1996). In Chapter 4 we see how these different types of memory can give rise to different types of memory structures. What is defined as an exemplar in Chapter 4 will make sense in the context of episodic memory, while what is defined as a schema will make sense in the context of semantic memory. Finally, a third type of long-term memory, called *procedural memory*, is also identified, which is used for holding instructions about how things proceed (such as algorithms governing motor action). What is defined as a script in Chapter 4 makes sense given the context of procedural memory.

Research suggests that judgments about people and social categories rely on episodic memory and semantic memory under different conditions. In particular, judgments are more likely to be based on the retrieval of particular behavioral episodes when we are unfamiliar with the individual or the group. However, as familiarity with the person or group grows, we develop abstract, semantic knowledge that is stored in memory separately from particular episodes. When asked to make judgments about these persons or groups, we may now retrieve the stored semantic representations, rather than particular episodes (e.g., Sherman, 1996; Sherman & Klein, 1994).

Complementary to long-term memory, the mind has a metaphorical monitor screen for displaying a subset of the concepts held in its long-term memory (i.e., those that become currently activated). This structure is usually called *short-term memory* or *working memory*. The analogy to a monitor screen lies in the fact that information currently residing in working memory is present to conscious awareness and subject to conscious processing (Jonides, 1995), but can be lost quickly and easily, especially if new information is retrieved (in keeping with the computer metaphor, when a new file is opened and the contents of the desktop have not been saved). Working memory has a limited capacity; only limited items of information are held and processed there each moment. Since only a small subset of the mind's concepts can occupy working memory at each moment, a time-sharing scheme has evolved; various concepts occupy working memory at different times (Higgins, 1996). Thus working memory is highly dynamic, with its contents refreshed and updated constantly. The cap on the total amount of information that can be simultaneously held and processed in working memory may be conceived of as indicating a type of cognitive resource or capacity, one that limits the operation of working memory. This resource or capacity is the kind most interesting to social-cognitive psychologists, partly due to its limited supply (Gilbert, 1998).

Consideration of alternative arrangements of the cognitive system may be informative not only about why the mind needs to have separate long- and short-term memories, but also highlight the advantages and potential pitfalls of the current system. An alternative arrangement would be to put everything in working memory (i.e., to let the mind be aware simultaneously of all the knowledge it has). This arrangement would save energy necessary for retrieving items from long-term memory. It would also eliminate the errors inherent in the retrieval. However, besides the obvious implementation problems (e.g., unrealistic demand for working memory's processing capacity), the simultaneous availability of one's entire knowledge base would interfere with one's current transactions with the world. At each moment, only a small subset of one's total knowledge base is relevant, depending on the situation one is faced with. Working memory allows the mind to prioritize items of information according to their relevance to the requirements of interacting with the current situation (Gollwitzer & Moskowitz, 1996). However, this advantage of the working memory comes with a new demand and new risks of failure (i.e., the necessity for selectively moving information from long-term memory to working memory). To receive conscious processing, information stored in long-term memory must be brought into working memory, through a process called *retrieval* (Higgins, 1996). The transportation of knowledge between long-term and working memories underpins a large part of thinking and reasoning (Higgins, 1996). The execution of this function is fallible; it is susceptible to errors.

Recollection versus Familiarity

The process of storing information in long-term memory involves a number of different mental operations that take place during and immediately after the presentation of information, such as rehearsing, noting, refreshing, and other operations that bind together the different facets of the information to form a memory trace (for a review, see Johnson, Hashtroudi, & Lindsay, 1993). Successful recollection of any given piece of information one has encountered in the past depends on the amount and quality of the information that was encoded in the first place. For example, one often encodes more than the information itself (its content), but also something about the original source of the information, or its context of acquisition (e.g., Johnson & Raye, 1981; Johnson et al., 1993). Interfering with the process of placing information in memory, or the fact that this process proceeded in only a shallow or partial way, can produce traces of the event in memory that are not well formed. For example, information about the context in which it was encountered may be lost, or information about the source of a piece of information may not have been encoded. When this occurs, it becomes difficult for people to make accurate decisions about where and when they heard a piece of information, or even whether it was true or not.

For example, Allport and Lepkin (1945) performed a study examining rumor transmission during World War II. In this study, the strongest predictor of belief in wartime rumors was simply repetition of the rumors. Of course, repetition of information from independent sources can be good grounds for belief—but in this case, sometimes the source of repetition was a special newspaper column designed precisely to warn people of unfounded, false rumors. People seemed to tell themselves, "I think I've heard this information before," and then once having determined simply that it felt familiar, they decided, "So it's probably true." Such inferences are not irrational, given the Gricean rules of communication reviewed above (e.g., norms dictate that communicated information should be true information). But a poorly formed memory trace led to errors that would have been avoided had there been clear recollection of the information's source. This type of error in memory, called *source confusion*, presents a real opportunity for problems in person perception. Consider the case of the eyewitness who believes he/she remembers having heard the accused suspect say something that is considered to be damning evidence by the prosecution. It is possible, however, that what the eyewitness recalls is a news report claiming the person said the "damning" statement, rather than an actual memory of having heard the information him- or herself.

Johnson (1988; Johnson et al., 1993; Johnson & Raye, 1981) and colleagues describe many instances in which people inaccurately recall the source of a piece of information. People label something that was imaginary as having really happened (perhaps mistaking a dream from 2 weeks ago for a real event, or a rumor heard from a gossip as an item seen on the news). Or they are confused about who said what. Johnson and colleagues (1993) claim that this happens because memories do not have abstract tags that indicate their source or original context (such as real vs. imagined, or true vs. false). Rather, people infer the source at the time of retrieval by evaluating the stored aspects of the memory trace along with its compatibility with prior knowledge. This allows people to be accurate in remembering *that* they have seen information before, but unable to identify the *context* in which they acquired the information. This is because memory for context can be selectively impaired by such things as divided attention, time delays, and aging. In sum, people may be very accurate in believing they have seen a piece of information before, but may be much less accurate about the details of its original context. These factors can determine whether memory is accurate and detailed, or false, or even something else—vague and unspecified. Rather than knowing they have seen something before and being able to recollect some (if not all) of the experience, people at times are left instead with only a "context-free" memory trace (Mandler, 1980), or a "feeling of fluency" that accompanies processing this information (Jacoby & Dallas, 1981)—that is, a feeling that the information is familiar, although they have no idea why. A false rumor feels familiar, and herein lies its danger. Familiarity is a form of memory, and people mistake their memories (even vague ones) for fact.

In line with this logic, Mandler (1980) proposed that there are two independent types of memorial information (see also Jacoby & Dallas, 1981). First, something may look familiar to you, so you recognize it as something you remember and have seen before. Second, you may distinctly recall the information—not merely recognizing it as feeling familiar to you, but having full knowledge of what it is, where you saw it, and all its associated details. Thus Mandler proposed a dissociation between two different types of memorial information: (1) *recollection*, or exact, detailed information that always leads to accurate reports of such details as the context of encoding and the source of the remembered information; and (2) *familiarity*, or vague information that signals "pastness" or prior contact. You may meet a person and have a distinct feeling you have met before, yet have no idea where or when. But you cannot shake yourself free from the feeling of familiarity. There is some trace of your experience with this person in memory, but this memory trace is not well developed and provides you with a type of recall that is more of a feeling (or sensation) of familiarity. Alternatively, every day you meet people for whom you have clear, strong, well-developed memory traces. Your friends and family are encountered, and you know immediately who they are. They do not feel familiar to you; you recollect every detail about them quite explicitly and easily. Furthermore, Jacoby (1991) proposed that recollection involves a controlled use of memory, but familiarity involves processes that are more automatic. Hence it is possible to disrupt recollection of all the details about a person without affecting the feeling that this person is familiar to you.

Retrieval as a "Horse Race"

Categorization has been defined as a process in which a stimulus triggers the retrieval of information from long-term memory and places it in short-term memory, where it is now described as activated. The "triggering" is the result of a silent (preconscious) series of steps in which the features of the stimulus are detected and then matched against stored representations. One final piece to the categorization puzzle must be addressed: What happens if there are multiple categories that fit a stimulus? When we encounter a Palestinian professor, do we have the category "foreigners" triggered, the category "professors" triggered, the category "Palestinians" triggered, or all of these (and other) categories triggered? According to Logan (1989), the retrieval of a category from memory when prompted by a stimulus unfolds over time. A path must be traversed from the stimulus cue to the category lying dormant in long-term memory; the category must then be delivered to consciousness and placed in working memory. The time delay for this process is determined by the strength of association between a stimulus and a category: "Memory retrieval takes time, and each trace has its own retrieval time distribution. The person can respond as soon as one trace is retrieved so the separate retrieval processes race against each other with the winner determining the response" (p. 65). The response elicited is essentially the end product of a race between constructs. The one retrieved more quickly is used to capture or describe the stimulus.

Thus the cue "Palestinian professor" has associations to various categories, each having its own retrieval distribution, with the category that claims the stimulus being the one that wins this horse race from dormancy to retrieval. Logan (1989) states that "the model does not require that absolutely everything that was ever associated with the object of attention be retrieved. It is sufficient that some proportion of the associations be retrieved" (pp. 70–71). This leaves open the possibility that multiple categories may be triggered by the same stimulus, but also leaves open the possibility that some categories may not be retrieved. We may categorize this individual as a Palestinian and a male, but not as a professor. Or we may use all three concepts. Or none.

Spreading Activation and Associative Networks

Knowledge in memory is associated; that is, there are links or connections among isolated pieces of information. Indeed, these connections are what constitute memory. What does it mean to say you know (or remember) that John Lennon was murdered in New York on December 8, 1980? It means that an association exists in your memory among the concepts "New York," "John Lennon," "Murder," and "December 8" (see Figure 3.1). The triggering of this memory activates associated memories, such as the gun-related deaths of other pop stars (e.g., the murders of Sam Cooke, Marvin Gaye, and Tupac Shakur, or the suicide of Kurt Cobain). Perhaps it triggers your beliefs about gun control. Anderson and Bower (1973, p. 9) inform us that "associationism has a tradition that extends over 2,000 years, from the writings of Aristotle to the experiments

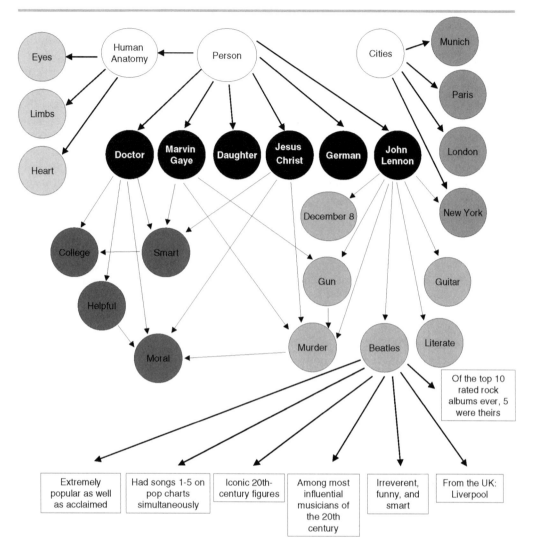

FIGURE 3.1. Associative networks connecting categories in memory.

of modern psychologists." Our goal here is not to attempt to review the complexity of the research of the last 30 years on associationism, let alone the writings of the last 2,000 years. All that we require for a discussion of person perception and social cognition is to accept that there is a network of associations in the mind between and within various knowledge structures. Anderson and Bower (1973, p. 10) identify four features shared among the long list of theories and writings on associationism, with the first feature being that "ideas, sense data, memory nodes, or similar mental elements are associated together in the mind through experience."

This definition of an *associative network* implies that knowledge does not reside in isolation, but is linked in memory to other bits of knowledge. In the metaphorical language cognitive psychologists use to describe this network, each isolated piece of knowledge being mentally represented is called a *node*. Thus, if you had knowledge about

John Lennon, it would be referred to as a *person node*. Just as a real net consists of knots that are tied together by rope or string, the mental network is a series of knots/nodes connected through associations. If you previously did not know who John Lennon was, you probably by now have constructed such a node that includes an association to Kurt Cobain, Tupac Shakur, and so forth, and it is likely to include the knowledge that John Lennon was a musician who was shot. Thus new nodes are constructed by creating links to existing nodes in the network, and such is the way in which we build our knowledge (and impressions) of other people. The behaviors people display are detected by us as perceivers, and we connect these to internal representations of the behaviors and traits that are deemed to be a good match to what is observed. Associated behaviors and traits then get triggered and perhaps linked to the observed persons as well, even if the persons do not act in the new ways. Thus you might infer that John Lennon was creative even if all you learned about him was that he was killed by a gun, just like the other musicians listed.

Thus, when a particular piece of knowledge is triggered, or when a stimulus has been categorized, the activation of that knowledge travels along the associative network to trigger associated concepts and knowledge, even those that have not been physically detected in the outside world. This process is called *spreading activation*. The stronger the association between concepts, the more likely they are to be activated, and the faster the activation is likely to spread. As an example, encountering one concept (e.g., an act of "kindness") facilitates the processing of associated concepts (e.g., thoughts about "morality") but not unrelated concepts. Activation starts at the node that has been triggered and will travel along whatever paths are present, flowing most easily and quickly along the paths that represent stronger associations. If activation rises above threshold, these concepts to which the activation has spread will also become triggered or activated.

Connectionism

In the period since the rise of network models of human memory (and in this period, many possible network accounts have emerged—prominent among them being Anderson's [1993] "ACT-R" model), a new form of network model has emerged that has been called *connectionism* (or *parallel distributed processing*). The major difference between former models and connectionism is that connectionism describes a more system-wide type of association than we have been describing. The network models described thus far posit individual nodes that are organized into sets of features and attributes, with some organizing principle being the heart of the node. Thus you have a person node for "John Lennon" with which all features relating to him are locally linked. With the connectionist metaphor of a networked memory system, there is no "John Lennon" node, nor any specific category around which a local organization exists (no "kindness" node, no "New York" node, etc.). Instead, there are distributed representations (not local ones) in which nodes are dispersed across a vast network of nodes. Your category for "John Lennon," rather than being a set of closely clustered nodes with direct links to each other (Figure 3.1), consists of a set of nodes that are simultaneously triggered (triggered in parallel) without needing to be conceived of as passing through a local system or shared space.

A good metaphor might be a scoreboard. For a scoreboard to function, many independent light bulbs must be turned on simultaneously in order to produce a perceptible sentence or series of numbers. It is only the simultaneous (parallel) activation of disparate bulbs among a vast and dispersed set of bulbs that allows the board to work. This is how a connectionist model imagines memory works. A category for "John Lennon" might be best thought of as a pattern of nodes being simultaneously triggered (perhaps node numbers 9 and 1,458 and 56,762 and 457, etc., all activated in parallel), even though they are not conceived of as being stored in a physically shared space with direct connections, to yield what you then experience as knowledge of "John Lennon." As stated above, we do not need here to get into a debate about connectionism versus other forms of associationism; nor need we review the details of such models (a vast task better left for a book dealing with models of categorization or cognitive psychology). We need only to accept the proposition that mental representations are connected through an associative network.

How Memory Informs Us about Category Structure

Having introduced the idea of knowledge being connected, we can begin to make assumptions about the manner in which knowledge is structured via these connections. According to Collins and Loftus (1975; see also Posner & Snyder, 1975), the concepts that internally (mentally) represent the knowledge we have of the world are spatially organized, such that, as illustrated in Figure 3.1, concepts that are associated with one another (e.g., "helpful–moral") are closer together than concepts that are not (or less closely) associated with each other (e.g., "literate–moral"). The path connecting them is shorter. In addition, concepts are marked not only by the distance that must be traversed to reach them from another concept, but by the number of links or associations made with other concepts. For example, in Figure 3.1, note the number of links associated with the concept "murder" relative to the concept "guitar." Stretching this illustration to the domain of concepts relating to people specifically, Figure 3.2 depicts a variety of unique ways in which the same information about a person could be organized within a mental structure.

Imagine you meet Erik and Roger at a party. Your interactions with them allow you to learn the following: Erik gives to charity, and Roger is a good basketball player. Erik returned a wallet he found in a store, and Roger surprised his girlfriend with a party for her birthday. Erik bought his girlfriend an expensive gift for no reason, and Roger won a local marathon. Erik told his employer exactly what he thought of some new policy that was instituted at work. How does this information get organized over the course of the evening? Is it according to traits (e.g., Erik exhibited two acts of generosity and Roger one)? Is it according to persons (Erik and Roger)? If it is according to persons, how do you organize the information about persons? Are the behaviors and traits and persons all interconnected (as in Figure 3.2A)? Or is only the behavior of each man stored, without traits stored as part of the representation, with any trait inferences needing to be derived later (through extra mental work) from the memory of the behavior (as in Figure 3.2B)? If the latter, are the behaviors connected to each other only through the higher-order person node (as depicted), or are there direct connections between the behaviors as well (this is not depicted, but could be by adding arrows between the behaviors in Figure 3.2B)? We could also imagine a structure similar to Figure 3.2A, in which traits are attached to each other and to a person node, and behaviors are each attached to the traits but not to each other (we would simply remove the interconnecting arrows that link the behaviors). Or we could imagine a highly interconnected network like that in Figure 3.2C, in which behaviors, traits, and persons are all stored together and linked to each other directly and indirectly.

Of course, the reason why we need to worry about detecting the structure of our person concepts is that how we structure the knowledge we have of people ultimately

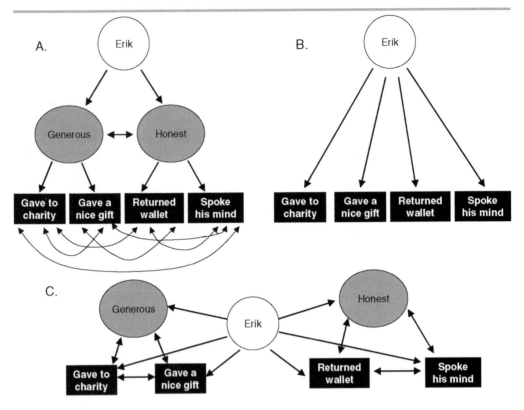

FIGURE 3.2. Different types of organization for information about people.

determines what comes to mind when we see them, how we interpret and organize new information about them, and what types of impressions we form (and later recall). With a brief review of memory structure and function behind us, we can now turn to discussing how person memory research has relied on memory-based research paradigms to illuminate impression formation processes and detect structure.

Increasing the Connections in the Associative Network

According to Anderson and Bower (1973), the components of a representation are recalled by traversing the pathways connecting them. This would mean that if your representation of Erik was structured according to the diagram in Figure 3.2C, there would be multiple ways to get access to the fact that Erik gave to charity: You could recall this directly by virtue of its being linked to your representation of Erik; you could recall it by recalling that Erik gave a nice gift; or you could access this by recalling that Erik is generous. The structure depicted in Figure 3.2B has fewer pathways that would lead you to this piece of information. For example, in the structure depicted in Figure 3.2B, recalling that Erik gave a nice gift could only lead to recall of the fact that Erik gave to charity if you first traversed the pathway up to the superordinate node to which each of these pieces of information is connected. If a representation has many different connections between items, as in Figure 3.2C, there is a shorter path from one item to another. The shorter the path between the items in the structure, the greater the likelihood that one item will be recalled, given that another item in the structure has already been recalled. Thus the more items that are added, the more connections (the richer the associative network), and the better the recall of any particular item in the structure—if, and only if, the structure is organized as in Figure 3.2C (e.g., Wyer & Gordon, 1984). Thus the structure of the category can have an impact on what we come to think and recall about a person. And, to flip this logic on its head, memory measures can be used to help inform us about how information about the people we interact with is structured and organized in the mind. If memory is richer as more information is learned, and if recall improves as we learn new information about the same person, it suggests that the information is organized using the person as a node, with associative links connecting the various features of the person.

Reaction Times (Speed of Retrieval)

The notion that associated concepts are more closely linked together in some sort of physical space suggests that the distance traversed along the link from one attribute to another has a shorter distance to travel when two concepts are more strongly associated. In terms of Logan's (1989) "race" model, this means we should be faster to respond to a piece of knowledge that is closely linked to a given stimulus item than to a piece of knowledge less strongly associated with the stimulus item; we should be able to respond more quickly to those items that have a shorter retrieval time distribution. Thus we might be faster to think that a person we have observed acting morally is also helpful than we are to assume that the person is literate, because "helpful" and "moral" are more closely linked than "moral" and "literate" are.

Collins and Quillian (1969) provided a clear illustration of this. They had participants read sentences and asked them to determine whether they were true or false. The sentences contained factual information, such as "A doctor is a college graduate," "A doctor has eyes," and "A doctor is a bird." The first two statements are obviously true (the third is obviously false), but what differentiates the true statements is the extent to which we might expect direct connections between the concept "doctor" and the concept it is paired with. "Doctor" and "college graduate" are nodes residing in the larger category "people." Various body parts are also connected to the node "people" and thus are connected to "doctor." However, the path from "doctor" to "eyes" can only be traversed by first going up to the higher-level category "people" and circumnavigating to the category "body parts" linked with "people" (see Figure 3.1). Thus we can determine fairly easily that doctors have eyes. But if the memory structure is organized through a series of hierarchical connections, then the connections at a more similar level of abstraction and linked more closely together in the spatial structure should be responded to more quickly. The path from "doctor" to "college graduate" is more direct, as this information is probably stored together and does not require passing through the node for "people" before making a response. Thus we can test notions about the structure of categories by examining the response times to various statements, as Collins and Quillian did. They found that their participants responded faster (they said "true" more quickly) to pairs of the sort "A doctor is a college graduate" than to those of the sort "A doctor has eyes." This finding ironically suggests that it is somewhat harder to retrieve the fact that doctors have eyes (something true of all people) than to determine that doctors have gone to college (something true of only a minority of people in the world).

Another illustration of retrieval time as a measure of category structure was provided by Meyer and Schvandeveldt (1971). Research participants were shown pairs of
letter strings, with the task of deciding whether each string was actually a word in the
English language. This type of task is known as a *lexical decision task*. Sometimes both
strings are words (e.g., "nurse" and "doctor," "nurse" and "butter"); sometimes they are
not (e.g., "nurse" and "grispe"). What is important is that in the cases where both letter
strings are words, there are some instances in which the words are associated (they have
some semantic link, such as "nurse" and "doctor") and other cases in which the words
are not associated (such as "nurse" and "butter"). If the structure is organized with connections from one category to another (with activation spreading through the associative network), then having first seen the word "nurse" should trigger related categories
in memory and make one faster to detect or respond to those items. This is precisely
what Meyer and Schvandeveldt found when they compared reaction times to word pairs
such as "nurse" and "doctor" versus word pairs such as "nurse" and "butter." When the
second word in a pair was semantically associated with the first, the speed with which it
took to perform the lexical decision task was reliably faster than when the second word
was unrelated to the first. Only the degree of association between the pairs of words
could account for this.

This suggests that we can use speed of retrieval as a measure of the strength of
association and structural connectedness between items of information about a person.
Indeed, the review earlier in this chapter of Rosch's (1975) work has indicated that if we
can respond more quickly to the item "A robin is a bird" than to the item "A penguin is
a bird," it tells us something about the way our category "birds" must be structured.
Rather than there being a set of necessary features, it suggests there must be an organization that involves a wide array of features, some of which are more central than others
(if the category was defined by a necessary set of features that all members possessed,
we would have no reason to be faster at detecting one member of the category than
another). "Robin," because it possesses more of the central features, is identified faster.
Thus we can learn something about the structure and relationship between various features by examining how quickly we can respond to one of the features after having been
exposed to the other. Do people store information about Jews as a category, and does
that category contain certain attributes? We could address this question by showing a
person the word "Jew" (or a picture of a Jew) and then measuring how quickly he/she
responds to attributes. If there are facilitated reaction times to some of these attributes,
it suggests that these attributes are organized in memory in an associative network that
links them to the concept "Jews" and to other attributes that are similarly linked to the
concept "Jews." Throughout this chapter (and this book), we will see examples of how
researchers use reaction time methodologies to make such inferences about mental
links between attributes and to learn about the structure of person categories.

Clustering in Recall

Let us ask a more basic question than the one relating to how concepts for people are
organized: Is Asch's (1946) assumption that perceivers form impressions, such that
traits are inferred from the information provided and this information is organized in a
person node (with the person serving as the organizing principle around which all the
traits and behaviors are now linked), correct? One answer is provided by using a methodology in which research participants are presented with a set of information about a
person and then their free recall for that information is examined. *Free recall* simply

means that people are provided with no hints, but must try to remember all of the information that was presented by their own devices. The researchers can then examine what participants have written down regarding what they can remember, in order to see how that information is clustered. Presumably, the way in which people remember information (how it is chunked together) may be an index of how it is organized in memory—it is pulled out of the system in a fashion that resembles how it is stored in the system (e.g., Bousfield, 1953; Shuell, 1977). In this case, the researchers are interested in seeing whether the information is clustered according to categories that represent clear personality types. What is essential in using such a measure is to make sure that when the information is initially presented, it is in a scrambled order. Then the researchers can analyze patterns in the recall to see whether it has been unscrambled and put together into meaningful clusters, with those meanings corresponding to personality types. For instance, has a participant delivered a recall of items in a way that now organizes them in a fashion that describes a "shy" person? Hamilton and colleagues (1980a, pp. 136–137) argue that "to the extent that such grouping is evident, the subject has imposed an organization on the stimulus items according to the cognitive schemas that were salient to him." (For discussions of how to actually compute clustering measures, see Ostrom, Pryor, & Simpson, 1981; Shuell, 1977.)

Perhaps the question of whether the information you receive about people is organized in memory around those people as person nodes may seem silly. After all, your intuition may be that there is no other way to organize information you see or hear about a person other than around the person, using that person as the organizing principle in memory. Ostrom and colleagues (1981), however, review several alternative ways of organizing information about people. One possibility is temporal organization: You may store information in the order in which it is learned or in the order in which it occurred, not according to the person who performed it. You may learn that "Roger acted rudely and Erik acted selfishly on Monday," "Roger acted sarcastically and Erik acted egotistically on Tuesday," and "Roger acted intelligently and Erik acted aggressively on Wednesday." This information may be organized according to Roger and Erik, but it may also be possibly organized around the day of the week on which it occurred (e.g., "On Monday there was rude and selfish behavior"). Think back to a time you were in a restaurant with more than one waiter or waitress serving your table. It is very likely that you have run into instances where you remember having asked for a beverage after you placed your initial order and before the salad arrived, but you were unable to remember which person you asked. The time sequence was encoded, but the event was not structured according to the person.

Alternatively, information may be blocked according to descriptors. Consider an experiment by Simpson (1979) in which research participants were presented with information about three different people—Dave, Tom, and John. They were told these things: Dave is a part-time usher; Dave is from Wichita (Kansas); Tom is from Richmond (Virginia); Tom collects beer cans; John collects coins; Tom is a part-time dishwasher; John is from Denver (Colorado); Dave tinkers with cars; John works part time on a farm. This information could be organized according to persons, but it could also be organized around one of several descriptors, such as hobbies, jobs, and hometowns. Half of the research participants were asked to decide how compatible they believed the three men would be as college roommates, and half were asked to decide which man would not fit well with the other men as roommates. After participants performed this task and then a filler task, their memory for the information was assessed (this came as a surprise to them). The clustering analysis revealed no evidence that participants were using persons as organizing principles for this information, but instead suggested that descriptor categories were being used.

The results of this experiment perhaps violate your intuition and justify the question posed above. In essence, if we take the findings of Asch (1946) that impressions seem to be structured in such a fashion that perceivers try to make information about a person "fit" and seem coherent, there should be a way to provide evidence that people do engage in this type of organizational structuring of information as they receive it (e.g., Hamilton et al., 1980a). The Asch method, of asking people what they think, perhaps forces people to try to formulate coherent clusters. Clustering is a procedure that provides a more natural way of detecting how people operate when they learn information about others.

Of course, your intuitions about how people function (as well as Asch's intuitions) are probably not unfounded. There must be instances in which people do naturally organize information around person nodes and form impressions about people that cohere together. Pryor and Ostrom (cited in Ostrom et al., 1981) set out to examine when this might occur. Once again, this question was answered by using clustering measures. The researchers reasoned that clustering would be promoted when there was a preexisting category representing the person in memory. Thus famous persons would be clustered by using the persons as organizing principles in memory, but strangers would not. To test this, research participants were exposed to lists of information describing four people, two familiar people and two strangers. The lists were created by taking the matrix of names and traits displayed in Figure 3.3 and creating descriptions of the form "Person X is/was Trait X." Participants were asked to learn the information provided, and their memory was later assessed. The clustering analyses revealed that no person organization existed for unfamiliar names, but it did exist for famous names. There were several trials conducted in this experiment where participants learned sets of information such as this, and person organization did appear to increase as the participants gained more experience with the materials and procedure. However, Ostrom and colleagues' conclusion seems to be that we should not assume that impressions of new people we meet are necessarily organized using the person as the integral unit:

	Mike Stadt	Howie Golden	Neil Hertzman	David Kramer	Paul Rizzo
Abe Lincoln	Tall	Honest	Self-taught	Leader	Bearded
Bob Hope	Golfer	Old	Conservative	Comedian	Hard-working
Muhammad Ali	Religious	Athlete	Champion	Black	Opinionated
Clint Eastwood	Tough	Actor	Handsome	Rugged	Virile
Jerry Brown	Outspoken	Bachelor	Politician	Californian	Independent

FIGURE 3.3. Traits associated with familiar and unfamiliar persons. From Ostrom et al. (1981). Copyright 1981 by Lawrence Erlbaum Associates. Adapted by permission.

Unfamiliar persons are not likely to serve as organizing foci for social information. Physical information such as age, race, height, and sex are all readily apparent when meeting a number of new people. . . . In such circumstances, one might remember that all the women were outspoken, but not remember which woman said what. (1981, p. 26)

Processing Goals and Free Recall

Srull and Wyer (1989) proposed a comprehensive model of person memory that consists of many postulates. The very first asserts that when a perceiver has the goal of forming an impression of another person, the spontaneous tendency is to use traits in one's impressions. That is, an impression of someone can be based on many things, with traits just one potential way of describing the person; yet traits are typically used to organize impressions of people when perceivers are explicitly trying to form impressions. If traits are being used to organize the impression, then an interlocking network of associations should develop between the traits that are being stored and the behaviors that they describe. This set of associations should make recall for the information easier, as each item provides access to all the others (as described above). Thus a coherent person impression that involves organization of traits and behaviors should be particularly well remembered, at least relative to a structure not characterized by such an organization (such as one where no traits have been inferred).

In addition, Srull and Wyer (1989) maintain that if perceivers are not asked to form an impression, they will not use traits to organize the information they have witnessed. This postulate is derived from the research of Srull and Brand (1983; see also Simpson, 1979). Srull and Brand asked some participants to anticipate that they would interact with another person (therefore implying that they needed to form an impression of what each person was like in order to prepare for this interaction). They argued that such a goal would initiate attempts by the participants to consider the behaviors in relation to one another. This was argued to make them more likely to infer traits and have a rich associative network than participants who were not asked to form an impression (and simply asked to memorize the set of information about the person). The traits, behaviors, and person, all supposedly integrated when forming impressions of the target, led perceivers to have superior recall for the information (especially as the amount of information provided grew and grew) relative to people without the goal of forming an impression. In fact, these people showed decreased recall as the amount of information provided grew, suggesting that they did not form a coherent structure with which to make sense and organize this information. Thus one method for testing how social perception is structured is to give people different processing goals and once again examine what they are capable of remembering. If people forming an impression organize information differently from people who are not, such differences would be evidenced by differences in the amount of information people are capable of remembering (e.g., Hamilton, Katz, & Leirer, 1980b; Srull, 1983; Srull & Brand, 1983; Wyer & Gordon, 1984). Ironically, people asked to remember information should remember less information than people who were not asked to remember it, but to form an impression. The benefits of the complex associative network formed during impression formation will yield superior recall.

For example, Hamilton and colleagues (1980b) asked research participants to read a series of sentence predicates (e.g., "rented an apartment near where he works," "played ball with his dog in the park," "went to a movie with friends Saturday night," "tries to keep informed on current events"). Half of the participants were asked to read these predicates with the goal of memorizing them for a recall test; the other half were told nothing of a recall test and were instead asked to read the sentences with the goal of trying to form an impression of the person being described. At the end of the experiment, all of the participants were asked to try to recall as many of the stimulus items as they could (and for the impression formation participants, this was a surprise memory test). The results found superior recall for the people asked to form an impression. This suggests that the two groups were structuring and organizing their impressions differently, with impression formation yielding a more complex and interconnected mental representation of the information that benefited recall.

As a side note, although such research should be taken as a nice illustration of how memory measures can be used to tell us something about structure, it should not be used to support the idea put forth by Srull and Wyer (1989) that impression formation goals are required for people to infer traits about others and to use those traits as a means for organizing information. Just because people with memory goals in this research do not appear to be inferring traits, this does not mean that people with memory goals never infer traits about others fairly spontaneously (Moskowitz, 1993b). As we can see, the stimulus items used in this research were not particularly diagnostic in terms of traits (e.g., "rented an apartment near where he works"), and sentence predicates were used *without mentioning actual people*. There would be no reason to expect people with memory goals to organize this information in terms of persons or traits when such information was not present in the stimulus set—no people were specifically mentioned, and the behaviors described did not imply traits. Impression goals, however, would force participants to think of these sentences in terms of persons and to try to generate traits. Therefore, it is not surprising that they used this type of information as an organizing principle once it became available, but this is hardly a good illustration of whether this is what happens naturally when interacting with real people. Chapter 7 reviews a literature that argues that even without explicit goals, impression formation occurs and traits are inferred.

Cued Recall

Relative to free recall, *cued recall* involves giving a person who is trying to remember something a hint or clue. This is a cue that is somehow connected to the thing they are trying to remember. Thus one way to test whether two pieces of information are associated in memory is to give someone one of the pieces of information as a cue and to see whether it helps the person get access to the other piece of information (e.g., Tulving & Thomson, 1973). The cue gives the person a node to start with, and activation can then spread from there and get him/her to the desired information (if it is associated with the cue that was provided). If sets of behaviors and traits about a target actor are connected, then any one trait adjective should serve as a retrieval cue for recall of all the behaviors connected to it in a person node. The likelihood of recalling a behavior will be greater if a trait associated with the same person node is also recalled (or provided as a recall cue). This logic was spelled out quite clearly by Carlston (1980, p. 95):

> Tulving and Pearlstone (1966) have shown that providing subjects with category cues facilitates the retrieval of items from a learned list. In the same way, the recall of prior trait inferences may cue the recall of observed events that imply those same traits . . . [because] they may correspond to the attributes spontaneously used to organize information about people in memory.

Therefore, the way in which information about people is organized can be examined under conditions in which trait-relevant behavioral information is presented (e.g., "Howard frequently erupted with bursts of anger on the slightest provocation"), and participants are asked to make inferences about the person based on such bits of information. The trait inference (e.g., "volatile") should serve as a cue that will help people remember the behavior if (and only if) that trait was stored with the information when it was read, so that they were organized as part of a structure that describes the person. Carlston (1980) provided such an illustration. Participants were asked to read a series of behaviors performed by a person named John. The behaviors were arranged so that they implied two clear traits (such as "cruel" and "kind"). The task was to make inferences about John based on some subset of the behaviors. For example, participants were asked to judge how kind John was (but not how cruel he was). After a time delay, they were asked to try to recall the inferences and then the behaviors. The results showed that people were quite accurate at recalling their previous inferences about John (even after a delay of 1 week), and that they were confident in the accuracy of their recall for these inferences. How did recall for the inferences affect recall for the actual behaviors? There was selective recall found for behaviors pertaining to the prior inference that had been made. Thus the behaviors that described the trait "cruel" were less likely to be recalled if a participant had earlier been asked to make an inference regarding how kind John was. But if the participant had made an inference about how cruel John was, these behaviors were now the ones better recalled. The trait seemed to be operating as a cue that delivered access to the behaviors associated with the trait. This suggests that traits and behaviors are represented together in memory, with a category structure including traits and behaviors organized around a person node.

WHEN CATEGORIZATION GOES AWRY: HEURISTICS AND BIASES

One problem that arises when perceivers are trying to categorize people (and objects) is that they use rules for making inferences, and these rules may not be the most accurate (e.g., Tversky & Kahneman, 1974). Categorization is essentially a process of trying to decide what mental representation (category) best fits a set of detected features in some observed stimulus. In social cognition, this involves detecting the behavior and features of a person and trying to assign these to a category. However, relying on rules of inference, rather than on an exhaustive search of all possible features against all possible categories, can lead to errors. It is true that such rules often work, and it is this functionality that explains their genesis and continued use. But they can also lead perceivers awry and cause them to make errors that might have been avoided with a more thorough analysis.

Of course, it may be that a perfectly thorough analysis is not possible (i.e., a complete examination of all the features of a person or object against all possible categories in the mind cannot be done). In essence, any judgment about whether a given object is an instance of a category contains *some level of uncertainty*, and no type of perfectly accurate inference is really possible. The task is probabilistic by nature. This is especially true of social cognition, where the properties of a person must be assumed from the behaviors a perceiver has observed, and are hardly as verifiable as the features that define an object (such as a pencil or a chair). Given the uncertainty of any type of person categorization, it makes sense that rules would evolve to provide guidelines for what seem to be rational and reasonable inferences about the person. Thus the use of such rules, or *heuristics*, is perhaps best seen as a rational resolution to the problem of having to make judgments under uncertainty. However, this rational choice turns into bias in situations where the rule is used even when uncertainty is minimized and evidence exists that would serve as a better basis for decision making (in this case, categorizing a person) than a simple reliance on the heuristic. "In making predictions and judgments under uncertainty, people do not appear to follow the calculus of chance or the statistical theory of prediction. Instead they rely on a limited number of heuristics" (Kahneman & Tversky, 1973, p. 237).

The term *heuristic* was imported into social psychology from the field of artificial intelligence. Computer models meant to mimic the way in which the human mind functions can be programmed with algorithms that exhaustively work on a problem until a correct solution is reached. Chase and Simon (1973) asserted that such algorithms have the problem of running endlessly and at times being unable to come to a solution. This is problematic, because this is not how humans think: Humans rarely just decide that there is no appropriate way to think or act, but end up generating some sort of solution. Why are humans able to think, categorize, and act in the absence of perfect solutions? *Because they do not try to find perfect solutions*. The analogy to algorithmic processing is not adequate to describe how humans think. Instead of engaging in a strategy of maximizing (seeking optimal solutions to problems), people instead can be described as using a strategy of *satisficing* (seeking adequate solutions). Approximations of optimal solutions can be arrived at, and this requires relying on shortcuts in processing rather than an algorithmic approach. These shortcuts are called heuristics. Liberman (2001, p. 294) has defined a heuristic as "a moderately diagnostic way to generate a judgment, known to be suboptimal, but relatively easy to use compared with more optimal judgment strategies. People use the heuristic as a proxy for more optimal judgment strategies." The phrase *moderately diagnostic* means that the use of a heuristic in making a judgment (such as judging whether a person whose behavior is being observed is an egalitarian person) provides a better basis for judgment than chance, but does not deliver the guarantee of a 100% correct judgment that an algorithmic strategy might deliver. For the most part, the heuristic is believed to produce accurate judgments most of the time. Their ease of use, relative to using algorithms, explains why people rely on heuristics.

Tversky and Kahneman (1974) provide some concrete illustrations to help us through this abstract notion of cognitive shortcuts, and also to reveal how the use of such shortcuts can produce errors in categorization. What we will see is that the rules people use are fairly rational ones, given limited information and decisions that need to be made when uncertainty abounds. But the rules are only useful if uncertainty exists or too much effort is required to arrive at a more complete and accurate judgment. When people rely on heuristics in cases where they could very well engage in more accurate types of analysis, and when uncertainty is reduced by the presence of useful data that would be relevant for the decision, then heuristics are a source of bias. We will review three such heuristics here: representativeness, simulation, and availability.

The Representativeness Heuristic

The *representativeness heuristic* is a rule whereby categorization is made based on overt appearance. People make decisions regarding the probabilities that govern relationships between entities (e.g., people and categories) based on the degree to which one is representative of the other. They follow a rule that seems to say, "If it looks like a duck, and quacks like a duck, it must be a duck." One need not observe the creature for weeks or conduct an internal examination to conclude it is a duck. The entity has an appearance that is representative of the category. Representativeness is observed when a judgment is made, or the probability that something is true is assessed, by how much it resembles one of the choices being considered in the decision. As Tversky and Kahneman (1974) put it, "When A is highly representative of B, the probability that A originates from B is judged to be high. On the other hand, if A is not similar to B, the probability that A originates from B is judged to be low" (p. 1124). Tversky and Kahneman provide a good example. If you hear that Bob is quiet and shy, reads a lot, and has an obsession with detail and orderliness, and then you are asked to decide whether Bob is a farmer or a librarian, you will make this judgment, or base your probability estimate, on how well the description of Bob matches your category for librarians or farmers. You then choose the one he resembles more closely, and decide that Bob is a librarian.

The problem with this strategy is that perceivers tend to use it in isolation and ignore other information that is relevant. The primary example of how this can lead to biases is by leading people to ignore base rates. A *base rate* is a prior probability, a factual description, or a statistical accounting that describes the situation. For example, if I tell you that Bob lives in a community where 80% of people are farmers, this is base rate information about the percentage of farmers. Your purpose should then be better served (that is, a more rational decision would be) to guess that Bob is a farmer, because the base rate is more descriptive than the extent to which the few features you know about Bob match a category you have. However, people are notoriously bad at paying attention to base rate information. If two events/people are similar to each other, or one seems to be representative of the other, people have a tendency simply to assume that this similarity indicates a real relationship. Thus, if Bob looks like a librarian, and I ask you to decide between "librarian" and some other concept, you may choose "librarian" because his actions and attributes are more representative of that category. This becomes a problem when this strategy is used despite the existence of better information that would allow for a more accurate (such as the base rate) response.

The ease with which people are willing to give up an effortful analysis and start to ignore prior probabilities and base rates was illustrated by Tversky and Kahneman (1974) in an experiment where research participants were asked to estimate the probability that a man was either an engineer or a lawyer. The man was said to be sampled at random from a group of 100 people described as engineers and lawyers. One experimental manipulation involved varying the probabilities that were associated with this group of 100 people. Some participants were told that the group consisted of 70% engineers and 30% lawyers. The rest were told that the profile was drawn from a pool made up of 30% engineers and 70% lawyers. The other experimental manipulation involved whether or not participants were provided with a personality profile of the man they were judging. When no personality profile was provided, the estimate reflected base rates. If people were told the pool had 70% engineers, they guessed there was a 70% chance the man was an engineer. However, getting a personality profile about the man altered the extent to which people made rational judgments. When a profile was provided, prior probabilities were ignored, even though the description provided did not sound like an engineer or a lawyer. A worthless description that provided no useful information led people to make judgments that essentially were 50-50—that is, to guess there was a 50% chance that the man was an engineer. (As an example of how useless the information was, participants were told: "Dick is a 30-year-old man. He is married with no children. A man of high ability and high motivation, he promises to be quite successful in his field.") If people abandon using probabilities at the behest of worthless information, imagine how easily they can be led to make categorizations that violate rational patterns when the information provided is not worthless, but superficially sounds representative of one of the categories (as with Bob, the supposed librarian)!

Actually, Tversky and Kahneman (1982) provided such an illustration when they examined people's responses to compound events. A *compound event* (or *conjunction*) is one in which two events happen together so that one event is contingent on the other, or is a subset of it. Consider an example of an event that is not conjunctive, where people need to make a prediction. In the spring of 2003, if you asked an American, "What is the likelihood that U.S. troops will be exposed to weapons of mass destruction in the next year?", you may have gotten an answer like "20%." Now consider the same question, but posed as part of a conjunctive event: "What is the likelihood that U.S. troops will be exposed to weapons of mass destruction in Iraq during the next year?" Rational thought would dictate that the odds of being exposed to such weapons (which would include being exposed to them in any country in the world, including Iraq) would have to be larger than (or at least equal to) the odds of being exposed to them in any one specific country. "One of the basic laws of probability is that specification can only reduce probability. Thus, the probability that a person is both a Republican and an artist must be smaller than the probability that the person is an artist" (Tversky & Kahneman, 1982, p. 90). Yet people routinely answer questions of the second type with responses larger than the number generated for the superordinate event. When I was a student, almost all of the students in my graduate course in social psychology made this error when Tory Higgins used it as an example, so this error is not limited to unsophisticated people! So why do people, even graduate students, think an event that is a subset of a larger class can be more likely than the class it is nested within? The answer is representativeness: People have a more well-defined image of the conjunctive event. In the spring of 2003, most Americans' picture of what having troops in Iraq looked like included the specific threat of chemical and biological weapons. Because the conjunctive event looked much more like the thing being asked about—it was representative of it—the estimate for the specific case (weapons and Iraq) was greater than estimates for the more general case (weapons anywhere). As Tversky and Kahneman stated, "the conjunction rule does not apply to similarity or representativeness. A blue square, for example, can be more similar to a blue circle than to a circle, and an individual may resemble our image of a Republican artist more than our image of a Republican . . . similarity or representativeness can be increased by specification of the target" (p. 90).

To illustrate representativeness at work, therefore, we need only illustrate that specification leads people to violate the conjunctive rule. We must show that people see the specific event as more probable than the more general case. This should occur when the specific event looks more like the thing being asked about than the general case. Tversky and Kahneman (1982) used categorization in person perception to illustrate this point. They asked participants to read a description of Linda: "Linda is 31 years old, single, outspoken, and very bright. She majored in philosophy. As a student she was deeply concerned with issues of discrimination and social justice, and also participated in anti-nuclear demonstrations." They then asked them to rate the probability that certain qualities were true of Linda—to assign a probability to her being in one category or another. One of the categories was "Linda is a bank teller." Participants did not see this as very probable. Another of the categories was "Linda is a bank teller and is active in the feminist movement." The laws of probability would dictate that she could not be more likely to be a feminist bank teller than a bank teller (the former is a subset of the latter), yet the majority of people rated the odds of her being a feminist bank teller as being higher. Even people sophisticated in the use of statistical reasoning (some of the participants were graduate students at Stanford) made this decision. This occurred because the description of Linda was not consistent with the image of bank tellers, but it was consistent with the image of feminists. Thus Linda did not seem likely to be a bank teller unless she was a feminist one! She may not look like a banker, but she can look like a feminist banker. The similarity occurring due to representativeness altered the categorization. In cases such as this, the subcategory, which according to the conjunction rule must be less probable than the superordinate category, is overturned by the use of representativeness. This is not necessarily an error or bad decision making. However, representativeness as a heuristic can explain a wide array of bad decision making. We examine some of these instances next.

First, it can explain why people assume their decisions are more valid than they really are. When a description of a person really sounds like a particular category or type, the high degree of overlap between the features and the category it looks like leads people not only to assume that the person belongs in that category, but to have tremendous confidence in this judgment. Thus, if Bob really sounds like a librarian, and Linda really sounds like a feminist, people will be superconfident in their categorization, even though other available information would be a better source for decision making and should undermine this confidence.

Second, representativeness explains problems people have in making estimates of chance events. If I ask you what the likelihood is that a coin will come up heads when I flip it (and it is not a two-headed coin), you are likely to answer, "50%." If I ask you the same question, but preface it by saying that I have just thrown the coin five times and it came up heads all five times, suddenly the answer you are likely to give changes drastically. It is hard for you to fathom that I can get six heads in a row, because this simply does not look like chance. Coin flips, being chance events, should look like chance. Thus, to get it to look like chance, you need tails to come up. So you may assume that tails will be more likely to come up, when in fact the chance on any one flip of getting heads is always 50%, and you should know this. Your representativeness heuristic gets in the way. Gilovich (1991) provided another great example of this, using basketball players and shooting percentage. If I asked you to tell me the chance that a great player such as Julius Erving (Dr. J) will make a shot, you might ask me, "What is his shooting percentage as a professional?" If I tell you it is 53%, you are likely to guess that his chance of making a given shot is 53%. However, what if I told you he just made three shots in a row and then asked you to guess the likelihood that he would make the next one? You might believe in a "hot hand" and assume that his chance is higher than his usual average, or you might assume that he is "due for a miss" and assume the chance is less than his usual average. What Gilovich found was that Dr. J's chance of making a shot (or that of any other member of the Philadelphia Seventy-Sixers team, whose shooting records were available) was no different when he had just made three in a row, made two in a row, made one in a row, missed one, missed two in a row, or missed three in a row. A player's shooting percentage is his shooting percentage, and prior instances do not have a real impact on current ones. We just think they should so that things will look like we think they should. We want reality to be representative of what we think it should look like.

Third, representativeness causes people to ignore the phenomenon of "regression to the mean." As just noted, an unusually great or poor performance is unusual; thus players (or other people being observed) can be expected to drift toward their more typical performance the next time they try the task at hand. However, because of representativeness, observers expect the next attempt to somehow look like the last attempt. The classic example is the *Sports Illustrated* jinx. The jinx is that after an athlete appears on the cover of this magazine, it has been noted that his/her performance usually declines. But what gets a person on the cover of a sports magazine? Usually it is exceptional performance, above and beyond what this athlete typically does (thus warranting special focus at this time). Observers then expect the athlete's future performance to be representative of the performance that warranted his/her being on the magazine cover. But such performance is unusual, and future performance is destined to drop back toward the mean (unless the athlete has drastically altered his/her skill level). Relying on representativeness can cause people to ignore something as basic as regression to the mean, and to generate all sorts of explanations (such as jinxes) to allow them to maintain a heuristic as valuable and useful.

The Simulation Heuristic

There are times where we all make decisions by running a simulation model: We act like experimenters and say to ourselves, "What would happen if this happened, versus what would happen if that happened?" In terms of categorizing people, we might want to simulate the different behaviors and features another person would possess and display in order to help us categorize. When we encounter Pat, a person whose gender we can't initially determine, these simulations could take this form: "If that person was categorized as a woman, I would expect to see Features X, Y, and Z" versus "If that person was categorized as a man, I would expect to see features A, B, and C." Or we could simulate the various behavioral ramifications of different types of categorizations. When we encounter someone at a party standing alone in a corner, we might run the following simulation: "If I were to categorize that man as an introvert, I would leave him alone" versus "if I were to categorize that man as bored, I would approach him." We simulate the outcomes of these "experiments" in our minds, and based on these predicted outcomes, we make decisions about how to interpret the person and act (Kahneman & Tversky, 1982).

We do not always do simulations beforehand to help us choose how to act, but sometimes we engage in these simulations after an event has occurred to help us understand the consequences and to imagine how we could have avoided it (Kahneman & Miller, 1986). Kahneman and Miller state that "reasoning flows not only forward, from anticipation and hypothesis to confirmation or revision, but also backward, from the experience to what it reminds us of or makes us think about" (1986, p. 137). This is the nature of regret. We look at an outcome and simulate an alternative reality; we say, "If only I had acted differently," and then depict how much better our lives would be if we had acted in that way. Feelings of regret will be intensified when we simulate or imagine an alternative (and better) reality. Thoughts that arise from thinking, "If only I had acted otherwise," are called *counterfactual thoughts*, and they are the products of mental simulations that we run. The extent to which we engage in counterfactual thinking is determined by the relative mutability of an event. The easier it is to imagine altering some mutable feature of reality that would undo the event, the greater the strength and psychological closeness of the alternatives, and the more likely we are to ruminate on them.

As an example, imagine you are attending a summer concert festival, and the festival is being held in a stadium with open seating (seating is on a "first come, first serve" basis). At the start of the day, it is announced that a large cash prize will be awarded to a lucky fan, and that the winner will be the fan sitting in a randomly determined seat number. Now imagine that your view of the stage has been blocked for an hour, and you see an opening in another part of the arena where some fans are departing. You switch seats. Later, when the winning seat number is announced, it turns out that the winner is occupying the seat you just vacated! What would your reaction be? You would be likely to feel as if you had almost won, simulating the alternative outcome. This would probably lead to the counterfactual thought "If only I had not moved, I would have won," thereby locating causality in your movement (Wells & Gavanski, 1989). You probably would feel a sense of disappointment and regret (Kahneman & Miller, 1986).

How does the use of the simulation heuristic affect the types of judgments that people make? Kahneman and Tversky (1982) demonstrated that mental simulation and considering the counterfactual realities surrounding an event produce amplification of emotional reactions. In one experiment, research participants were asked to read about two men who missed their scheduled flights when their taxis, having been delayed in traffic, arrived at the airport 30 minutes after the scheduled departure times. One man's flight was described as having left on time, whereas the other man's flight was described as having been delayed for 25 minutes and had left just 5 minutes before the man arrived at the airport. Participants were asked to rate the reactions of each of the men to their situation. The results showed that they rated the latter man as being more upset. For him, catching his flight seemed more possible; that is, it was easier for him to imagine and to simulate making up the necessary 5 minutes than it was for the other man to imagine making up 30 minutes. The event was more mutable. Although the expectations and the objective situation of both men were identical (both men expected to and did miss their flights), the intensity of each man's emotional reaction was presumed to be different. Thus the simulation heuristic alters the way in which events are experienced. As another example, Medvec, Madey, and Gilovich (1995) found both increased joy and increased regret, depending on the salient counterfactual alternatives, among the reactions of Olympic athletes. Athletes who won silver medals were rated as appearing less joyful than athletes who won bronze medals, despite the better objective finish for the silver medalists. Medvec and colleagues explained this effect by noting that for the silver medalists the salient counterfactual alternative was winning a gold medal, whereas the salient counterfactual alternative for bronze medalists was not receiving any medal.

Wells and Gavanski (1989) illustrated that mental simulation can have a strong impact on forming impressions and reaching conclusions about people. They presented research participants with a story of a paraplegic couple who was denied a cab ride. The couple then decided to take their own car, and the car ended up plummeting off a bridge that had collapsed, killing them both. What did research participants think about the cab driver? The answer to this question depended on whether participants engaged in mental simulation or not. In one version of the story, the cab driver was described as driving over the very same bridge—however, doing so moments before its collapse and hence avoiding any harm. In another version of the story, the cab driver's car met the same fate as the paraplegic couple's car, but the cab driver was able to swim to safety and did not die in the accident. In these two versions of the story, the outcome for the paraplegic couple was the same: They were denied a cab ride, they took their own car, and they died. However, in one version of the story, the outcome was highly mutable. It was easy to imagine the couple's having survived if they had not been denied a cab ride, because they would have made it over the bridge before it collapsed if the cabbie had just agreed to take them. Mutability is essential to mental simulation. The couple would not have died if the laws of gravity had not been in effect, but the laws of gravity cannot be undone. However, the behavior of the cabbie was mutable and could have been undone. Thus it was easy to simulate this alternative reality.

In essence, one version of this story undid the negative event. What was the impact of being able to simulate the alternative outcome, or easily imagining the event being undone, on how participants evaluated the cab driver? The driver was rated as more responsible, and his decision to avoid the couple as more causal in their ultimate death, when participants read a story in which the cab driver successfully navigated the same bridge on which the paraplegic couple met their untimely demise. Despite the same outcome for the couple and the same behavior on the part of the cab driver in the two versions of the story, the ease of simulating an alternative reality altered the way in which participants categorized, interpreted, and assigned blame. In an instance such as this, learning about someone's death evokes thoughts about how it could have been avoided, and the alternatives are entered into a mental simulation to see how they might have altered the outcome and thus change the conception of responsibility assigned to the various players. Consider the implication of such a finding for a wrongful-death lawsuit. A doctor might be seen as more guilty for having let a patient die (or as being more directly responsible for the death itself) if mental simulations can produce alternative realities in which the person might have lived. Perhaps getting jurors to engage in mental simulation might alter the degree to which they find a doctor guilty, or perhaps it could reverse their decision altogether. Preventing such simulations would be a good defense strategy.

The Availability Heuristic

When some information comes to mind quickly, this ease of retrieval is usually thought to signify something. We believe that things that are easily called to mind are things that we encounter frequently, that happen often, and that are likely to be true. This is often the case; the most common explanations or the most common examples of a particular situation or thing are typically the ones that come to mind first. A robin is a common representative of the category "birds" and is one that we are fast to respond to and to generate. If someone asks us to judge the percentage of the bird population made up of robins versus the percentage made up of owls, we are likely to judge robins to be the more frequent birds because Robins are more available to us in memory, and we would be correct.

When an example is easily made available in memory, and this availability in memory is then used as a proxy for something meaningful about the example, we are using a heuristic. It is a heuristic that associates the ease of retrieval of information with the frequency with which this information is encountered and the probability that this information is true. Tversky and Kahneman (1982, p. 164) labeled this the *availability heuristic*: "That associative bonds are strengthened by repetition is perhaps the oldest law of memory known to man. The availability heuristic exploits the inverse form of this law, that is, it uses strength of association as a basis for the judgment of frequency." This quote explains the rationale behind the availability heuristic. Experience in life teaches us that the things we frequently encounter are things that we easily remember, so we assume that if we can easily remember something, it must be because we frequently encounter it. However, a problem with this strategy is that the ease with which we can recall something—the extent to which something is accessible to us—is not always a reflection of its actual frequency in the world outside of our limited experience. Frequent exposure may make a person, behavior, place, or object easily remembered, but ease of memory does not guarantee frequency of exposure. Thus the availability heuristic may lead to biased estimates for two clear reasons.

First, there are many reasons we can easily remember something other than the fact that we frequently encounter it, and these reasons have nothing to do with its actual probability. Some such reasons are reviewed in Chapter 10; two of them are *familiarity* and *salience*. For example, when we are familiar with something it may come to mind quite readily, and we may think it is more probable than it really is because of familiarity, not actual frequency in the population. As an example, a recent class that I taught had 50 students, 43 of whom were women. If I were asked to guess what percentage of college students were women, my experience would have led me to provide a biased estimate. Relying on what was available would not have provided an accurate basis for estimation, because availability was overdetermined by familiarity. The frequency with which I think about something makes it accessible to me, but this increased accessibility may lead to overestimation of its real frequency. In addition, something may be highly memorable because of its salience—its extremity, vividness, or novelty—and not because it is frequently encountered or likely to be true. If asked whether Americans are more likely to be killed in plane crashes or in bathroom accidents, people will typically answer, "Plane crashes." Why? Is it because they have data informing them that this is true? No. It is because a plane crash is easier to call to mind than a bathroom accident. Is it called to mind more easily because it happens more often? Most likely not. It is called to mind more easily because it is a highly vivid and spectacular (in a tragic way) event that garners much media attention. However, people use the fact that it comes to mind to signify that it happens frequently, when all it signifies is that it is vivid and easily recalled. People tend to overestimate the occurrence of salient things (e.g., deaths by fire, auto accidents, and murders) and to underestimate the occurrence of events that are less talked about and less accessible. It is for this reason that witnessing a car accident will increase the belief in the likelihood of such crashes occurring, relative to reading about a crash. Seeing is more vivid than reading.

Second, the fact that we frequently encounter things is not necessarily a good reflection of the extent to which those things are encountered by others or in the world at large. In essence, the availability heuristic is a rule informing us as perceivers to make judgments using the first examples, explanations, or estimates that we can bring into mind. However, we tend to recall absolute numbers and not relative numbers. We bring to mind specific examples, but not the context they occur in. If asked whether psychology majors are more likely to become medical doctors then English majors, we try to recall the number of people we know who are English majors and psychology majors who are pre-med students, and compare the absolute numbers. We fail to adjust for the fact that we know a far greater number of psychology majors, so obviously we can recall more pre-med students who are psychology majors. Absolute numbers are accessible, and we use them to guide judgment.

As a first empirical illustration of the availability heuristic, let us examine an experiment conducted by Tversky and Kahneman (1973), where research participants were asked to memorize a list of names. The names contained famous persons of both genders; however, in some cases the names of the men were better known than the names of the women (e.g., Richard Nixon vs. Lana Turner), and for other participants the list contained names of women who were relatively more well known than the men (e.g., Elizabeth Taylor vs. William Fulbright). Some of the participants were asked to judge the numbers of men and women in each list. In actuality they were equivalent, and all that differed was the fame of one of the groups. Other participants were asked simply to recall as many names from the list as possible. The results revealed that the gender that had the more famous names was judged to be the more frequent one in the list, and was more likely to have members of its group recalled. When men were more famous than women, participants thought the list had more men and actually remembered more men. In fact, recall was extremely advantaged for famous names, with 50% more names being remembered. Fame made the names salient; increased salience made those names easier to recall; and this made people overestimate the frequency of the group with which those names were associated.

What causes the effects associated with the availability heuristic? Two possibilities are suggested by the Tversky and Kahneman (1973) experiment. First, the absolute number of names recalled could have led participants to use this number as a proxy for the real list. More male names recalled would mean more male names on the list. Second, the experience of being better able to recall male (or female) names could have made participants use the ease of retrieval as an index of the real list. The feeling of being able to retrieve male names easily would make it reasonable to assume that ease of retrieval was associated with frequency. A problem in teasing these two possibilities apart is that most procedures that make it easy to retrieve information also make people likely to recall more absolute amounts of that information. However, Schwarz, Bless, and colleagues (1991) conducted a clever experiment that maneuvered around this problem. In this experiment, people were asked to list assertive or unassertive behaviors from their own past, and then were asked to judge their own assertiveness. If content is what causes the availability heuristic, then the more cases of their own assertive (unassertive) behavior participants could list, the higher the ratings of their assertiveness (unassertiveness) would be. However, what if people pay attention to subjective experiences that go along with recall (such as ease of retrieval)? If something is difficult to recall, it might lower ratings (e.g., these participants might reason, "If I have such trouble listing assertive behaviors, I must not be that assertive"). Indeed, recalling many instances of assertive behavior from one's past (12 examples) is hard to do and is experienced as difficult. However, recalling a handful of experiences from one's past (six examples) is relatively easy. Given this fact, Schwarz, Bless, and colleagues had a way to pit ease of retrieval against the absolute amount of recall to see which one drives the availability heuristic. Recalling 12 behaviors gives many examples of the behavior, but also yields a feeling of difficulty of retrieval. Which of these two sensations drives the effect?

Participants were asked to describe either six or 12 examples of past behavior that was either very assertive or very unassertive. If content only drives the availability heuristic, then the more assertive (unassertive) behaviors participants listed, the higher their self-ratings on that dimension were expected to be. However, if subjective experience plays a role, a reversal could be expected: Ratings would get lower as participants listed more items (because they were struggling to recall relevant examples). Schwarz, Bless, and colleagues (1991) found that in the easy condition, participants rated themselves as more assertive when they described six assertive versus six unassertive behaviors. However, people in the difficult condition showed the reversal: Those who described 12 unassertive behaviors rated themselves as more assertive than those who described 12 assertive behaviors. These findings support the idea that ease of retrieval is what guides the availability heuristic.

Heuristics as Bounded Rationality

Liberman (2001) asserts that biases such as the ones reviewed above often give the appearance that people are irrational: They use rules of thumb that apparently do not work and that lead them to make seemingly stupid decisions. However, these are not irrational choices. They are rational choices, in that they represent useful strategies that often work. It is true that they do not provide maximal efficiency, but they meet a standard of satisficing. Thus it is not that people are irrational creatures; they are creatures who attempt to rational, but are bounded or limited in their ability to act perfectly in this way.

To help us all make judgments, particularly under uncertainty when we require help, we have rules that we use—ones that we have learned over the course of our lives. These rules or shortcuts help us to predict and estimate what is likely to be the best solution to the task in front of us, whether it be judging/categorizing people or making decisions. The rules that we implement are called *heuristics*, and they are typically described by contrasting them with an elaborate and exhaustive examination of the features of the situation we are in. Rather than expend this type of mental effort, we use our heuristics because they generally lead us to acceptable judgments that we are confident with and happy with. The problem is that sometimes these heuristics do not fit the situation we are in; sometimes the heuristics bias the way we interpret information, so that we make errors. We often stray very far from what statistical reasoning and probabilistic models would suggest. Particularly in person perception, rationality often seems to be left in the lurch; a heuristic that may have been rational under conditions of uncertainty or minimal information is clung to even after the informational richness has developed to the point where the heuristic is no longer needed, and the data would provide better information than the rule of thumb. However, Liberman (2001) argues quite convincingly that the use of heuristics is often functional, and that if a heuristic serves a function it should be conceived of as a rational choice, rather than a source of bias. Although they are shortcuts, and certainly represent a case of minimal mental effort, these shortcuts develop because they help us in navigating through the social world.

CODA

Miller, Galanter, and Pribram (1960, p. 92) asserted that "All of us are cognitive gamblers—some more than others, but most of us more than we realize." In essence, each time we encounter a person, object, or event, we are engaging in a gamble. We are making an inference about the likelihood that the observed person/object/event fits with some mental representation that provides us with our particular knowledge of that class of people/objects/events. The gamble is often a good one, because the categories we have developed have emerged from experience and have been taught to us by the culture. However, at times we call on the wrong categories. Not all features are equally central to defining a category, and the features that are not central reside at fuzzy borders between categories. A consequence of this is that it may at times be difficult to state where the border between one category and another can be drawn. This is what makes it possible to categorize incorrectly. An Indian Sikh may be miscategorized by the person with an underdeveloped category as an Islamic cleric. A Canadian traveling abroad may be mistaken for a U.S. citizen. At other times we call on the correct categories, yet these are not guaranteed to be filled with accurate information. In each of these cases, our gambles have been bad ones. Yet regardless of the potential errors, categorization is ubiquitous and often occurs implicitly.

In social perception, the importance of categorization is illuminated by work on both the functions and the structure of categories. Much of this work has relied on assessing memory for people to provide a window into the impression formation processes of the perceivers. One important methodological procedure has been deliberately ignored in this chapter, and this involves examining recall for information that is consistent versus inconsistent with perceivers' categories (related to research on the relationship between what information perceivers remember about a person vs. what information is used in their impression of a person). This research will be used in the next chapter to help us discuss a central question regarding the ubiquitous use of categories: Does a reliance on categories reflect the fact that perceivers are by nature lazy, or that they are by nature seeking to be economy-minded and efficient in their allocation of mental effort? This is essentially a question of why people decide to operate in a fashion that is subject to errors, such as mistaking a person as being in one group versus another, treating different groups as the same, disregarding differences between people while focusing on similarities, and using a previously learned heuristic when either a more exhaustive analysis or a reliance on base rates would suggest otherwise. The next chapter describes people as needing to make a trade-off between two opposing needs: the need to avoid making errors, and the need to have inferences/knowledge about other people so they know how to act. As Lingle and colleagues (1984, p. 75) state, "the trade-off is resolved more toward maximizing inferences than toward avoiding errors." Because categories are functional, people use them despite occasional errors.

4 On Schemas and Cognitive Misers

MENTAL REPRESENTATIONS AS THE BUILDING BLOCKS OF IMPRESSIONS

Imagine that you are walking down the street and you hear the sound of bells coming out of a white truck. This experience need not be evaluated in detail for you to ascertain why the truck is making music. Instead, you can quickly and easily fit this experience into clusters that exist in your memory. Chapter 3 has defined this process as *categorization* and has explored why categorization is important for person perception. However, that chapter has not explored the question of why many conclusions about other people are arrived at so "quickly and easily." Categorizing other people has been described as a pervasive process necessary for making sense of these others, but there is nothing likely to justify the idea that much of this sense making not only begins with categorization, but ends there as well. We have reviewed the functions of categories in Chapter 3, but this is not meant to imply that categories constitute or determine final judgments of others. For instance, knowing that a person is a woman or a man may be very functional in guiding your interaction with this person, but should the prior knowledge you have of women serve as a filter through which all of your more sophisticated impressions pass?

This is a question at the heart of *stereotyping*—a form of categorizing people that shapes the impressions we make about them, not merely the initial categorization. When we stereotype, we recognize that perceiving others through the lenses of categories is a "miserly" thing to do (in terms of cognitive energy expended). That is, we realize that a stereotype may be a problematic way of thinking—not only because the content of the stereotype may be wrong (and in such instances it would be a faulty basis for judgment), but also because we are hardly thinking about the content of a person's character when using a stereotype. Instead, we are being stingy with our thinking, using prior knowledge as a tool for arriving at a fast judgment instead of thinking deeply about a person. What we may not realize is that we are constantly using a variety of mental structures, not just stereotypes, as lenses through which sophisticated inferences are filtered. A question to keep in mind throughout this chapter is whether we should characterize this reliance on categories as a miserly way for people to think.

However, before addressing the question of why we use mental representations throughout the many stages of the impression formation process, we will first examine the many forms taken on by these clusters of knowledge (our mental representations). As an example, we might think of a category as containing typical features, traits, and behaviors believed to be common among a group of people; these are partially based on our experience with specific people from the group, but those specific people do not need to be part of the mental representation. This possible structure for a category is called a *schema*. Thus experience with Willie Mays, Mickey Mantle, Barry Bonds, Don Mattingly, Ken Griffey Jr., Reggie Jackson, Alex Rodriguez, Derek Jeter, Sammy Sosa, and Thurman Munson may be used to give us an abstract mental representation of the category "baseball players" that includes the features and qualities of baseball players, even though those specific players may not be part of the structure of the category. Alternatively, we might conceive of categories as collections of specific examples of types of people belonging to the class. Thus my category "baseball players" may simply be the list of players named above, and from that list I distill traits and behaviors that these people exemplify if I am asked to form an impression of how well a new person fits this category. This possible structure for a category is called an *exemplar*.

You can easily examine, from your own experience, the variety of possible ways in which information you have about people can be structured (and hence can affect how you make sense of a particular person). When you encounter an African American, this triggers a category for "African Americans." But what constitutes this category? Naturally, the answer to this question will have important implications for the impression formed and the behavior enacted. Does the category comprise traits and attributes, each of which is assumed to be characteristic of the individual members of the group? Is it structured according to abstracted features and traits, some of which we assume will have a probability of being present in the current person? Does a prototypical "Black person" come to mind—a composite person who seems to capture the group best, based on your own past experience? Or do specific Black people come rushing to mind as the category is triggered? Perhaps what is triggered is a set of rules that dictates how you should behave. Let us return to the example at the start of the chapter to illustrate these various possibilities.

The phrase "ice cream truck" is never mentioned above, but you have probably categorized the object briefly described as such. When you hear and see an ice cream truck, what sort of mental representation is activated—what do these structures look like? You might rely on an abstract type of structure that conjures up for you a wide set of features and behaviors found in a typical ice cream truck, culled from your past experiences with many trucks. This set of typical features would provide you with expectancies that could guide your interaction with the truck and the person inside it. You might use a more concrete cluster that labels this as a specific type of ice cream truck: one driven by "the Good Humor man" or "Mr. Frosty." This can provide for you specific types of expectancies unique to each example of an ice cream truck (Mr. Frosty will have soft ice cream for you, the Good Humor man will not, etc.). Finally, your cluster might not provide for you a mere list of features (such as "has soft ice cream"), but instead provide a script that instructs you how to interact with the driver of the truck. After all, the manner in which you purchase ice cream in a store is different from the manner in which you purchase ice cream from a truck. You know, thanks to your category, that you are not supposed to enter the truck through the door as you would in a store, but to approach a window and order the ice cream from there. Given that structure will have a clear impact on function, it is important to examine the many forms that these clusters of knowledge, our categories, take on (and for our interests, we focus on categories of person types).

TYPES OF MENTAL REPRESENTATION REGARDING PEOPLE

Schemas

The term *schema* is typically first attributed to Bartlett (1932)—a cognitive psychologist who was doing research on how stories are transmitted from person to person, especially stories from a culture different from that of the people communicating the story to each other. When stories come from foreign cultures, it is possible that the content and form of the story are unusual to the perceiver. Bartlett specifically chose such unusually structured stories and observed that the stories seemed to evolve as they were transmitted, eventually becoming more coherent to the perceivers, but losing some important details from the original transcript. Bartlett reasoned that people had prior knowledge about the form and structure of stories, and that the new information was interpreted and recalled in the context of their prior structures. These schemas were said to alter the way the information was encoded and remembered, thus leading to the production of stories that were more consistent with the perceivers' schemas and further removed from the original "foreign" form. This sounds similar to what the Gestalt psychologists were telling us (at approximately the same time) about emergent meaning and perceptions seeking to find a coherent and meaningful structure. The schema was said to be an abstracted set of prior knowledge about a class of events—in this case, a story—that provides emergent meaning to comprehension and memory of the events (just as had been observed in perceptual organization).

A *schema*, in the modern use of the term, is a proposed organizational structure for the knowledge that comprises one's categories. A schema is defined by the fact that the features making up the category are stored in an *abstract form*, rather than a simple collection of specific examples drawn from past encounters and specific behaviors and attributes observed during interactions with specific people (or objects or events). It describes generalized *types* as well as specific instances. Thus we may have a schema for college students that calls to mind a set of abstracted behaviors and attributes, rather than simply calling to mind specific examples of college students we have known (i.e., it implicates declarative knowledge and information stored in semantic memory). Instead of a stockpile of relevant examples, the information we have about the category is conceived of as a list of possible attributes and behaviors that may be evidenced by a member of the category. In addition, the schema is assumed to contain within it the *relationships* that are known to exist among the features (Fiske & Linville, 1980; Fiske & Taylor, 1991; Taylor & Crocker, 1981). In this way, schemas provide more than a taxonomy of features, but an understanding of the connections between the features and *the rules that govern the features*. Finally, schemas are said to guide the manner in which new information is processed, and to selectively dictate what information is retrieved from memory (e.g., Fiske & Linville, 1980). What we see and what we think we have seen are determined in large part by schemas.

The definition above is not meant to exclude concrete examples from being contained within schemas. Rather, the schema is meant to hold all of one's knowledge about a person, object, or event. Taylor and Crocker (1981) assert that a schema should be thought of as

> a pyramidal structure, hierarchically organized with more abstract or general information at the top and categories of more specific information nested within the general categories. The lowest level in the hierarchy consists of specific examples or instances of the schema (e.g., specific people or events). The schema is connected to other schemas through a rich web of associations . . . one event may be represented in each of several schemas, with connections among the schemas, indicating these cross references. (p. 92)

Thus one may have a specific example of a person—say, one's mother—that can be represented (or linked to) several schemas. One may have a schema for one's parents, which would obviously include one's mother. One may also have a schema for kindness, in which one's mother is stored as a relevant example of a kind person. Furthermore, one may have a schema for lawyers, to which one's mother is linked (obviously, this would only be true if one's mother is a lawyer, or constantly in need of one). As an additional example, one may have a schema for the attribute of "egalitarianism." However, the attribute itself may be a lower-level component of another schema—perhaps for one's schema of social activists, or defense attorneys, or liberal politicians. In this last example, a lower-level attribute of one schema ("social activist") is seen to be capable of being the organizing principle around which a different schema is based (see Figure 4.1).

One fairly intuitive effect of having a schema is that it will influence the processing of information about a person in a way that *leads one to see and remember information about the person in a manner consistent with the schema.* This is known as *schema-consistent processing.* We have already seen a good example of a schema-consistent bias in how peo-

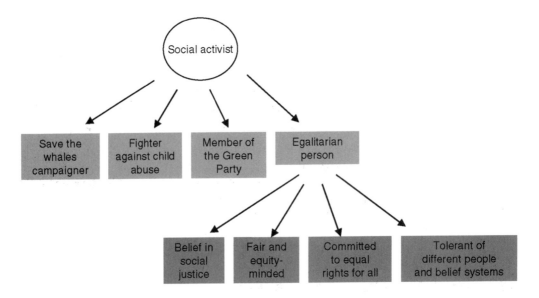

FIGURE 4.1. A lower-level attribute of one structure is itself an organizing principle for another.

ple process information, in the Hastorf and Cantril (1954) experiment described in Chapter 1. People came to interpret the information presented to them about a football game in drastically different ways, depending on the schema that they brought to the situation. Zadny and Gerard (1974) illustrated a similar effect of schemas on memory. (For a fairly comprehensive review of how schemas influence memory, see Alba & Hasher, 1983; also, read on, as the story gets more complicated later in this chapter.) Research participants were told that a person they were going to read about was a college student with a particular major. Some of the participants were told that this person was majoring in chemistry, and others were told that the student was majoring in music. Each of these majors was represented in memory by a schema, one that most people could readily identify in their own minds. The participants then received information to read about the person's life on campus, and recall for this information was later tested. The information that was consistent with the schema was better recalled. People who were told that the person was a chemistry major were more likely to recall information about the person's course enrollments that reflected the person as taking a preponderance of science courses. Even small details about the person that were consistent with the schema were better recalled, such as objects the person was carrying and the titles of the books he owned.

Similarly, Anderson and Pichert (1978) found that schemas influenced what people remembered about a house that was being described, with the schemas being ones relating to the persons who were looking at the house. Research participants were asked to read information about a home with the task of imagining that they were either burglars "casing the joint" or prospective homeowners. Each of these categories brought to mind schema-relevant information, which then guided what people noticed when they were scanning the information and subsequently what they were able to recall. The results found, again, a schema-consistent bias in recall: Imagining themselves as burglars led participants to recall more "theft-relevant" items than imagining themselves as homeowners.

Before we start to discuss specific types of schemas, let us return to a point raised in the Taylor and Crocker (1981) quote above. What does it mean to say that information is structured hierarchically? A hierarchical structure requires a "single-ancestry relationship" to exist (Lingle, Altom, & Medin, 1984, p. 98). This means that if one category (e.g., "doctors") is nested within another category (e.g., "helpful people") which is in turn nested within another category (e.g., "people"), the members of the lowest level in this link (doctors) must also be members of the highest level (people). In addition, all of the features associated with the higher-level categories in the hierarchy must also be true of the more specific instances. Our knowledge of Catholics does not need to contain the fact that they have limbs, because the category "Catholics" is embedded within the category "persons," which has connected to it links to the fact that people have limbs (see Figure 3.1 in Chapter 3). Thus, if there is a hierarchical organization, we do not need to store information true of all members of a category at each node embedded within the superordinate category, since all members of a category have the features associated with the levels above it in the hierarchy. This hierarchical structure makes sense if we are trying to imagine a way to describe the mental system that does not involve great redundancy and inefficiency.

Now that we have argued for the hierarchical nature of knowledge representation, let us back away from these claims! Although there is certainly some degree of embeddedness of information, there also is a great deal of overlap between categories. Thus not all categories are nested within other categories in a hierarchical relationship.

Some categories are linked to many categories in an overlapping fashion (see Chapter 3). This too is clearly stated in the quote from Taylor and Crocker (1981) above, as well as evidenced in Figure 3.1. Concepts that have many connections and that get used frequently can perhaps develop strong associations to other concepts, and these strong associations may account for why people respond so quickly to one concept when given an associated concept, rather than the distance that is being traversed from one node to the other. The speed with which people reply that "Catholics believe in Christ" may simply reflect a strong association between these two concepts that allows for the signal to travel faster, rather than to the fact that "Christ" and "Catholics" are stored close together in a hierarchical structure. People may have less experience relating other concepts, such as "Christ" and "limbs," and this may be reflected in a weaker association that needs greater time for spreading activation to occur across the net.

Perhaps the structure consists of some combination of hierarchically arranged nodes in a network, as well as overlapping nodes and categories that have many associations to each other in a network, with varying strengths of association attached to each pathway. Our point here is simply that schemas are relationships among pieces of knowledge, with some of those relationships being stronger than others. This includes relations between abstract knowledge as well as specific instances. The exact structure of mental representations (if there is just one structure) is still a topic of debate (e.g., Chen, 2001; Sherman, 2001). It is discussed here only to illustrate that knowledge about people is among the categories organized in the mental network of associations, and that the way we conceive of the structure of the "person node" influences what we believe may get triggered when we encounter individual pieces of information linked to the node. A lack of a clear-cut resolution on this issue of category structure does not stop us from postulating the existence of schemas and other types of mental representations, or discussing the impact they have on how we think about people and form impressions.

Self-Schemas

Schemas are proposed to exist for all of the knowledge we possess, and this would by definition include the knowledge we have about ourselves! Markus (1977) put forward the idea that our self-concepts are in effect schemas in which all the information we have about ourselves is organized and linked. This information includes abstract conceptions of ourselves that represent our most cherished values, aspirations, and beliefs, as well as specific examples of behavior from our past that are central to these attributes. A self-schema is probably made up of the attributes listed most easily if any of us were to respond to a test that asked us to complete the following thought: "I am _____." The features/attributes that immediately come to mind (e.g., "smart," "hard-working," "a good mother," "pretty," "athletic," "honest") are then linked to more specific attributes and behaviors associated with each feature. According to Markus,

> self-schemata will be generated because they are useful in understanding intentions and feelings and in identifying likely or appropriate patterns of behavior. [Note that some authors have used "schemata" as the plural of "schema."] While a self-schema is an organization of the representations of past behavior, it is more than a "depository." It serves an important processing function and allows an individual to go beyond the information currently available. The concept of self-schema implies that information about the self in some area has been categorized or organized and that the result of this organization is a discernible pat-

tern which may be used as a basis for future judgments, decisions, inferences, or predictions about the self. (p. 64)

Markus (1977) performed what is usually considered the first examination of how schemas influence the processing of self-relevant information—in other words, that self-schemas have real processing implications for how individuals see and remember the world. The prediction was that *self-schemas will allow people to make judgments about a schema-relevant behavior or attribute fairly easily and quickly, to make predictions about future behavior relevant to that attribute or behavior fairly readily and accurately, and to resist discovering information about themselves that is contrary to that which their self-schemas would suggest to be true.* (These and other hypothesized functions of schemas, prototypes, and so forth are being given in italics and will be summarized later in the chapter.) In this regard, when a trait or behavior is said to be relevant to a person's self-schema, it must be one that is more than a trait/behavior the person might like to possess or thinks is good. A self-schema consists instead of traits and behaviors with which the person has real experience, and to which the person has acquired a meaningful attachment as part of his/her self-definition.

Research participants were selected who rated themselves as having either (1) self-schemas concerning traits relating to independence; (2) self-schemas for dependence; or (3) no self-schemas relating to the trait domain of independence–dependence (Markus called these participants "aschematics," to signify that this dimension of behavior was not relevant to their self-definition). These ratings were done at the start of the semester and were far removed from the time period in which the actual experiment occurred (so the "schematics" did not know the experiment had anything to do with their self-schemas). Participants at the experimental session were exposed to a set of traits (one at a time) on a screen and were asked to determine whether the words were self-descriptive or not (by pressing a button marked "me" or "not me"). Reaction times for the responses were recorded. The traits that were being presented on the screen were selected so that 15 were related to independence, 15 were related to dependence/conformity, and 30 were related to creativity–noncreativity (these were included as control words, and responses to these were compared with responses to the independence–dependence words). After this task, a subset of the words from each category was presented to participants; they were asked to indicate which words were self-descriptive, and then to describe why they were self-descriptive by providing evidence from their past behavior.

The results revealed, first, that people schematic for the trait of independence were more likely to say that a word relating to independence was self-defining than people who were schematic for dependence. Meanwhile, people schematic for dependence were more likely to say that words relating to dependence were self-defining than people schematic for independence. More interesting (since we would really hope that if persons were schematic, they would choose words relevant to that dimension as self-relevant) were the results concerning the speed of responding. People schematic for dependence were faster to make decisions regarding whether a word was descriptive of "me" or "not me" when those words were relevant to dependence (as opposed to words relevant to independence and to control words). Similarly, people schematic for independence were faster at making decisions when the words were related to independence than when they were dependence-related or control words. Aschematics did not differ in their responses to any of the types of words. The main finding was that schematic participants not only could accurately choose words that are self-descriptive, but were faster at detecting and reacting to those words. In addition, people who were schematic were better able to provide behavioral evidence to support their assertion that a trait was self-descriptive if that trait was relevant to their self-schemas (they could back up their assertions with facts). For example, people schematic for independence wrote more descriptions for independence-related words than did aschematics and people schematic for dependence. They did more than claim to be independent (which people not schematic for independence did as well); they remembered having lived lives full of behavioral evidence of independence (which aschematics did not do).

In a second experiment, Markus (1977) illustrated that people who are schematic for a particular set of self-relevant traits will interpret information given to them as a form of self-feedback differently from people who are not schematic. Specifically, *people with self-schemas are resistant to receiving information that is counterschematic.* The participants in this second study were asked to take a test (actually bogus) said to assess levels of suggestibility. Obviously, people schematic for independence would not include notions of being susceptible as part of their self-definition, and they should be more likely to reject feedback suggesting that they had scored highly on this test. This was precisely what Markus found. The aschematics found the test to be more accurate and to provide a better description of them than did the schematics, who were more likely to question the validity of the test scores. Feedback about themselves that the aschematics found to be credible was rejected by the schematics. Thus Markus's research illustrates two of the fundamental influences that schemas have on information processing: Individuals are faster to detect and respond to schema-relevant information, and they are more likely to reject and see as invalid information that is inconsistent with their existing schemas. Perhaps most importantly, the work illustrates the usefulness of conceiving of self-knowledge as being a schema.

Rogers, Kuiper, and Kirker (1977) provided further evidence of the processing implications of self-schemas. They posit that one function of a self-schema is to help a person process self-relevant information and personal data: "The central aspect of self-reference is that the self acts as a background or setting against which incoming data are interpreted or coded. This process involves an interaction between the previous experiences of the individual (in the form of the abstract structure of self) and the incoming materials" (p. 678). The individual's vast reservoir of self-knowledge can help him/her to embellish self-relevant material by filling in the blanks and providing extra descriptive richness. Rogers and colleagues' experiment sought to illustrate how linking information to the self makes the encoding of that information richer and more complex. To do so, their participants were exposed to words that were to be judged. Some of the judgments involved invoking the self; others did not. For example, sometimes participants were asked to make semantic ratings relating to the words by deciding whether the words were similar in meaning to target words. Other times they had to make structural ratings relating to the words by deciding whether the words were printed in a larger typeface than target words. And sometimes the participants were asked to make self-reference judgments by deciding whether words were self-descriptive or not. The participants were then given a surprise memory test. As reviewed in Chapter 3, better memory on a surprise free-recall test is presumed to indicate a deeper, more complex memory structure. Thus, if self-reference has benefits for the processing of words, words should have been better remembered when they were presented as part of the self-referencing task as opposed to any of the other tasks. This was precisely what was found. The data suggest that the self is used as an organizing structure for interpreting new information, altering the way in which that information is processed (in this case, giving it a deeper, more thorough memory trace).

Role and Relational Schemas

Schemas relating to specific types of people (the self, dependent people, egalitarian persons, etc.) are not the only types of representations relevant to social cognition. We also possess mental structures that capture the features (and relationships among those features) for the various roles people play, as well as for the various types of social relationships people enter into (and perhaps we can conceive of a particular relationship, such as husband, as a type of role that people play with specific others). According to Fiske and Taylor (1984, p. 159), "a social role is the set of norms and behaviors attached to a social position, so a role schema is the cognitive structure that organizes one's knowledge about those appropriate norms and behaviors." Role schemas provide for us our knowledge of the rules, norms, and expected behaviors associated with broad social categories such as gender, age, and race, as well as the norms and behaviors associated with more specific types of categories relating to social positions, such as occupations (doctor, journalist, garbage collector, etc.) and relationship status (lover, brother, friend, etc.). For example, the role of friend requires listening to others when they are complaining and dejected, being supportive and helpful, helping generate fun experiences and enjoyable times, being stimulating and engaging, and *not* harboring feelings of lust (in which case the role has shifted from that of friend to that of secret admirer or unrequited lover).

Once again, memory measures have been used to illustrate that role schemas are at work. Cohen (1961) asked research participants to watch a videotape that depicted a woman engaged in a variety of behaviors (e.g., having dinner with her husband). The interest was in what sorts of detail participants would recall about the video and how memory for details would differ as a function of role schemas. Some of the participants watched the video with the understanding that the wife was employed as a waitress; others believed that she held the occupational role of librarian. The details recalled were found to differ between the two groups in a schema-congruent fashion. The librarian was more likely to be remembered as having glasses and liking classical music than the waitress, who was more likely to be recalled as being a beer drinker. In addition, such schema-consistent information was more likely to be recalled than schema-inconsistent information (such as a librarian owning a bowling ball).

Baldwin (1992) proposes that relationships are internally represented, such that one's prior interpersonal experiences can exert an impact on how information relevant to one's relationships is perceived, interpreted, and remembered. Baldwin (1992, p. 461) has defined *relational schemas* as "cognitive structures representing regularities in patterns of interpersonal relatedness . . . the focus, then, is on cognition about relationships, rather than about the self or the other person in isolation." These cognitive structures include action sequences and behavior patterns that define the relationship between two (or more) social entities (such as self and mother). A relational schema includes not only summaries of typical action patterns, but thoughts, feelings, and motivations that permeate the relationship. The logic is that the triggering of the schema will trigger these related emotions, goals, cognitions, and behaviors, making them more likely to have an impact on one's current information processing. Thus feelings toward one's mother might influence how one thinks about some new person if something about the current environment triggers the relational schema for the mother (e.g., if someone bears a physical resemblance to one's mother, this could trigger a relational schema and affect how one interprets this new person, without the realization that one's mother is influencing current thought and behavior).

An illustration of this idea was provided by Baldwin, Carrell, and Lopez (1990). Their goal was to determine whether internally represented interpersonal information in the form of a relational schema could be activated outside of awareness and influence people's evaluations of personally relevant information, without their realizing this. In one experiment, they investigated the relationship between graduate students and their professors (a very significant relationship for students aspiring to get a PhD, as personal success is significantly tied to the tutelage of advisors). In a second experiment, they examined the relationship of individuals to the Catholic Church (as best represented by an image of the Pope). For example, participants in the second experiment were Catholic women. They were shown disapproving images of either the Pope or an irrelevant person (a stranger) below the level of conscious awareness (subliminal presentation). The participants were then asked to evaluate their own performance on a task to see whether the triggered relationship would affect their self-evaluations. Self-ratings were reliably lower following the disapproving face of the Pope as compared to a stranger, despite the fact that the face was never consciously detected. This result cannot be explained by notions that general disapproval was triggered, because in both groups disapproval was being observed (albeit subliminally). The best explanation for the finding is that specific relationship patterns were being triggered, and disapproval as it related to the Catholic women's relationship with their church would be quite different from disapproval more generally. Thus this relational schema, and the meaning of disapproval within the context of the schema, were what had an impact on responses. The knowledge structure was unconsciously triggered, and with it the emotions and motives associated with that relationship, which then altered information processing.

Event Schemas: Scripts and Frames

Baldwin (1992) asserts that relational schemas include specific action patterns associated with specific relationship partners. An extension of this logic is that specific sets of action patterns are associated not only with relationship partners, but with environments. We have schemas that dictate specific ways of behaving for specific situations. At the start of this chapter, it has been noted that you probably know how to purchase ice cream from an ice cream truck as opposed to a store. This is made possible by the fact that existing cognitive structures specify how to behave with an ice cream vendor, at the dentist, in a fast-food restaurant (how you act and get food in McDonald's is different from Denny's, which in turn is different from fine dining), and so forth. Such knowledge is referred to as a *script*. Schank and Abelson (1977) defined a script as a "predetermined, stereotyped sequence of actions that defines a well-known situation" (p. 41). By their nature, scripts specify procedures (how to act), as well as semantic knowledge that defines the situation and the elements within it. Thus they contain information that specifies more than just expectations about what events will occur, but the order of events as well (and thus implicate procedural memory). Scripts are conceived of as a series of IF-THEN clauses that dictate responses in the presence of certain conditions. For example, IF there is a row of cash registers at the front of the restaurant, THEN you go up and order food there rather than sitting down and waiting for a waitress.

When do people perform in a scripted way? After all, not every situation will trigger a predetermined manner of responding; nor should it be assumed that any time an inference is made about a situation, a script has been invoked. One must be able to bridge the gap from the script as a cognitive structure to behavior. This is done by choosing to enter the script if a particular set of preconditions are met. One establishes an action rule that specifies when and where certain actions can be initiated simply by the presence of features in those environments signaling that the script (and the action dictated by the script) is appropriate. In this way the script is triggered by the situation, but only after experience in such situations has allowed one to develop an action rule dictating that it is appropriate to behave in a predetermined way in that situation (Abelson, 1981). Therefore, the preconditions for scripted behavior are the attachment of an action rule to a script; a context that will trigger the script; and a mental representation that can be triggered in memory, given the appropriate context. Chapter 2 has described the studies of mindlessness performed by Langer, Blank, and Chanowitz (1978)—studies where scripts were being automatically triggered by the situation and guiding the manner in which people responded. The participants acted mindlessly not because they were ignorant, but because the appropriate way to act was specified by the script, and the triggering of the script surrendered the decisions about what to do (and when to do it) to the IF-THEN clauses specified by the procedural nature of the script.

The script concept bears a resemblance to work on *frames* in cognitive psychology. Minsky (1975), who introduced the term, defined a frame as a mental representation that contains information about stereotyped setting or situations, such as attending the opera, taking an exam, or going to work in the morning. Minsky proposed frames to be hierarchically structured, with the top levels specifying unwavering truths about the situation, such as the fact that one's office will be there when one arrives. The lower levels of the frame have what are referred to as *slots*. The slots specify the specifics of this particular instantiation of the frame. Thus, if one arrives at work to find that one's boss is away on a business trip for the week, a different set of specific behaviors would be entered into the slot than if one arrived to find that one's boss wanted one to lead a group meeting in an hour. The slots can be replaced with the specific information that the current instantiation of the script invokes, but there is also a default value for the slot that specifies how one typically behaves when nothing unusual is happening within the situation that day. In our office example, the default value might be first to get a cup of coffee as one's computer is booting up. The frame, therefore, not only tells one how to act in this situation, but has built-in flexibility to tell one how to act in different versions of this situation, including how to act if the typical expectations are disconfirmed (such as when one arrives to learn that one is leading a meeting in an hour). In this regard, it must be noted that even the unwavering truths at the top of the hierarchy may occasionally yield unexpected findings (such as when fire or terrorism has destroyed one's place of work overnight), and the frame still specifies appropriate ways to act under this version of the situation.

Prototypes versus Exemplars

Kihlstrom and Klein (1994, p. 159) provide a definition of a *prototype* by reminding us first that Rosch (1975) and others "proposed what has become known as the *probabilistic view*, which argues that the summary descriptions of category members take the form of some measure of their central tendency with respect to salient features." Rather than a list of required features that are singly necessary and jointly sufficient, the structure is best represented by a central tendency, or a list of features that are present in most members of the category. A prototype is a representation detailing a typical category member, summarized by the set of most common features that are most probable to be found in a category member. "Thus, birds tend to fly, sing, and be small, but there are a few large, flightless, songless birds. The category prototype is some instance, real or imagined, that has a large number of these typical features" (p. 160). Person categories are also likely to be prototypes—abstractions about the categories culled from experience. Cantor and Mischel (1979, p. 11) remarked: "Clearly it would be difficult to find a set of necessary and sufficient features shared by all members of any particular person category that one would want to use as the definitive test of category membership. For example . . . some extraverts seem primarily dominating and active rather than warm and sociable." Because prototypes are abstractions of sets of likely characteristics derived from personal experience, two individuals can have different prototypes for the same category (different mental images of what the typical category member looks like, or what the central tendency of the category looks like). Despite the fact that prototypes can differ in content from person to person, they do not differ in function. The role of prototypes in how perceivers think is equivalent for different perceivers.

Perhaps the classic illustration of the role of prototypes in person perception was provided by Cantor and Mischel (1977, p. 39), who proposed that "the prototype seems to function as a standard around which a body of input is compared and in relation to which new input is assimilated into the set of items to be remembered about a given experience or list of stimuli." The goal of the research was to demonstrate that traits exist and operate as prototypes—in other words, that personality traits are defined in people's heads as having certain characteristics. If a trait gets activated or perceivers label someone as being of a certain type (e.g., geek, jock, princess, misfit, delinquent), then they think that this person has the other central features that make up the prototype for that personality trait. If people learn and remember information by categorizing according to their prototypes, *they will use prototypes to generate missing information (fill in the gaps in their knowledge) and to generate additional information (inferences).* If a prototype is activated, then all of the features of this representation will be activated, thus altering how the information is interpreted, and altering what people remember as having seen. Thus information not explicitly observed will be confused with information actually presented because of their association in the mental structure. We should expect to see these types of errors in recall where people mistakenly identify information that was not present as part of their memory for what was present.

Cantor and Mischel (1977) asked research participants to read about some people who were described either as extraverted or introverted, in order to see whether the participants would remember these people as having other traits that were not described, but related to being either an introvert or an extravert. For the extraverted and introverted descriptions, six of the 10 sentences used to describe each person had adjectives in them that described the person as moderately extraverted (or introverted). The other four were traits that were unrelated to this dimension. Next, participants were given a memory test after a short delay. They were provided with a list of traits, and their job was to decide which ones were actually in the earlier stories. For example, relating to the extraverted person, participants were given 15 words to choose from. Of these 15, five were moderately related to extraversion, and only two of them were actually in the original story; five were highly related to extraversion, and none of those were in the original story; the remaining five were unrelated to extraversion. The pattern was the same for the introverted person. The participants' task was to read each of the words on the memory test and rate how confident they were that it had been in the actual story. The results showed that participants were more confident in thinking that they saw words that actually *were not* presented but that were *related* to extraversion (or introversion), compared to words that *were not* presented but *unrelated* to extraversion (introversion). They remembered seeing information that was not there because of the relationship between the behaviors and traits in the prototype. The data suggest that when people form impressions of others, they use the features detected to help them "type" the person. The features of the prototype that match the person are then activated and used to describe the person further, thus biasing perceivers' memory of the person.

Just as the classical view of categories was challenged by the prototype view, the prototype view of categories was challenged by the *exemplar* view of category structure. Medin (1989) suggests that categories do not consist of summaries of highly probable features of the typical member, but of specific examples of actual members (thus drawing on the information stored in episodic memory). Thus, rather than there being an abstracted sense of the sorts of features a typical extravert might possess, the category "extravert" would instead be conceived of as a set of actual extraverts one has encountered in one's experience—*exemplars*. Smith and Zarate (1992) define an exemplar as a cognitive representation of an individual that can range from being a fairly complete list of the features of a specific person to a list including only a few key features that are seen as descriptive of the person. For instance, your conception of your mother is likely to be a fairly detailed and complete exemplar, whereas your conception of Charles Manson is probably inhabited by only a few central attributes. Each exemplar, however, is clearly stored in your mind, as the mere reading of those words "mother" and "Charles Manson" has probably brought specific images to mind.

Thus, when categorizing takes place, if the current person matches or fits the exemplars from a given category, that category is used to describe the new person. According to Lingle and colleagues (1984, p. 91), "a new item will be identified as a category member if it cues the retrieval of a critical number of exemplar representations from the category and does so before cuing the retrieval of a criterial number of exemplar representations from some contrasting category." The process is one of comparison between specific instances or examples. Murphy and Medin (1985) argue that the exemplar view better represents category structure, because it can go beyond the prototype view in explaining how categories function. They argue that variability within a category is not captured well by prototypes. For example, restaurants differ in terms of how the bill gets paid, with sometimes the money going to the server and other times being brought directly to the cashier. People know that when a restaurant has a counter with stools, it is likely to be one where the cashier gets paid, but when a restaurant has candles on the table, it is likely to be one where the server will collect the money. This type of variability is easily captured by a mental representation that stores examples of restaurants one has encountered, but not by one that has an abstracted list of typical features of restaurants (which discards such specifics).

Smith and Zarate (1992) have proposed the most comprehensive model of exemplars in social judgment and mental representation. They suggest that exemplars are stored representations of specific events and people (representing certain types or attributes) that are accessed, typically preconsciously, and influence judgment. This view is best summarized with the assumption that "the perceiver has many cognitive representations of persons (exemplars). Each representation includes not only encoded perceptual attributes of the person, but also the perceiver's inferences, attributions, and reactions. When the perceiver encounters a new target person, information from stored representations that are similar to the target will be used to make judgments" (Smith & Zarate, 1992, p. 4). Which exemplar is retrieved and used is determined by many contextual factors, and the way in which a person is judged and treated, therefore, will be dependent on the exemplar to which that person is being compared. For example, a Palestinian professor (an example offered in Chapter 3) is someone who can be categorized according to relevant exemplars of Palestinians or relevant exemplars of professors. The context can help to determine which category is most likely to be triggered and what types of exemplars will influence processing. If the person is encountered at a statistics lecture in front of the class, perhaps the "professor" exemplar will be most salient and determine how this person is categorized and ultimately evaluated/judged. We will reserve our discussion of the impact of exemplars on judgment for Chapter 10, where this issue is discussed in detail.

As we will see in Chapter 10, these distinctions between categories as prototypes and categories as exemplars are not mere theoretical points. Whether an exemplar or an abstracted list of traits (a prototype) is triggered in the mind can dramatically alter how people interpret the behavior of the person they are observing (e.g., Moskowitz & Skurnik, 1999; Stapel & Koomen, 2001). The debate as to whether schemas are best described as prototypes or exemplars is one we will not resolve here. In fact, it might be best to side with Lingle and colleagues (1984), as well as Cantor and Kihlstrom (1987), who proposed that mental representations of people contain a blend of each, shifting between them. Certainly, the work reviewed in Chapter 10—which reveals that people can have both types of structures activated, with differing effects on how people form impressions—would support the idea that both abstractions and specific examples are stored as part of a given person category (as does the review of semantic vs. episodic vs. procedural memory in Chapter 3). It is beyond the scope of this book to provide a detailed account of mixed models of exemplar/abstraction use. There are some specific models that suggest when each will form the basis of category knowledge, and the interested reader is directed to those sources for a thorough treatment of these issues. In the social domain, the work by Klein and colleagues on impression formation (Klein, Loftus, Trafton, & Fuhrman, 1992; Sherman & Klein, 1994), and Sherman and colleagues' work in the domain of stereotype representation (Sherman, 1996; Sherman, Lee, Bessenoff, & Frost, 1998), offer mixed models that show the same developmental sequence in determining whether exemplars or prototypes are used. These researchers find that when familiarity with a target is low, exemplars are used. As familiarity with a target grows, abstractions are created and are used instead of exemplars. In this way, exemplars serve as the basis for prototype formation, and until a well-developed prototype emerges, some mixture of the two can be seen in mental representation.

THEORY-BASED MENTAL REPRESENTATIONS

The discussion of mental representations thus far has suggested that categories are activated and used as a function of feature matching. Categories have been described as containing features, and categorization as dependent on the number of matching features between some stimulus and a category. The more features that are matched between a stimulus and a category, and the fewer the mismatches, the greater the chance the stimulus will be seen as an instance of that category. However, several theorists have offered alternatives to these feature-based approaches to schemas and categorization (e.g., Murphy & Medin, 1985; Rips & Collins, 1993; Wittenbrink, Gist, & Hilton, 1997). As Chen (2001, p. 130) noted,

> a critical problem with featural similarity as an organizing principle is that it is unclear how the particular set of features that makes members similar, or that determines categorization, is decided (Medin, 1989; Murphy & Medin, 1985; Medin et al., 1993). There is an infinite number of features that make two stimuli similar or dissimilar to one another, or a new instance similar or dissimilar to the members of a category. As such, the assumption that categories reflect feature lists, and that categorization is based on some function of the number of shared and unshared features between an instance and a category, falls short because knowledge beyond features is needed to constrain what features are relevant to category membership (e.g., Murphy & Medin, 1985). Perhaps the clearest examples of this shortcoming are categories that group together instances that share little or even no obvious featural similarity, such as the category for "things to take out of one's house in case of a fire," which might include pets, money, jewelry, and photo albums as members. (example cited in Murphy & Medin, 1985; see also Barsalou, 1983; Medin, 1989)

Alternatives to feature-based structures posit that mental representations include *theories*. By *theories*, it is meant that mental representations contain "explanatory or causal forms of knowledge" (Chen, 2001, p. 125). When scientists try to make sense of some phenomenon that they are studying, they develop theories about the phenomenon. These theories play a facilitating role in generating explanations for the phenomenon. What the theory notion suggests for social cognition is that people operate in a similar fashion to scientists: The phenomenon in question is the behavior of other people, and perceivers develop theories about behavior to explain it (e.g., Gopnik & Wellman, 1994; Heider, 1958). In developmental psychology, the child's use of theories to explain behavior is referred to as a *theory of mind* (e.g., Wellman, 1990), whereas in social psychology, researchers speak of *implicit theories* that people use to understand behavior (e.g., Bruner & Tagiuri, 1954; Clore, Schwarz, & Conway, 1994; Dweck & Leggett, 1988; Kelley, 1972b; Nisbett & Ross, 1980; Wegener & Petty, 1995; Wegner & Vallacher, 1977; Wilson & Brekke, 1994). Why did he act that way? Why did she say that? The answer a perceiver arrives at (the way in which he/she categorizes the behavior) may involve a theory the perceiver has about those particular types of people or the types of situations in which those people find themselves.

This position, which is sometimes called the *theory theory* (because it is a theory that people rely on theories), assumes that laypeople have knowledge much like scientific theories that they apply to explain behavior. In this view, categories are not simply lists of features or examples, but theories that make these features coherent, relate them to one another, and can be used for explanation and making inferences about causality (e.g., Murphy & Medin, 1985). As an example, Gopnik and Meltzoff (1997) propose some very general theories used by even extremely young children. First, newborns seem to possess a theory about what it means to be human versus nonhuman, displaying an ability to distinguish between people and objects. A newborn knows to imitate people but not machines. Second, newborns look to their immediate environment (what is physically contiguous) to see whether there is an effect of their actions; this behavior is seen as reflecting the existence of the infants' theory about mechanical causation.

As a child grows, theories evolve about the nature of personal causation—what causes people to act as they do. The theory of persons as distinct and independent entities evolves and acquires the notion that people have distinct wants and desires relating to the external world. Wellman (1990) referred to this as a child's developing a *desire theory*, and the explanations the child generates to account for the behavior of others are usually seen in light of this theory. The child ponders, "Why did Billy act that way?" The answer returned is "Because he wants to." The desire theory is later modified to a *belief and desire theory*, in which explanations for behavior can now include beliefs as well as wants. The theory acquires the notion that people are not only objects of impulse that act according to wants and desires, but creatures of cognition who have beliefs about the world and who can internally represent the external world. The theory is then adapted again later (with maturity) to include the notion that other people have their own sets of beliefs about the world that are different from one's own (what is usually referred to as *perspective taking*). By the time one is an adult, the theory has grown to link the behavior of others to stable traits, which are more enduring than wants, and which provide better causal explanations for behavior (a point to be discussed in more detail in Chapter 6 on attribution). According to Wellman (1990, p. 114), "specific beliefs and desires are often explained as springing from such larger traits (the desire to wear pretty clothes may spring from a vanity or, perhaps, from an insecurity about one's attractiveness). Because of this grounding of specific beliefs and desires in traits, traits figure prominently in causal explanations of actions."

The theories discussed thus far have been extremely broad. In social psychology, especially in person perception, the idea that perceivers use theories has been meant to imply that they have highly specific knowledge structures that are related to particular social groups and persons. This chapter will not provide an exhaustive review of all the specific theories that people use in making sense of one another. Instead, let us review a few examples here, and note that other relevant examples of "theory use" are highlighted throughout this book where relevant. For example, Dweck (1996) posits that people hold implicit theories about performance and ability. For some people, ability is theorized as being a fixed entity that is stable, with the implication that it reflects some underlying trait or enduring quality of a person. For other people, ability is theorized to be something malleable and dynamic, and suggests that people can change and grow in a particular domain. These theories would dictate whether a person doing something dumb is characterized as being stupid with a flawed character or as having been caught up in bad circumstances or a momentary lapse of reason. This is reviewed in Chapter 9. Kelley (1972b) provides a set of fairly specific theories perceivers employ when attempting to ascertain the cause of another person's behavior. These theories (*causal schemas*) are reviewed in Chapter 6. Finally, as already discussed in Chapter 3, categories become socially shared because the culture teaches all members of the culture the same theories. These different theories then dictate the degree to which perceivers see the behavior of others as having been caused by the traits of the person or by the power of the situation. Perceivers in Western cultures differ in their implicit theories (and consequently in their attributional style) from perceivers in non-Western cultures. This culture-based theory about how to understand behavior is a topic reviewed in some detail in Chapter 7. Let us now review in detail three theories relating to person perception.

Implicit Personality Theories

We have already discussed how the retrieval of a category from memory will not merely lead to the accessibility of that category; its activation will spread from that specific concept to related constructs. What may be considered as part of the associative network linked to a given category? One such factor that links various mental representations together are implicit theories about types of personalities. For example, perceivers have theories describing certain types of people or sets of traits that usually co-occur in people (e.g., Cantor & Mischel, 1979; Leyens & Fiske, 1994; Rosenberg & Sedlak, 1972; Schneider, 1973).When one of these traits is made accessible through the retrieval of its category from memory, the rest of the traits can be triggered without the individual's consciously thinking about person "types" or relationships between traits. This set of beliefs about the relationships between traits that leads to their association and spreading activation is known as an *implicit personality theory*. According to Grant and Holmes (1981), "an implicit personality theory can be viewed as sets of clusters of traits that form cognitive schemas representing clear-cut exemplars or prototypes of different personality types" (p. 108). An implicit personality theory is related to cognitive structures such as stereotypes. Eagly, Ashmore, Makhijani, and Longo (1991) describe stereotypes as implicit personality theories in which group membership is one trait thought to covary with other traits. Prototypes are also closely related to implicit personality theories, as we discuss next.

Some views of the ways traits are related to each other in the mind posit a strictly associationistic view in which people think about others in terms of correlations among traits. Other views conceive of traits as being related along specific dimensions; traits that fall within or along the same dimension (e.g., friendly–unfriendly, adventurous–reckless, confident–conceited, persistent–stubborn) are expected to covary. Implicit personality theories, however, should not simply reflect correlations among semantically similar adjectives. There must be unique person-specific components of the inferred *relations* among traits (De Soto, Hamilton, & Taylor, 1985). Implicit personality theories should reflect a more typological approach in which people are said to think of others in terms of "person types," such as prototypes (e.g., Ashmore, 1981; Hamilton & Trolier, 1986; Taylor & Crocker, 1981). The traits that compose the same "person type" will be seen as related and causally interconnected (Anderson & Sedikides, 1991; Cantor & Mischel, 1977; Schneider & Blankmeyer, 1983; Sedikides & Anderson, 1994). When perceivers view an individual exhibiting certain traits and behaviors, they try to match these to a prototype. If the observed behaviors and traits match well with the prototype, missing information about the person is filled in by using that prototype (Schneider & Blankmeyer, 1983). Thus an implicit personality theory is an *organizational structure that contains the attributes associated with a specific person type and the relationships (causal interconnectedness) between those attributes*. Triggering one of the attributes can trigger them all through their association together via the theory.

Theories about Significant Others

As noted earlier in regard to relational schemas, one group of people for whom we have mental representations stored in memory are significant others. Whereas implicit personality theories are theories we have about generalized types of people (e.g., women, extraverts, egalitarians, geeks), we also have cognitive structures for specific people—most notably those people who are central to our everyday lives and those who occupy a favored status in our hierarchy of people (friends, parents, spouses, siblings, grandparents, lovers, mentors, etc.). Thus these are exemplars. So, we may ask, what is so special about exemplars that denote significant others? Andersen and Cole (1990) propose that mental representations of significant others have rich associations. Significant-other representations have feelings, motivations, and roles related to them; they contain more knowledge about internal states than representations of nonsignificant others do (e.g., Andersen, Glassman, & Gold, 1998; Prentice, 1990). In addition, perceivers will spontaneously list a greater number of distinctive features to characterize a significant other. These features are distinctive in that they are less likely to be associated with stereotypes and traits, but characterize something unique about the person. Finally, given how relevant such individuals are to perceivers' own emotional and motivational outcomes, perceivers are likely to try hard to make sense of and understand their significant others (e.g., Read & Miller, 1989). This richness and distinctiveness in significant-other representations suggest that they have greater structural complexity than other types of mental representations (e.g., Andersen & Klatzky, 1987).

Chen (2003) argues that perceivers are particularly likely to have theories stored about their significant others, and that these theories play an important role in person perception. First, what evidence is there for theories about significant others? Chen examined whether mental representations of significant others are best thought of as lists of features about a person (e.g., "Dad is outgoing and extraverted") or as theories about why a person has certain features (e.g., "Dad is outgoing and extraverted because he likes to have fun"). The existence of theories as part of one's mental representation was measured by examining the extent to which certain types of IF-THEN relations are present in the cognitive structure. By IF-THEN relations, Chen refers to the notion that a causal relationship exists between some state (IF) and some response (THEN). For example, the mental representation would not simply contain the knowledge that "Dad likes to have fun" or "Dad is extraverted." It would contain a relational clause that says, "IF Dad is at a party, THEN Dad likes to have fun." IFs are the situations people encounter ("IF at a party . . . ," "IF at work . . ."), and THENs are the responses observed in those situations (" . . . THEN he is extraverted," " . . . THEN he is focused and serious"). What is important here is that not all IF-THEN relationships are considered theories. Simply noting an association between two events does not make a theory. It requires the inference of a psychological state as a mediator and cause of the relationship. A theory specifies not only what the trait or behavior is, but when and why the trait or behavior can be expected to be elicited. When an IF-THEN relationship is mediated by psychological states that serve as the causal link between them, a theory is said to exist. "IF Dad is at a party, THEN he is extraverted" is turned into a theory when feelings, goals, and expectancies about "Dad" serve as the causal link connecting the IF and the THEN. Thus, to test for the presence of a theory, Chen looked to see the types of causes people would generate for IF-THEN statements about significant others (versus nonsignificant others).

Chen (2003) asked research participants to read a list of "IF" statements that specified specific situations, such as "IF at a party . . . ," and asked participants to complete each sentence with a response ("THEN . . ."). They were asked to do this with a significant other as the person whose behavior was being described, with a member of a stereotyped group as the person whose behavior was being described, and with a nonsignificant other as the person being described. This produced sets of statements such as "IF at a party, THEN Dad talks to everyone." If they could not think of a relevant response, the statement was to be left blank. Next, participants were asked to read each IF-THEN observation they had listed, and to provide a reason for the behavior they described. That is, they were asked to provide a BECAUSE phrase for every behavior (e.g., "IF at a party, THEN Dad talks to everyone BECAUSE . . ."). These served as causal explanations that could then be evaluated to determine the extent to which people implicated psychological states, such as feelings and goals. Chen hypothesized that if participants had theories, psychological states would be listed as the reasons (the BECAUSE) for the link between the IF and THEN. As an example, a BECAUSE reflecting a mediating psychological state (and hence a theory about the person) would be "IF at a party, THEN Dad talks to everyone BECAUSE he is worried that others do not like him." The psychological state of insecurity is the theoretical link between the situation and the behavior observed. An example that would not reflect a mediating psychological cause would be "IF at a party, THEN Dad talks to everyone BECAUSE it is his job to do so." The results revealed that participants generated more BECAUSE statements (explanations) for significant others. More importantly, the reasons offered in the explanations for significant others mentioned psychological states a greater proportion of the time than responses made for stereotyped and nonsignificant others.

This work illustrates that people seem to include theories in their mental representations of significant others to a greater extent than they do for nonsignificant others. The next question that logically comes to mind is this: What consequences of having such theories exist for social cognition? Chen (2001) posits that these theories of significant others can be triggered by strangers. *People who for some reason call to mind significant others will be reacted to in a way that is influenced by theories about these significant others!* If a person reminds you of your mother, you may assume this person has traits, features, and behaviors associated with your mother that have not been revealed. Why? Your theory of "mother" gets triggered and applied to the new person. You transfer the qualities that define your theory of "mother" to this new person. Andersen and Glassman (1996) have referred to this process as *transference*, using a term borrowed from clinical psychology (e.g., Freud, 1912/1958) but giving it a social-cognitive twist. In this context, *transference* refers to the perceiver's activation of a mental representation of a significant other containing features and theories about that person, which then causes the perceiver to rely on those features and theories when interpreting the behavior of the new person. The perceiver acts in a fashion consistent with how he/she would act toward the significant other, perhaps displaying unusual affection or disaffection to someone the perceiver barely knows. As the Lyle Lovett song goes, "I married her just because she looks like you."

Chen (2001) describes research that illustrates this transference effect. Research participants were asked to list features describing a significant other, such as "Dad is an extravert." Then, later in the year, so as to remove any possibility for the participants to link the two experimental sessions, participants were brought back to the lab for an ostensibly different experiment. The participants were then asked to "meet" several fictional target persons by being presented with a series of descriptions. However, some of the fictional targets were described as having some of the features matching what a participant had earlier said about a significant other (thus the materials were prepared specifically for each person in the experiment). These were believed to trigger the representation of the significant other and the accompanying theories one has about that significant other. Chen then tested to see whether those representations of the significant other were used in describing the fictional person. A procedure similar to that used by Cantor and Mischel (1977, described earlier) was used. Participants were asked to complete a memory test about each fictional target person. They were presented with a series of descriptive sentences and asked to rate how confident they were that the description was one they had earlier learned about the fictional person. Some of the statements were ones that were actually presented earlier; others were not presented earlier, but were statements a participant had listed as being descriptive of his/her significant other. Participants had greater confidence in statements about a fictional person that were true of a significant other but that were never stated as being true about the fictional person when the fictional person had previously been described using other features known to be true of the significant other. Transference of traits was occurring from a significant other to a fictional person via the theory a participant had about the significant other.

Action Identification

Any given behavior can be identified at various levels of interpretation, ranging from detailed descriptions of behavior focusing on the mechanics of the action (i.e., explaining how the act was completed), to more abstract identities explaining why a behavior was conducted and with what effect (i.e., explaining the consequences of the action). For example, "putting a stamp on an envelope" is a lower-level identity than "sending a message," yet each is equally valid in explaining the very same action. The same act can mean very different things to two different people, and can even mean two different things to the same person at two points in time. One may start with the categorization of one's behavior as "sending a message," only to have that categorization turn to "putting on a stamp" as one searches in vain for the stamp that one needs to send the message. Categorizing behavior starts with the realization that any action can be categorized in multiple ways according to the level of specificity with which the action is described. Vallacher and Wegner (1985) referred to this process of categorizing an action at a certain level of specificity in some hierarchy (from detailed to abstract identities) as *action identification*. Essential to this categorization is the notion that only one identification for an action is made at any moment. That is, people adopt a single, prepotent identity for an action.

The level at which behavior is categorized, and the meaning attached to the behavior as a result of that categorization, are often dependent on one's naive theories about what the appropriate level of analysis/identification is. Is it best to focus on the most mechanistic level, the most abstract, or somewhere in between? One's theory of the appropriate level of action identification is said to be linked to the difficulty of the action (Vallacher & Wegner, 1987). Effortful and difficult actions are typically identified in low-level terms, whereas practiced and effortless actions are typically identified in higher-level terms. Thus naive theories specify that it can be advantageous to use lower-level action identification when one is learning a new task. Thinking about the mechanics of one's action on an unfamiliar and difficult task will make it easier to perform the action. When learning to dance a waltz, one must focus on the exact movement of each foot at each point in time. Identifying the behavior at this mechanistic level is necessary to perform the behavior successfully, even if the behavior is not enacted smoothly (my own wedding video provides evidence of this!). However, using an inappropriate theory of action identification can result in a debilitated performance. One skilled at the waltz will suffer if focused on mechanics. For example, self-focused attention, while advantageous for a novice, can be devastating when one is already skilled in a domain (e.g., Vallacher, Wegner, & Samoza, 1989). Baumeister and Steinhilber (1984) have proposed that this is what sometimes causes athletes to commit unusual errors and to "choke" under pressure. The pressure causes one to focus attention on the self, which in turn leads one to an unnatural (for skilled behavior) attention to the mechanics and details of one's behavior. This shift in action identification causes behavior that is normally routine to become strained and disrupted. An experienced tennis player, for example, is better off concentrating on "beating the opponent" (a higher-level action identity) than on "hitting the ball" (Vallacher & Wegner, 1985).

People prefer to think about behavior at a level that provides comprehensive psychological meaning, and low-level action identification does not provide a very satisfying way of thinking about one's own behavior or as providing sufficient meaning (Vallacher & Wegner, 1987). Indeed, when experimenters force people to think about behavior in low-level terms, people seem to seek out cues of higher-level meaning in the environment (Vallacher & Wegner, 1987). Higher-level action identities can define the actor as well as the action, and essentially tell us about the superordinate goals of the actor. For this reason, naive theories of action identification point the person toward a somewhat more abstract level of identification. Theories that point to lower-level identities can be prompted in certain contexts and with certain behaviors, but naive theories more generally point away from a focus on the lowest levels of abstraction. Rather than "moving our lips" or "making utterances," we are "being supportive" and "providing words of comfort." This level of identifying action—not too abstract, not too focused—is what people use.

COGNITIVE EFFICIENCY OR COGNITIVE MISERLINESS?

We begin with what seems a paradox. The world of experience of any man is composed of a tremendous array of discriminably different objects, events, people, impressions. There are estimated to be more than 7 million discriminable colors alone . . . [and even subtle differences] we are capable of seeing, for human beings have an exquisite capacity for making distinctions. But were we to utilize fully our capacity for registering the differences in things and to respond to each event encountered as unique, we would soon be overwhelmed by the complexity of our environment. . . . The resolution of this seeming paradox—the existence of discrimination capacities which, if fully used, would make us slaves to the particular—is achieved by man's capacity to categorize. To categorize is to render discriminably different things equivalent, to group the objects and events and people around us into classes and to respond to them in terms of their class membership rather than their uniqueness.

—BRUNER, GOODNOW, and AUSTIN (1956, p. 1)

In the quote above, the stimulus world is characterized as millions of items that bombard our senses; without limiting the intake, imposing structure on it from within, we will find our experience chaotic and meaningless. James (1907/1991) had earlier put forth these sentiments when he described experience as "a motley which we have to unify by our wits" (p. 76). Lippmann (1922, p. 55) similarly stated that our senses are met by the "great blooming, buzzing confusion of the outer world" and echoed James's notion that we must limit the intake. We handle the confusion of the stimulus world not by scrutinizing each element in it, but by choosing what to attend to, that "which we have picked out in the form stereotyped for us" (p. 55). Allport (1954, pp. 169–170; emphasis in original) summarized this perspective: "Outer reality is in itself chaotic—full of too many potential meanings. We have to *simplify* in order to live; we need stability in our perceptions. At the same time we have an insatiable hunger for *explanations*. We like nothing left dangling."

Yet if we hunger for explanations, why not pursue the best ones? If we have the power to make extremely subtle discriminations between objects, distinguishing among 7 million colors, why can some of us not distinguish between a Sikh and a Muslim? Why rely so much on schemas to make sense of the world and to make inferences/predictions about the people we encounter, when we have the cognitive ability to think in much finer-grained detail and complexity? We focus next on two principles that help to explain why we are not always "accuracy seekers" and why we instead rely heavily on inferences about new stimuli made from prior knowledge.

The Principle of Limited Capacity

We humans are *bounded* in our mental abilities. The stimuli present in any situation are too numerous and complex for total representation by the information-processing system. We only have the ability to process a subset of the total amount of stimuli from the "great blooming, buzzing confusion of the outer world." Most of the information striking our senses must be filtered out (see Broadbent, 1958; Bruner, 1957; Deutsch & Deutsch, 1963; Treisman & Geffen, 1967), leaving only a fraction of the total stimuli to be consciously considered. However, just because some information passes through this attentional filter, it does not guarantee that this information will be analyzed and exhaustively deliberated upon. It may not be feasible to deliberate upon this information because we lack the cognitive *capacity* to do so. We humans have only so much mental energy we can devote to performing a task. As discussed in Chapter 3, working memory is limited in its capacity. Many cognitive tasks, such as making complex judgments, require mental effort that usurp this limited processing capacity. If the limits of the system are taxed, performance deficits may result, because the requisite capacity is unavailable (e.g., Gilbert, 1989). Time spent working on one cognitive task usurps energy that could be spent working on another task.

Cognitive Load

This state where so much mental effort has been allocated to a cognitive task that it taxes mental resources, diminishing the ability to process information relating to other cognitive tasks, is known as *cognitive load* (it is also called *being cognitively busy* or *cognitive busyness*). Taking the time to assess each new person in his/her full complexity is simply too taxing of mental resources to allow us to perform other tasks needed to prepare behavior. Because we do not have the mental resources to process all the information we desire, we use schemas to help us. Allport (1954, pp. 8–9) asserted:

> Overcategorization is perhaps the commonest trick of the human mind. Given a thimbleful of facts we rush to make generalizations as large as a tub. . . . There is a natural basis for this tendency. Life is so short, and the demands upon us for practical adjustment so great, that we cannot let our ignorance detain us in our daily transactions. We have to decide whether objects are good or bad by classes. We cannot weigh each object in the world by itself. Rough and ready rubrics, however coarse and broad, have to suffice.

If it is in fact the case that processing capacity is bounded, there should be clear, observable effects that signal this state of affairs. If you had previously been exerting mental effort toward evaluating the qualities of a person with whom you were interacting, cognitive load should constrain your ability to continue to operate in this fashion; the resources you would need to perform a task by exerting mental effort would not be available. To function adequately, you would have to develop the ability to perform such tasks using less effort, with, perhaps, a loss of accuracy. Schemas are used as a response to a bounded processing system limited in its capacity.

Seeing Is Believing

Kruglanski and Freund (1983) provided an illustration of the point that a reliance on categories increases when processing capacity is taxed. Participants in their experiment were student-teachers in Israel who were told that the experiment was examining one aspect of a teacher's job, grading students. Instructions informed them that they would evaluate a composition written by an eighth grader for literary excellence, using a scale from 40 (failing) to 100 (excellent). Given that teachers, particularly those who believe that this task is part of their training, need to be explicitly objective and accurate when grading students, one would think that full mental effort would be dedicated to the task, and categorical expectancies would have little to do with the teachers' performance. However, what would happen if teachers, despite having the goal to be objective, were *unable* to exert the processing capacity required to grade accurately?

To test this, the availability of cognitive resources for performing the task was manipulated. Half the participants were told that because of scheduling problems, they only had 10 minutes to read and grade the composition (not enough time to perform the accurate and effortful type of analysis required by the task). The other half were told that they would have an hour, giving the teachers enough time to pursue their goal of providing accurate assessments of the student. The composition participants were asked to grade were identical, except for one thing. Half of the participants were given information suggesting that the student who wrote the composition was an Ashkenazi Jew (a lighter-skinned person of Eastern European descent), and half were led to believe the student was a Sephardi Jew (a darker-skinned person of Spanish descent). Prevailing schemas associated with these categories specified that superior performance should be exhibited by Ashkenazi Jews. The researchers hypothesized that these schema-based expectancies would have little impact when no cognitive load existed, but when capacity was restricted, participants would begin to see what they already believed to be true (rather than what was specified by the actual information). Even though the participants were teachers grading papers, they would be biased. The results revealed that participants rated the Ashkenazi student as better than the Sephardi student, but only when faced with limited capacity. A dramatic difference in grades (80 vs. 64) emerged when time pressure created a situation of bounded mental resources. No difference existed when capacity was available (65 vs. 64).

In summary, strains on our ability to give time and effort to our judgments lead to an increase in schema use. A consequence of this is that we come to see new information in a manner that is consistent with the expectancies provided by our schemas. Thus the old saying "Seeing is believing" takes on new meaning. Rather than meaning that we need to see something in order to believe it, the phrase in this case instead means that we tend to see things in a way consistent with what we already believe. This tendency is exacerbated when we are under cognitive load. However, this raises two important questions: Do we only show an overreliance on schemas when under cognitive load, or do we have as a default way of thinking a tendency to use schemas in describing new information? Second, if this is a default strategy, what does this say about human thought processes—are we lazy or highly evolved (adaptive)?

The Principle of Least Effort

The *principle of least effort* was the label provided by Allport (1954) to describe the fact that, as perceivers, we seek to maximize our outcomes with the least amount of work possible. Chapter 3 has referred to this as *satisficing*. This principle, therefore, provides an answer to the first question posed above. It states that the information-processing default is to use simplifying strategies. Yet this does not mean we are doomed to think only categorically. As Chapter 5 will address quite explicitly, we are certainly capable of altering the amount of cognitive effort we choose to dedicate to a task, and do so quite readily when goals and circumstances dictate. However, the default position seems to be that when we could either exert more or less energy in thinking about our social world, we choose to exert less. We typically choose to lean on the prior knowledge that we have gathered through a lifetime of experience.

Throughout this chapter, the various ways in which schemas (and prototypes, exemplars, scripts, and theories) help people to produce reasonable (sufficient) judgments have been given in italics. These functions of schemas have revealed how they allow perceivers to accomplish many, if not all, of the goals of person perception with relatively little effort. Schemas do the following:

1. Allow people to detect, identify, and make judgments about schema-relevant behavior or attributes. They provide a structure or framework on which to hang new experiences.
2. Allow people to identify and react to schema-relevant information easily and quickly.
3. Lead people to see and remember information about people in a schema-consistent manner.
4. Are resistant to change and deflect the reception of information that is counterschematic. People resist information that is contrary to what their schemas would suggest to be true.
5. Allow people to make predictions about future behavior readily and accurately.
6. Lead people to act in ways consistent with the predictions and inferences afforded by the schema (such as when transference occurs).
7. Allow people to generate missing information (fill in gaps in knowledge) and to generate additional information (inferences). Thus information not observed can be confused with information found in a schema.
8. Often operate implicitly, and can even be applied to making sense of processes that are themselves implicit and undetected.

However, the fact that people rely on schemas and follow the principle of least effort does not address the second question posed above: *Why* do they rely on minimal amounts of effort in thoughts about the social world (given that humans have minds capable of thinking with much greater complexity)? Two opposing answers to this question have been suggested. The first makes use of the principle of limited capacity. It states that because limited cognitive resources are available to dedicate to mental tasks (such as thinking about what other people are like and why they act as they do), this default style of thinking has emerged "in the service of cognitive and emotional economy" (Jones & Thibaut, 1958, p. 152). This poses a functional account of how people cope with limited resources: They seek to be economical in the use of limited mental resources by avoiding effortful expenditures of cognitive energy (by developing simplifying strategies). In this account, least effortful processing is an adaptive response to limited capacity, an evolutionary step that promotes survival by providing needed information quickly.

However, an equally plausible explanation as to why people seem to use as little effort as possible when thinking about others (and to rely overly on schemas and preconceived conceptualizations) is that people are simply lazy. Laziness would be a viable account for why people seem to use very little effort, if it could be shown that such minimal processing is used even when sufficient resources exist to process information. That is, labeling it as "economical" when people exhibit a failure to use resources for a task and those resources *are available* seems to be a poor choice of labels. Responding with minimal effort when it is possible to act in a mindful, deliberate, and systematic fashion would seem to be better characterized as acting in a fashion that is stingy and miserly in the use of their cognitive abilities.

Let us review each of these accounts as to why people follow the "principle of least effort": laziness/miserliness versus efficiency. Then let us close this section by considering yet a third position, summarized by Sherman (2001). Rather than attempting to explain why people use the least amount of effort possible, Sherman proposes that people do not use the least amount of effort possible, proposing instead that using least effort is something that occurs rarely. People are described as almost always trying hard in their attempts to understand other people, and they apply different strategies and knowledge structures to achieve this. Because of the demands being placed on the processing system or because of the goals individuals may be pursuing, it is often the case that they cannot exert the amount of effort they would desire to exert. But people are described as reacting to these resource constraints and goal constraints by attempting to maximize the information gained for the effort expended. This is the essence of efficiency.

Cognitive Misers

Fiske and Taylor (1984) coined the term *cognitive misers*. The notion of being a cognitive miser implies that because effortless processing is so often needed to cope with situations of stimulus overload, people become overdependent on it. By *overdependence*, it is meant that people exert minimal amounts of mental effort even in situations where they could easily exert more effort and arrive at better, more accurate conclusions about the people with whom they interact. Even when stimulus overload does not abound and perceivers can exert their powers of rationality and analysis quite freely, they think and act as if they are bounded in their rationality, simply because this type of responding has become a habit.

Relying on Rules of Thumb Rather Than Thorough Analyses

Consider the case when we categorize someone as attractive. Often we will use our prior expectancies and theories about attractiveness to guide how we interpret what the attractive person is saying. We will do this in lieu of evaluating the content of the person's message. Chaiken (1980) noted that rather than exert the effort to evaluate a message from an attractive person, we instead rely on simple rules of thumb that are associated with a schema about attractive people. In this case, the rule of thumb (theory) is that attractive people are more trustworthy; attractiveness is seen as representative of the communicator's accuracy. This is one reason advertisers choose celebrities to endorse products, even if the reason for a person's celebrity has nothing to do with the service provided by the product! For instance, it is assumed that the attractiveness of

Tiger Woods will allow him to be effective as a car spokesman, leading people to trust his opinion of the quality of the product. This should occur despite the fact that a good-looking golf star does not necessarily have expert advice to offer on the topic of cars.

If such simple rule-based reasoning is capable of guiding our responses, rather than the effortful evaluation of what a person has to say, we should agree more with an attractive person regardless of the content of what that person says (and even if we are not under cognitive load when hearing it). To examine this possibility with another form of attractiveness—likability—Chaiken (1980) asked research participants to listen to a message that came from either a likable or an unlikable person. The likable person was a college administrator who praised the undergraduates from the home institution of the research participants; the unlikable person insulted these same students. In addition to varying how likable the messenger was, Chaiken varied the content of his message—the quality of what he had to say. The person presented either a strong message or a weak message. The results showed that participants were using the likability of the messenger as a proxy for message strength. If they liked the messenger, they agreed with his position, regardless of its quality. If they disliked the messenger, they were unmoved by his position, regardless of its quality. Thus the very same message was either liked or disliked, based on the category to which the speaker had been assigned. Message content was seemingly ignored. Chaiken concluded that people rely on simple rules of thumb, rather than exerting more effort to actually examine the information being put forth.

A Bias for Seeing Expectancy-Congruent Information

We not only have a tendency to rely on schemas when deciding whether to agree with others; we also tend to see information as skewed in a way that supports what we already believe to be true. Several examples of this fact have already been discussed (e.g., Hastorf & Cantril, 1954; Lord, Ross, & Lepper, 1979). In fact, Ross, Lepper, and Hubbard (1975) found that a schema perseveres even when the original basis for the schema is found out to be blatantly false. People were provided with a false belief (e.g., "Our special test reveals that you are a socially sensitive person, much more than the average person"), and a schema surrounding this belief was developed. Later, participants were told that the test serving as the basis for this self-belief was totally bogus. Yet people still believed that they held the attribute in question. Presumably, although no evidence to support this schema had been provided and disconfirming evidence had been provided, participants generated their own confirming evidence by selectively scanning their past for examples that would confirm the schema. They saw what the schema said they should, and continued to believe this was characteristic of them, even when they discovered that the basis for the schema was a blatant lie.

A bias to favor information congruent with expectations (i.e., information consistent with existing schemas) can be seen in many different ways in which people think about the reasons for other people's actions. Let us focus here on two demonstrations. The first illustrates how impressions of other people are biased by schemas; the second illustrates how the type of information people seek to find out about others they plan to meet is biased by schemas.

Biased Impression Formation. Wyer and Srull (1989) proposed that if perceivers learn information about a new person and are then asked to form an impression of this person, "they will search for a general trait or an evaluative concept that is relevant to this judgment. If they find such a concept, they will use its implications for the judgment without reviewing the specific behaviors on which the concept is based" (p. 59). Thus behaviors incongruent with prior expectancies may not be used in judgment, which instead tends to rely on the gross application of the category. Exceptions to this tendency naturally exist (it is a tendency, not a law), and the conditions under which people do not apply categories and do consult the specific behaviors the new individual exhibits (including those incongruent with the schema) are discussed in Chapter 5. Here we focus on the pervasive tendency to rely on existing categories to shape impressions.

A classic demonstration was provided by Darley and Gross (1983). Research participants were asked to watch a videotape of a young girl named Hannah. Half of the participants first saw Hannah playing in an affluent neighborhood where she was said to live; the other participants saw Hannah in what appeared to be a poor neighborhood. This (along with information about her parents' occupations) served to manipulate the schema that Hannah was associated with (rich vs. poor). Schemas, in turn, led half the participants to have a set of expectancies associated with affluent children and the other half of the participants to have expectancies associated with poor children. Participants then saw another videotape of Hannah at school, taking a test said to assess academic ability. Importantly, the performance that was observed provided no conclusive evidence regarding Hannah's abilities. She was seen correctly answering both difficult and simple questions, as well as failing to answer such questions correctly. As we would expect if people were relying on schemas to make judgments, the people who had categorized Hannah as wealthy formed an impression of her as having above-average academic ability, based on her test performance. People who categorized her as poor formed an impression of her as having below-average academic ability, despite using the same videotape on which to base this impression.

This reliance on schemas in describing others is seen not only in the types of broad judgments people make about the nature of others' character and abilities, but in the subtle ways in which people describe others' behavior. Maass, Milesi, Zabbini, and Stahlberg (1995) have demonstrated that schema-consistent behavior is described in a more abstract way than behavior that does not fit a schema. The reason for this is believed to be a bias people have to confirm what they expect and to maintain their schemas. Maintaining schemas can be accomplished by the types of impressions people form and the manner with which people describe the behavior they observe. An impression that relies on abstract descriptions is harder to overturn and more resilient than one based on concrete descriptions. Therefore, consistent information is more likely to be described in abstract ways relative to inconsistent information, thus making it more resilient.

Maass and colleagues (1995) suggest that if one observes an undesirable behavior from a person for whom one has a negative expectancy, this behavior is consistent with an existing expectancy. Such expectancy-consistent actions are then described as being caused by reasons that are more abstract than when a behavior that is inconsistent with the expectancy (a positive behavior) is observed. For example, let's say you observe exactly the same behavior from two different people at two points in time: Each person is driving 110 miles per hour on a dark, wet road that has a 55-mile-per-hour speed limit. Let's also assume that you think this is negative behavior. If you have a negative expectancy about the first person, such as thinking he/she is a reckless person, you would be likely to maintain that expectancy in the manner by which you describe the behavior. You would use an abstract description, such as "That person was being reckless." However, if you had no such expectancy for the second person performing the very same behavior, or if you had the opposite expectancy (such as "That person is very responsible"), the type of description you might use would be different—more concrete, such as "That person was driving excessively fast."

Wigboldus, Semin, and Spears (2000) have further illustrated the schema-confirming nature of the way in which we describe behavior and form impressions. Wigboldus and colleagues noted that when a person acts in a manner consistent with our schemas, we describe that behavior as being caused by stable personality traits (thus confirming our expectancy about the person), more so than when we observe the same person acting in a manner inconsistent with our schemas. Research participants who were asked to communicate a message about a person for whom they had an existing expectancy tended to phrase messages about the expectancy-consistent behavior of this person in terms of traits (more than they did with messages describing the person's inconsistent behavior). Resulting from this communication style, communicators, as well as message recipients, used traits to describe expectancy-consistent messages more than they were used to describe inconsistent messages. The restriction of explanations for consistent behavior to descriptions in terms of stable traits led to further support for the existing expectancy. Hence, it led to expectancy maintenance.

Biased Hypothesis Testing and Information Gathering. *Biased hypothesis testing* refers to the tendency to seek evidence that confirms one's existing expectancies (hypotheses) and to neglect the gathering of evidence/information that would disconfirm one's expectancies. This is a "bias" because it is a less than advantageous way to gather information if one is concerned with diagnosing whether one's expectancies are correct. The best way to test whether an expectancy is correct is to see whether it can be proven wrong. It only takes one instance of opposing evidence to conclude that the hypothesis/expectancy is wrong; yet one could gather supportive evidence all day, and it would not necessarily mean that the expectancy is true. If people were indeed cognitive misers, this would suggest that they would prefer not to exert the effort to revise and update their expectancies, and would instead choose a strategy of biased hypothesis testing. Instead of using a strategy that would actually help them accomplish the goal of finding out whether an expectancy is correct or false, a strategy that would leave them anchored to the existing expectancy would be used.

Evidence for just such a bias was provided by Snyder and Swann (1978), who asked participants to test the hypothesis that a fellow student, who was supposedly waiting in the next room, was an extravert. The participants were then given a short profile to read that described the category "extraverts" and established a set of expectancies regarding extraverted people. The participants were next given a list of questions to read that were designed to elicit evidence that a person was either an extravert (e.g., "What do you like about parties?") or an introvert (e.g., "What factors make it hard for you to open up to people?"). From these questions, the participants were to select 12 to use in testing the hypothesis that the person in the next room was an extravert. The results showed that participants tended to choose questions that would provide evidence in support of the hypothesis, rather than those that would contradict it. They did not try to find out whether the person was an introvert (which could provide direct evidence that the person was not an extravert); they instead chose questions asking the person to describe instances in which he/she acted in an extraverted fashion. The answers received to these questions generally provided evidence in support of the hypothesis, regardless of whether the person answering the questions was actually an extravert. The tendency to seek confirmatory evidence when testing a hypothesis was found even when participants were offered cash prizes for the most diagnostic questions.

However, it should be noted here that people are apparently not doomed to only seeking information that confirms their schemas and expectancies. Although people may avoid seeking evidence that proves the very opposite of what they already believe (such as testing to see whether someone is an introvert when he/she is already believed to be an extravert), they are capable of seeking information that is more diagnostic, rather than merely trying to support what they already expect. Trope and Bassok (1982) suggest that people often use what these authors call *diagnosing strategies* (or *diagnostic hypothesis testing*) when testing their expectancies. A diagnosing strategy is one in which people attempt to ascertain the probability that a behavior is caused by an underlying disposition. Rather than merely seeking to confirm the underlying disposition, the focus is on the probability that the disposition exists. A diagnostic strategy for hypothesis testing would be one where a question that is asked, or evidence that is examined, is capable of discriminating between the given hypothesis and some alternative. Thus a question that will provide an answer in which an extravert is likely to respond one way and an introvert is likely to respond another way is a diagnostic question. Trope and Bassok provided research participants with a hypothesis to test: "Is the person you are going to meet an 'analytic' person as opposed to an 'intuitive' person?" They then provided participants with a set of information to be used in testing this hypothesis. Some of the information was diagnostic, in that an analytic person would answer one way while an intuitive person would answer another way. Some of the information was confirmatory, in that it seemed to be true of analytic people. Thus the participants could differentiate between information that merely confirmed the expectancy and information that was diagnostic (helping them distinguish between the two types of people). The results suggested that people prefer diagnostic information over information that is simply confirmatory.

One might detect an immediate concern with this research. Snyder and Swann (1978) looked at how people tested whether a person was an exemplar of a well-known schema—extraverted people. Trope and Bassok (1982) looked at how people tested whether a person was a member of some schema that might not be so well defined (analytic people vs. intuitive people). It could be that because this schema was so poorly defined, people needed to use some other strategy to test their hypothesis in order to feel as if their judgments were reasonable ones. Diagnosing may be more likely when schemas are weak, and a confirmatory strategy may be the norm when schemas are better developed and resistant to change. Trope and Bassok conducted more experiments that were closer in nature to those of Snyder and Swann, in order to examine the types of hypothesis-testing strategies people would use. Participants had to test the hypothesis that a given person was an extravert. This time, the results were mixed: People did choose diagnostic questions. When such questions were of a highly diagnostic nature (participants could easily distinguish between the two alternative categories), they were embraced. However, there still was a tendency for people to prefer hypothesis-confirming questions to ones that disconfirmed the hypothesis. The findings suggest that people seek to confirm hypotheses, though they do not totally disregard information that might be inconsistent with the hypothesis if it seems to be highly useful and diagnostic. Otherwise, inconsistent information is not sought out.

Seeing What Isn't There

We not only have a tendency to see what we expect to see, to focus on the available evidence that is consistent with what we already believe to be true; we also have a tendency to see evidence for the things we believe to be true *even when such evidence does not exist.* As an example, if you believe that women are less skilled at computational tasks than men, then you might start to believe you see evidence that the women you work with are actually less able to solve problems that involve computation than the men. If this evidence actually exists, your observation might be considered astute, but if this evidence is "imagined," then you have incorrectly shown bias toward the women in your office.

This is particularly likely to occur when certain conditions are met. For example, if you are a computer programmer, the likelihood of bumping into a woman at work is small, and the likelihood of a programmer's having problems performing simple computations is small; women and errors of simple computation are rare events at computer-programming jobs. When two rare events happen at the same time, we have a tendency to see them as being linked. Thus, even if a woman in your office makes an error as often as a man, because the presence of female programmers and errors of simple computation are rare events, you will be more likely to see these two events as linked and more likely to remember the woman's failure than a man's failure. Thus you come to see a relationship that does not exist and for which there is no evidence. Such bias is experienced by women and ethnic minorities quite frequently in the workplace.

Chapman (1967) called the incorrect assumption of a high correlation between two things that are unusual or rare an *illusory correlation.* The initial evidence for this effect was provided in an experiment where research participants were presented with pairs of words as part of a learning experiment. Chapman found that when attempting to remember the word pairs, the participants overestimated the frequency of presentation for word pairs that contained two exceptionally long words. The conclusion was that the unusual length of the words attracted attention. This increased attention led to increased memory for these words, and the subsequent assumption that if these words were more memorable, they must have been seen more frequently. In actuality, these words were presented in pairs no more often than any other pair of words. Hamilton and Gifford (1976) argued that similar processes account for why members of a majority group associate negative behaviors with minority groups. Both are infrequently encountered (or at least negative acts are encountered less than positive ones, and members of a minority group are seen less often than those in the majority group). Thus, if a negative behavior is performed by a minority group member, this pairing of unusual events makes it especially memorable and produces the illusory correlation that they frequently co-occur. Minorities are seen as performing more negative behaviors than others, even if base rates do not warrant this conclusion. Majority group members see a relationship that is not real.

Hamilton and Rose (1980) used the phenomenon of illusory correlation to demonstrate how people distort evidence to fit their expectancies—to see what isn't there. They asserted that a stereotype (or at least an incorrect stereotype) is essentially an illusory correlation in which a perceived relationship exists between membership in a particular group (e.g., women) and a set of traits (e.g., being emotional, sensitive, and poor at math). They predicted that because of illusory correlations, if one of the items in the correlation is activated (such as group membership), then people will pay more attention to the other item in the correlation—the traits and behaviors that are expected to accompany it. Thus, when people encounter a member of a stereotyped group (e.g., a woman), this leads them to think that the behaviors and traits supporting the stereo-type (e.g., poor math skills) are more prevalent than they really are—even if stereotype-consistent behaviors occur just as often as, and no more often than, stereotype-irrelevant behaviors. Similarly, even if the person acts in a manner inconsistent with the stereotype just as often as in a way that is irrelevant to the stereotype, the stereotype-inconsistent behaviors will come to be seen as less prevalent than the irrelevant behaviors. People will perceive a correlation (albeit a negative one) where one does not really exist. Illusory correlation leads to a manipulation of the available evidence on which people base their impressions of others, so that they (1) see what is not there, and (2) do not see what is there (when what is present is contradictory to stereotypes).

Hamilton and Rose (1980, Experiment 2) illustrated this in an experiment in which information about two people was presented to research participants. The two people were members of groups for which stereotypes exist—doctors and salesmen. The infor-mation that was presented was either neutral/irrelevant in regard to the stereotype (such as a doctor being described as "humorous") or consistent with the stereotype (such as a doctor being described as "helpful"). Hamilton and Rose reasoned that ste-reotypes would lead the participants to see an illusory correlation between doctors and traits consistent with the stereotype (e.g., being helpful). Participants received informa-tion that supported stereotypes, yet they distorted the information so that it came to be seen as even more prevalent (and thus providing strong evidence to confirm the stereo-type) than it really was. For example, for some of the participants the trait "helpful" was presented six times over the course of the experiment, and in four of the six cases it was used to describe the doctor (and twice to describe a salesman). Thus "helpful" was asso-ciated more closely with the doctor than with the salesman. The same procedure was used for presenting neutral information. The trait "humorous" was presented six times over the course of the experiment. For some participants it was used to describe the doctor in four of the six cases, and was thus used more often in describing the doctor.

What is critical about this experiment for our current discussion is the fact that the stereotypic trait (e.g., being helpful) appeared no more often in describing one of the people (e.g., the doctor) than the neutral trait (e.g., being humorous). Yet the findings were strikingly clear: There was a bias toward remembering that the doctor was helpful rather than humorous. The actual information in no way suggested that one of these traits was more prevalent than the other, yet the stereotype-consistent trait was remem-bered as being more prevalent. Although it was true that "helpful" was used more often to describe the doctor than the salesman, so too was "humorous." Thus it was accurate to remember the doctor as more helpful than the salesman, but it was inaccurate to recall the doctor as more helpful than humorous. And it was also inaccurate to assume that the evidence that the doctor was helpful (four of six traits) was more prevalent than it actually was (such as remembering "helpful" as being presented five or six times instead of the actual number, four).

Cognitive Efficiency

The principle of least effort need not imply that people choose not to be accurate and effortful in expenditure of mental capacity because they are lazy. It is possible that least-effort processing is an adaptive/functional response to the everyday realities of having limited capacity. Just as natural resources need to be conserved, mental resources must not be wasted. This is not to suggest that being accurate is bad or wasteful. But pursuing accuracy in a fashion that is demanding of mental energy is not economical. If cognitive load disables the ability to engage in effortful processing, and life is essentially a state of cognitive load, then to get through life people need to be able to operate well on automatic pilot. They must be able to rely on prior experience and well-learned patterns of responding at the cost of exerting greater mental energy, especially when the over-allocation of attention and mental effort to some tasks drains cognitive resources. As Bruner (1957, p. 142) stated, "the ability to use minimal cues quickly in categorizing the events of the environment is what gives the organism its lead time in adjusting to events. Pause and close inspection inevitably cut down on this precial interval for adjustment."

Thus maybe people are being efficient in their allocation of attentional and processing resources; they are being economical and conservationist. Tajfel (1969) stated that the effort used to pursue meaning "works within the limits imposed by the capacities of the individual" (p. 79), and "for reasons of cognitive economy [meaning] will tend toward as much simplification as the situation allows for" (p. 92). However, despite its being described as economy-seeking, the mind is not like a nation's economy. A national economy can spend more than its resources and exist in a state of debt. The mind must always operate within a balanced budget. People do not have more resources to expend than those they are born with, and those must be utilized to their fullest extent. Thus people evolve strategies that tend to work (even if these are not the most accurate). They attempt to get solutions and make judgments that are sufficiently good, that allow them to act appropriately—and to the extent that less effort can accomplish this, it is utilized. But if people are being economical, surely there must be some *savings* that can be observed. The resources not used for working on one task must be available and able to aid in the performance of a second task. This is the type of mental economy that truly would be adaptive, where the savings from categorical thinking could be spent in effortful processing elsewhere.

The functional account for categorical thinking, therefore, claims that schema use has benefits to the perceiver: Mental energy and resources are available to be put to use elsewhere. For example, when a person is working on two tasks simultaneously, the cognitive load associated with this multitasking makes it difficult to succeed on either task. This is a resource allocation problem. If schemas could be used to work on one of the tasks, this would "free up" energy that could help with the other task. Mental effort saved on one task could be transferred to the other. Thus, particularly under cognitive overload, schemas are "tools" used to facilitate processing.

Efficiency Is Evidenced by Increased Performance on a Secondary Task

In support of this functionalist account, Macrae, Milne, and Bodenhausen (1994) asked research participants to perform two tasks simultaneously. The first task was to watch a computer monitor and use the traits that were being presented about a person to form an impression of that person. The second task had them simultaneously listening to a tape-recorded description of the geography and economy of Indonesia—a topic that they did not know much, if anything, about (so they would need to listen closely). It was arranged so that 10 traits about a person would appear, and then 10 traits about another person would appear, and so on. For each set of traits, half of the traits provided were consistent with a schema. For example, all participants were be told to form an impression of John and were given these traits: "rebellious," "aggressive," "dishonest," "untrustworthy," "dangerous," "lucky," "observant," "modest," "optimistic," and "curious." However, half of the participants were provided with a category label—for example, "John is a skinhead"—to help them with the impression formation task, while the other half were not given a category label. Therefore, for half of the participants the category label would serve as an organizing structure to make sense out of those traits (i.e., to make them seem as if they go more naturally together). The researchers predicted that, given this set of events, two things should occur. First, people with category labels should be able to remember more traits, since they would have their schemas to help them. Second, even though they were doing better on this first task, they should also do better on the second task. The savings in effort from relying on the schema could be used to put toward the other task of learning about Indonesia.

To examine this, the research participants were asked both to recall the traits that had been presented about a given person and to answer questions in a multiple-choice test (20 questions) on Indonesia (e.g., "Jakarta is found on which coast of Java?"). The results showed the predicted effects: People with category labels performed better on the unrelated, second task. They got over two questions more correct than people who were not using schemas. The savings from having used a schema was spent on the task that cost more mental effort.

Efficiency Is Evidenced by Better Recall for Seemingly Discarded Information

The evidence presented in support of the cognitive miser view has asserted that people are biased toward using information that is congruent with their existing schemas. Srull and Wyer (1989, p. 61) have summarized this point in Postulate 5 of their person memory model: "Once an evaluative concept of a person is formed, the person's behaviors are interpreted in terms of it. The ease of interpreting behaviors in terms of the concept, and therefore the strength of their association with it, is an increasing function of the behaviors' evaluative consistency with the concept." This conclusion is consistent with the pioneering work of Asch (1946), where individuals were shown to be skilled at taking disparate sets of traits about people and forming a coherent impression. One might assume that such research illustrates that incongruent information is discarded. After all, it is not used in judgment. However, just because information consistent with schemas is used in judgment does not by itself provide evidence that information incongruent with schemas is ignored. In fact, exactly the opposite may be true: Perhaps incongruent information is actually focused on quite intensely, thought about deeply, and carefully considered. Srull and Wyer address this in their Postulates 6 and 7:

> If a clear evaluative concept of a person cannot be extracted on the basis of the initial information received, people who are uncertain about the person's traits will think about the behaviors they have encoded in terms of each trait in relation to one another. . . . Behaviors of the person that are evaluatively inconsistent with this concept are thought about in relation to other behaviors that have evaluative implications in an attempt to reconcile their occurrence. (pp. 61–62)

Inconsistent information needs to be explained. Rather than ignoring it, people start attending to and thinking about such information, to figure out how it is possible that a person can perform such incongruent acts. When the information conveyed by the observed behaviors is consistent with a schema, then people do not need to exert the effort of contemplating these behaviors too deeply. It is easily assimilated to the structure. However, inconsistent information is problematic. As Asch (1946) claimed, perhaps people try to make the inconsistencies "fit" so that they do not seem inconsistent and a coherent impression can be formed. However, imagine the cognitive work required of Asch's research participants to be able to unify a set of disparate traits in a meaningful way. It was presumably quite strenuous, especially if the observed traits and behaviors were evaluatively inconsistent with the schema (such as when a cheap person acted generously, or a violent person acted tenderly). This discussion suggests two important points. First, if people are cognitive misers, then they should be unlikely to process inconsistent information. If we can establish that people are processing inconsistent information, then it would suggest that people are not acting miserly and that this is not the appropriate metaphor for describing social cognition. Second, if this process of considering inconsistent information is strenuous, then if people are under cognitive load or taxed, then they should be unable to do it (thus perhaps giving the appearance that they are being miserly and wanting to use least effort, when in fact they are wanting to be effortful and nonmiserly, but are blocked from doing so).

The emerging argument here is that using schemas in producing a judgment is easy, while integrating the incongruent pieces of information is difficult and requires effort (Stangor & Duan, 1991). Though discarded from judgment, schema-incongruent information may not be totally discarded. Perhaps effort has been spent on making sense of and thinking deeply about the inconsistent information (as specified in Srull & Wyer's [1989] Postulates 5, 6, and 7). That is, the bias for using only congruent information in judgment may mask the fact that people do try to make sense of incongruent information. *They spend the mental effort saved from using categories in the judgment task on analyzing the inconsistencies.* If this is true, the integration and coherence making that Asch (1946) discussed—while not reflected in people's use of the inconsistent information in their judgments—should be reflected in their recall. Evidence of increased memory for the inconsistent information discarded from judgment should show that these judgments are not miserly. Instead, people have in fact spent a great deal of effort thinking about the incongruent information (simply choosing not to use the spent effort to incorporate the inconsistencies into judgment). This would result in their processing that information more deeply and making more associative links between the observed behaviors. Following the logic of the associative network models reviewed in Chapter 3, this would deliver superior recall for schema-incongruent information. Thus evidence that schema use is efficient (not miserly) would be provided by a disconnect between what people recall and the judgments they make: Judgment would be biased in a schema-congruent way, recall in a schema-incongruent way.

Consider an example. When your extremely cheap friend Joe decides to buy lunch for the gang, this triggers mental energy aimed at attempting to figure out what accounts for his shortened pockets. A consequence of this greater effort in attempting to resolve the cause of this unexpected event is the increased memory you will have for it—it has been elaborated upon and linked to other items in your mental representation of your friend. However, if your cognitive resources are crunched (say, you are simultaneously thinking about why your date called to cancel for Friday night), you should be unable to expend the effort to note the uniqueness of Joe's current behavior. Your "cheap" friend will suffer the indignity of having his act of generosity going largely unnoticed and unavailable to be recalled at a later point in time. He will forever be seen as a penny-pinching moocher. Conversely, if you have a schema available for making sense of why your date for Friday night cancelled (e.g., "Those liberal, vegetarian, hippie types are so flighty, free-wheeling, and irresponsible"), then the effort saved from thinking about the one task may now free you to once again contemplate Joe's inconsistencies. Even if your impression of Joe does not change, and he still is judged to be a cheap bastard, at least you will have salient memories of the one time he opened his wallet and violated the schema.

The Disconnect between Judgment and Recall. Hastie and Kumar (1979) asked research participants to study six sets of lists of behaviors, with each list containing 20 sentences. Prior to the presentation of the 20 sentences in each set, traits were presented that summarized the gist of the sentences (i.e., they established the trait that the majority of the sentences implied, such as intelligence). In each set, 12 of the sentences implied the same trait, four implied the opposite trait (inconsistent information), and four were neutral pieces of information. The participants were asked both to memorize the behaviors and to form an impression of the person they described. The major finding was that although the judgments made of the person were based on the 12 sentences consistent with the schema, superior recall was found for the items incongruent with the schema (relative to neutral and consistent items). A person characterized by the trait "intelligent" was described to participants. Their memory for this person was more heavily weighted by the information that was *inconsistent* with the trait "intelligent," while the person was at the same time judged to be intelligent. These results indicate a disconnect between what is recalled and the judgment made to characterize a person (e.g., Anderson & Hubert, 1963).

It is important to note a caveat to the finding just reported about the disconnect between the traits that are used in forming a judgment and the traits that are later recalled. In the Hastie and Kumar (1979) experiment, the research participants were asked to form an impression prior to receiving the traits. Therefore, the traits were processed with the goal of forming an impression, and with that impression serving as a means by which to organize the incoming information. Thus the inconsistent traits were processed more deeply because they failed to fit with the impression. But what happens when we do not have the goal of forming an impression, and therefore may not have a schema ready to interpret the incoming information? In such cases, judgment and recall should be very similar: The traits used in judgment should be the same as those we recall. Why? If we have not been forming an impression as we receive the information about the person (what is called *online impression formation*), then the only way we can form an impression is to try to recall what the person is like (what is called *memory-based impression formation*), increasing the likelihood that recall and judgment are similar. Hastie and Park (1986) examined the evidence for this assumption. Research participants were instructed to make a judgment regarding a person's suitability for a job. Half of them knew about the judgment task before receiving any information; the other half found out that they needed to make a judgment only after hearing the information. Thus the latter group needed to construct a judgment after the fact, while the former group formed an impression online. The results revealed that when participants formed judgments online, there was not a positive correlation between what they remembered about the person and the type of judgment they made. However, when they found out about the judgment task after having already heard the information about the person, they were forced to form a memory-based judgment, and a positive correlation between judgment and recall was found.

The Effortful Nature of Inconsistency Resolution. The assumption is that processing information inconsistent with a category is more effortful and less automatic than processing information congruent with the category. Thus using categories in online judgment should make available extra processing resources to be used for resolving inconsistencies. If this is indeed the case, and the recall advantage for inconsistent information is due to this increased depth of processing, people unable to exert the requisite processing should no longer show a recall advantage for inconsistent information.

Bargh and Thein (1985) focused on this question by presenting research participants with information about another person that predominantly favored a particular impression's being formed (e.g., "This person is honest"). Twenty-four sentences describing the person were presented, 12 of which described one trait (e.g., honesty), six of which described an incongruent trait (e.g., dishonesty), and six of which were neutral. The participants were told that their task was to form an impression of this person, thus making the task up to this point nearly identical to that of Hastie and Kumar (1979). However, Bargh and Thein added a factor (as well as one other factor not relevant to the current point) that extended the work of Hastie and Kumar: Participants were to read the sentences either while under a state of cognitive load or without being encumbered by load. As might be expected, the participants who were not faced with cognitive load performed quite similarly to those people in the Hastie and Kumar research; a greater percentage of incongruent behaviors were recalled relative to congruent and neutral behaviors. However, this pattern changed for participants under cognitive load; the advantage recall previously seen for incongruent information disappeared. Participants apparently did not have the resources free any more, despite having used categories in their judgment, to engage in the effort required to make sense of and attempt to integrate the inconsistent information.

Macrae, Hewstone, and Griffiths (1993) replicated this point, using social stereotypes as the categories that participants used in making their judgment, and behaviors congruent (or incongruent) with these stereotypes as the descriptions of the person. They asked research participants to watch a videotape of two people interacting. One of the people was categorized as either a doctor or a hairdresser. This person then proceeded to exhibit some traits that were consistent with the schema, as well as some traits that were not consistent with the schema. The prediction was that participants would attempt to make sense of the person's behavior, which would include incorporating the inconsistent items into the overall impression. However, to do so would require spending significant mental effort on making sense of the inconsistencies. If a cognitive load was placed on the participants while they were attempting to integrate these disparate pieces of information, they presumably would not have the capacity to engage in the effortful process of inconsistency resolution. Thus their recall should selectively delete the parts that were difficult to incorporate and make sense of—the information inconsistent with the schema. Load was manipulated in this experiment in an extremely simple manner: Participants were asked to recall an eight-digit number while watching the videotape. Remarkably, this simple task, which was no greater than any of the many tasks people perform while interacting with others, was able to alter the type of information that participants attended to while forming their impressions. Category-consistent information was recalled to a greater degree when cognitive load was present, whereas the absence of cognitive load presumably allowed people to analyze the inconsistent information, thus giving it an advantage over congruent information on the recall test.

Is There Always Better Recall for Incongruent Information? The conclusion that people recall incongruent information best (given sufficient cognitive resources) seemingly opposes the earlier-discussed tendency for people to better remember information that is congruent with their schemas (e.g., Anderson & Pichert, 1978; Cohen, 1961; Zadny & Gerard, 1974). We will see this point emerge again in Chapters 11 and 12, which discuss how and when information consistent with stereotypes is better remembered (e.g., Rothbart, Evans, & Fulero, 1979). One simple way to resolve this question would be to point out that many of the experiments that show how wonderful recall for schema-consistent information is simply do not present perceivers with schema-inconsistent information. Thus it is not surprising to see that when perceivers are presented with some information consistent with a schema and some information irrelevant to a schema, recall is better for the consistent information. What is intriguing is the fact that even when both schema-consistent information and schema-inconsistent information are present, there does not seem to be one simple rule specifying that one of these types of information is better remembered.

Whether people recall information that is congruent or incongruent with a schema depends on several things: (1) whether the schema being used is strong/well learned or weak/still developing (e.g., Klayman & Ha, 1987); (2) whether the incongruent information is attributed to the person's personality or is seen as being caused by uncontrollable pressure in the situation (Crocker, Hannah, & Weber, 1983; thus, if it is caused by the situation, it really isn't all that inconsistent with the category, since a person forced to lie isn't really being inconsistent with being an honest person); and (3) which type of recall task is used (free recall vs. recognition vs. frequency estimation), since this may determine which type of information has an advantage in memory (e.g., Garcia-Marques & Hamilton, 1996; Hastie, 1981). Rather than elaborate on each of these points here, let us return to this issue in Chapters 11 and 12.

Efficiency and Accuracy: A Tug of War?

The notion of *cognitive efficiency*, as described above, suggests that to be efficient is to be a minimalist in allocating cognitive resources. Such a definition of efficiency would present a conflict or competition between striving to be accurate and striving to be efficient, as accuracy would seemingly require effort aimed at examining all relevant data. On the surface, the conclusion would seem to be that striving to be efficient would mean that people categorize rather than seeing the uniqueness of the individual; they use shortcuts instead of being deliberate; they exert less rather than more effort whenever they can get away with it. The default response to the stimulus world is not to be as accurate as possible. It is to categorize it, to understand it, to gain meaning from it so that people know how to behave, and to do this in the least effortful way.

But are efficiency and accuracy necessarily at odds? Need we assume that when people use categories in processing information, this comes at the expense of accurate and effortful processing? Sherman (2001) suggests that this need not be the case. For example, Hastie and Kumar (1979) found that using categories in judgment promoted greater accuracy for recall of category-inconsistent information, and that this was accomplished through efficient processing promoting greater/deeper analysis of such information. Similarly, Macrae, Milne, and Bodenhausen (1994) found that the energy saved from relying on a stereotype allowed for greater accuracy in an unrelated and stereotype-irrelevant task (answering questions about Indonesia). Findings such as these have led Sherman to propose that rather than opposing accuracy, efficiency in processing can lead to greater accuracy.

Sherman's (2001) model argues that to maximize the efficiency of information processing, people rely on two types of information: detailed behavioral information about specific individuals, and abstract categories. Similar to miser models, this model proposes that the use of schemas makes consistent behaviors easy to comprehend, especially when processing resources are scant (because they match information already stored in the schema). However, unlike strict miser approaches (which would assert that schemas are crutches allowing people to do less), schemas are not seen as a filter that narrows all subsequent information processing to fit the category. Instead, it is argued that because information congruent with the category is understood so easily, it provides an energy "savings" that can then be directed toward the processing of detailed behavioral information, even information that is inconsistent with expectancies. With such a model, the use of schemas allows for the *flexible distribution of resources*, thus creating both stability and plasticity in information processing. By *plasticity*, it is meant that the system is able to revise schemas in light of new information. Though this is difficult to do while people are under cognitive load, the fact that they have continued to process inconsistent information while under load, and stored this information in memory, allows them to return to this information at a later time when resources are available (e.g., Nosofsky, Palmeri, & McKinley, 1994; Schank, 1982). At that time, they can make adjustments to their concepts that allow these concepts to develop as new, relevant information is gathered (e.g., Sherman, Klein, Laskey, & Wyer, 1998).

According to Sherman (2001), the very fact that people lose the ability to recall inconsistent information when they are being taxed by cognitive load is evidence of their efficiency; that this efficiency is used in the pursuit of accuracy; and that people are not cognitive misers! How so? Because the processes of inconsistency resolution are effortful and difficult, they require cognitive resources to be carried out. If such resources are not available, then the process cannot occur. The very fact that these processes had been occurring in the absence of load, and the fact that load eliminates it, suggests that in the absence of load people are exerting effort. Such processing is efficient not because it promotes miserliness, but accuracy. People are working hard to consider the inconsistent information, and this argues against the idea that people do not usually work hard, or that they are misers who rely on least effort. In fact, this desire to work hard and not simply to see new information in a way consistent with expectancies can still be seen when people are under cognitive load. Although it is true that such people no longer have the resources available to engage in inconsistency resolution (and therefore they are forced to rely on the consistent information when attempting to remember the information presented to them, because they have not been able to thoroughly encode the inconsistent information), it can also be shown that they *want to* analyze the inconsistent information. Although the lack of resources prevents them from being able to do it, there is evidence that people at least focus attention on this information when under load, thus indicating that they intend to analyze this information, but just do not have the fuel in the tank to get the process home.

To illustrate, consider a series of experiments conducted by Sherman, Lee, and colleagues (1998). Research participants read stereotype-consistent and -inconsistent information about a target person (Bob Hamilton) who was first identified as belonging to a stereotyped group (he was labeled as either a skinhead or a priest). Half of the people read the behavioral descriptions while under cognitive load, while half had full access to their cognitive resources. A first experiment assessed the amount of time participants spent reading the information provided for them. The results revealed that people spent a greater amount of time reading inconsistent information (a priest who shoved his way to the center seat in a movie theater) than consistent information (a priest who gave a stranger a quarter to make a phone call) when under cognitive load.

No differences were found when load did not exist. Participants seemed to be directing attention toward the inconsistent information when they were under load, devoting greater resources to the encoding of inconsistent information. A cognitive miser model would predict the exact opposite. In another experiment, Sherman, Lee, and colleagues once again had participants, half of whom were under cognitive load, read stereotype-consistent and -inconsistent information about a person (e.g., "swore at the salesgirl"). Participants were then asked to identify words flashed very briefly on a computer screen. The extent to which participants had attended to details was measured by their ability to identify words that had appeared in the sentences they had seen (e.g., identifying the word "salesgirl"). Once again, attention to details of the inconsistent information (when a priest was swearing at the salesgirl) was evident, even when participants were under cognitive load. In opposition to what cognitive misers would do, people experiencing a depletion of mental resources were found to have better attention to details for incongruent information.

Thus, just because people under load have better recall for consistent information, this does not mean that they are attending to the consistent information more carefully or encoding it more thoroughly than inconsistent information. In fact, when under load, people *attend more carefully* to inconsistent information, and more thoroughly *encode the details* of inconsistent information (Sherman & Frost, 2000; Sherman, Lee, et al., 1998). These findings compliment those of Bargh and Thein (1985), who showed that the recall advantage for inconsistent information evaporates under load. At the same time the recall advantage for inconsistent information is evaporating under load, recognition accuracy for that information increases, and attention is still focused on the inconsistent information. Nonetheless, people do not recall this information well. Instead, in the absence of being able to think deeply about information, schema-consistent items benefit from people's ability to use a schema as a source of guesses or as a retrieval cue (e.g., Carlston, 1980; Snyder & Uranowitz, 1978). But the fact that recall under load diminishes for inconsistent information does not mean that people stop attending to it. Sherman (2001) takes increased attention to such information as a sign that even under load, people do not want to be misers and instead want to exert the effort needed to think about inconsistencies; the will is there, but the ability is not.

CODA

Schemas are used to ease the complex task of forming impressions of others. By springing to mind effortlessly and silently, they guide new information into the cognitive system and provide the much-needed inferences and meaning that allow us to plan our behavior. However, why do we need to fit new information to old categories in order to derive meaning? Why can't we be taught what an object is de novo at each encounter? After all, relying on inferences about what category an object or person belongs to can result in incorrect inferences. Would it not be more accurate, and our judgments of others be more precise (and thus more adaptive), if we exerted the effort to analyze the uniqueness of each new stimulus we encounter? Certainly this would have prevented several Americans from conducting racist attacks against Sikhs following the destruction of the World Trade Center and part of the Pentagon. At the time of the attacks on Sikhs (in the days following September 11, 2001), this destruction was assumed to have been perpetrated by members of an entirely different religious group (Muslims), who happen to be superficially similar in a few respects to Sikhs. Generalizing from the Muslims who were believed to have committed the attack (al-Qaida members) to *all Muslims* is a severe enough error of incorrect categorization. But to generalize to an entirely different religious group based on superficial matching of features (articles of clothing, skin tone, etc.) reflects an extreme form of rigidity in categorical thinking. Erroneous categorization does not always lead to such dire consequences, but why ever get it wrong if we have the ability to get it right?

Some characterize the human reliance on schemas as evidence that we humans are cognitive misers. This notion assumes that schemas have become a means of avoiding potentially meaningful experiences and staying dug into the same old grooves. However, category use, while at times resulting in a loss of accuracy, need not be equated with a decrease in accuracy. Although we rely on schemas even when there is no cognitive load, and we should perhaps be exerting greater mental effort, this tendency to act like cognitive misers is matched by a competing tendency to show remarkable plasticity in processing and to be able to process and fit together seemingly inconsistent pieces of information. Indeed, schema use can be quite efficient and may allow for increased effort dedicated to information that is not easily subsumed by the schema. This ability to flexibly allocate our attentional and processing resources, limited as they are, allows us to reduce the effort we expend on some tasks so that we may increase our ability to process other tasks (and produces what on the surface seems like a paradoxical finding: The information used in making a judgment is different from the type of information most likely to be remembered). Importantly, such flexibility in processing allows for plasticity in the mental system. Categories can be revised and updated with the addition of new knowledge. This process may not happen online, especially if resources are depleted. But unexpected and incongruent information can be processed and stored, to be retrieved and evaluated another day.

This has led some to argue that rather than being cognitive misers, we humans are cognitively flexible, efficient, and adaptive. We use categories effortlessly in the face of limited resources, but we are not doomed to rely on the knowledge learned when we were young and our categories were first developed. The mental system evolves—and this occurs not despite of, but perhaps in concert with, the efficient and effortless use of categories. Indeed, the plasticity of the mental system when we are contemplating other people is the focus of the next chapter. When do we rely on schemas, and when do we go beyond schematic processing?

5 Dual-Process Models

Nonviolent direct action seeks to create such a crisis and foster such a tension that a community which has constantly refused to negotiate is forced to confront the issue. It seeks so to dramatize the issue that it can no longer be ignored. My citing the creation of tension as part of the work of the nonviolent resister may sound rather shocking. But I must confess that I am not afraid of the word "tension." I have earnestly opposed violent tension, but there is a type of constructive, nonviolent tension which is necessary for growth. Just as Socrates felt that it was necessary to create a tension in the mind so that individuals could rise from the bondage of myths and half-truths to the unfettered realm of creative analysis and objective appraisal, so must we see the need for nonviolent gadflies to create the kind of tension in society that will help men rise from the dark depths of prejudice and racism to the majestic heights of understanding and brotherhood.

—MARTIN LUTHER KING, JR., "Letter from Birmingham Jail" (April 16, 1963)

Woven into King's (1963) eloquent jail-cell wake-up call to America are many of the key elements that contribute to modern-day psychological models of social cognition. As we have been reviewing in the early chapters of this book, people have a tendency to rely on "less effort" and categorical thinking when evaluating others. Thus the categories people rely on, and the lack of effort exerted in drawing conclusions about others, can lead them to apply faulty and inaccurate categories—to lean on stereotypes, schemas, and prior expectancies. This is what we might assume King meant when he described people as being held bondage by "myths and half-truths." People often fail to arrive at the "unfettered realm of creative analysis and objective appraisal," and in Chapters 3 and 4, we have examined why this might be the case. Whether it be due to limited capacity or to the fact that people prefer to "think less" and rely on the least-effort principle, they often fail to reach the heights of objective and creative analysis of others.

But King's assumption is not that people are incapable of breaking free of these bonds. Instead, people are seen as having the cognitive flexibility to rise above this simplistic way of thinking about others and to embrace an objective appraisal. This belief that people may typically rely on categorical thinking, but can exert the flexibility of will and mind to be more objective and effortful, is the basic premise of *dual-process models*. Thus, on the one hand, processes of social cognition involve a reliance on stereotypes, heuristics, categories, schemas, and "half-truths." Because in these instances people rely on general, preexisting theories about others, and from these theories make inferences about specific individuals, this type of processing is generally referred to as *top-down* or *theory-driven processing*. On the other hand, people can exhibit quite a good deal of "creative analysis" and "objective appraisal" in thinking about others. We have already seen evidence of this in Chapter 4, in discussing the type of mental work that is triggered when information inconsistent with an expectancy is encountered. It is not merely ignored and dismissed; in fact, significant cognitive work may be exerted toward resolving the inconsistency. In these cases, people do not rely on prior theories, stereotypes, and heuristics, but examine the qualities of each individual when constructing an impression. Dual-process models use several interchangeable terms to refer to this type of effortful and elaborate processing of information about an individual: *personalization*, *elaboration*, *systematic processing*, and *attribute-oriented processing*. More generally, because impressions are being built from the observed data (the behavior of another), such processing is referred to as *bottom-up* or *data-driven processing*.

A second ingredient in King's (1963) analysis is also of central interest to dual-process models: Namely, what is it that motivates people to shift from the comfort and ease of top-down processing to exerting the effort required of systematic processing? In King's words, the answer is that a tension in the mind motivates people to rise from the "depths of prejudice" to the "majestic heights" of understanding. Tension (psychological, not physical) forces them to analyze others carefully and reanalyze their own prior views. Psychologists have had much to say about the motivational powers of a state of psychological tension. Tension, as reviewed in the Introduction to this book, is a psychological state people find aversive and are motivated to reduce. In this case the tension arises from top-down thinking's being deemed unacceptable. This tension can be reduced through engaging in more elaborate processing of information relevant to the person who had previously been judged in a top-down fashion.

A final ingredient in King's (1963) letter also maps quite closely onto dual-process models of impression formation: Namely, what triggers tension in the mind of the perceiver and initiates the shift from schematic and stereotypic processing to individuating and attribute-oriented processing? In King's approach, tension is initiated by the behavior of the person being perceived. If the person being perceived by others can act in a manner that is opposed to the prevalent biases, stereotypes, and expectancies, then it forces the people doing the perceiving to confront the fact that their theory-driven approaches to understanding this person are not working. Regarding the application of this idea to King's involvement in the civil rights movement in the United States, King chose to advocate nonviolent protest—a challenge to the existing stereotype that African Americans were more violent and less intelligent than Whites. By consistently challenging the stereotype, King believed that the members of the majority group (White Americans) would be forced to reevaluate their stance and think more deeply about the issues and about African Americans. Dual-process models recognize this as a viable form of tension induction. Consistent behavior that is clear, diagnostic, and counter to prevailing stereotypes (such as when a supposedly violent group of Black men, according to a stereotype, responds to brute force with nonviolent protest and peaceful pleas for change) can motivate a shift away from stereotypic processing and can trigger elaborate and detailed thinking about an issue or person. Although this is not the only manner tension can be produced, King (operating without the benefit of the research we will review here) struck upon one good method available to him.

Martin Luther King, Jr., famously dreamed of a world where people are judged not by the color of their skin (categorical/stereotypic processing that is characteristic of being "theory-driven"), but on the content of their character (personalized and systematic processing that is characteristic of being "data-driven"). The latter requires perceivers to rise up from the "depths" of categorical thinking to a more elaborate and systematic analysis of another person as an individual. To do so requires that perceivers have the flexibility to shift from being theory-driven to data-driven. If capable of doing so, people are perhaps best viewed not as cognitive misers, but as *flexible interpreters* (Uleman, Newman, & Moskowitz, 1996) or *motivated tacticians* (Fiske & Taylor, 1991): They have a tendency to rely on preexisting theories, but can be motivated to utilize the flexibility of their cognitive system and think about others in a more elaborate fashion. As we will see, being more effortful in evaluating others may not guarantee being objective and fair in thinking about others. After all, people can exert considerable effort to uphold an existing bias against someone and to cling to stereotypes. Rationalizations are often a quite effortful way to maintain whatever beliefs people wish to maintain (e.g., Kunda & Oleson, 1995). But although exerting mental effort does not guarantee thinking objectively and rationally, dual-process models at least view people as having the capability to approach the objective appraisal of others of which King dreamed.

A SAMPLER OF DUAL-PROCESS MODELS

With enough time and testing of defining cues, "best fit" perceiving can be accomplished for most but not all classes of environmental events with which the person has contact. There are some objects whose cues to identify are sufficiently equivocal so that no such resolution can be achieved, and these are mostly in the sphere of so-called interpersonal perception: perceiving the states of other people, their characteristics, intentions, etc. on the basis of external signs. And since this is the domain where misperception can have the most chronic if not the most acute consequences, it is doubtful whether a therapeutic regimen of "close looking" will aid the misperceiver much. . . . But the greatest difficulty rests in the fact that the cost of close looks is generally too high under the conditions of speed, risk, and limited capacity imposed upon organisms by the environment.

BRUNER (1957, pp. 141–142)

Dual-process models describe people as having a default strategy in which inferences are formed and impressions are made via heuristics, schemas, stereotypes, and expectancies. This strategy at the effortless end of the information-processing continuum has been described in Chapter 4 as having evolved out of a need to manage the complexity of the environment using a cognitive system with limited resources. The restrictions to one's cognitive resources can arise from conditions in the environment such as these: working on many tasks at once, which places people under cognitive load ("limited capacity"); working on tasks under a deadline, where time pressure limits how long you can deliberate about the qualities of others ("speed"); and working on tasks that, in and of themselves, are complex and difficult. Bruner asserts that interpersonal perception is an example of such tasks: Person perception is a domain where the thing being perceived (another individual) is highly equivocal. Even with all the time and capacity in the world for effort and analysis, people may never come to truly understand the character of another person by observing his/her behavior. Thus they often simply rely on the strategy of using the cognitive shortcuts that their prior theories and categories supply. However, Bruner paved the way for dual-process models by asserting that people are sometimes willing to pay this cost and engage in the effort of what he called a "closer look" at the information. The important psychological questions concern when, why, and how they are willing and able to pay such costs.

Brewer's Dual-Process Model of Impression Formation

The term *dual-process model* was coined by Brewer (1988) in describing a comprehensive theory of the processes involved in impression formation (depicted in Figure 5.1). Although theories that are now categorized as dual-process models had existed in social psychology prior to that point (e.g., Chaiken, 1987; Kunda, 1987; Neuberg & Fiske, 1987; Petty & Cacioppo, 1986; Trope, 1986a), Brewer's model built an important bridge between research focused on how people use schemas, categories, and heuristics in judging others in a fairly effortless and automatic way, and much earlier research focused on the rational and methodical processes that people employ when forming

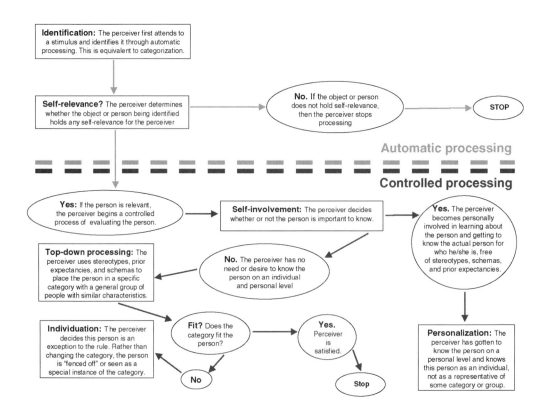

FIGURE 5.1. Brewer's (1988) dual-process model of impression formation. From Brewer (1988). Copyright 1988 by Lawrence Erlbaum Associates. Adapted by permission.

attributions of others (reviewed in Chapter 6). For many years, it was known that people use each of these processes in their social cognition. However, the conditions that delineated when social cognition would be marked by an overreliance on categories and fairly automatic processes, and when it would involve an attention to details and fairly effortful processes, had not been established. Several integrative models emerged between 1986 and 1990 that attempted to specify the conditions governing when and why people shift from the more automatic type of processing to the more systematic type (e.g., Brewer, 1988; Chaiken, Liberman, & Eagly, 1989; Devine, 1989; Fazio, 1990; Fiske & Neuberg, 1990; Gilbert, 1989; Kruglanski, 1990; Kunda, 1987; L. L. Martin, 1986; Petty & Cacioppo, 1986; Trope, 1986a; Wyer & Srull, 1989). These models share a set of assumptions in which impression formation is organized according to stages that occur sequentially, such that the "miserly" perceiver will not expend resources for further processing unless certain conditions are met.

The attempt to integrate the two types of cognitive processes that had been the focus of impression formation research helped to reintroduce the notion of motivation—a concept that had been diluted (though not absent altogether) in the cognitive revolution—to mainstream social psychology. In research studying the automatic nature of these processes, goals were often held constant, rendering them almost obsolete. In research of the 1960s and early 1970s on attribution (see Chapter 6), motivation was usually treated as an explanation for why people are biased and why these typically rational processes break down. Rather than being seen as central to the process, it was viewed as sending the process awry. However, when researchers began attempting to integrate different forms of thinking within a given perceiver, they soon rediscovered that motives and goals play a central role requiring that they be integral in any model of social cognition. The first volume of Sorrentino and Higgins's (1986) *Handbook of Motivation and Cognition* helped to awaken the field to this issue, and dual-process models soon sprung forth. As a case in point, Brewer's (1988) dual-process model views the role of motivation as central to determining the type of social cognition perceivers will engage in: "The majority of the time, perception of social objects does not differ from nonsocial perception in either structure or process. When it does differ, it is determined by the *perceiver's* purposes and processing goals, not by the characteristics of the target of perception" (p. 4; emphasis in original).

Identification

Brewer's model specifies that both automatic and controlled processing contribute to our ultimate impression of another person. At the automatic level, the model begins with processes of attention and identification not unlike the silent process of categorization that Bruner (1957) described and that we have reviewed in Chapter 3. When a person enters our social environment, we perceivers must first focus attention on that person and identify the person as being present, as having certain features, and as having performed certain types of behavior. Brewer (1988) referred to these automatic processes that allow us to capture the presence of a target stimulus (in this case, a person) and identify the basic features that the target is eliciting as *identification*. Thus, without any conscious effort by us as perceivers, some form of information is perceptually salient enough to cue a social category. The model suggests that a few social categories are used often and consistently enough to be triggered automatically (e.g., age, ethnicity, race, and sex). Exactly which of these categories becomes the superordinate category label that may organize subsequent impression formation and processing depends on features of the context, the perceiver, and the target. Fiske and Neuberg (1990) assert that qualities that "possess temporal primacy, have physical manifestations, are contextually novel, are chronically or acutely accessible in memory, or are related in particular ways to the perceiver's mood will tend to serve the role of category label" (p. 10).

Sometimes the categorizations we make by using this process of matching observable features of a target to our existing mental representations of "person types" are wrong. We may assume that a person who speaks fluent English without accent is an American, when in fact the person is Cuban; we may assume that a person with fair skin is not an African American, when in fact many people with one White parent and one Black parent identify themselves as African Americans regardless of their skin color. As Allport (1954, p. 20) says, "Sometimes we are mistaken: the event does not fit the category. . . . Yet our behavior was rational. It was based on high probability. Though we used the wrong category, we did the best we could." For reasons elaborated in Chapter 3, categorizations are an essential and functional part of our understanding of the world, and this feature-matching process allows us to label and type each stimulus we encounter in a fast, efficient, economical, and relatively (if not 100%) accurate way.

Determining Relevance

The primary outcome of this initial identification stage is a preconscious decision as to whether further processing is necessary. Our categorization will allow us to detect whether the person is relevant or irrelevant to us. If a person we have encountered is irrelevant to our current goals and purpose (e.g., a stranger passing us on the subway platform, a driver stopped at a red light as we walk down the street, a clerk at the market placing Ring Dings on the shelf), then further processing, and the expenditure of cognitive effort to think about this person, are not necessary. Impression formation processes are halted. However, if the person is deemed somewhat relevant—and this can range from a minor degree of relevance (such as a store clerk who is placing Ring Dings on the shelf when we want Ring Dings) to a major degree of interest (such as a stranger passing us on the subway platform who attempts to mug us)—then impression formation processes are triggered. At this point, a critical choice is made between the two alternative processing modes described in the model. Thus even the initial, preconscious decision that determines whether we dedicate any energy to thinking about a person and process further information about the person depends on goals (i.e., the relevance of the target).

Once a target has been deemed relevant, processing that is automatic (preconscious automaticity) is no longer engaged. There is a shift toward processing that fails to meet all of the criteria for an automatic process, if only because such processing is goal-dependent. As discussed in Chapter 2, any processing that requires a goal for its initiation, as opposed to the mere presence of a stimulus in the environment, is not considered automatic. This is not to say that such processing cannot occur with extremely little effort, or even without our awareness. But processing from this point onward does require a goal—the goal of needing to know more about the person because of his/her potential relevance to us. The degree to which conscious effort and awareness are engaged by subsequent processing is now what distinguishes the subsequent stages of information processing and establishes the two broad modes of processing (categorization vs. personalization) that comprise the dual processes in the model.

Categorization/Typing

Motives do not only determine whether we proceed to think about others; they also determine *how* we proceed to think about them. The decision to gather further information about a person does not mean that it will always be an effortful, deliberative, rational, and objective process. We can produce judgments of others in a categorical way, relying on schemas, heuristics, and prior expectancies about the category of people the particular individual being judged belongs to (e.g., stereotypes). Brewer (1988) has referred to this relatively effortless type of thinking, which is anchored by and directed exclusively by the categories that have been (rather passively) triggered, as *categorization* or *typing*. In this type of impression formation, our judgments about a person are based on available "person types" or schemas that are matched to the information at hand about the person being evaluated. An iterative, pattern-matching process is conducted until an adequate fit is found between one of the person types or categories stored in memory and the stimulus characteristics. The process starts with a rather general category, and if there is no match, subtypes of the general category that provide more specific types are compared against the target person. Brewer offers a concrete example of an abstract superordinate category and the more concrete subtypes within that category. The superordinate category "older men" is fairly abstract and contains a wide range of features. Within that superordinate category is the more specific category type "businessmen," which is still relatively abstract, but less so than the category label in which it is nested ("older men"). Moving downward in the category hierarchy, we arrive at even more specific subtypes of the category "businessmen" that have fine-grained sets of features, such as an "uptight authoritarian boss who is a tightwad and a stickler for detail" (Brewer, 1988, p. 12).

Given these different levels of category types, Brewer has concluded that the exact manner in which a given person is categorized depends not only on the features of that person being matched against a category, but on the level of abstraction within the category structure the feature matching process begins. Exactly where in a perceiver's category system this process begins can be determined by several factors: what categories are automatically triggered during identification, cues in the current situation, and the processing goals of the perceiver. For example, if a person is initially classified according to age as a teenager, and then information is attended to that indicates a counterstereotypic role (e.g., the teenager is a writer for *Rolling Stone* magazine), then his/her role as a writer will probably be organized as a specific type of teenager (e.g., a "whiz kid"). However, if age is not salient in the initial categorization—for example, if the editor of *Rolling Stone* magazine called the manager of the band Led Zeppelin and said he could expect Cameron (an age-unspecified writer) to come and tour with the band—then the initial impression will start with a more general category, "writer," rather than "whiz kid."

These categorizations are important for several reasons. First, category-driven impressions might be the sole contributor to one's final judgment of the person, constituting the entire basis for one's opinion. That is, there are times when perceivers are perfectly happy to rely on their categories to supply them with broad overgeneralizations that can extend from the category level to individual members of the category. Allport (1954) provides an excellent example of this when discussing how stereotypes of groups can be extended to an individual member of a group once he/she is categorized by the perceiver as a member of that group. The very first sentences of

Allport's seminal book make this point: "In Rhodesia, a white truck driver passed a group of idle natives and muttered, 'They're lazy brutes.' A few hours later he saw natives heaving two-hundred pound sacks of grain onto a truck, singing in rhythm to their work. 'Savages,' he grumbled" (p. 3). Second, even if the impression one forms evolves and is transformed in later stages of information processing, the category-based judgment will still serve as an anchor and input (starting point) for any subsequent judgment (e.g., Park, 1989). Finally, categorical processing not only serves as an anchor around which future, effortful judgments shift; it also anchors the effortless processing that occurs during categorization. That is, during the process of trying to match "person types" against a given person's characteristics in order to categorize him/her, the initial categorization, even if not successful at categorizing the person, has an impact on how the subsequent feature mapping and person typing proceed. If the initial match between a category and a person's features is not successful, this first attempt will not be discarded for a new, perfectly irrelevant schema/person type to match against the target person. Instead, if the initial fit is not adequate, "the search for an appropriate categorization will be directed downward, among subtypes of the original category, rather than horizontally among alternative categories at the same level of abstraction. . . . Thus, initial category activation sets in motion an iterative process that constrains the final category selection" (Brewer, 1988, pp. 18–19).

Individuation and Personalization

The processes of categorization seem to involve no more motivational impetus than trivial levels of self-involvement. If a person is somehow relevant to us, category-based processing is initiated. But as our needs and goals as perceivers dictate, we can engage in more detailed, elaborate, and effortful types of cognitive processing. This is not to say that all category-based processing must be relatively effortless. At times we expend quite a good deal of energy and effort to maintain our categories. Chapter 4 has discussed how we process information that is inconsistent with (or incongruent with) an expectancy or category that has been triggered; we often work quite hard to continue to process in a categorical way (because, despite this effort, it is still less effortful than reorganizing our whole category structure and changing an entire mental representation). Brewer (1988) provides another example of fairly effortful, category-based processing, in a process labeled *individuation*. In this type of processing, information we receive about a person that is inconsistent with the category label is not disregarded; nor is a more specific subtype of the category called into play to describe the person. Instead, the individual is treated as an isolated case or a specific instance of the particular category. Thus the qualities of the individual are processed in detail—not for the purpose of making that individual fit well with the existing features of the category, but to create a specific and detailed novel instance of the category. Brewer provides a good example: "The first anchorwoman that appeared on a national television news program was no doubt highly individuated as a member of the category of news broadcasters" (p. 21).

There are times, however, when no form of category-based processing is deemed appropriate by us as perceivers. It is at these moments that the model suggests a wholly different form of processing in both format and organizational structure. At this point in the process, the individual becomes the basis for organizing information. Here the category label is no longer superordinate, and the individual's attributes serve as the organizing framework for understanding that individual. Brewer referred to this type of information processing as *personalization*. Brewer (1988, p. 22) asserts that "the new organizational structure is a sort of mental flip-flop of the category-based structure," and provides an example via analysis of the statement "Janet is a nurse." This information can be organized and analyzed in a category-based way, with Janet being treated as a type of the category "nurse." Alternatively, it can be organized and analyzed in a way that treats "nurse" as subordinate to, and a feature of, the properties of an individual named Janet. In one case, the category "nurse" is the organizing structure around which the emerging mental representation is built; in the other case, it is the individual, Janet. "The concept of 'nurse' as a feature of Janet would contain only those aspects of nursing that are characteristic of Janet in that role, and would be disassociated from the prototypic representation of nurse as a general category, which may contain many features not applicable to Janet" (p. 22).

Exactly what sort of conditions lead us as perceivers to conclude that no form of category-based processing is appropriate? Brewer (1988, p. 25; emphasis in original) asserts that "personalization implies some degree of *affective* investment on the part of the perceiver, either because of the target person's relationship to the perceiver's personal or social identity, or because of the target's relevance to the perceiver's personal goals." Thus, if someone is similar to us, we are less likely to rely simply on category-based processing and more likely to expend the mental energy to personalize him/her. Similarly, if a person is linked to important goals that we seek to attain (e.g., a coworker whose work on a joint project will also determine how we are evaluated, a manager whose evaluation of us will determine whether the company decides to promote us), we are more likely to move beyond simple category-based processing and form impressions of this individual based exclusively on the attributes and features we have taken the time to detect.

The Heuristic–Systematic Model

The heuristic–systematic model (HSM; Chaiken et al., 1989) provides a fairly comprehensive account of the mechanisms that drive social cognition. According to the HSM, people's thinking about themselves and others can be described in terms of two broad information-processing strategies. These two strategies are often described as endpoints on a continuum of processing effort that can be exerted in forming judgments (see Figure 5.2).

Two Processing Modes

At one end of the continuum is the relatively effortless *heuristic processing*—a reliance on prior knowledge such as schemas, stereotypes, and expectancies that can be imposed on information so it will easily fit into existing structures. Instead of exerting effort toward thinking carefully about content (whether it be the content of a person's character or the content of a message), people instead preserve their processing resources by relying on superficial assessment. That is, people rely on heuristics, shortcuts, and rules of thumb in thinking about their social world. Such rules of thumb, categories, and expectancies are learned through experiences in the social world, and are readily called to action when people encounter a cue in the environment that signals the relevance of one of these previously learned rules or responses. As an example, past experience indicates that a person whose point of view achieves a wide consensus among others is often a person whose point of view is correct. Armed with this "Consensus implies correct-

There are two general strategies for processing information about people. These can be conceived of as opposing ends of a continuum. The continuum represents the amount of mental effort one exerts when thinking about others. Many believe the human default is to exert less, rather than more, effort.

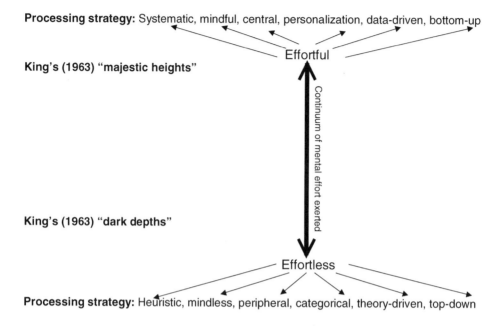

FIGURE 5.2. Two processing modes.

ness" heuristic, perceivers may react to future encounters with a majority position on an issue in a heuristic fashion. They can superficially assess the situation by relying on the rule of thumb, forming an opinion in a top-down fashion without scrutinizing the actual arguments used by the majority in advocating their position. Thus, if most people agree with something, these perceivers will agree with it too, using the consensus as the basis for their opinion.

On the other end of the continuum is *systematic processing*. Systematic processing involves a detailed evaluation of the qualities and behaviors of others, as well as the reexamination of personal thoughts and prior beliefs about the stimulus. Individuals will attempt to formulate a judgment through reconciling the current data that they have analyzed quite closely with their reexamined beliefs, using processes such as integration (Kelman, 1961) and validation (Moscovici, 1985b). Because perceivers are actively thinking about how some stimulus information relates to other knowledge they possess, systematic information processing requires a sufficient amount of their limited cognitive capacity or processing resources in order to be carried out, as well as some degree of motivation to instigate such effortful processing.

Consider the example used above. If past experiences indicate that a person whose point of view achieves a wide consensus among others is often a person whose point of view is the correct one, then perceivers develop expectancies and heuristics not only about what it means to be in the majority, but also about what it means to be in the minority (Moscovici, 1985a). Armed with these "Consensus implies correctness" and

"Lack of consensus implies incorrectness" heuristics, people may react to future encounters with both a majority and a minority position on an issue in a heuristic fashion. In particular, they may simply react with disdain and disregard for what the minority has to say. However, as was the case with the nonviolent protests of the civil rights movement in the United States, the perceivers can be shaken from "top-down" thinking so that they no longer are imposing their previously held theories, heuristics, and biases. If people doubt the reliability and validity of their heuristic thinking (the stereotypes about the minority seem out of place or incorrect), this will trigger thought processes whereby the minority's position is deeply evaluated and thoroughly appraised, and their own positions (and biases) are reevaluated. The perceivers will examine the data, building a judgment from the bottom (the facts), rather than imposing one from on high.

This assumption of two processing modes raises two further questions: Why assume that one of these is the default mode, and what are the appropriate motivational conditions that lead one to shift from the default to the other mode of processing? The HSM presents two principles that answer these questions—the least-effort principle and the sufficiency principle. Each should be familiar by now, as they reflect principles already discussed earlier in the book.

The Least-Effort Principle

Whereas Allport (1954) put forward the principle of least effort (reviewed in Chapter 4), the HSM puts forward the least-effort principle! As you might expect, these are one and the same idea. Recall that the least-effort principle asserts that when performing cognitive tasks, people prefer less mental effort to more mental effort. This suggests that the default processing strategy will be the one requiring the least amount of effort and usurping the least amount of capacity—the heuristic route. How can we detect whether the use of heuristics is the default way of processing information? By examining whether heuristic processing is found to occur even when there are no specific motivating circumstances to engage in this processing mode. Such processing should merely require the presence of the appropriate cues in the environment to trigger the use of the heuristic. For example, if perceivers are evaluating the positions of a minority by relying on heuristics, the recognition that the minority lacks any consensus should be a cue that will trigger relevant rules of thumb, which the perceivers then will rely on if not motivated to think "harder."

Petty, Cacioppo, and Schuman (1983) provided an illustration of people using heuristics as a default strategy. Their research examined why people are persuaded by celebrities who endorse a product in a commercial. The logic was that seeing a celebrity leads people to rely on simple rules of impression formation, such as "Famous people are trustworthy" or "Attractive people know a lot about dietary and cosmetic products," rather than evaluating the details about the product. Petty and colleagues had research participants read about a razor that was being endorsed by either a sports star or an unknown person. There were two potential sources of influence in this situation. Participants could read the text of the endorsement carefully and evaluate the product based on its merits, or they could superficially evaluate the product and rely on the word of the endorser. If participants were using the former strategy, they should find the product equally good, regardless of whether the celebrity or the "regular guy" was the person endorsing it. If they were relying on heuristics, the celebrity should be much more persuasive at selling the product than the "regular guy," even if the text of their sales pitch was the same. The results revealed that rather than using the text to guide impressions, the participants did indeed use a heuristic about the person delivering the text. Thus instead of evaluating people and products in detail, scrutinizing their qualities, people rely on simple and easy rules.

The Sufficiency Principle

The sufficiency principle asserts that for whatever task people are confronted with—whether it be forming an impression of someone, planning how to act toward someone, forming an attitude, making a decision, or simply comprehending some information—there is a point at which they feel that their task is completed and they can move on to the next task at hand. This point is said to be achieved when the individuals feel *confident that they have sufficiently performed the task* that was set before them. This point of sufficient confidence that allows for a feeling of task completion can be conceived of as a threshold—a *sufficiency threshold*. That is, in almost all things, people desire to feel somewhat confident about their thoughts, feelings, and actions. And when they are gauging their sense of confidence in the validity of their own beliefs, attitudes, and actions, this can range from not at all confident to extremely confident. People may not (in fact, it is likely that they typically do not) always desire to have extreme confidence in what they say and do. They are sometimes happy simply to have moderate amounts of confidence in their judgments and feelings, so long as they feel it is *enough* confidence to warrant relying on those judgments/feelings in their interactions.

This sufficiency principle allows us to conceive of the point at which we perceivers feel confident enough in our thoughts and actions as a threshold that can be set anywhere we choose, and as a point that is subject to change from situation to situation. For example, when we are evaluating a TV commercial or a stranger at the market, we may feel relatively confident in the opinion we form, despite barely listening to what is being said to us. Yet when evaluating a love interest, we may cling to the person's every word with an effort and detail that we might not have known we possessed. We seek to feel extremely confident that our responses to this person are accurate and appropriate, so we set the threshold for deciding when our thoughts and deeds are sufficient quite high.

The Relationship between Effort and Sufficiency

The sufficiency principle asserts that although people prefer least effort, they must exert *enough* effort to reach the sufficiency threshold. If people desire the feeling that their judgments are good enough, they will only rely on heuristics in forming judgments if those heuristics deliver to them a sense of *judgmental confidence*. For the most part, heuristics provide sufficient responses to allow people to navigate through social interactions. The *product* of heuristic processing is a judgment based on relatively little effort. To the degree that relying on little effort yields a sufficiently good product—judgments and behaviors that leave people feeling sufficiently confident that they have acted in a reasonable manner—then they are happy to rely on such heuristics and do not need to engage in any further processing of information. If heuristic processing is experienced as producing inadequate actions, judgments, or feelings—that is, the level of confidence in the judgments that heuristics produce falls short of the threshold—people will exert more effort and continue working on the task at hand until a feeling of sufficiency is achieved and the threshold is surpassed. Thus the least-effort principle exists because using less effort (relying on heuristics) typically gives people a sense that they have formed judgments in which they are sufficiently confident (see Figure 5.3).

For example, experience may teach one that people who are politically conservative are against abortion. If this position opposes one's own feelings, one may try to avoid discussing the topic with a conservative who attempts to discuss it. A cue—the other person's conservatism—triggers a heuristic in the mind ("Conservatives have extreme views, so don't bother arguing with them; they will not yield"). The heuristic, in this case, works. It allows one to have inferences that seem reasonable enough, and allows one to plan behavior that will yield a smooth and trouble-free encounter. Thinking less has produced sufficient inferences to generate successful social behavior. However, if one's confidence in relying on this heuristic is not sufficient, one will be forced to increase processing effort; that is, when one encounters a conservative, one may deem a sole reliance on heuristics to be inappropriate. It may be true that conservatives typically oppose abortion, but this given individual may have been expressing a dissenting, pro-abortion view that one's heuristic processing did not allow one to detect. One must initiate more elaborate forms of evaluating this person until one has produced a judgment that one feels is sufficient (is reasonable enough to rely on). At what point is effort frozen (rather than continually increased)? When one's current confidence in a judgment has catapulted over the sufficiency threshold.

In this hydraulic-like model, the energy that drives the shift from effortless to effortful thinking about other people is a pressure to have greater accuracy and to remove feelings of doubt. If least-effort processing produces judgments, behaviors, and evaluations that perceivers have relatively little confidence in, a problem exists. They desire a certain level of confidence in the cognitions that their processing system produces (this is said to be the sufficiency threshold). When relying on "least effort" yields

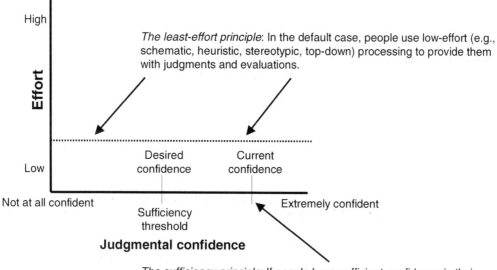

FIGURE 5.3. The least-effort principle and the sufficiency principle.

judgmental products that are not sufficient—that fall below the sufficiency threshold—a *confidence gap* is said to exist (see Figure 5.4A, Time 1). This is said to be experienced by the perceivers as an uncomfortable and displeasing state of psychological tension. Because the tension state is not pleasant, the perceivers are motivated to reduce the state and eliminate the gap between their current level and desired level of confidence. How can this be accomplished? The pressure from the experienced confidence gap pushes processing effort upward. Because of the hydraulic-like relationship between confidence and effort, lacking confidence in judgments generates increased effort in the processes that yield or produce these judgments. Thus the confidence gap can be reduced as one makes the transition from the least-effort principle's reliance on minimal processing effort to expending more effort. Perceivers will now process information in a more systematic fashion (see Figure 5.4).

In Figure 5.4B, the left-hand side of the figure illustrates how an initial increase in effort (as represented by the gray arrow) can lead to a reduced confidence gap (as represented by the black arrow). However, in this instance the moderate amount of increased effort is not sufficient to produce a judgment in which the person feels "confident enough." Existing confidence at this point (Time 2), though higher than at Time 1, is still below the desired amount of confidence (the sufficiency threshold). Therefore, the individual still experiences a confidence gap and the pressure to reduce this gap. This, once again, is accomplished through exerting even greater processing effort

A. The cognitive system experiencing psychological tension (at Time 1).

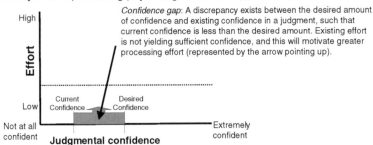

B. Processing effort is increased to reduce psychological tension (Times 2 and 3).

Systematic processing: Effort is expended to elaborate on a stimulus until judgment is "good enough." At left, the effort exerted at Time 2, though increased from Time 1, produces a confidence level at Time 2 that is not sufficient; a confidence gap (though reduced from that existing at Time 1) persists. At right (Time 3), effort increases and confidence in judgment is now sufficient.

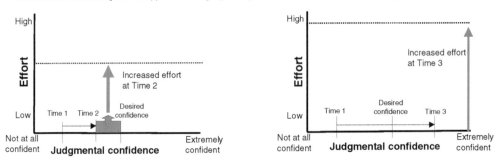

FIGURE 5.4. Dual-process models and the relationship between effort and confidence.

until the products of this data-driven analysis of the stimuli are finally recognized as sufficiently good. The increased effort has yielded an increase in confidence, such that at this point (Time 3) the processing effort has yielded judgmental products that surpass the desired amount of confidence (as evidenced on the right-hand side of Figure 5.4B by the dashed black arrow moving past the sufficiency threshold).

The Motivation to Make the Transition from Less to More Effort

The HSM suggests that the impact of heuristic processing on judgments will be greatest when motivation for systematic processing is low. Some trade-off must be struck between the goal of exerting least effort and the goal of having judgments one is sufficiently confident in. Although heuristic processing more fully satisfies the least-effort principle, systematic processing is more effective at producing greater amounts of confidence and is thus better able to satisfy the sufficiency principle. The assertion that humans process heuristically by default suggests that on balance, the trade-off between less effort and sufficiency is adequately met by heuristic processing; the sufficiency threshold is set low enough that it can adequately be reached by heuristic processing alone. Determining when people shift from heuristic to systematic processing revolves around the issue of when heuristic processing is *insufficient*. When the motivation for systematic processing exists, the impact of heuristic processing on judgments will be somewhat attenuated. In these instances, judgments based on information gathered through a deliberate and effortful strategy should be more reliable and trustworthy than those produced by a reliance on simple decision rules.

The next logical question arising from this discussion is this: What motivational circumstances are required to instigate systematic processing? We have already provided one type of answer to this question. The shift to systematic processing will be dependent on the existence of a gap between actual and desired confidence. This confidence gap is then experienced as an unpleasant tension state: People are now motivated to reduce the tension through systematic processing. However, the best answer to this question requires identifying *how* a confidence gap is produced or *how* to get people to experience their current judgments as insufficient. To alter what is experienced as "sufficient," to experience a confidence gap, and to have motivation to engage in systematic processing, one of two things must happen. First, people's confidence can be undermined, so that a judgment that was once firmly accepted is called into doubt. Here, the sufficiency threshold itself does not change; people's existing level of confidence in their previously accepted heuristic changes so that it slips below the sufficiency threshold (e.g., Maheswaran & Chaiken, 1991). Second, desired confidence can be raised by a shift in the sufficiency threshold—a raising of the amount of effort needed in order to feel confident.

Undermining confidence. Confidence in a judgment (or attitude or belief or action) is not a fixed entity; it can change. At one point in time people might be confident in their use of a stereotype or a heuristic, only to feel unsatisfied with the judgments based on such minimal processing at a later point in time. In fact, this can occur (1) without a desire for any greater confidence than before, and (2) when the amount of confidence desired is quite low. For example, imagine you are meeting a woman, Jane, on Monday morning, and she shows up 40 minutes late without an explanation. You might feel confident in your opinion that Jane is unreliable, even if that opinion is based on a heuristic (such as "People who are extremely late for an appointment are unreliable"). In fact, you might have a very low sufficiency threshold that allows you to be perfectly satisfied with this conclusion, despite giving minimal thought to evaluating Jane. However, on Tuesday afternoon you find out from a mutual friend that Jane is poor, and is embarrassed that she cannot afford a car or a watch. And these issues related to her being poor are what made her late (and to fail to tell you why she was late). In this case, you may no longer be confident in your heuristic-based judgment that Jane is unreliable.

Note that in this example, it is not the case that you desired a judgment that was based on better processing, or that you desired greater confidence than your original heuristic provided. You were initially perfectly satisfied with using little processing effort and relying on your heuristic. It was that the confidence you had in the conclusion your heuristic provided for you was later undermined, and your confidence then fell below the sufficiency threshold; your conclusion no longer provided a sufficiently good explanation for Jane's behavior (see Figure 5.5). Jane might be unreliable, but you are no longer confident enough in this heuristic-based conclusion, because new information (Jane's poverty caused her lateness; her pride caused her failure to explain this) has introduced doubt and lowered your confidence in the conclusion. As Maheswaran and Chaiken (1991, p. 15) have stated, it is "possible to promote systematic processing even when sufficiency thresholds are low by undermining perceivers' confidence in their heuristic-based judgments."

To illustrate this mechanism through which people are motivated to process systematically, an experiment will next be reviewed—one illustrating that systematic processing is initiated when conclusions drawn from a heuristic are subsequently challenged. Thus, while heuristic-based judgments and conclusions may be initially experienced as valid and sufficient (at Time 1 in Figure 5.5), a subsequent event can shatter confidence in these conclusions, lowering such confidence so that it falls below a personally defined threshold of what constitutes a sufficiently good judgment (at Time 2 in Figure 5.5). This triggers a switch to systematic and effortful processing that was previously not necessary (at Time 3 in Figure 5.5).

Maheswaran and Chaiken (1991) examined this point by looking at how consumers respond to advertising messages. Participants in their experiment were asked to read about and evaluate a new product, the "XT-100" answering machine. The participants first received information about how the product had performed in prior consumer tests; they were told that a sample of consumers who had been previously surveyed liked the product very much ("81% of 300 western consumers who had used the XT-100 were extremely satisfied," p. 16). Thus these participants in this experiment were now probably ready to evaluate the product fairly positively, regardless of what information they were actually given about the product. However, there was one proposed catch to this logic. If it turned out that the information describing the product was fairly negative, this would undermine participants' confidence in the heuristic. Most people were said to like the product, yet the information participants received about it would be highly incongruent with this claim. This unexpected information, inconsistent with the heuristic, should induce doubt and uncertainty in participants who were simply relying on the heuristic. Confidence in the heuristic should be lowered so that it fell below the sufficiency threshold. Contrast this with what should happen when participants received fairly positive information about the XT-100. In this case, they had an expectancy that the product will be good; they were predisposed to like the product because their heuristics informed them that it would be a good product; and a superficial assessment of the information provided (minimal processing effort) should inform them that all of this was correct—the product was fairly positively reviewed. Thus, in this case peo-

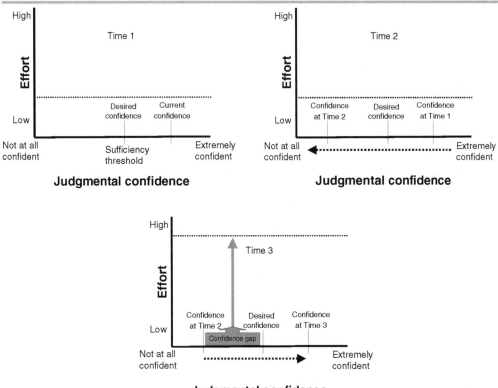

FIGURE 5.5. Instigating systematic processing by undermining judgmental confidence.

ple should have no need to exert too much effort in evaluating the product, relative to the people who were led to lack trust or confidence in their heuristic-based processing.

Maheswaran and Chaiken (1991) examined these hypotheses by manipulating whether participants received information about the XT-100 that was consistent or inconsistent with their heuristic-based expectancies. The information was said to have been provided by a product-testing agency's report that compared the XT-100 with competing brands. People receiving congruent information (a positive report on the XT-100) should feel free to process heuristically and exert relatively little processing effort when doing their evaluation of the product. People receiving incongruent information (a negative report on the XT-100) should lack confidence in heuristic processing and engage in more systematic processing (exerting greater processing effort). How could the researchers detect whether people were using heuristic versus systematic processing, exerting little versus much processing effort? The report had detailed information about how the product performed, as well as quite general, overall summary statements about the quality of the product. The logic of this experiment hinged on the idea that if people were systematically processing the message, they would pay much more attention to the details in the report, thinking about the XT-100's performance on these specific dimensions. Heuristic processors would focus instead on more general thoughts that summarized the overall quality of the product.

The results provided support for the notion that when confidence in a judgment falls below a sufficiency threshold, systematic processing is triggered. First, people who received the unexpectedly negative report about the XT-100 reported having significantly less confidence in their rating of the XT-100 than people who saw a report that coincided well with the consensus information. Second, when people were asked how much confidence they *desired* to have, people who received the unexpectedly negative report about the XT-100 and people who saw a report that coincided well with the consensus information both expressed similar amounts of desired confidence; their sufficiency thresholds were equal. Combining these two points, the groups had equal amounts of confidence they desired to have in their judgment, and the members of one group (the people with confirmed expectancies) had an actual level of confidence that was sufficient in that it did not differ from the confidence they desired. The members of the other group, however, desired a level of confidence they lacked (because of the inconsistency between the report and the consensus of the people surveyed). Finally, the most important question of the experiment addressed what type of information processing was used. As predicted, people who lacked sufficient confidence in their judgment engaged in more thinking about the qualities and attributes of the product being evaluated. They gave more attention to and thought more explicitly about the details of the report than people who had sufficient confidence. They were also better able to remember these details when unexpectedly asked to try to recall the details of the report at the end of the experiment. Lowered confidence in the product of their heuristic-based processing triggered a confidence gap that motivated people to process systematically, despite the fact that the amount of confidence they desired was fairly stable. Actual confidence merely slipped below this sufficiency threshold and motivated people to think more deeply.

We have just seen how information incongruent with people's expectancies can lead them to alter the manner in which they think about and evaluate a novel and relatively uninteresting product (no offense to the XT-100). To what extent can these same ideas be moved outside the context of measuring attitudes toward objects and into the domain of person perception? When perceivers think heuristically and stereotypically about others, can their confidence in those stereotypes and heuristics be undermined by exposure to information contrary to the stereotype/heuristic? If so, is this sense of insufficient confidence enough to alter the manner in which perceivers think about the people they interact with?

Chapter 12 reviews one line of work examining what is called *minority influence*, which is focused on the perceptions of, attributions toward, and attitudes formed toward members of minority groups (and the strategies used by such groups to alter people's heuristically based perception, attributions, and attitudes). Over the past 30 years, there has been a growing body of empirical support for the idea that a minority that expresses opinions and behaviors incongruent with how the majority group expects others to think and act is able to force the majority to reexamine the expectancies previously held (e.g., Baker & Petty, 1994; Bohner, Erb, Reinhard, & Frank, 1996; de Dreu & de Vries, 1996; Moscovici, 1980, 1985a; Moskowitz, 1996; Mugny, 1975; Nemeth, Mayseless, Sherman, & Brown, 1990). Behavior incongruent with what perceivers expect, especially from members of a minority group, initiates an alteration in the thought processes of the perceivers. Similarly, the "person memory" literature reviewed in Chapter 4 has illustrated how exposure to information about others that is incongruent with prior expectancies leads people to think more deeply about those others and engage in more elaborate processing effort. The dual-process notions we are reviewing here allow us to examine the question of why and how incongruent behavior observed in a minority causes perceivers to shift from effortless to effortful thinking—it creates a confidence gap in which judgmental confidence is undermined. Chapter 12 provides a more detailed review of minority influence as being caused by the undermining of judgmental confidence. The basic point is that behavior from a minority that is inconsistent with the majority's expectancies relating to that minority will trigger systematic processing. This increased level of analysis creates the possibility that perceivers' confidence in relying on heuristic processing will be undermined, thus opening the door for the perceivers to change the way they think about that minority.

In sum, one way to trigger systematic processing, and to shake perceivers from the comfort of thinking heuristically and effortlessly about others, is to present those perceivers with information (behavior) that is so inconsistent with their prior expectancies that they can no longer rely on those expectancies alone. Such behavior removes the perceivers' ability to ignore or superficially assess the stimulus, and undermines the confidence they once held in the judgments yielded by their stereotypes and heuristics. This basic tenet of dual-process models was offered decades ago in Kelley's (1973) description of the terms governing the use of schemas: "Perhaps there is an indication here of a preference for simple explanations—a preference that manifests itself only when the hypothesis of simple causation is not too strongly contraindicated by the data" (p. 122).

One problem with relying on behavior that violates an expectancy as a way in which to motivate people to be more "thoughtful" and systematic is simply that behavior often is not so clear-cut. Typically behaviors are complex and multifaceted, open to interpretation. It is difficult to maintain a behavioral sequence that is so concrete and clear that it prevents the possibility of negative interpretations, especially given that people are often predisposed by their prejudices to find them. In addition, this strategy of motivating people to attend carefully to others requires that the burden be placed on these others not only to articulate valid and engaging ideas, but to worry about how these valid and engaging ideas are being presented. Rather than having perceivers motivate themselves to think deeply, it asks others, the targets of these perceptual processes, to metaphorically shake perceivers from the slumber of their heuristic processing. In Allport's (1954, p. 384) terms, this state of affairs places a "preponderance of responsibility" on other people. But must the motivation to engage in systematic processing be initiated by the behavioral strategies of others? Let us examine next how perceivers can, of their own accord, be motivated to engage in systematic processing.

Raising the Sufficiency Threshold. Rather than being overpowered with clear and unexpected behavior initiated by others, which forces perceivers to process systematically, the perceivers can *adopt goals* that promote systematic processing. In this case, the "close looks" of which Bruner (1957) spoke are willfully chosen as a strategy: People are motivated to initiate elaborate processing because they desire greater certainty in their judgments than least-effort processing will allow. Instead of having a low sufficiency threshold (and desiring to exert minimum amounts of processing effort), people are described as being flexible enough to occasionally set high sufficiency thresholds that require elaborate processing. In this case, a confidence gap is created because *perceivers' desired level of confidence drifts upward*. When perceivers have set a high sufficiency threshold and desire a great deal of confidence in their judgments, then it is likely that the judgments produced by heuristic processing will not be experienced as good enough, and a confidence gap will exist. It is the perceivers' own goal to be highly confident in their judgments, evaluations, and actions that instigates systematic processing (see Figure 5.6).

Thus, in instances where people do not desire extreme accuracy, minimal processing effort can deliver judgments that surpass the sufficiency threshold (as seen at Time 1 in Figure 5.6). However, when the judgment matters, they are then motivated to set higher sufficiency thresholds and demand greater judgmental confidence. When desired confidence drifts upward, it may be set at such a high point that current confidence in a heuristic-based judgment falls below the sufficiency threshold and is no longer experienced as "good enough" (Time 2 in Figure 5.6). The higher sufficiency threshold will create a confidence gap if heuristic-based judgments are no longer sufficient. This gap will increase processing effort and require perceivers to engage in systematic processing to deliver a sufficiently good judgment (Time 3 in Figure 5.6). The natural question that follows is this: What goals are capable of producing this upward drift in sufficiency thresholds?

One such goal that leads to increased sufficiency thresholds is the goal of having a vested interest or increased *personal involvement* in the outcome of the judgment. For example, egalitarian individuals might set a high sufficiency threshold and demand to have accurate and confident judgments when interacting with members of socially stigmatized groups, because this situation is personally relevant to them—it addresses an important goal for them. The role of personal relevance in the use of heuristic, top-of-the-head, effortless processing was examined by Borgida and Howard-Pitney (1983), focusing on this motivation's impact on the effects of perceptual salience. Salient things

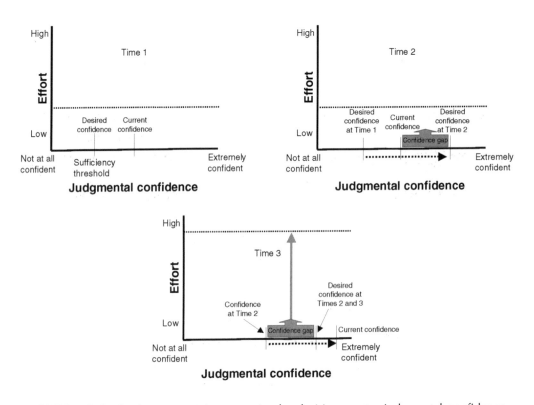

FIGURE 5.6. Instigating systematic processing by desiring greater judgmental confidence.

attract our attention. As reviewed in Chapter 1, we assume that the things on which we are focused are more likely to be the causes of what goes on around us (Taylor, Crocker, Fiske, Sprinzen, & Winkler, 1979), and we accord more weight (and perhaps more ability to influence us) to the people on whom we focus attention. The use of such heuristic and effortless processing leads to effects such as our being more likely to agree with people who sit at a head of a table, and to assign greater responsibility to the actions of people who stand out in a crowd (even if they stand out for reasons that have nothing to with the behavior we are judging). But do these effects of attention and salience slip away when personal relevance is involved?

Borgida and Howard-Pitney (1983) had perceivers listen to a debate on a topic that they believed was either relevant or not relevant to them personally. Specifically, personal involvement was manipulated by varying whether the participants (all college students) believed they would be personally affected by a proposed change in the undergraduate course requirements. Their attention was focused on one person in the debate whom they heard arguing for one side of the issue. When personal involvement was low, students rated the salient person more favorably, regardless of whether that person argued in favor of or against the proposed changes. Perceivers seemed to be using a heuristic that dictated giving preferred status to salient people. When involvement was high, the ratings of the salient person now depended on what position the person took regarding the curriculum changes, rather than simply where the students were focusing their attention. Thus, when perceivers had heightened motivational concerns regarding a topic (i.e., a vested self-interest in it), salience effects were attenuated. Raising the sufficiency threshold so that the perceivers desired greater confidence in their judgment shifted their processing strategy from top-of-the-head processing to more systematic processing.

Similarly, individuals with the goal of not appearing foolish in public might be motivated to set a high threshold for their desired judgmental confidence. This type of goal, where people are motivated by public scrutiny and evaluation of what they think, say, and do, is called *accountability*. For example, if you are reading about a topic for a public presentation that you need to give, you may attend more closely to the material and be more careful in the conclusions you reach than if you were reading the same material for private consumption. Or, if a supervisor evaluates your performance, the amount of time and effort you put into the product you put forward is likely to be greater than if you were not being held accountable for your work. It should be noted that accountability does not always lead to more accurate thinking, but it leads to the kind of thinking desired by the audience to which the cognizer is accountable. Thus accountability could lead to self-serving thinking, outcome-directed thinking, or the like. But often, being accountable means that others are observing cognizers to see how accurate they are. Tetlock (1983) examined the impact on judgment of being held accountable by assessing the degree to which people engage in heuristic versus systematic processing in situations where they are held accountable versus not accountable.

Tetlock (1983) focused on a particular form of effortless processing—the tendency to maintain an already established belief, even in the face of evidence that might suggest revising that belief. In Tetlock's research, the focus was on *primacy effects*. As reviewed in Chapter 1, this is the finding that early information has a greater impact on judgment than later information. Thus beliefs about a person tend to be formed quickly from the initial information received, and later information is not given the appropriate weight, effort, and evaluation required to incorporate it fully into the final judgment. The key assumption of the study was that accountable participants would be less susceptible to primacy effects because of how they encoded information. Accountable, as opposed to unaccountable, participants should be more cautious about drawing inferences from incomplete evidence. This should lead them to attend to more information and analyze that information more carefully. Because of such vigilance in processing, they should be able to recall more of the information at a later point in time. Consistent with these predictions, unmotivated people exhibited primacy effects in forming impressions, placing greater emphasis on information presented early. However, people who were told prior to receiving any information that they would be accountable for their impressions were immune to being influenced by the order in which that information was presented. In addition, measures of how much information was recalled revealed that accountability led to better memory for information.

One final example of a goal that leads people to raise their sufficiency thresholds is the goal of being accurate. Sometimes the situation explicitly calls for this goal, such as when people serve as jurors (where a judge might instruct them to pay close attention and to be objective and accurate) or work as teachers (where evaluating students requires accurate assessment of exams). Other situations merely suggest (imply) that accuracy is important, such as working with other people to attain some mutual goal (e.g., you have a partner for a joint project, and being rewarded depends on the performance of your partner). When one person is dependent on another individual to obtain a desired outcome, and that outcome cannot be attained through the person's own effort alone, the person is said to be in a state of *outcome dependency*. In the example just given, it is useful to form accurate judgments about what your partner is able to contribute, so you can best utilize those skills; you need to assess him/her accurately.

Neuberg and Fiske (1987, Experiment 2) examined how outcome dependency alters people's reliance on heuristic, categorical, and effortless processing. They reasoned that when a negative expectancy is associated with a particular category, people typically evaluate members of that category by using the negative expectancy as a guide. For example, most people hold negative expectancies about what it would be like to interact with a person who has schizophrenia. Thus they would be likely to form judgments of a schizophrenic person that are fairly negative, despite not thinking too carefully about or attending much to the behavior of that person. The person is treated not as an individual, but as an instance of the category. However, individuating and systematic processing could perhaps break this habit of categorical processing if the perceivers had sufficient motivation to perform this effortful type of processing (if their sufficiency threshold drifted upward). Neuberg and Fiske asked participants in their research to volunteer for a purported program on "patient reintegration" in which patients would be released from the hospital and need to start preparing for life on the outside. Thus nonthreatening interactions, in which the patients with schizophrenia worked on tasks with others (the participants), were said to be required. For some participants the patients were said to be schizophrenic, and thus negative expectancies were introduced via this category. Other participants had no category-related expectancies. The participants were then led to believe that they were either outcome-dependent on their partners in this interaction, or fairly independent of the partners. Participants were said to be outcome-dependent when they were told that their joint performance with their partners could win them a cash prize if their teams performed better than other teams. Finally, supposedly in an effort to help strangers work together in this fashion, the participants were told that they would be exchanging some personal information with their partners before working together on a series of tasks.

The main question of interest was whether being outcome-dependent would make the participants evaluate the information they received about others more closely. If there was no category label, then no negative expectancy would exist, and people should form impressions of their partners that were based on the details of the information they received (there would be no heuristic cue to suggest a heuristic, expectancy, or stereotype that could easily guide judgment and explain the behavior). If there was a category label, impressions of the partners should be based on relatively effortless processing, derived from the expectancy rather than from a detailed evaluation of the information provided. However, participants should not simply rely on their expectancies if they had a motivation to be accurate when judging someone for whom a category label had been provided. And having their partners linked to their outcomes should make people want to be accurate, so they could work best together and get the money. Thus the researchers predicted that if positive information was provided, participants would form a positive impression of their partners. If negative information was available, ratings would be negative—not because people were simply using their expectancy and were heuristically processing, but because they had raised the desired amount of confidence they needed in the judgment of their partners, had spent time thinking about these persons, and had obtained negative information. Therefore, it was predicted that effortless processing should only occur if the partners were identified (labeled) as being part of some group to whom negative expectancies were linked and if the partners were not outcome-dependent. These predictions were supported by the research results. The experimenters timed how long it took perceivers to form their impressions of their partners and used this measure as a proxy for the amount of processing effort. As predicted, when people were made outcome-dependent on persons labeled as having schizophrenia, they took twice as much time to form their evaluation of those persons as the people who were not outcome-dependent did.

The Theory of Lay Epistemics

As noted in the Introduction to this book, *epistemology* is the study of knowledge and knowing. The theory of *lay epistemics* (Kruglanski, 1980, 1990) is a theory of how laypeople come to know what they believe they know. According to the theory, the acquisition of social knowledge occurs through two phases or processes. In the first phase, people generate hypotheses about the reasons for (causes of) the events in their social world. In the second phase, people then test and validate these hypotheses. The first process presents an intriguing problem. A potentially infinite number of hypotheses may be generated to explain any given event; therefore, the process of generating hypotheses must somehow be stopped so that people can select, and feel confident in the selection of, one of those hypotheses. Once they have settled on a hypothesis, the persons have now arrived at social knowledge in which they feel confident and that they can use as a sufficient explanation for the event (and to plan how to act). They have moved from deliberating endlessly about the possible reasons why an event has occurred to having a satisfactory answer.

Let us consider an example. You and your colleagues/friends are trying to decide who to admit into your ranks as an employee/friend (e.g., to admit someone into your basketball team, work group, company, social club, etc.). Your colleague Angelika argues strongly against one candidate and strongly in favor of another, and you, as the lay perceiver, try to understand why she has argued as she has. The social event that needs to be explained is Angelika's comments. A number of hypotheses may rush to mind to explain her remarks. First, maybe Angelika truly thinks one candidate is the best and another is the worst. Second, it is instead possible that she believes that most candidates will polarize the group and create too much dissension between group members (some of whom like one person, while others despise that person); thus Angelika has chosen to advocate for the person she believes everyone will agree is acceptable, rather than the person she really thinks is the best. Third, perhaps Angelika is aware that the ultimate responsibility for the decision lies in you, and wants nothing more than to help make you look good (and has chosen candidates that will bring prestige and honor to the group and to you). Fourth, perhaps she knows that responsibility for the decision lies in you and wants nothing more than to humiliate and embarrass you, so she has tried to manipulate the situation so as to produce the worst possible solution. Fifth, maybe Angelika has a personal agenda. She knows that such decisions are complex, and wants to admit someone to the group who helps the group on some dimension that she feels is important, even if the criterion she is using to make her decision is not one valued by you or the rest of the group (e.g., most group members want someone who is highly creative, but Angelika disregards that criterion and instead wants someone mathematically inclined and technologically savvy, regardless of the candidate's creativity). Finally, perhaps social pressures external to the actual decision are exerting an impact, such as affirmative action policies (e.g., "We must hire a Black person") or prejudice ("We must not hire a Black person"). As this example demonstrates, almost any social event poses many possible causes. As perceivers we begin immediately, and somewhat automatically, to generate such explanations. The theory of lay epistemics focuses on when and why and how people shift from generating and deliberating over a multitude of hypotheses to confidently adopting a specific, single explanation.

Thus, in order for a person to arrive at a judgment, the epistemic process must be brought to a halt. In the language of Gestalt psychologists, the stream of hypothesis generation must be "frozen" so that the cognitive system attains a state of equilibrium, or *closure*. As discussed in the Introduction to this book, when people have uncertainty or doubt, a state of psychological tension associated with lacking closure is experienced. People are motivated to reduce this tension, put an end to doubt, and attain closure; they arrive at a sufficient explanation for why an event occurred. Thus, while generating many hypotheses regarding why an event occurred can be perceived as a good thing, it also introduces an extension of a period of uncertainty, doubt, and lack of closure. At some point, this period of uncertainty must be brought to an end and closure attained. Kruglanski's (1990) theory of lay epistemics focuses on the factors that determine when people attain closure—that is, when they stop generating hypotheses and decide they have sufficient confidence in an hypothesis that has already been generated and validated.

The theory of lay epistemics outlines two general categories of factors that determine when hypothesis generation will stop. One factor is related to *cognitive capability*. People's capability to generate hypotheses involves their knowledge of the person/topic/event at hand, as well as momentary factors in the situation that promote one hypothesis over another. For example, one may not be able to generate multiple hypotheses about an event because one knows relatively little about the event. One's capability to generate hypotheses is not determined solely by what information is or is not available. The situation one is in may also limit the number of hypotheses one is capable of generating by making some hypotheses more salient than others. In the running example, if something in the current situation reminds you how selfish Angelika can be, you may generate only hypotheses that are related to her being self-ish or opposed to you doing well, and you may lack the capability to generate hypotheses that would allow you to consider her as trying to be fair or to help you do well. The situation can restrict what comes to mind by making hypotheses that are related to the current situation more likely to be generated, while unrelated hypotheses do not come to mind.

A second factor that determines when hypothesis generation will come to a halt is perfectly unrelated to whether people are capable of generating hypotheses; it is the *motivation to engage in hypothesis generation*. People's goals dictate how willing they may be to suspend having closure while considering all the possible alternatives and generating hypothesis after hypothesis. Certain motives lead people to deliberate effortfully about an event, with many possible hypotheses being generated and evaluated. At other times, people are simply not motivated to exert the effort of generating hypothesis after hypothesis and evaluating each. Instead, they are motivated to stop thinking fairly early in the hypothesis generation process and to arrive at a fast solution, with relatively little cognitive effort being exerted. Thus goals serve to energize and deenergize the epistemic process. What sorts of goals does the theory of lay epistemics suggest control the type of thinking in which people are willing to engage? Two broad classes of goals determine whether the epistemic process will be frozen early after consideration of only a few hypotheses, or thawed over a longer period of time after a systematic examination of many hypotheses. The theory describes these as goals that promote a *need for structure* (in later versions of the theory, this terminology has been changed to a *need for closure*) and goals that promote a *desire for validity* (or a *fear of invalidity*). A need for structure/closure will promote attempts to attain closure quickly, while a desire for validity/fear of invalidity will lead people to suspend attaining closure until the best possible conclusion is reached.

Need for Structure/Closure

Need for structure is characterized by quick cessation of the epistemic process; it elevates the costs associated with lacking cognitive closure, leading people to seek the quickest route to closure. It instigates a search for "an answer on a given topic, any answer, as compared to confusion or ambiguity" (Kruglanski, 1990, p. 337). It promotes a state where alternative hypotheses are less likely to be generated, information inconsistent with what is expected is less likely to be attended to, and ambiguity is avoided (making it conceptually similar to Frenkel-Brunswik's [1949] notion of intolerance of perceptual ambiguity, which describes people as thinking in a manner marked by "perceptual rigidity, inability to change set, and tendencies to primitive and rigid structuring," p. 122). Neuberg, Judice, and West (1997) make an important conceptual distinction between different forms of closure seeking—*seizing* and *freezing* processes. They assert that there are two largely independent epistemic motives relating to halting the epistemic process. The first is called *seizing*, and is determined by the desire for what is called *nonspecific closure* ("Any decision will do"). By this it is meant that perceivers are motivated to have an answer quickly, but it can be any answer that is reasonable and makes sense. They seek closure, but it need not be one specific type of closure. Independent to this is a process called *freezing*, where the focus is on attaining one form of specific closure—the desire to make a decision consistent with an existing (even if recently obtained) structure.

If a heightened goal to attain structure leads people to arrive at quick and easy answers (grabbing at the first reasonable explanation for a given social event), Kruglanski and Freund (1983) reasoned that people's judgment would be more likely to be influenced by expectancies or inferences that were formed early in a judgment task. Such information should have a greater impact on people with a heightened need for structure, because their lack of generating and examining alternative hypotheses makes it less likely that their initial judgments will be modified in light of other information that might be later encountered. Thus the impressions of persons with a high need for structure should be more predictable from the evaluative implications of traits presented early in a sequence than from the evaluative implications of traits presented later (a primary effect). To manipulate need for structure, Kruglanski and Freund placed some of their research participants under "time pressure" by asking them to make judgments within an extremely short time frame. Kruglanski (1990, p. 337) stated that an important cost of lacking fast structure is "failing to act or decide on an issue in time to meet an important deadline." Under time pressure, the threat of missing such deadlines presumably looms large and is assumed to heighten need for structure. After half of the participants were placed under time pressure and half were not placed under time pressure, they were presented with pieces of information about another person and asked to rate that person's qualifications as a job candidate. Presumably, if participants were playing the role of an employer evaluating a job candidate, they would be motivated to form an accurate and valid judgment and to consider all the information being presented equally well. But if need for structure promoted fast closure and settling on the first satisfactory conclusion, then the information presented earlier in the list of information provided should be more influential in the ratings of the participants. To test this prediction, half of the participants received positive information about the candidate followed by negative information, while the other half received negative information followed by positive. As predicted by the theory, participants exhibited a higher degree of primacy effects when there was a high need for structure: People under time pressure who saw negative information first formed more negative impressions than people who saw negative information first who were not facing a deadline. A similar pattern emerged when positive information was presented first: More positive impressions were formed when people had high need for structure.

Desire for Validity (Fear of Invalidity)

A danger of reaching a conclusion too quickly (such as when one has a high need for structure) is that the judgment may not be a valid one. *Fear of invalidity* is the fear of committing oneself to an invalid position (especially if negative consequences are associated with invalid judgments). The processing initiated by a fear of invalidity is characterized by an epistemic thaw (avoidance of early closure) and an extension of the epistemic sequence, so that one has a prolonged examination and extensive processing of relevant information. Fear of invalidity can motivate people to be energy users—cognitive philanthropists rather than misers. It can be instantiated by a desire to be accurate, by the association of punishment with being inaccurate, and by a desire to avoid the dullness and predictability associated with relying on whatever thoughts come to mind first. Mayseless and Kruglanski (1987) manipulated desire for validity by telling some research participants that the task they were performing was one that had "considerable functional significance, and constitutes a component of general intelligence" (p. 176). Essentially, they were led to believe that reaching a decision too quickly on the task, without examining the relevant information extensively, could reveal that they lacked intelligence. Thus, with this negative consequence associated with forming an invalid judgment, participants were assumed to be motivated to avoid reaching closure too quickly. Other participants were told nothing about how the task related to their intelligence. The task that they were asked to perform involved looking at enlarged pictures of common objects that were taken from unusual angles. This made the objects difficult to identify. Participants were asked to list all the conceivable hypotheses they could generate regarding what type of object represented in a given picture. Relative to the control condition, participants who feared making an invalid judgment and were motivated to avoid early closure generated significantly more hypotheses.

Thus the theory of lay epistemics describes two processes of hypothesis generation and cessation that people use in attempting to reduce doubt. The theory posits that individuals perceive a stimulus, generate hypotheses about what the appropriate category to "capture" that stimulus might be, test (validate) the hypotheses, freeze the hypothesis testing when an appropriate solution has been arrived at, and then make inferences and plan action accordingly. The particular course (i.e., the evidence attended to and the weight given a piece of evidence) and termination of the validation process are directed by whether the persons desire an answer quickly (their willingness to "live with" uncertainty).

Correction or Dissociation Models

In the dual-process models reviewed thus far, we have seen one type of effortful mental process that people employ: They think more deeply, reassess prior beliefs, and analyze features and details more closely, engaging in counterargument generation and attempts to validate, through close inspection of the veracity of the information at hand, the data before them (whether these data are the qualities and behaviors of another person, the issues and arguments heard and observed in a commercial or political speech, or their own prior beliefs). We turn now to another type of mental task that requires effortful/systematic processing—correction processes.

Some dual-process models share the assumption that people are sensitive to and nervous about biases that may be influencing their judgments and impressions of others. People like to think that their impressions are fair, sufficient, and accurate, regardless of whether this is actually the case. What truly matters to them is their ability to believe firmly (with confidence) in the appropriateness of their thoughts. When they become suspicious that an unwanted bias is affecting their thoughts, it triggers an attempt to correct their judgment and remove this unwanted influence. The desire to have an uncontaminated and appropriate set of cognitive processes initiates mental effort bent on delivering this "purity" of thought. Thus the motivation to be accurate and fair, to have uncontaminated and unbiased judgments and decisions, will lead people to exert increasing amounts of mental energy and effortful processing.

Typically, these types of models assume that by default, people engage in a more effortless, categorical type of information processing. Such processing, as we have been exploring, is susceptible to many types of bias. People rely overly on heuristics; they overgeneralize from categories to individual members of those categories (often without sufficient justification); they disregard information incompatible with their expectancies and place undue judgmental weight on information that confirms what they already believe; and they allow person types and salient exemplars to limit how a novel person is evaluated. So long as people remain blissfully unaware of these contaminating forces, they are satisfied with their judgments. In addition, even if they were aware of these category-based processes, they might still be satisfied with their judgments so long as the categories were felt to be warranted, useful, and accurate enough. However, when people (1) become aware of these effortless processes and (2) also begin to suspect that the processes are exerting an unwanted influence on judgment, it is then that they feel the motivation to increase processing effort to rid their impressions of these intrusions.

In essence, an initial, category-based judgment anchors an impression, and a subsequent, effortful process of correction/dissociation adjusts that impression away from the anchor and toward a more "objective" accounting of the other person. Several models in social psychology adopt this "anchor and adjust" processing logic in accounting for social cognition, and subsequent chapters review several of these. Chapter 7 examines the dual-process models of Gilbert (1989) and Trope (1986a), which account for how and when people rid themselves of an attributional bias arising from effortless inferences about the traits and qualities of those they perceive. Chapter 10 examines the "set–reset" model of L. L. Martin (1986), which accounts for a bias in impression formation linked to the overuse of concepts and exemplars that one has recently been exposed to (information that is perceptually ready). Chapters 11 and 12 present a model of stereotyping suggesting that stereotypes are effortlessly triggered and then consciously removed from evaluations and judgments (Devine, 1989).

These models share a set of assumptions about correction processes that also reveal the delicate nature of such processes. Debiasing one's responses, so that they are corrected for an unwanted influence, depends on one's possessing (1) awareness that one is biased, (2) motivation to remove this influence, (3) theories about what that influence is and how it pushes judgment, and (4) cognitive resources for carrying out these effortful processes. Because of these contingencies, one may have an imperfect ability or desire to engage in the effortful processing that allows judgments to move beyond category-based and heuristic processing.

Awareness

Even when people desire to be accurate in judging others and to have no unwanted influences from their effortless inferences about others, they may simply fail to recognize that such influences exist. Defeating bias by being systematic, effortful, and deliberate requires the knowledge that a potential source of bias exists! Chapter 1 has been dedicated to expounding the idea of naive realism—a phenomenon that, by definition, tells us that people simply are not aware of the fact that they are biased, clinging instead to the false belief that their perceptions are based on some "absolute truth." This is particularly troubling in the domain of stereotyping, because people often do not know that they use stereotypes. For instance, they think the problem of racism is caused by some troublesome group of racists "out there" somewhere, not by them. This naivete in typical persons' recognition of their own biases was described in an address entitled "In Search of a Majority" delivered by James Baldwin to the Kalamazoo College class of 1960 (and later printed in the 1961/1993 collection of essays called *Nobody Knows My Name*):

> Presumably the society in which we live is an expression—in some way—of the majority will. But it is not so easy to locate this majority. The moment one attempts to define this majority one is faced with several conundrums. Majority is not an expression of numbers, of numeri-

cal strength, for example. You may far outnumber your opposition and not be able to impose your will on them or even to modify the rigour with which they impose their will on you, i.e., the Negroes in South Africa or in some counties, some sections, of the American South. (p. 127)

I want to suggest this: that the majority for which everyone is seeking which must reassess and release us from our past and deal with the present and create standards worthy of what a man may be—this majority is you. (p. 137)

Motivation to Correct

For correction processes to be engaged, people must be motivated to stop the bias from exerting an influence once they become aware of the bias. This may seem obvious, but there are many instances where people may simply not care that they are biased (or at least care enough to do anything about it). For example, prejudiced persons are unlikely to stop using stereotypes once they become aware that their stereotypes may be affecting them. Partisans are unlikely to change how they evaluate the members of an opposing political party if made to realize that party membership may be biasing their views. A parent is unlikely to stop giving the benefit of the doubt to his/her child, even if there are many signs that doubts should exist. Thus, in addition to being aware of bias, perceivers must, through goals linked to things like outcome dependency and accountability, be motivated to remove the bias.

Naive Theories of Bias

If one is aware of a bias and motivated to attempt to remove that bias (correct for it), one still requires some set of beliefs concerning what the nature of the bias is and how to best eliminate it. One must have some theory of the manner in which those biases exert an impact. Once a theory has been identified, one can then attempt to implement an appropriate correction strategy. Theory-guided corrections work in a "do-the-opposite" manner—identifying the direction of the bias and attempting to shift judgment in the opposite direction (thus restoring judgment to "normal" and undoing the impact of the theory). Consider the following snippet from an article by Elisabeth Bumiller about President Bush's reasons for going to war in Iraq, which appeared in *The New York Times* on September 16, 2002:

Last week the president drove the speculation even further when he referred obliquely at the U.N. to an assassination attempt against his father, saying, "In 1993, Iraq attempted to assassinate the emir of Kuwait and a former American president." A senior official later told reporters, "Obviously, one doesn't want to appear to personalize this." In fact, only two men know for sure how much the father is influencing the son on Iraq. But interviews with Bush family friends and senior White House advisers produce a consistent belief: not much. The 41st president would never so directly tell the 43rd what to do, they say. They also insist that President Bush is able to distinguish between his feelings as a son and his responsibilities as commander in chief. "I promise you, he has the ability as a human being to disassociate any personal emotions with the job he is doing as president," said Ron Kaufman, a Buh family friend and a close adviser to the 41st president. (p. 15)

This quote reveals several assumptions (by a variety of people) about what happens when people suspect that they are biased, or that someone or something in the environment is biasing their responses. The first assumption is that people "know for sure" what influences them. Others may not know, but the persons being influenced can detect bias and can accurately deduce the effects of that bias. The second assumption is that a person who becomes aware of bias has the ability, "as a human being," to dissociate that bias from responses. Thus if President Bush had personal feelings that drove him to desire revenge for his father's attempted murder, he could detect those feelings and accurately know how to adjust his reaction so that his decision about whether to attack Iraq (the nation responsible for the alleged murder attempt) was not influenced by these personal feelings. Are such assumptions accurate? What actually happens when people think they are being influenced by some unwanted agent (either internal or in the environment)?

According to Wegener and Petty (1995), the answer to this question is that people try to correct for this bias, to prevent themselves from being influenced. This is precisely what the quote above describes. How can they accomplish this? People hold *naive theories* about the nature of the influence (theories about the magnitude and direction of some biasing force) and take steps to correct for that perceived influence by countering the impact that these theories claim exists: "People might use a subjective reaction to a target but adjust that initial reaction in light of a theory" (Wegener & Petty, 1995, p. 39). Thus, in the quote above, this is reflected in the fact that President Bush was said to "distinguish between his feelings as a son and his responsibilities as commander in chief" and to dissociate these personal emotions from his professional decisions. The subjective reaction of the President might be rage at Iraq's leader and desire for revenge, but he could detect this influence, had a theory about how it was influencing his decision whether to initiate a war, and could remove that influence (adjust the subjective reaction to account for the detected bias). Wegener, Dunn, and Tokusato (2001, pp. 281–282) have summarized this succinctly: "[The perceiver] will evaluate the potential biasing effect(s) of salient factors in the judgment setting. . . . This is accomplished by consulting naive theories of the bias(es) associated with the salient factor(s)." However, just because people suspect they are being influenced and take steps to try to prevent it, this does not necessarily mean that they are correct in assuming an influence exists or that they are taking the appropriate steps to fix it if it really does exist.

For example, a teacher, Mr. Vance, who has his own child in class might worry that his positive affect for the child could be influencing his evaluation of the child's ability as a student. When concerned with contamination of this sort in one's subjective reaction, one attempts to correct it. One holds a naïve theory about that influence, and this theory then shapes the type of correction that is attempted. In this example, Mr. Vance has a theory that he is being too lenient toward his own child, so he acts in an opposite fashion: He starts being extra critical of the child and using harsher standards than those he uses for other students. However, these are referred to as *naive theories*, because such theories of influence need not be accurate. What triggers the use of theories of influence is the *perception that one is biased or is being unduly influenced*, not an actual influence. Even if Mr. Vance is not being biased in favor of his own child, he could still believe this bias to exist and still hold a theory about the nature of the bias and how to rectify it. Nisbett and Wilson (1977) describe an experiment that provides an excellent illustration of how people perceive an influence on their mental processes where none really exists. Research participants watched a film either with or without a distracting background noise. When participants in the background-noise condition were asked whether the noise influenced their ratings, most reported that it had. However, the actual ratings of the film did not differ for these two groups. Their theory that they had been influenced by the noise was simply incorrect.

One may not only be using a theory of influence when one is not really being influenced; one may end up using the wrong theory (e.g., Wilson & Brekke, 1994). Thus one may really be biased, but have the wrong naive theory about how strongly one is biased (the magnitude of bias) or in what way one is biased (the direction of bias). In our example, Mr. Vance may truly be biased toward his child, but only in that he has a moderately positive predisposition. If he then acts in an extremely harsh way to compensate for the bias, his theory has overestimated the magnitude of the bias. Alternatively, he could have a flat-out incorrect bias: He could actually be more harsh toward his child, but he may have a naive theory that he is probably too lenient on the child. He may then use the theory to trigger even harsher treatment. Bias does indeed exist, but the naive theory Mr. Vance uses to inform him of the nature of the bias is wrong (or in the wrong direction). In the President Bush example, the intuitions expressed in *The New York Times* about how the President might deal with his emotions toward Iraq were partially correct. As a human, he would try to detect the bias and correct for it. However, the assumption that he would detect the correct bias and accurately dissociate this bias from judgments he made as commander in chief was not a good one. Let us now provide a few empirical examples of how people use naive theories to try to correct their judgment, and as a result produce what may be bad judgments.

Wegener and Petty (1995) assert that people hold naive theories reflecting an idiosyncratic view of how they are being influenced. If true, then the manner in which people attempt to correct their judgments should reflect the underlying theory of how they are being influenced. If one has a theory that one is being influenced by having one's judgments pushed in a positive direction (such as Mr. Vance's favoring his own child), then one should try to make corrected judgments that are in a more negative direction (such as Mr. Vance's judging his own child more harshly). If one's naive theory is that judgments are perceived to be influenced in a negative direction, then one tries to be more positive to counteract the perceived bias. Wegener and Petty use a more precise language, distinguishing between *assimilative* and *contrastive* biases. In this terminology, there is a context, and one has a naive theory that one is being influenced by this context in one's judgment of some target. If the target is made to seem similar to the context as a result of this influence, this is said to be an *assimilative influence*. If the target is made to seem more unlike the context than it would had the context not been present, this is a *contrastive influence*.

For example, Wegener and Petty (1995) asked participants how they thought that thinking about the weather in exotic locations like Jamaica and Hawaii would influence their ratings of less exotic places (Midwestern cities like Indianapolis) as vacation spots. They predicted that most people would believe it to have a negative impact, or a contrastive influence (they would have a theory specifying that less exotic places will seem extra undesirable in comparison to Hawaii). They also asked participants how desirable the jobs were perceived to be in beautiful weather locales, like Hawaii. In this case, an assimilative influence was predicted such that because of the great weather, people would believe that others probably love working and living there. A first experiment revealed that these were precisely the naive theories that research participants held—the same context (thinking about the weather in Hawaii) led to a perceived contrastive influence on one judgment target (Indianapolis) and an assimilative influence in another (working in Hawaii). Once having identified these theories, the researchers could now explore the real question of interest to us: If people have different theories about how they are influenced when judging different targets, do they correct for the influence, and do the corrections taken differ when judging each of the targets (according to the theory of influence specific to that target)? Wegener and Petty expected that the negative impact on ratings of Midwestern cities from having contemplated the exotic locales would be corrected for. These cities should increase in attractiveness if people were aware of the bias and were using naive theories to correct for it (recognizing the impact of the biasing agent and removing that influence from judgment). To assess this, participants were asked to rate the desirability of vacationing in Midwestern cities, and to be sure not to let their ratings of exotic locales influence them (thus making sure that they would use their naive theories). The results revealed that the more negative the theories of influence (such as theorizing one would harshly judge a Midwestern city after thinking about Hawaii), the more positive subsequent ratings of these Midwestern cities became. People adjusted their judgments, using their theories of influence as a guide.

Wegener, Petty, and Dunn (1998) illustrated this point further, using people as the targets (rather than cities). For example, research participants had to rate how violent Arnold Schwarzenegger was. Some of the participants made this rating after first making a similar rating about extremely nonviolent people, such as Gandhi and the Pope. Other participants made this rating after first making a similar rating about extremely violent people, such as Hitler and Stalin. The logic was that the initial ratings of either extremely nonviolent or violent people would serve as a context that could introduce bias. Perceivers would detect this potential source of bias and worry that their ratings of Schwarzenegger would be influenced by the previous ratings. One group would hold a theory specifying something like "Next to the Pope, Arnold is pretty violent," whereas the other group would hold a theory with exactly the opposite implications: "Next to Hitler, Arnold is not violent." Thus the same target (now Governor Schwarzenegger of California) would be reacted to in extremely different ways if people followed their theories. Participants who first rated Gandhi would worry that they would be biased by Gandhi's nonviolent shadow and rate Arnold as extra violent. Thus, to be nonbiased, they would have to make sure they rated Arnold as nonviolent. Participants who first rated Hitler would worry that they were being biased by Hitler's genocidal nature and would underestimate Arnold's violence as a result. Thus, to be nonbiased, these people would have to rate Arnold as extremely violent. This was precisely what was found. When asked to try not to be biased and to correct for any unwanted influence on their evaluations, people holding opposing theories about how they might be influenced judged the same person in diametrically opposing ways. Naive theories of influence exist, and they guide judgment. With such naive theories in hand, and the motivation to use them, people can now correct. Or can they?

Cognitive Capacity

Even if people are aware of bias, motivated to eliminate that bias, and in possession of a theory about how (and how much) that bias is influencing them, they may still end up not engaging in correction processes. Why? Because such processes are effortful and require the systematic reevaluation of an already existing impression. As we have discussed in several places in this book, such processes require processing capacity to be available. If cognitive load is present in the current situation, the requisite capacity to engage in theory-based correction may simply be unavailable. Thus people may have the desire to correct, but lack the cognitive capability to do it. Bruner (1957) summarized this irony of social life quite nicely: "It is doubtful whether a therapeutic regimen of 'close looking' will aid the misperceiver much. . . . [The] greatest difficulty rests in the fact that the cost of close looks is generally too high under the conditions of speed, risk, and limited capacity imposed upon organisms by the environment" (pp. 141–142). By *close looks*, Bruner refers to attempts by perceivers to analyze the data closely. Such attempts are blocked by the ever-present perils of social life—the need to think and act quickly (speed) and the bombardment of information that must simultaneously be processed (limited capacity). The processes required for correction are simply too strenuous, given the other, simultaneous processing demands. In fact, the lack of such abilities is one reason we have claimed that categorical and other forms of effortless processing have developed in the first place.

The Timing of the Goal

The discussion of how goals affect cognitive processing in the dual-process models reviewed above must also include an examination of the question of the timing of the goal's instantiation. Tetlock and Kim (1987) suggested that goals are most successful in defeating passive influences on judgment by making people more vigilant in the way they *encode* information. That is, if you are going to exert effort in thinking about a person, it is best to do so at the moment that you are receiving that information and actually interacting with that person. This is not to say that goals cannot have an impact on your *reprocessing* of information, or on your attempts to retrieve information about a person from memory and engage in systematic processing on this stored information. However, the systematic processing of information from memory requires you to have stored enough information about that person in memory that you can later retrieve it and process it elaborately (Thompson, Roman, Moskowitz, Chaiken, & Bargh, 1994). Obviously, the inclusion of this extra step will mean that systematic reprocessing is at a relative disadvantage to systematic processing that occurs at encoding (online).

For some types of categorical/heuristic/schematic processing, specific influences on information processing can be demonstrated by varying when goals are provided. For example, in the research of Tetlock (1983) reviewed above, accountability goals triggered systematic processing that was able to overturn judgments that were more effortlessly formed. However, Tetlock also found that this effect was restricted to instances in which people were told they were accountable *before* receiving information about the person. When they received the information first, and only later found out that they were accountable for their impressions, categorical impressions persisted (people were still heuristically processing).

However, other research has found that "when" the goal is introduced is not an important factor. Accountability triggers systematic processing when it is introduced before perceivers meet a person, as well as when it is introduced at some point after perceivers have met the person and have already formed an impression (e.g., Thompson et al., 1994). Goals (such as accountability) introduced after initial inferences have been drawn should have a *harder* time debiasing or correcting inferences, but this does not rule out debiasing altogether. If this is the case, why then does some research suggest that correction is only possible when the goal is presented in time for online correction, allowing people to generate complex and multifaceted inferences that can defeat passive influences as the information is being interpreted? Some speculation is offered.

First, perhaps some types of categorical processing are weaker than others and are more easily overturned, even after an impression has already been formed. Second, perhaps the nature of the goals needs to be particularly self-involving in order for reprocessing to be successfully initiated. Third, perhaps this has to do with judgmental confidence. Judgments that result from some types of categorical processing may be held more confidently than those resulting from other types of categorical processing. For these confidently held judgments, people may feel so confident that they do not feel as if they need to go back and reexamine the information. Fourth, perhaps the time itself is the key issue. If the goal is introduced after people have already formed an impression, but the time between having formed an impression and being told that they will need to be accurate is short, people will still have the ability to recreate the original information from memory and alter their impressions accordingly. But if the time interval is longer, it is possible that people's ability to recall is interfered with, so that the information is simply not available in memory any more. As previously stated, capacity alone may not be enough to instigate control over passive processes, but neither may be having intent. Regardless of what people intend to do, they must have the capacity and the ability to carry out those intentions. Perhaps these limiting conditions for correction (a goal, capacity, and ability) are more constraining at recall and make retrieval-based influences from intent more difficult to produce.

EFFORT AND ITS RELATIONSHIP TO ACCURACY AND CONFIDENCE

Biased Systematic Processing

Increased effort in thinking about a person, issue, or event is not necessarily the same thing as more accurate thinking—a fact labeled by Chaiken and colleagues (1989) as *biased systematic processing*. Systematic processing can be biased for at least two reasons. First, we perceivers may be motivated to come to a particular conclusion, expend effort to defend that conclusion, and make sure it is the result that is attained. Kunda (1987) has referred to this as *motivated reasoning*. Second, we may simply try to be accurate, but have false knowledge and incorrect theories that we use in our detailed analysis. Try as we might to be fair, if we are armed with bad information, we will end up with a false conclusion. This is called *misdirected decontamination*.

Misdirected Decontamination

Even if we become aware of a bias in our judgment, and we have the desire and ability to correct for this bias and "decontaminate" our thoughts, we may have an incorrect naive theory of what that influence is (e.g., Nisbett & Wilson, 1977; Wilson & Brekke, 1994). Thus, rather than "correcting" judgment, we adjust it (according to this wrong theory) in a manner that makes it biased in a new and different way. This is discussed further in Chapter 10. For now, let us simply highlight the fact that greater effort in thinking about people and events does not guarantee that we will have greater accuracy in our final judgments, decisions, and evaluations. One reason for this is that we service our cognition with incorrect theories about what is influencing us. In trying to fix our cognition, we pull a faulty tool out of the cognitive toolbox. For example, President Bush relied on faulty intelligence information in deciding to invade Iraq in 2003.

As another example, in his second term as President of the United States, Bill Clinton was constantly receiving negative press: He was impeached by Congress, accused of having an affair with a White House intern named Monica Lewinsky, found to have lied to a grand jury (and to the American public in a famous, finger-wagging denial) regarding that affair, and subjected to scrutiny regarding potential illegal activity in a real estate deal (Whitewater) and in campaign financing. Ironically, the public loved him (if we use approval ratings as an index). Many people felt that despite all these troubles, he still would have defeated George W. Bush for President in 2000 if he could have run for a third term! One possible explanation for this Clinton love may have been the use of a bad theory of bias. People may have assumed that the negative affect they felt toward Clinton resulted from the intense media scrutiny and unyielding attacks of partisan Republican foes. Rather than these attacks' being successful, they may have backfired on Republicans by allowing people to develop a false theory that their negative feelings toward the President were caused by the attacks of the media and partisan opponents. Instead of a theory that attributed their negative feelings to the President's actual misconduct, people may have used a naive theory that led their thinking about the President in a totally different direction. Note that in this example people were not thinking effortlessly or categorically. They were using a theory to help them effortfully sort out their cognition about a complex target (President Clinton). It was just that in their effort to drive toward an accurate end, they were using a bad map.

Motivated Reasoning

Not all bias is due to the "innocent" inability to hold an accurate theory of influence. Some bias is quite motivated. To assume that the only motive that drives us to think deeply about information is one that specifies a drive for accuracy is to grandly underestimate ourselves as perceivers. Chapter 1 has identified a myriad of motives and goals that provide the energy driving human social cognition. The consequence of having so many motives that may potentially drive the way in which we think about others is that the energy and effort we expend on systematic processing is not always spent on gathering the best and most objective data. Instead, we rationalize, spin, and self-deceive; we selectively attend and evaluate; and we engage in a variety of mental gymnastics aimed at using our effortful cognition to prove what we want it to prove and what we desire to believe is true. This type of motivated reasoning, capable of producing bias in impression formation, is the focus of Chapter 8, so let us limit discussion of these issues here to a few relevant examples to illustrate the point. Chaiken and colleagues (1989) explored three general types of motivated reasoning.

The first type of motive that directs systematic processing is *accuracy motivation*. It is represented by goals, already discussed, that lead people to seek to be accurate: fear of invalidity, desire for self-assessment, outcome dependency, accountability, and increased responsibility. People motivated to be accurate in evaluating their own behavior are said to have *self-assessment* motives (e.g., Trope, 1986b). When accuracy-motivated, systematic processing proceeds in a more objective and unbiased fashion in an attempt to seek the "truth." Illustrations of accuracy-driven processing have already been provided in connection with the theory of lay epistemics (e.g., Mayesless & Kruglanski, 1987) and the HSM (e.g., Maheswaran & Chaiken, 1991).

Other motives besides accuracy, however, can bias perceivers. A second class of motives detailed by Chaiken and colleagues (1989) is *impression motivation*. This is the desire to maintain beliefs, attitudes, judgments, and actions that allow others to form a specific type of impression of one in accordance with one's interpersonal needs in a social situation. It is the motive to produce a certain premeditated set of consequences in one's interpersonal relationships and to project a certain image. This is typically accomplished by trying to take into account the qualities, views, and disposition of one's partners in a social situation. Such an impression management (e.g., Schlenker, 1980) or self-presentational (e.g., Jones, 1990) goal allows one not only to anticipate the characteristics that others wish to see, but to produce the desired outcomes from another person by displaying those desired characteristics for them. Need for approval, fear of rejection, desire for power, ingratiation, communication goals, and social role needs are all motives capable of triggering impression-motivated systematic processing. Such processing is often selective and strategic, aimed at assessing the social acceptability of beliefs and judgments.

For example, Sedikides (1990) gave some research participants the goal of communicating a particular type of impression to other people, asking them to tailor their message to suit the audience who would be receiving it. Others were given no such instruction. The perceivers who were busy attempting to match their own behavior to the qualities of the people they would be interacting with were more systematic in their evaluation of these other people. When participants had no such goals, they were shown to judge other people according to whatever concepts came most easily and readily to mind. This top-of-the-head type of processing was abandoned by people who were concerned with having others form a specific impression of them. Participants were not aware of the fact that they typically process in an effortless fashion. Thus, their failure to rely on such processing was not due to a correction process or to decreased confidence in their judgment. Instead, they increased their desired confidence, with the impression goal raising their sufficiency threshold, making them want to think more deeply.

Finally, the last class of motives discussed by Chaiken and colleagues (1989) includes those aimed at protecting and maintaining self-esteem; this class is labeled *defense motivation*. The defensively motivated systematic processor scrutinizes information in a directional, selective manner, so as to confirm the validity and prevent the falsification of important, self-relevant knowledge, beliefs, and relationships. The goal of the defense-motivated person is to preserve, verify, and enhance the self-concept and those aspects of the world in which the self is personally vested. These motives reflect a desire to form and defend conclusions that are consistent with prior knowledge (including self-knowledge), as well as to form and defend conclusions that promote self-esteem. Thus, within defense motivation are two distinct types of motives—one geared toward consistency and one toward ego defense/enhancement.

Consistency Motivation and Self-Verification. Two decades prior to the rise of dual-process models, social psychology was replete with another group of models, the *cognitive consistency* theories. These theories are far too numerous and complex to review in detail here. However, the premise of such theories is that humans are fundamentally driven to avoid inconsistency among their cognitions. Festinger's (1957) *theory of cognitive dissonance* is perhaps the best known. Its premise is this: When a person has two cognitions that are inconsistent, this arouses an aversive drive state, similar to hunger. As with physically derived drives, people are motivated to reduce the discomfort associated with the drive state (the dissonance). They are motivated to restore consistency among the discrepant cognitions to reduce their discomfort. As discussed in the Introduction, such inconsistencies are experienced as doubt, and in an attempt to reduce doubt people try to attain certainty, predictability, and control over the dissonant cognitions. This excessively brief review of consistency theories highlights the current point: People expend mental energy not only to attain accurate information, but also to attempt to maintain existing beliefs. These attempts at maintaining consistency occur even in the face of dissonance-arousing information that is inconsistent with and potentially damaging to those beliefs. As reviewed in Chapters 3 and 4, rather than overhauling their existing belief systems, people instead engage in elaborate processes (consistency resolution processes, rationalizations, data twisting) that will eliminate the dissonance while maintaining the old views. Swann (1990) has referred to such attempts to maintain existing beliefs concerning the self as *self-verification* (for a review, see Chapter 8).

Darley and Gross (1983) and Snyder and Swann (1978) provided classic illustrations of belief preservation, consistency seeking, and expectancy verification in the manner in which people evaluate and test hypotheses. People exert effort aimed at arriving at a specific conclusion that maintains a prior belief. Darley and Gross referred to this type of verification in hypothesis testing as the *perceptual confirmation effect*. Darley and Gross reasoned that when people have a particular expectancy, hypothesis, stereotype, or prior belief triggered, it will serve as an anchor that guides subsequent information processing. This research, reviewed in detail in Chapters 3 and 11, illustrates that people subsequently gather information in a manner bent on confirming their existing hypotheses. This can involve not only seeking out information consistent with what they already believe, but, as in the case of the Darley and Gross experiment, twisting the perception of existing data that are not actually consistent with their hypotheses so that what they perceive is a set of confirming evidence—perceptual confirmation.

Self-Esteem Defense/Enhancement. Sedikides (1993) recognized the importance of the motives to assess (accuracy) and verify (consistency), but argued in support of Allport's (1937, p. 169) claim that a person's "most coveted experience is the enhancement of his self-esteem." As reviewed in the Introduction, the maintenance of a positive view of the self is a powerful motive that drives cognition. When we are thinking about our social world, we are biased toward interpreting the information and events around us in a way that bolsters self-esteem and wards off negative self-evaluations. But self-esteem enhancement is not only attained through the way in which we think about ourselves; it is also determined by how we evaluate others. The self is not an island, but a complex array of *social identities* that link an individual to various social groups (what Brewer, 1991, called the *social self*). To maintain a positive sense of self requires us not only to be biased in how we evaluate self-relevant information, but to maintain positive views of the groups to which we are linked. This fact is the essence of *social identity theory* (e.g., Tajfel & Turner, 1986), which details how esteem enhancement affects evaluations of others:

> 1) Individuals strive to maintain or enhance their self-esteem: they strive for a positive self-concept, 2) Social groups or categories and the membership in them are associated with positive or negative value connotations. Hence, social identity may be positive or negative according to the evaluations, 3) The evaluation of one's own group is determined with reference to specific other groups through social comparison. (Tajfel & Turner, 1986, p. 16)

Thus evaluations of others are biased because these others are linked to us through social/group bonds.

In support of this idea, Tesser (1988) proposed a model of self-evaluation suggesting that we can be systematically biased in how we evaluate others, ranging from those with whom we share to those with whom we do not share a relevant social bond. In this *self-evaluation maintenance model*, it is assumed that others often play the role of "comparison standards." When we seek to evaluate ourselves—to come to understand whether we are performing well or poorly on a particular dimension—we look to others for information. For instance, if students want to evaluate their performance on an exam, their objective scores are usually not enough. In addition to knowing the grades they received on the exam, individuals want to know how well they did relative to others! We all use others as a standard of comparison against which we evaluate and judge, engaging in what Festinger (1954a) called *social comparison*, for the purpose of attaining self-knowledge. Festinger stated that "there exists, in the human organism, a drive to evaluate his opinions and his abilities. . . . To the extent that objective, non-social means are not available, people evaluate their opinions and abilities by comparison respectively with the opinions and abilities of others" (pp. 117–118).

When we engage in social comparison, who do we choose to compare ourselves against? We select people whom we expect to be similar enough to yield useful information about our abilities. If I want to know whether the present book is successful, I will not compare the sales figures against the top book on *The New York Times* best-seller list. I instead will turn to similar books written by psychologists (or other academics). Additionally, since comparison to others is done to help one feel positive about one's self, there is another factor to consider: the direction of the comparison. We sometimes engage in *upward social comparison* with someone who is superior to ourselves, because such comparisons can set standards to strive for and may provide surprisingly positive results that can really boost our self-esteem. However, a surer strategy for boosting self-esteem is to engage in *downward social comparison*—a comparison with someone whose performance is inferior to our own. Downward comparisons will typically yield a positive view of ourselves, but if we go too low, we may be providing false feedback about our ability because we are comparing ourselves to people far worse than us. We will feel good about how well we do, but the comparison may not be informative about our true abilities.

In this way, even relative strangers provide information about ourselves, through processes of social comparison, if those others have performed in the dimension for which we desire feedback and self-evaluation. In an attempt to bolster our self-views, we can compare ourselves to others and reflect on the qualities and achievements of others in a biased way. The variety of ways in which cognitive flexibility and effort can be used to promote positive self-views and to ward off negative self-views is a focus of Chapter 8, and we will review only Tesser's (1988) self-evaluation maintenance model at this point for the purpose of providing one illustration.

The self-evaluation maintenance model recognizes that the manner in which we compare ourselves to others depends on just how close those others are to us and just how relevant their behavior is to our own self definition. Others can range from being complete strangers to people with whom we share important social ties/bonds. The behavior of others can range from being extremely relevant to us (they have the same career) to being totally irrelevant (they achieve in a domain that has nothing to do with us). Even people with whom we share social ties—through kinship, political affiliation, friendships, social groups, ethnic groups, religious groups, alma maters, hometowns, and nationality—can vary in closeness to us and in the degree to which their behavior is relevant to us. The self-evaluation maintenance model asserts that sometimes we evaluate ourselves, via the performance of others, through a process of *reflection*. We can bask in the reflected glory of the achievements of people with whom we share a social bond, even when the bond and the achievement are fairly trivial (e.g., our college football team wins a game, or someone from our hometown makes the news or achieves success in music or movies). In these examples, reflection helps to bolster self-esteem because the success of others becomes a ray of light that illuminates our self-evaluation. However, reflection is really only a useful way to boost self-esteem if the behavior of others is not overly relevant to us (is not threatening to us) and if we have some social tie to the person. If we have no aspiration to be movie stars, pop stars, or football heroes, then the success in these domains of other people can reflect on us. But it is hard to bask in the glory of someone who is succeeding in the very area in which we were hoping to succeed. In addition, reflection makes far more sense when we have some form of a social tie to the person. Reflection is not a very useful way to evaluate ourselves if the person is someone to whom we have no social tie.

Instead of reflecting on the glory of others, Tesser's model also specifies that we evaluate ourselves through social comparison. Social comparison is especially likely if the person we are comparing ourselves against is performing in a domain relevant to us and in which we desire feedback. Whereas the negative performance of others may allow comparison processes to provide a boost to self-esteem, the positive performance of others can threaten self-esteem (particularly if it is someone with whom we share a social bond). It is here where biased systematic processing can come into play. We should be motivated to see ourselves positively through social comparisons, even if the objective evidence might not warrant such a conclusion. For example, a Democrat might exert a good deal of mental energy to convince him-/herself that the Democratic candidate in a debate performed better than the Republican. The employee up for a promotion might use all his/her powers of rationalization to believe that his/her performance on the job is superior to that of other employees in line for the same promotion. In sum, social comparison processes can be used to allow us to maintain and enhance a positive view of ourselves, and this can occur through the biased systematic evaluation of and comparison to the behavior of others who are behaving in a self-relevant domain.

CODA

Dual-process models address how and when people stop being cognitive misers and start engaging in close looks. This involves discovering what factors cause people to experience doubt—a lack of confidence in their judgments. There have been two general responses to this question. One has been that this occurs when the data are so inconsistent with the prior structures stored in memory (e.g., expectancies, stereotypes, schemas) that they force people to abandon a reliance (or strict reliance) on such theory-driven processing. Unambiguous information about a person—information that is counter to expectancies and stereotypes—challenges perceivers' perspective. The ability to force prior conceptualizations onto the currently encountered person is rendered impractical. A second has been that "close looks" are willfully chosen as a strategy by flexible processors: People are motivated to initiate elaborate processing because they desire greater certainty in their judgments than least-effort processing will allow. They can desire to be accurate.

The link between motives and information processing is developed from this inter-play between people's striving to exert as little mental effort as possible, yet simulta-neously to hold judgments in which they feel sufficiently confident (ones that surpass a sufficiency threshold). The processing strategy that is utilized depends on where the sufficiency threshold is set and how much effort is deemed necessary for a judgment to be confidently held. There are two distinct motivational assumptions suggested by this dual-process logic. One is that motives are capable of establishing and shifting the suffi-ciency threshold. A variety of motives can be successfully implicated in this shifting and setting function, which serves to create gaps between actual and desired confidence. The second motivational assumption is more fundamental. It is that the existence of a gap between actual and desired confidence, the experience of feeling that a judgment is not sufficient, is in itself an aversive state that people seek to reduce. People are said to desire confidence, and lacking a sufficient experience of confidence is in itself motivat-ing.

The dual-process notion can be seen as far back in the psychological literature as James's (1890/1950, p. 451) belief that effortless processing predominates, but more effortful processing can occur under the appropriate conditions:

> The stream of our thought is like a river. On the whole, easy simple flowing predominates in it, the drift of things is with the pull of gravity, and effortless attention is the rule. But at intervals a log-jam occurs, stops the current, creates an eddy, and makes things temporarily move the other way. If a real river could feel, it would feel these eddies and set-backs as places of effort.

James (1907/1991) warned that people are neither purely theory-driven (using "princi-ples") nor data-driven (using "facts"); rather, they possess qualities on both sides of the line:

> Each of you probably knows some well-marked examples of each type, and you know what each example thinks of the example on the other side of the line. . . . Most of us have a han-kering for the good things on both sides of the line. Facts are good, of course—give us lots of facts. Principles are good—give us plenty of principles. The world is indubitably one if you look at it one way, but as indubitably is it many, if you look at it in another . . . your ordinary philosophic layman never being a radical, never straightening out his system, but living vaguely in one plausible compartment of it or another to suit the temptations of successive hours. (pp. 9–10)

This is a clear exposition of the idea that the "temptations of successive hours"—fluctua-tions across time and situations in needs and goals—can lead people to shift from a theory-driven approach to processing the world, to a data-driven approach.

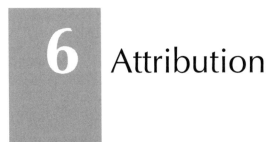

6 Attribution

In the United States, people who commit assault (or murder, or a variety of other crimes) can be punished more severely if their crimes are designated as "hate crimes." Many Americans (usually of either a conservative or libertarian political affiliation) often wonder what purpose this designation serves. They ask, "If a person is brutally attacked, what does it matter if part of the reason for the attack is that the attacker does not like some group that person belongs to (e.g., the victim is gay, or Black, or Hispanic, etc.)?" Their logic is that the consequences of the act should stand alone as an indication of the crime and as a designator of punishment. They argue that the best we can do when assigning punishment is to punish according to the damage caused and to the intent of the criminal, as inferred from the damage caused, and that this should not depend on what race (or sexual orientation) the victim happens to be. This logic captures two truisms of how people think about the American legal system: The punishment should suit the crime, and it should reflect the (inferred) intentions of the criminal. First, if one shoots another person and the person lives, it does not matter in defining the crime if one was trying to kill that person. One should not be on trial for murder if the victim was not killed (even if one intended to kill). The punishment (and definition of the crime) should suit the crime committed, not the one intended. However, this does not mean that intent is not factored into the system. The former basketball player Jayson Williams was recently on trial for having shot and killed a man. Yet this occurred while he was "showing off" a gun from his collection, with the gun being fired accidentally and the man being killed unintentionally. The question of intent here was very important in terms of how he was treated by the law. (He was, in fact, acquitted of manslaughter but found guilty of trying to make the shooting look like a suicide.) Thus intentions can make a very large difference in how we interpret the meaning of an act (in this case, a crime), altering how we assign blame and how severely we punish.

233

The question in many criminal cases is reduced to one of jurors needing to ask themselves "What did this alleged criminal intend to do, given what has been documented as having happened?" But how can jurors judge intent? It is not observed. It is the psychological state of the alleged criminal that we need to infer from his/her action. To the degree that we can infer intent, the more confident we are that a crime was intended, the more harsh we may be when deciding on the "just deserts" for that person. Thus we may answer those Americans who ponder the purpose of designating an attack as a "hate crime" with a reference to the fact that what we seek ultimately is to understand the person's intent. However, the intent of another person is not an observable, measurable entity, but needs to be inferred. When we make inferences about a person, we can do so with varying degrees of confidence. We can never be 100% certain that we have made a correct inference, because we are never going to have access to the internal workings and thoughts of another person. To the extent that we can increase our confidence in the inference we make about another person's intent, we can make better decisions about how to act (in this case, how to punish him/her for a crime). Finally, to the extent that we can establish a crime was a hate crime, we have been able to gain strong information about the intent of the criminal. We now know not only what consequences the perpetrator caused, but for what *motives* the person intended to kill and perhaps how strongly he/she intended those consequences to come about. Intent matters—and a hate crime differs in intent from other violent crime. Designating something as a "hate" crime gives us information that can affect our degree of confidence in our inferences about the person's intent.

Indeed, intent matters not only in the American legal system, but in the moment-to-moment lives of people. We observe others' actions and the consequences brought about, and we attempt to infer what caused these events. Once we have such inferences, we know what to think of these people and how to act toward them. We do not want to act solely in response to consequences, but rather to others' intentions. Imagine, for example, that you are at a concert, standing near the front of the stage, and the person next to you pushes you with such force that you fall to the ground. If you acted solely on the basis of consequences, you might stand up and shove that person, or engage in a violent and profanity-laced outburst (or if you are in a mosh pit, you might just stand up and shove right back). However, if you acted on the basis of intent, you might first want to answer two questions: "Did the person act intentionally?" and "What were the person's specific intentions?" The latter is often equated with the question "What were the person's motives for acting?" or "Why did the person act that way?" This is really the type of question that attribution theory primarily tries to address. In answering the first question, you might look to see whether the person pushing you had intended to shove you, or whether that person was being violently shoved into you by a throng of people storming toward the stage. The person who shoved you unintentionally should certainly not be treated in the same way as the person who shoved you intentionally. Once you have answered the first question, you would then want to make inferences about the specific causes of the intended act—what motivated the person to shove. And such is the nature of almost every waking moment we spend in the presence of other people. We are constantly needing to infer why people act and talk as they do, focusing not only on the consequences, but the intent. We make attributions about the reasons for events we observe.

The Introduction has defined an *attribution* as the end result of a process of classifying and explaining observed behavior in order to arrive at a decision regarding the reason or cause for the behavior—a decision as to why a person has acted in the fashion that we have witnessed (or heard about, imagined, etc.). Though working long before dual-process models had been articulated in the literature, Kelley (1967, 1972a) outlined a model of attribution that included the ways in which causal schemas are used in making judgments of others (and inferences about their intentions), as well as the influence from a systematic analysis of relevant information. Like Allport (1954) before him and the developers of the dual-process models who followed him, Kelley (1972a) assumed that effortless and schema-driven processing comes naturally and represents an information-processing default.

Before reviewing Kelley's (1967) model, let us begin by examining work that influenced Kelley's thinking, including that of his contemporaries as well as the work of psychologists working in the two decades prior, who were interested in analyzing the way in which we think about others. Perhaps the most influential figure in the field of person perception (and attribution theory more specifically) was Fritz Heider (1944, 1958). Though contemporaries of Heider, such as Ichheiser and Michotte, expressed extremely similar ideas, Heider's (1958) book entitled *The Psychology of Interpersonal Relations* served as a rallying call and departure point for a generation of social-psychological research. Heider's approach was actually quite elemental and (with the benefit of hindsight) intuitively obvious: It assumes that to understand the manner in which we think about people in our social world, we should analyze the language we use to talk about people. Through examining the words we use to describe why people act as they do, we can get a sense of the types of reasons and motives that we use to categorize and explain others. Heider's contribution to social psychology is largely assumed to be associated with an examination of "surface" matters, as he called them in his 1958 book, employing the common-sense language used by lay attributors to naively make sense of the actions of other people: "Our concern will be with 'surface' matters, the events that occur in everyday life on a conscious level, rather than with the unconscious processes . . . the discussion will center on the *person* as the basic unit to be investigated" (Heider, 1958, p. 1; emphasis in original). This general approach was called *common-sense psychology*—not as a knock on its simplicity, but as a description of rules we all follow.

HEIDER'S COMMON-SENSE PSYCHOLOGY

The study of common-sense psychology is one of value for the scientific understanding of interpersonal relations . . . in the same way one talks about a naïve physics which consists of the unformulated ways we take account of simple mechanical laws in our adapted actions, one can talk about a "naïve psychology" which gives us the principles we use to build up our picture of the social environment and which guides our reactions to it.

—HEIDER (1958, p. 5)

The starting point for Heider's (1958) common-sense psychology—his analysis of the types of causes people ascribe to the actions of others—was to ask what *potential* causes exist. Heider discussed two global forces that can account for why people act as they do: those emanating from the *person* (the stable character, disposition, or essence of the person, as well as temporary states, motives, goals, and sentiments) and those emanating from the *situation*. An example can illustrate this point. When a person is seen performing a dishonest behavior, we can attribute the cause of that behavior to the person (e.g., he/she is a dishonest person; he/she is a person who has temporarily adopted the intent to be dishonest) or to the situation (the person is seen as having been forced to perform an action that could be described as dishonest). Heider meant by the word "person" what he called *personal causality*, which is *intentionality*. He used the word "situation" to refer to *unintentional* events, which fell under his label *impersonal causality* (Malle, 1999). Thus with person causes, a perceiver comes to see the behavior as intentionally chosen by the person, and the perceiver's attributional task is to determine the reasons for that choice—why did he/she intend to act as such? With situation causes, the person produces a behavior that was not intended, and the perceiver's attributional task is to determine what causes would lead a behavior that the person did not will to happen to come about. Psychologists have come to refer to the person–situation distinction as the rather simplistic distinction between an internal, personal force and an external, environmental force. Somewhat lost is Heider's original distinction between intended verus unintended behavior, and personal versus impersonal causality.

Person as Cause

In Heider's analysis, the force emanating from the person that gives rise to behavior is labeled the *effective force of the person*. Although this can include temporary states of the person as well as one's stable disposition, the disposition of the person is assumed to be especially powerful in determining how perceivers ascribe the cause for why a behavior was performed. This point was illustrated in responses to a film that Heider and Simmel (1944) showed to research participants. In the film, a series of geometric shapes were shown in motion. When asked to describe the motion, participants tended to display anthropomorphism, describing one of the shapes as chasing the other and attributing the reason for the pursuit to dispositional qualities. As Malle (personal communication, 2003; emphasis in original) has put it, "perceivers use the language of agency and intentionality even when describing (and explaining) abstract movements, as long as they *look* like agentic behavior." This tendency to rely on describing behavior as intended is also seen in our explanations as perceivers of the actions that people perform. Heider (1958) suggested that there is a tendency to attribute an observed behavior to the personality of others. If we observe a person acting in a dishonest fashion, what explanation seems more logical or springs to mind more easily than asserting that this behavior was intended by the person and caused by a dishonest disposition?

Why might it be that the personality of the person is so readily assumed to be the cause of behavior? Heider (1958) provided two explanations. First, *behavior engulfs the field*; by this, he meant that the behavior another person performs draws attention to the person and makes the behavior (and the person performing it) far more salient than the context in which it occurs. Therefore, even if pressures in the environment cause a person to be dishonest, the behavior is so salient that it makes it hard to see the more abstract situational pressure. Second, Heider (1944, 1958) believed that the best, most complete explanations (for anything, but especially for the behavior of people) are those that provide a stable, clear, and concrete cause. Given that people dislike uncertainty and doubt, an end to doubt that is optimally comforting can be provided by assuming stable causes for the events in the world. Attributing the cause of behavior either to the person's stable personality or to the person's mental and motivational states (derived from the person's somewhat stable values, intentions, and needs) provides the clearest, simplest, most certain type of explanation. As Heider (1958, pp. 79–80) stated, it is an important principle of common-sense psychology, as it is of scientific theory in general, that man grasps reality, and can predict and control it, by referring transient and variable behavior and events to relatively unchanging underlying conditions, the so-called dispositional properties of his world. . . . Dispositional properties are the invariances that make possible a more or less stable, predictable, and controllable world. They refer to the relatively unchanging structures and processes that characterize or underlie phenomena.

Social psychology since Heider's time has perhaps overemphasized the importance of other people's traits as a form of intentionality, to the relative exclusion of other types of person causes (temporary goals, moods, etc.) that could explain the reasons for their behavior (perhaps because of Heider's assertion of the power such an explanation offers). However, Malle (1999) reminds us that Heider did not mean for a "person cause" to be limited to assuming that the traits or personality of the person must be seen as the cause for an observed behavior.

Situation as Cause

Although people obviously are performing their own behavior, they are not always in direct control of or able to choose those behaviors. We can say that a person acted dishonestly without meaning to imply that he/she is a dishonest person. People act dishonest for a host of reasons, some of which are temporary and not linked to their long-standing personality (other person causes), and others of which are caused by the situation they find themselves placed in (situational causes). Attributing a behavior to the situation is easy to do (perhaps) when the situational force that pressures the person to act in this way is strong and clear—such as when a person is being held hostage and is forced to lie to authorities at gunpoint. Few people would label such a person as a liar or dispositionally dishonest. But situational pressures are not always so strong and clear. Take, for example, the person who acts kindly to his/her boss. The cause for this behavior may be a kind disposition, or it may be because the pressure of being promoted requires that one act in a pleasant way toward one's superiors. Such situational causes are subtle and hard to see, but they can be just as responsible for the behavior as those that are more salient or more intuitively obvious.

Whereas Heider (1958) specified that there is a tendency to attribute behavior to person-based causes, he also detailed that people are able to consider the extent to which social pressure causes the behavior. Heider called this the *effective force of the environment*. If perceivers were scientific and rational-minded, they would consider the joint effects of the effective force of the person and the environment, weighing them against each other to arrive at a logical conclusion.

Attribution and Language: The Words "Try" and "Can"

When a person is seen as the cause of an effect (with an *effect* meaning the consequence of an action), this means that the person is being perceived as having the ability to have performed the action, as well as having put forth the effort to bring it about. This insight was arrived at through Heider's realization that the language people use when talking about intentional action makes heavy use of two words—"try" and "can." Examine these illustrative examples of cause and effect.

Effect: The baseball ends up in the dugout. Cause: He *can*not throw the ball from second base to first base accurately.

Effect: The man pushes the woman to the sidewalk. Cause: He is *try*ing to protect his wife from an out-of-control car.

Effect: She goes to the dance with William. Cause: She *tried* to make it known that she wanted to go with him, so that he would ask her.

Effect: The assistant manager gets promoted to manager. Cause: He *can* do the job better than the other candidates.

In Heider's analysis, these two words ("try" and "can") are commonly used in describing behavior because they reflect two important underlying dimensions that capture how we think about the relationship between the behavior of others and their disposition—ability and effort. Heider (1958), therefore, further broke down the effective personal force, assuming that it was determined by the underlying concepts of *effort* and *ability*.

Effort is related to one's intentions—what one is *trying* to accomplish. Ability, on the other hand, addresses the question of what one is capable of doing. "Try" is determined by internal, motivational factors. The extent to which one tries is purely a force of the person. "Can" (whether one has the capability to accomplish something), however, is more complicated. Part of the concept of "can" comes from the personal factor of ability. However, another aspect of the concept of "can" depends on features of the environment. Thus what one can do is jointly determined by the personal force and the situational force. One may have lots of personal ability, but if prevented by forces in the environment from acting on that ability, one will not be able to act. This has already been evidenced in our discussion of cognitive load in Chapter 4. One has the personal ability to process information quite complexly; yet if other tasks that make one cognitively "busy" are simultaneously present, the ability to process information is disrupted. But personal ability is not only undermined by the presence of a cognitive load. Sometimes the very nature of a task is so complex and challenging that, despite having high levels of personal ability, one may be forced to admit that one "cannot" perform this task. This does not undermine the point that one has ability; it simply means that the features of some tasks make the situational pressure too great to allow one to be able to act on that ability. For example, one may have high aptitude in mathematics, but an extremely difficult calculus problem may not allow one to display that high ability. One may be an excellent hitter throughout the course of a baseball season and one's career, but Pedro Martinez as an opposing pitcher may prove to be too great a challenge, even for one of high aptitude. Thus "can" is dependent on both the personal and situational force.

Related to "can" is the concept of "may." "May" presupposes that one has the ability to perform an act (one "can" do it) and asks the related question of whether there is any external pressure that blocks the performance of what one can do. In this case, the external pressure is in the form of social sanctions. One requires permission from some social agent that exerts power over the individual. Once this sanction is provided, one may act. But it is wholly possible for one to be *able* to act, yet despite the fact one can act, one does not because they *may* not. Consider the teenage girl who wishes to date, yet her father refuses to allow her. She has both the ability and the desire to go out with a particular boy who has asked her out, yet she does not, because she may not: There is a social agent with power over her who specifies what she may do. A correct attribution and an incorrect one have drastically different implications. If the boy fails to realize that the girl's problem is that she *may* not date, he will assume he is being rejected and potentially give up his pursuit, as well as feel depressed. If he realizes that she may not date, he knows that the problem lies in an external and powerful agent, and that he is not being rejected. The emotional consequences are very different, and the strategy he takes could potentially change (from giving up pursuit to figuring out what would change the father's mind).

Thus far, attributions, have been discussed in terms of one dimension—the *locus* of the cause. A behavior is attributed to a cause that is located either inside the person (a person attribution) or outside the person (a situation attribution). However, Heider's (1958) analysis of the use of "can" points out another dimension along which attributions vary. Behavior may be attributed either to *stable* or to *unstable* (varying from one point in time to another) forces. "Can" involves both the person's ability and the forces from the environment. The former is stable and unchanging: One either has aptitude in mathematics or not; one is either an excellent offensive baseball player or not. However, the component of "can" that comes from the environment can be either stable or unstable. For example, one type of situational pressure was said to come from the difficulty of a task (such as solving a hard calculus problem, or facing Pedro Martinez). This is a stable feature of the environment—a hard problem will always be hard, and Pedro will always be unhittable. However, another type of situational pressure is said to exist in temporary conditions, such as when one is asked to solve a problem while busy working on a secondary task. In this case, the presence of a secondary task fluctuates, so that it may prevent being able to solve the problem at one point, yet may fail to be present at another point in time. Such unstable forces from the environment are most similar to what we would commonly call chance or luck. One may have the bad luck of facing Pedro Martinez in one inning, but given this is the Red Sox, one is sure to face a lousy pitcher the next!

Does this analysis of the dimension of stability apply to the concept "try" as well? Earlier it has been stated that to "try" is an internal force. But not all internal forces, like ability, are stable. Effort is something that emanates from a person, but it is not a stable force of the person. One tries harder at some points in time than others. The motivation to act fluctuates over time.

In this review of a piece of Heider's analysis of the language we use to describe behavior, we see a simple categorization scheme developing that captures the types of explanations we use for making sense of human behavior. This scheme relies on two dimensions of causes—those that vary in stability (stable vs. unstable), and those that vary in locus (those located in the person vs. those located in the situation). If we analyze an example, such as bad performance on a math test as the behavior we observe, this suggests that there are four possible causes for the behavior, and we attribute the cause for the behavior to one of these four (see Figure 6.1). The performance may be

	Internal locus (person attribution)	External locus (situation attribution)
Stable	Ability	Task difficulty
Unstable	Effort	Luck

FIGURE 6.1. The possible causes for a behavior, based on Heider's analysis of "can" and "try."

due to something stable about the person, such as his/her low aptitude for math (ability). It may be caused by something unstable about person, such as his/her lack of studying (effort). The cause may be located within the situation, but to something unstable, such as loud noise in the hallway during the exam (an instance of bad luck). Finally, the cause may be something stable in the environment, such as the poor quality of the teaching or the extreme difficulty of the tests this teacher is known to give (task difficulty).

Unintended Behavior Attributed to the Person (as Opposed to the Situation)

When we perceive an intention to act in the actor whose behavior we are observing, the cause for the behavior, as Heider (1958) asserted, is clearly in the person. However, *unintended actions* can also be caused by the person. For example, an unintended action, such as breaking someone's thumb when trying to block his/her shot in a basketball game, was clearly caused by the actor, despite being incidental to the true intention. Most psychological theory has focused on persons as causes for intended actions only (Malle, 1999). It is as if an unintended action must be seen as caused by the situation. However, as noted above, people can be the causes of their own unintended actions and outcomes as well.

Malle (1999) has argued that Heider (1958) used the term *situation* to refer to unintended acts, and that by *situational attribution* he meant that the cause for the behavior was due to an unintended factor. But the term situation attribution has been (mis)taken by researchers to mean that external forces led to the behavior. This has had two results. First, researchers have neglected the fact that the causes for some unintended acts are not in the situation, but within the person. Second, researchers have assumed that the perceiver's primary goal in person perception is to determine whether the cause for behavior is internal or external; they have ignored important questions of whether cause is intended or unintended, and whether the reason for an event is personal or impersonal. Drawing from Heider, Malle posits that intended and unintended actions are distinct types of events, and that people explain intentional and unintentional behavior in different ways.

What we have lost by missing this piece of Heider's (1958) framework is that people use distinct types of explanations for a person's behavior when it is seen as intended or unintended. In Malle's (1999) analysis, *reason explanations* (arriving at the reason a person intended to perform an act) are used for describing intended actions, and *causal explanations* are used for describing unintended actions. For example, if perceivers use reason explanations for intended behavior and cause explanations for unintended behavior, then presenting some people with reason explanations for some observed behavior and others with cause explanations should lead to very different reactions regarding the observed person's intent. People should see the behavior described to them via a reason explanation as an intended behavior, and the behavior described to them via a cause explanation as unintended. Imagine reading that a person was driving 25 miles over the speed limit. The cause for this behavior can lie within the person and be clearly intended (because he/she wanted to get to the beer store before it closed at 10:00 P.M.) or it can lie within the person and be unintended (because he/she failed to read the speedometer). Which type of explanation people receive has been shown by Malle to alter their descriptions of the person's intentionality.

THE JONES AND DAVIS THEORY
OF CORRESPONDENT INFERENCE

Heider (1958) provided a framework for examining how perceivers think about the causes of actions when they are consciously attempting to think about and discern such things. When perceivers consciously attempt to understand action, there are still a host of strategies they can use to accomplish this goal. As Chapter 5 has pointed out, at the broadest of levels we can discuss strategies that involve a systematic analysis of the behavior versus those that involve a schematic, top-down analysis. Jones and Davis (1965) introduced the first formal model of attribution processes—one examining the specific rules perceivers follow when engaging in an effortful and systematic analysis of the behavior of others (attempting to make inferences about the traits, personality, and disposition of the observed person). The model is called the *theory of correspondent inference*, because the basic question being examined is this: What factors cause a perceiver to infer that an actor's behavior corresponds with some underlying disposition? Thus a *correspondent inference* is an inference or attribution asserting that the behavior of another person corresponds with stable personality traits of that person. It is a dispositional attribution. "Correspondence refers to the extent that the act and the underlying characteristic or attribute are similarly described by the inference" (Jones & Davis, 1965, p. 223).

The link that can be drawn from the theory of correspondent inference to Fritz Heider's analysis (and back to the Gestalt theorizing that influenced Heider) is seen in a fundamental assumption of the Jones and Davis (1965) theory: "The person perceiver's fundamental task is . . . to find sufficient reason why the person acted. . . . Instead of a potentially infinite regress of cause and effect . . . the perceiver's explanation comes to a stop when an intention or motive is assigned that has the quality of being reason enough" (p. 220). Jones and Davis assumed that the goal of perceivers is to attain closure—merely to understand why the observed persons have acted as they have. Rather than seeking accuracy, perceivers seek an end to doubt, to have "reason enough." The question then becomes one of discerning what rules people follow when systematically and elaborately trying to arrive at a "sufficient reason" for others' behavior.

In trying to make attributions for an intended action, a perceiver's goal is to ascertain the reasons why a person behaved as he/she did. *One* possible reason is that the person has a trait leading him/her to act in this way, and Jones and Davis's (1965) model focuses on this particular type of reason explanation (if we can call this a reason—in reality, all a correspondent inference tells us is that a person intended to perform a behavior, not really the reason why the behavior was performed or what his/her intentions were). Although the model is explicitly concerned with how people make inferences about what *trait* can explain an observed effect arising from someone else's behavior, the processes described in the model are also quite applicable to other, similar types of questions. The principles Jones and Davis describe may also be used to describe how people decide whether a reason or a specific intention was responsible for an observed behavior (and the consequences of that behavior). For this reason, although the Jones and Davis model focuses almost exclusively on trait inference, the examples used in this chapter to illustrate the principles Jones and Davis reviewed will often stray from simply discussing how people infer traits. Instead, the examples provided will often show people arriving at reason explanations (or inferring specific intentions/reasons in other people). (To further justify using such examples, it should be noted that Jones and Davis asserted at the start of their chapter that their model is about how people reason about the causes of events—although they did not really follow up on this point in the rest of their model, outside of the inference of a "trait" as a cause).

Multiple Effects

The Jones and Davis (1965) model is based on a perceiver's analysis not only of the observed behavior, but of the consequences that arise from the person having performed the behavior. An act can typically have many consequences—or, in the language of the model, an act can have multiple *effects*. Clearly, the behavior caused the effect, but the question of interest is this: What caused the behavior to produce this effect? Was it an unintended consequence, or did the person mean to produce this effect? Not all of the effects that follow actions are intended; some even oppose what the actors intended to accomplish. Perceivers use the consequences of the actions they observe to help them make inferences about the intent of the actors. The trick for the perceivers is to discern what consequences (effects) were intended versus unintended, and what intended effects carry causal weight (as not all intended effects reflect a cause for the action).

Consider an example. Two people end a relationship. One of them needs time apart without speaking to the other. This is intended to help him/her get over the pain that is associated with the breakup. Therefore, while this person does intend to ignore the former partner, this consequence does not carry much causal weight. The reason the person has adopted this strategy is not to accomplish the goal of ignoring the former partner, but to accomplish a higher-order goal of feeling better and getting over emotional turmoil. If the ignored "ex" attributes causal weight to the act of getting ignored, the act of ignoring the ex can now have the unintended effect of insulting the ex or making him/her feel even more unwanted. It can also have the unintended effect of making the ex dislike the person who has chosen to engage in this strategy of ignoring. And making the ex start to experience extreme dislike may be exactly the opposite effect of what the person had intended by undertaking the course of action. This example is meant to illustrate the initial point of the theory of correspondent inference. Namely, in attempting to understand behavior, perceivers not only categorize behavior and make inferences from that categorization about why the other persons acted as they did; in addition to the behavior, there are the many effects of the behavior, and perceivers analyze the multiple effects that emerge from the behavior. From an analysis of multiple effects, the perceivers can make better inferences about the internal state of the actors. Without being able to see into the minds of other people, perceivers can observe the results that the others' actions bring about and make inferences about why they would want such effects to come about. To Jones and Davis, the basic problem for a perceiver during interpersonal perception is to make an inference about the traits of an actor from an analysis of the multiple effects of his/her behavior (and, from those effects, make inferences about what the person had intended).

Three Ingredients for Making Correspondent Inferences from an Analysis of Effects

In order for a perceiver to judge intentionality (whether a behavior was performed intentionally or an effect was brought about intentionally) by looking at the consequences of a person's action, the perceiver needs to know three things aside from what the behavior is and what the consequences (multiple effects) of the behavior are. First, does the actor have knowledge of the consequences of the action? For a person to have intended a consequence, the person must be aware that his/her actions will have the consequences that they do. If the actor is unaware that a particular effect would have come to pass as a result of his/her behavior, the perceiver should be unlikely to assume the person was trying (intending) to have that effect.

Second, the actors not only must be aware that a particular effect will result from the behavior, but must have the desire or intention to bring about those consequences (the motivation to bring about the effect). If the actor does not want a consequence to result from an action, it makes little sense for a perceiver to infer that the action or consequence was intended. Third, the actor must have the capability to bring about the desired consequences. These three ingredients allow a perceiver to make inferences about a person's intent, and such inferences about intent are needed if the perceiver is to determine that the person's action reflects his/her disposition. But this leads naturally to the next question of interest. Once the perceiver knows the ingredients that allow him/her to examine whether the person intended a consequence, how does the perceiver then go about analyzing the consequences (the multiple effects) to determine whether a correspondent inference is warranted? What are the factors that promote a correspondent inference's being formed by the perceiver?

Factors That Promote Correspondent Inference

How Desirable the Consequences Are

The *desirability* of an effect is essentially the measure of how much the actor would enjoy it, deriving pleasure or gain from the effect coming to pass. It makes sense that if a person is likely to enjoy the consequences of an action, this would tell us that the person must have intended to produce that consequence. After all, aren't we all likely to intend to produce consequences that benefit us? But the issue for our current analysis is not merely whether the person intended the behavior and its effect, but whether the effect has any causal weight. Does the fact that the person performed (and intended to perform) a behavior that has desirable consequences tell us anything about the disposition of the person?

In fact, the desirability of the consequences of an action is *inversely related* to the probability that the perceiver will form a correspondent inference. This statement may sound complicated, but the logic is simple. If an effect is one that all people want, then knowing that an actor attempted to bring about that effect really tells us very little about that specific person's disposition. It tells us only that he/she likes and wants what most people like and want.

> As the perceiver considers the multiple effects of action, he will usually assume that some of the effects were more desirable to the actor, and therefore more diagnostic of his intentions than others . . . upon observing that an action leads to a normally desirable effect, the perceiver usually will believe that most persons, including the present actor, find that effect desirable . . . attribute–effect linkages based on universally desired effects are not informative concerning the unique characteristics of the actor. (Jones & Davis, 1965, pp. 226–227)

Consider an example. You drink a lot of beer at a party, and this has multiple effects: You get less inhibited; you are more likely to approach a stranger you find attractive; you might be lucky enough to arrange a date; you ignore the friend you came to the party with, who is not having luck meeting interesting people; the friend is mildly annoyed at you; you wake up with a hangover the next day. As perceivers, we look at the multiple effects of your action and assume that the desirable ones were the intended ones and the undesirable ones were unintended. However, we learn relatively little about your personality and disposition from the fact that you intended these desirable effects. Certainly, if you say drinking at a party makes you more sociable and less inhibited, it tells us perceivers a little about you (you are not likely to be an extravert; otherwise, you would be able to act that way without alcohol). But the bottom line is that if a desirable act is universally desired, it is relatively uninformative about you as a person.

Noncommon Effects

We have already established that the behaviors actors engage in have multiple effects. To understand which of those effects signals the real reason for a particular action, perceivers engage in a naive analysis of what the effects were for the chosen course of action and what the consequences would have been for the nonchosen course of action (i.e., if the person had acted differently). When the consequences of one choice of action overlap with the consequences of another, Jones and Davis referred to those shared consequences as *common effects*. When the consequences of one choice of action do not coincide with the consequences of another, those are *noncommon effects*.

Consider President Clinton's denial of having an adulterous affair. Many people remember him striding to the podium, wagging a finger at the camera, and saying, "I did not have sexual relations with that woman." His chosen course of action in that situation consisted of defiance and telling a lie (since he did actually have sexual relations of some type with "that woman," Monica Lewinsky). Perhaps at the time, the President believed that the possible effects of his chosen course of action included (1) convincing people that he was not an adulterer; (2) rallying the support of his political party; (3) creating outrage (if his lie was ever discovered) that he had lied about the affair at two points in time—both during his deposition for the Whitewater scandal and during this trip to the podium; (4) putting to rest a scandal that would have marred his image and the Presidency; (5) saving his marriage; and/or (6) protecting his daughter from embarrassment associated with the accusation's being true. His *nonchosen* course of action in that situation consisted of honesty, remorse, and humility. Thus the President could have strode to the podium, looked people in the eye, and said, "I made a mistake. It involved some type of physical/sexual relationship with a woman who is not my wife, and it did not involve the act of sex itself. More than that you do not need to know, except that I regret my indiscretion and the shame it brings on my family, myself, and my office." This action could have had effects associated with it that included (1) convincing people that he was an honest yet flawed man; (2) rallying the support of his political party; (3) creating outrage at his immoral behavior; and/or (4) creating outrage that he lied during his deposition for the Whitewater scandal, further igniting a scandal that might unseat him from the Presidency. What we would call common effects in the current analysis were those consequences that were shared by both courses of action (in this example, they included rallying the political party and creating outrage at the fact that he lied during the Whitewater deposition). Noncommon effects are those consequences uniquely associated with one course of action but not with the other. In this case, there were many.

Jones and Davis (1965) have asserted that perceivers make inferences about the personality of another person not merely by looking at the consequences of that person's actions, but by examining how those consequences compare to the consequences that would have resulted if the person acted in a different fashion. "As perceivers of action, we can only begin to understand the motives prompting an act if we view the effects of the act in the framework of effects that other actions could have achieved" (Jones & Davis, 1965, p. 223). If the consequences of one choice do not coincide with the consequences of other choices of action, then those noncommon effects can be particularly useful in attempting to understand why a person acted in one way versus another, as they indicate the different consequences resulting for the person as a function of the different behaviors he/she could have performed (see Figure 6.2). If there are a few noncommon effects, that means there are lots of overlapping reasons between two courses of action, and only a small handful that make one option distinct. Thus it is likely that the person acted in a particular way because of these distinctive consequences. Too many noncommon effects, however, reduce the distinctiveness of any given effect and make attribution less clear-cut. As Jones and Davis put it, "An inference from action to attribute is correspondent as an inverse function of the number of noncommon effects following the action" (1965, p. 228). Thus, as the number of noncommon effects increases, the likelihood of correspondent inference decreases.

An example might help to illustrate the inverse relationship between noncommon effects and correspondent inference. Imagine you are trying to understand the reasons why your friend Mark from Poughkeepsie, New York, has chosen to go to one university (McGill) over another (Columbia). Let's list the effects your friend associates with each course of action (attending one university versus the other). Columbia has the following consequences for Mark: He will live in an urban setting, get prestige, be in a great academic environment, be linked to an only adequate tradition of athletic teams, and spend an extreme amount of money. Mark decides that attending McGill will have the following consequences for him: He will live in an urban setting, get prestige, be in a great academic environment, be linked to an only adequate tradition of athletic teams, spend relatively little money, and live in a foreign country with a multicultural setting. If you eliminate the common effects (excellent academics, urban settings, prestige, only adequate sports) and list the noncommon effects, you are left with the fact that McGill is less expensive and offers a multicultural environment. You would then assume that these noncommon effects correspond with the disposition of the person—that Mark has chosen McGill because he is concerned with being thrifty and avoiding debt, as well as with gaining valuable experience in a foreign country with a different culture.

Now consider the same task, but replace Columbia with the University of Florida. The effects listed for Florida include living far from home, spending relatively little money, having great weather, having select departments that are among the best in the country, being better than Florida State, and having an excellent tradition of sports

1. Examine the situation for the nonchosen actions that were available.
2. Look at the overlap of the consequences for chosen and nonchosen actions (common effects).
3. Eliminate common effects as having causal weight.
4. Be more likely to see effects that are noncommon (not the same between a chosen and a nonchosen act) as causal; this is heightened if the number of noncommon effects is small.

FIGURE 6.2. How perceivers determine whether an inference is correspondent from the effects.

teams. Once you eliminate the common effects, you are left with at least five noncommon effects associated with attending McGill (urban setting, excellent academics, prestige, adequate sports, and a multicultural environment). Given all these unique consequences associated with going to McGill (the increased number of noncommon effects), it is harder to reach conclusions about what factors correspond to Mark's underlying disposition and are responsible for his choice of McGill. In summary, a few distinct (noncommon) effects unique to one course of action, and several overlapping (common) effects with other courses of action, provide the clearest case for correspondent inference.

Situational Constraint

We have just discussed how, to understand the underlying reason for an act, we need to consider what other potential actions could have been taken and what other consequences could have been brought about. Related to this question is still another: To what extent does the situation promote one particular interpretation? To the extent that the situation constrains what the actor is able to do, and reveals that there were no other options available, perceivers would be less inclined to regard the actor's behavior as an indicator of his/her personal qualities. If an actor is free to choose among many courses of action, perceivers are more likely to assume that the actor intended the observed behavior and that a dispositional cause is at the root of that intention. "Correspondence of inference declines as the action to be accounted for appears to be constrained by the setting in which it occurred" (Jones & Davis, 1965, p. 223).

Once again, we will use an example to illustrate this point. Say the President (a Republican) is planning to send the country to war and needs the support of Congress. Let us further assume that a Republican senator is threatened with losing the financial backing of her party in the next election if she does not support the President (publicly) on this issue. Her vote is now constrained by the situation in which it occurs, and her true position on the issue is now, according to the model, more difficult to infer than if we assumed absolute freedom for her to vote her conscience. In the language of Jones and Davis (1965), we are examining her behavior in the context of the consequences (effects) that would have emerged had another action been performed. Had she voted against the war, she may have lost her job. The roles we all play in life have a similar constraining effect. A professor is constrained by what is acceptable behavior in his/her position, as is a sanitation worker. Just because someone collects trash from your home, you would not assume he is a clean person, tidy by disposition. His role demands that he clean up, thus constraining what he/she does, and this leads you to decrease the probability of a dispositional inference. Similarly, just because a professor offers lots of criticism, it does not make this person domineering or controlling by disposition. Her job has forced her to act in these prescribed ways.

Finally, the meaning of an act cannot be solely attained by the consideration of the presence of situational constraint. If a person is constrained by the situation, then the fact that he/she acts in a domineering way is not informative. It may very well be the situation that causes the behavior. However, it may very well be the disposition of the person as well. The fact that the person's job leads him/her to act in a domineering way does not rule out the possibility that this person is a domineering person (maybe domineering people even seek out jobs that allow them to dominate). A person who is forced to act friendly because of normative constraints (such as when the situation requires that you meet your boyfriend/girlfriend's parents) may still be a friendly person. Situational constraint is not enough to rule out a disposition; it simply should make perceivers less likely to infer a disposition, or have less confidence in their correspondent inferences.

How Normative (versus Unique) the Behavior Is

The more different your actions are from how the average person would act in the same situation, the more likely it is that your behavior will be seen as having been dispositionally caused. If you act in a normative fashion, then your action is (as is the case with desirable consequences following from your behavior) not highly informative. Performing a behavior that most people would perform tells us little about your personality. However, when your behavior is distinctive and unexpected, then it is more likely that the behavior corresponds to your underlying, stable disposition. "Correspondence increases as the judged value of the attribute departs from the judge's conception of the average person's standing on that attribute" (Jones & Davis, 1965, p. 224).

Some caution should be used in thinking about behavior in terms of how unexpected or surprising it is. As Kelley and Michela (1980) point out, there are two reasons why a behavior can be unexpected. The first is that it violates the norms specified by the situation. However, the second can be that as perceivers we have expectancies about the person (not about the situation), such as those provided by both a stereotype and a history of experience with the person. These types of violations of expectancies do not lead to dispositional inferences, but to situational ones. When we expect a particular person to act a certain way, and he/she does not, we are likely to assume that something about the current situation has caused the person to act in the unexpected way—a situational attribution being associated with unexpected behavior. In summary, if behavior is unexpected because it is not what most people would do in that situation, then a dispositional attribution is likely. However, if it is unexpected because it violates what that particular person would normally do, then unexpected behavior leads to a situational attribution.

The Hedonic Relevance of the Action

The *hedonic relevance of an action* refers to the extent to which the behavior addresses the motives and goals of the *perceiver*. If an observed behavior helps to promote the values, goals, and desires of the person observing that behavior, then that action is said to have hedonic relevance for the perceiver. The model predicts that as hedonic relevance increases, so too does correspondence of inference. Why? It posits that when behavior produces its effects, a perceiver for whom those effects are relevant will have experience with these types of outcomes (and behaviors) because they are so closely tied to the individual's own goals and wishes. This familiarity with the effects may lead the person to see two effects as being highly similar to each other (as both address his/her needs). The identical effects seen by a person for whom the effects lack hedonic relevance may be seen as very different from each other. Thus, one person interprets a set of effects as essentially several instances of the same outcome, whereas other people see these effects as several distinct outcomes. The consequence of this is that as hedonic relevance increases, the number of noncommon effects decreases. What to others may seem like many noncommon effects appears like a smaller set of noncommon effects to the person whose goals are related to the effects. The result of this reduction in noncommon effects is an increase in correspondent inference.

THE KELLEY MODEL:
SCHEMATIC AND ANALYTIC ATTRIBUTION PROCESSES

Kelley (1967, 1972a), in developing his theory of attribution, derived a set of assumptions from Heider (outlined above) concerning the locus of causality: The cause for an effect or an outcome is believed to be located either within the person acting or within the environment he/she is acting in. This is also generally referred to as an internal or external (respectively) attribution. The person, as cause, is a fairly straightforward concept. The cause of the behavior could be some attribute of the person who performed it. An external attribution is slightly more complicated. Some researchers speak of an external attribution as the case where the cause for an act is the situation. But the word "situation" is a little misleading, because in the common use of the word, we think of a particular geographic location—a place. Thus, if Paul gets drunk at a party, the party would be the situation, and it is possible that something about the party caused Paul to be drunk (a spiked drink, extreme social pressure, beer with high alcohol content).

But another example illustrates why use of the word "situation" in describing the locus for an attribution can cause some confusion. It is possible for *other people* to be a "situation" when we are talking about external attributions. For example, when Princess Diana was killed in a 1997 car crash, most of us probably attempted to form an attribution to understand this well-publicized event. This would involve attempting to understand why the driver was going so fast in a Paris tunnel that he lost control of the vehicle. The person whose behavior we are attempting to explain is the driver, and the action was the driver crashing the car. But the external cause, the situation that was placing pressure on him and potentially causing his behavior, was not the geographic location—the tunnel. This may have been part of the situation, since had he been on an open, straight stretch of road, he might not have lost control. But the external forces that were most responsible for determining his behavior stemmed from other people— the photographers' pursuit of the car, and Diana's demands that the photographers be avoided. The situation, therefore, was Diana's desire to elude the paparazzi. Thus the external cause here was other people. One last example to illustrate would be our learning that Benjamin experiences true joy when he is looking at Van Gogh paintings. The action we want to understand is Ben's experience of joy; the Van Gogh painting is the situation.

In these examples, we see that "situation" is a confusing word to use to capture the locus of the cause in attributions. Instead, Kelley (1967, 1972a) used the word "entity" or "entity attribution" to refer to situational causes. So what did Kelley mean by this? An *entity* is the particular object, event, person, or place that could potentially be seen as the locus of causality for the action that the perceiver is trying to understand—something or someone that could be seen as drawing out the action and causing it to occur.

Causal Schemas

As Chapter 5 has shown, systematic and effortful examination of behavior is not always conducted. Sometimes such analysis is simply too difficult for people. At other times there simply is not enough information provided to engage in a systematic analysis. Yet people still make attributions under such circumstances. How? Kelley posited that in such circumstances, people arrive at valid judgments through the use of schemas associated with attributional reasoning—schemas developed over a lifetime's worth of experience at making causal judgments:

> The mature individual has a repertoire of abstract ideas about the operation and interaction of causal factors. These conceptions [enable perceivers to make] economical and fast attributional analysis, by providing a framework within which bits and pieces of relevant information can be fitted in order to draw reasonably good causal inferences. (1973, p. 115).

Given that schemas are assumptions about how the world is organized and the relationships between events, they specify how particular causes and effects are related to each' other, thus allowing perceivers to assume the presence of a cause if they observe an effect. For example, one might develop, over the course of one's experience, a schema specifying that failure on an exam is usually associated with lack of proper preparation. Thus, if one learns that someone else has failed on an exam, one might immediately use this schema to provide an attribution that explains the behavior: The other person failed to prepare appropriately. Schemas need not always specify specific relationships between causes and events, but also rules for making inferences about causes from effects (and in fact the schemas discussed by Kelley are hardly this specific, but are abstract ones, more like logical rules). Kelley detailed two such rules: *discounting* and *augmenting*.

The Discounting Principle

We begin with the question of how people form attributions about isolated instances of behavior. According to Kelley (1972b), what occurs when an attributor observes a single behavior, toward a single entity, performed by a single person, and is then faced with the task of deciding which of several potential causes is responsible for the behavior? When there are several potential causes that can explain an effect, this is said to be a state where *multiple sufficient causes* exist. For example, when George W. Bush ran for President in 2000, he used the term "compassionate conservative" to describe himself—supposedly dissociating himself from what he believed to be the American people's view of conservatives in general as lacking in compassion. He wished to be seen as a compassionate conservative, unlike the rest. This label outraged many politically conservative people, who believed that Bush was allowing liberals to claim that their policies were more compassionate than those of conservatives (it also outraged liberals, who found him not compassionate at all!). As one man put it to me, "What makes a liberal who gives and gives and gives more compassionate than a person who does not give because he believes 'tough love' is the appropriate way to show compassion to people?" That is, this conservative felt that, despite not giving, he was extremely compassionate, and the "coddling liberals" were misguided and not being very compassionate at all, simply worsening problems with their bleeding hearts. This is a question of attribution: Why is the person who gives seen as compassionate, whereas the person who expresses compassion by not giving seen as the very opposite of what was intended—selfish? The answer lies in the notion of multiple sufficient causes. When a man expresses support for policies he would label as "tough love," there are many causes a perceiver could use to sufficiently account for that behavior (he is selfish; he does not believe in charity; he harbors prejudice toward the groups that would be receiving aid; he seeks to maintain the status quo in society and keep some groups superior to others; he is expressing tough love, etc.).

If there are multiple sufficient causes, as in this example, yet only one instance of observed behavior (e.g., finding out that this person strongly opposes welfare), how does one choose from among all the possibilities when deciding what caused the behavior? One answer Kelley has provided to this question is reminiscent of what Jones and Davis (1965) said about noncommon effects: "If [the perceiver] is aware of several plausible causes, he attributes the effect less to any one of them than if he is aware only of one as a plausible cause" (Kelley, 1972a, p. 8). This has come to be known as the *discounting principle*. In this example, in the absence of more information, seeing a person decry giving seems superficially selfish, thus making this explanation more plausible than the others, and allowing the perceiver to discount the other possibilities and feel confident in the conclusion that the observed person is selfish.

As another example of discounting, in one episode of the TV series *Seinfeld*, the characters are outraged by an act that Jerry labels as "regifting." It turns out that Elaine had given a gift to a mutual friend, and the very same item was then received by Jerry as a gift from that mutual friend. He had taken the gift Elaine gave him and recycled it as a gift for Jerry. Why should their reaction turn to outrage when they learn it was "regifted"? What changes when Jerry and Elaine learn that the gift Elaine gave to someone else was apparently unwanted by that person and was given instead to Jerry? The behavior (Jerry getting a gift) and the consequence (the degree to which Jerry likes the gift) have not been altered at all. The reason the reaction shifts from gratitude to outrage is that although the behavior and its consequence are constant, the attribution associated with this instance of behavior changes because *the number of sufficient causes for having received the gift changes*. In general, when you receive a gift, you typically believe there is one cause for the person's having given it to you—it is meant to be a genuine and distinctive expression of the person's affection. Thus the one plausible cause is the disposition of the person giving the gift; that person likes you enough to take the time and effort to find a gift you would like. When you find out it is a recycled gift, it suggests another sufficient cause for the action other than the person caring enough about you to think about what you would want. Perhaps the person simply felt obligated to get you something, and could do no more than unload some unwanted item. The presence of this alternative sufficient cause (that the person does not take time to think about you at all) discounts the other plausible cause (that the person either is generous or likes you). As Kelley (1972a, p. 8) stated, "the role of a given cause in producing a given effect is discounted if other plausible causes are also present."

In effect, the logic for the discounting principle comes directly out of Jones and Davis's (1965) discussion of correspondent inference, as Kelley (1973) himself made clear: "Much [of] the present formulation of the discounting principle owes to Jones and Davis. They have clearly stated the key idea of several versus one (many versus few) plausible reasons and have asserted that the case of one or few reasons permits more confident inference from behavior to person properties." The main difference is that whereas Jones and Davis said that correspondent inference is inversely related to the number of effects uniquely associated with the act (noncommon effects), Kelley said that people examine the number of plausible causes for the act.

The discounting principle describes the type of causal schemas people employ in the presence of a *facilitative cause*. By *facilitative cause*, it is meant that some cause is present (perhaps among other plausible causes) that is sufficient to promote the behavior (effect). If a perceiver observes (or infers) the presence of a cause that can account for the effect and that would facilitate the occurrence of the effect, the perceiver uses a simple rule for making the inference: Discount all other plausible/possible causes and assume that the effect is caused by the observed, facilitative cause. In the *Seinfeld* example, when Jerry learns he has received a "regifted" item, there is now a facilitative cause that is present; the person did not spend time shopping for him and thinking about him, but has handed over an unwanted item. Because the presently observed cause (wanting to quickly fulfill an obligation to give a gift) would facilitate the behavior (the effect of giving a gift), Jerry and Elaine discount other sufficient and plausible causes that are not observed that would also facilitate and cause the behavior—such as the person's being generous or having affection for Jerry. Behavior does not always occur in the presence of a facilitative cause. In many instances, a behavior occurs in the presence of some force that works against the occurrence of the behavior; this is called behavior occurring in the presence of an *inhibitory cause*. When behavior occurs despite an inhibitory cause, it suggests to the perceiver a totally different schematic rule of inference than when a facilitative cause is present. We turn to this next.

The Augmentation Principle

Think once again of the TV show *Seinfeld*. In one episode, the character named George is interviewing for a job with the New York Yankees, and he is introduced to the principal owner of the team (another George, Steinbrenner). The character George proceeds to tell Steinbrenner that, as an owner, he is an arrogant oaf whose decisions have crippled the team (obviously this was filmed prior to the team's playing in six World Series between 1996 and 2003). Or consider once again the example of a President of the United States who engaged in extremely scandalous, indiscreet, and immoral actions with a college-age woman. The behavior occurred despite the fact that (1) opponents were already accusing him of scandals and scrutinizing his behavior closely, (2) there were role constraints associated with his being a moral leader, and (3) there was heightened attention to his actions because he was running for reelection. These are examples of behavior occurring in the presence of an inhibitory cause. An external cause exists that can account for the behavior *not to be performed*. One should usually not insult people, but this is especially true when one is being interviewed for a job by the owner of the company. The situation suggests that one instead be ingratiating. One should not have extramarital affairs, but this is especially true if one is a moral leader whose every move is closely observed.

What type of inference do we make, and what type of schematic rule do we use, when the situation should inhibit the response that was given (e.g., when the situation calls for ingratiation, but the response is rudeness)? In these instances, our judgments of the person's disposition as responsible for the action seem to be heightened, because the action occurs in the presence of an inhibitory cause. If an inhibitory cause (or something that would prevent the act from occurring) is present, but the act occurs anyway, then the behavior is perceived as having been enacted with such conviction that it was able to overcome the thing blocking it. This is called the *augmentation principle*, because when a behavior occurs in the presence of some constraint, cost, or risk, the behavior is attributed to the actor even more strongly than it typically would be (internal attribution is heightened or augmented). According to Kelley (1972a, p. 12),

> When an effect occurs in the presence of a plausible inhibitory cause, a reverse version of the discounting principle, which might be called the augmentation principle is required.

This can be stated as follows: if for a given effect both a plausible inhibitory cause and a plausible facilitative cause are present, the role of the facilitative cause in producing the effect will be judged greater than if it alone were present as a plausible cause for the effect.

Multiple Necessary Causes

There are times at which there are not merely multiple possible causes for some effect, but multiple necessary causes. By *multiple necessary causes*, it is meant that the effect will not occur at all unless each of the multiple causes is present. This creates a very simple causal rule for us as perceivers: If the behavior (effect) is present, then each of the necessary causes must be in place. If the effect does not occur, then we must be able to conclude that one of the necessary causes is not present in this situation. For example, if we know that to do well on a statistics test (the effect) requires both being extremely good at math and studying extremely hard (multiple necessary causes), then we can form an attribution, given only limited information. If a person does well on the exam, then he/she must have studied hard and have high ability at math.

Evidence for Causal Schemas

An excellent empirical illustration of the discounting and augmentation principles (though these were not yet named as such at the time the experiment was conducted) comes from Jones, Davis, and Gergen (1961). The logic of the experiment was that behavior conforming to the expectancies associated with a specific role is not informative about a person's disposition, whereas behavior that breaks free from such situational constraint should be attributed to disposition, since out-of-role behavior carries much information.

Research participants were asked to listen to an audiotape of a job interview with one of two men. Some participants heard a tape where the man being interviewed was applying for a job on a submarine, while others heard a man applying for a job as an astronaut. They were to make judgments about the person being interviewed—a prospective astronaut or submariner. On the tape, the person doing the interviewing began the session by describing the ideal candidate for the job. For the submarine job, the ideal candidate was described as friendly, outgoing, cooperative, and obedient. For the astronaut job, the ideal candidate was described in an opposite manner—as one who did not need other people and was inner-directed. In each of these two scenarios, the person being interviewed then proceeded to respond in a manner making it clear that he either possessed the very traits that the job required, or failed to possess those traits. So half of the participants heard an interviewee respond in a way perfectly consistent with the role he was asked to play: When asked to interview for a job, this person proceeded to tell the "employers" that he was exactly like the type of person they wanted to hire. However, half heard a person do the opposite: He performed in a way inconsistent with the role, telling the employers that he was nothing like the ideal candidate for the job. That is, the submariner applicant described himself as a person better suited for the astronaut job, and the astronaut candidate described himself as someone perhaps better suited for the submariner job (see Figure 6.3).

The results showed that when the "interviewee" conformed to the constraints specified by the role, participants' ratings were not very dispositional and not confidently held. However, when the interviewee responded with out-of-role behavior, he was rated

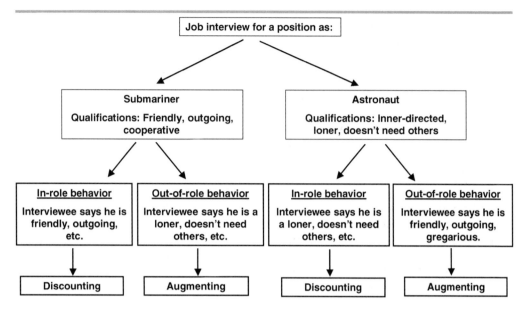

FIGURE 6.3. Augmenting and discounting due to conforming to and violating expectations.

as having a high likelihood of possessing the traits he claimed to possess during the interview, and participants were quite confident in assigning these correspondent inferences. How does this research illustrate discounting and augmenting? A person interviewing for a job on a submarine who claimed to be extraverted was plausibly stating this because it was a trait consistent with the interview situation (a plausible, present external cause). This plausible external cause led to discounting of the internal cause, and the person was not seen as truly possessing the traits he described. The pressure of the situation (telling the interviewer what he wished to hear) was a more face-valid explanation for the behavior, the more plausible of the possible causes. The alternative causes were discounted. Thus, when the behavior conformed to the expectations of the role, discounting of the person's disposition as the cause for the behavior occurred, and no correspondent inference was formed (and the person was probably seen as disingenuous and fake).

However, when behavior occurs in the presence of an inhibitory cause, such as when the situation dictates acting one way and a person acts in the opposite manner, this should augment the attribution made to internal causes. In the Jones and colleagues (1961) study, when a person being interviewed for a job as a submariner responded by saying he possessed the very traits better suited for an astronaut, this should have augmented the attribution that he really possessed the traits of being inner-directed and not needing other people (and, of course, the same would have been true of the person being interviewed to be an astronaut who claimed to have the traits better suited for a submariner). Knowing what traits were needed for the job served as an inhibitory cause to the person's saying he possessed the opposite traits. Saying this would have suggested he had overcome the obstacle of what the situation would dictate him to do, and this would have augmented the likelihood of the perception that he truly possessed the traits described (and that he was an honest person). In Jones and Davis's (1965, p. 236) language,

> in-role behavior does not lead to confident, correspondent inferences because such behavior has multiple consequences. . . . Each of these effects is a "plausible reason" for in-role behavior. . . . On the other hand, plausible reasons for out-of-role behavior are comparatively scarce. One of the few noncommon effects of behavior at variance with role demands is the satisfaction of expressing one's true nature.

An Attributional Analysis of Persuasion

Eagly and Chaiken (1975, 1976) examined the use of causal schemas in attributions formed about a messenger delivering a speech. The logic was that if an expectancy exists about what position that messenger will take in the message, this expectancy should function as a cause for explaining the behavior (the position advocated in the actual message). For example, if a person is delivering a speech about the topic of gun control, and if the person is delivering that speech to members of the National Rifle Association (NRA), an expectancy is established. The attribution formed is dependent on whether or not the position advocated in the message is discrepant or consistent with the position the message recipients *expect* will be advocated.

If the person delivers a speech that is favorable toward gun control, then the expectancy has been confirmed by the behavior; therefore, the expectancy is a facilitative cause. If the person delivers a speech that is against gun control, then the expectancy is disconfirmed by the behavior, and the expectancy in this case is an inhibitory cause. Behavior that violates an expectancy should augment (lead to greater amounts of) person attribution, and behavior that is congruent with the expectancy should discount (lead to weaker degrees of) person attribution. However, as Wood and Eagly (1981) point out, when behavior occurs in the presence of a facilitative cause, we cannot rule out the possibility that this is still a behavior caused by personal (as opposed to situational) forces. Despite the fact that the communicator appears to be biased by the situation, the possibility that this person is actually expressing his/her true opinion in this instance still exists (it could be that this individual really does happen to agree with the audience). This creates attributional ambiguity. In order to eliminate this doubt, the message recipient may be motivated to process the message systematically. The perceiver is likely to desire more information and to want to think more about causes for the action than the person who has seen the behavior in the face of an inhibitory cause. This would also have been true of the participants in the Jones and colleagues (1961) study described above. Although a person who said he had all the traits of an astronaut might only have been saying what he expected others wanted to hear during an interview for an astronaut job, it could also have been true that he really did have these traits. Presence of a facilitative cause could not rule this out. Thus perceivers might have been likely to judge the person as not really possessing these traits, but might have been willing to look at more information if they were given the opportunity (relative to someone who saw out-of–role behavior).

In research testing the use of such causal schemas (Eagly & Chaiken, 1975, 1976; Eagly, Wood, & Chaiken, 1978; Wood & Eagly, 1981), research participants were presented with information prior to hearing a message that induced them to form an expectancy that a messenger was biased. For example, research participants were provided with information suggesting that the messenger's willingness to express accurate positions in his/her speech had been compromised by the situation (such as giving a speech about gun control to the NRA). Using such an approach, Eagly and Chaiken (1975, 1976) and Eagly and colleagues (1981) found that when the actual message *disconfirmed* the premessage expectancy, participants perceived the message as unbiased (they believed the person was expressing a true opinion). In explaining such findings, Eagly and colleagues invoked the augmentation principle. The presence of a plausible inhibitory cause (that the situation would bias the person to say one thing) served to strengthen or augment the other sufficient cause—that the messenger's position on the issue might be true. However, if the message *confirmed* the expectancy, participants were more likely to perceive the message as biased. Here, the discounting principle was invoked. The expectancy of bias served as a sufficient and facilitative cause; participants then discounted the possibility that the message reflected the person's true beliefs. (However, as predicted above, Moskowitz [1996] also found that although discounting had occurred, participants were more likely to engage in systematic processing of the message.)

Finally, the reason this is known as an *attributional analysis of persuasion* is that the schemas used for arriving at attributions also determine how persuasive the message is. If a message is perceived to be an accurate reflection of someone's true opinions, and there is no reason to suspect those opinions are biased, then that person will be persuasive. The positions they are advocating in the message should sway the message recipient and lead the recipient to shift his/her attitudes so they fit with the positions advocated in the message. Conversely, if a recipient attributes a message to the pressure of the situation the messenger is in, such that the positions espoused are perceived to be biased, that message will not have persuasive impact. Thus schemas allow perceivers to form attributions of others that in turn shape perceivers' opinions.

The Causal-Calculus/Analysis-of-Variance Model

Kelley (1967) also believed that despite using simple schemas in situations where the amount of information available is low, people at times engage in a systematic analysis of various factors that allow them to make decisions about where to place the locus of causality. Kelley's model of the attribution process described a perceiver's processing of attribution-relevant information as being similar to a scientist's use of the statistical procedure known as *analysis of variance* (ANOVA; see also Försterling, 1989). The similarity to ANOVA lies in the fact that there is a dependent variable (the action, outcome, or event being analyzed), and there are independent variables (the various factors [dimensions of information] or potential causes that people consider when making attributions). These dimensions or factors, just like independent variables, have levels associated with them; the perceived act can be described as either high or low on a given dimension. Perceivers then analyze the pattern among these independent variables to calculate an attribution. When the action is high on Dimension 1, low on Dimension 2, and high on Dimension 3, this pattern suggests to the perceivers a particular type of attribution (the content of or definitions for these dimensions will be reviewed shortly). Försterling (1992) adds that the strength of the attribution to a particular cause is like the F statistic in ANOVA, while the certainty of the attribution is akin to the significance level. While perceivers do not always follow this rational, *causal calculus* for arriving at attributions, the model begins with this description of the ANOVA-like approach that perceivers take when they are attempting to be deliberate, systematic, and rational in producing attributions.

Covariation

The ANOVA model presents a rational account of how people deliberately and systematically use information in order to make the decision about where the cause for an observed action is located. The model revolves around the notion of *covariation*. If two events occur in tandem (or fail to occur in tandem), they can be said to be varying together. Thus the variance in one event is linked to the variance in another. The *covariation principle* asserts that an effect is attributed to the one cause with which it covaries over time. An example can illustrate the point. Imagine that in your office parking lot, "cute" little pictures of cats are being anonymously left on your car windshield (and not on anybody else's). They appear on some days and not others. The occurrence of the pictures varies. Imagine, as well, that of all the people you work with, you notice that one person (Employee X) appears to be out of the office many days a week, yet in the office on others. The presence of the person at work varies. Finally, imagine that you have noticed a covariation: The pictures seem to appear on your windshield on the same days that the person in question shows up at the office. The variance in the one event is linked to the variance in the other. Using the covariation principle, you would probably assume at this point that (make an attribution that) the cause of the effect (cats on the car) lies within the thing with which it covaries (Employee X's attendance). As Kelley (1967) stated, "the effect is attributed to that condition which is present when the effect is present and which is absent when the effect is absent" (p. 194). Naturally, actual covariation is not what really determines attribution. So long as a perceiver thinks two events covary, a causal link will be made between them.

However, the nature of this causal link will not be fully explicated by merely relying on covariation. You may now know who is responsible for the pictures of cats that have appeared on your car, yet you still do not know *why* they have appeared. Kelley's (1967) ANOVA model addresses this issue by pointing to several dimensions of causes that people analyze to flesh out their attributions. The causes can be in the disposition of the person, in the power of the situation, or in the timing with which the event occurs. According to Kelley, there are three dimensions of information (factors in the ANOVA) that people typically utilize to assess the covariation of each of these possible causes with the action: *consensus*, *distinctiveness*, and *consistency*. These dimensions (defined below) draw from, and can be traced to, the factors discussed by Jones and Davis (1965). This might be partly responsible for why, as the story goes, E. E. (Ned) Jones found the early draft of Kelley's manuscript that crossed his desk to be one of the most important pieces of social-psychological writing that he had ever read. (Its impact suggests that he was not alone in this assessment, though undergraduates who read the piece might struggle to agree while struggling to comprehend it!) The story also has it that Jones thought the analogy to ANOVA to be so accurate and descriptive that he "kicked" himself for not making it himself.

Consensus

Consensus is one dimension of information that perceivers must consider for them to determine whether the person or an entity is responsible for an observed behavior. What type of information comprises the dimension known as *consensus*? Consensus information describes how people other than the actor would react in the same situation or toward the same entity. As with all three dimensions of information that make up the causal calculus, there are two levels to the independent variable (dimension) known as consensus—high consensus and low consensus. *High consensus* means that the action generalizes across other actors (is not specific to one person, but is something that many other people would do). *Low consensus* means that few (if any) others act the same way the person being observed has acted. Essentially, consensus tells us what other people would do, if everything else was held constant.

Let us return to the examples used earlier. If we know that Benjamin enjoys Van Gogh paintings, what question would we need to ask to determine whether there is high or low consensus? It would be "Do many other people like Van Gogh paintings?" If we know that Princess Diana's limousine driver was speeding to get away from photographers, what would we want to know to determine whether the driver was exhibiting high or low consensus? It would be "Do many other limousine drivers of the rich and famous use high speed to elude photographers?"

Low consensus suggests that the circumstances do not cause the outcome (since they would lead others to act the same way); although it does not rule out the possibility that the entity has something to do with drawing out the behavior from the actor, it suggests that the situation is not the primary cause. High consensus suggests that the entity is responsible for the action. If many people like Van Gogh paintings, this does suggest that something about Van Gogh paintings appeals to people. However, high-consensus information alone does not rule out the possibility that something about the person is involved. Other people may like Van Gogh paintings, but this does not rule out that something about Ben's disposition makes him a particular lover of Van Gogh. We need further information to make adequate judgments. This can be provided by conducting a similar analysis of the remaining two dimensions.

Distinctiveness

Whereas consensus is a dimension providing information about the person, distinctiveness is a dimension providing information about the entity. *Distinctiveness* information describes how the same person (the actor) reacts to different entities. *High distinctiveness* means that the action does not generalize across other entities, but is specific to this particular entity. The actor behaves this way only in this particular situation (with this particular entity). *Low distinctiveness* means that the actor behaves the same way to many entities. Notice an important difference between consensus and distinctiveness: Being able to generalize on consensus means that lots of people do the same thing, and this is high consensus. But generalizing on distinctiveness means that lots of entities produce the same reaction, and this is low distinctiveness. In other words, distinctiveness is about the distinct nature of the entity. Having similar reactions to many entities does not make a given entity very distinctive.

For example, if Ben reacts the same way to Klee, Picasso, Warhol, and Michelangelo as he does to Van Gogh, we cannot say that Van Gogh is particularly distinct when we are attempting to understand Ben's reaction. There is low distinctiveness. If it is unlikely that the distinct love of Van Gogh in particular is what causes Ben's enjoyment, we would be less inclined to make an external attribution to Van Gogh and more likely to make an internal attribution to Ben's love of art. What type of questions would we need answered to determine whether the actions of Princess Diana's limousine driver at the time of her death had low or high distinctiveness? Since the entity in this situation was Diana's desire to evade the paparazzi, we would need to ask how the driver acted with other entities—did his behavior generalize across other entities? If the driver never drove at such high speeds or so recklessly when he was with other celebrity passengers or when he was driving by himself with his family, it would suggest that the response was something distinctive to the entity. This high distinctiveness would make us more inclined to make an external attribution and less inclined to blame or hold responsible the driver for the outcome of the action (even though he was the one who performed the action and crashed the car).

In the ANOVA model, therefore, one dimension of information alone does not provide for an adequate attribution. We need to consider the combination of distinctiveness and consensus information. What would the combination of high consensus and high distinctiveness suggest? For Ben and Van Gogh paintings, it would suggest that many people besides Ben like Van Gogh paintings, and that Ben likes only Van Gogh paintings and not art in general. This would suggest that something particular about Van Gogh paintings causes Ben's response, and that it causes this response in most others as well. We would make an external attribution to the entity. What would the combination of low consensus and low distinctiveness suggest? It would suggest that very few people like Van Gogh paintings, and that Ben experiences joy from looking at works of art by other artists. This would suggest that something particular about Ben causes the response. We would make an internal attribution to Ben.

Distinctiveness is somewhat related to Jones and Davis's (1965) discussion of situational constraint. High distinctiveness means that the behavior occurs only in a particular situation (it fails to generalize across entities). This could occur because in the specific situation in which the behavior emerges, one has no other options. Of course, it also could occur because one has other options, but there is something special about the situation that draws out a particular type of reaction. Thus, while lacking choice is not the only way for a situation to be distinct, it can be conceived of as one way of producing a highly distinctive response. Low distinctiveness, however, implies a person attribution, because many situations elicit the same behavior. This can only occur if one has the freedom to act as one wishes in those situations. In such cases, the same behavior across these diverse situations suggests that one is acting in a way reflective of one's underlying disposition. This analysis also suggests that distinctiveness is somewhat tied to Jones and Davis's notion of noncommon effects. A noncommon effect means that the consequences of a behavior occur only with one particular choice of action (they fail to generalize across other actions). This is a type of distinctiveness—one in which the consequences of an action are distinct to that action. Kelley took the concept of distinctiveness and applied it to the action's being distinct to a particular entity. Just as noncommon effects require perceivers to think about the other consequences that may emerge if one acts in a different way (if the consequences of one's behavior generalize across different actions), distinctiveness requires perceivers to think about other actions that may emerge if one is faced with a different entity.

Consistency

So far, the ANOVA model only allows us to determine whether the cause is internal or external to the person. But Heider (1958) focused our attention on a second dimension that helps determine causality and understand an action—stability. Kelley (1967) captured the stability dimension by yet a third piece of information perceivers were said to consider in their causal calculations. The final dimension is the consistency of the action. *Consistency* refers to the stability or duration of the action—its ability to generalize across time, given that the entity and the person are held constant. *High consistency* means a recurring action and suggests a stable attribution; the same action is produced by the same person when the same entity was encountered. *Low consistency* means there is instability in the person's reaction to the entity over time.

For example, suppose we observe one person interacting with another person at lunch over a period of time. In one instance, the person is bossing around the other and providing all sorts of unsolicited feedback. In other instances, this type of behavior is not observed. The person is considerate and seems to be a good listener. This might suggest that the person has many possible ways to act, and selects from among them at different points in time (although in the same situation). The conclusion would be that the person is not domineering, since that is a stable trait, but acts in a way that lacks consistency. High consistency would suggest a stable attribution, while low consistency would suggest an unstable attribution. Keep in mind, however, that low consistency does not tell us why in a particular situation the person chooses to act in a domineering way. It would simply allow us to conclude that whatever the reason, it is something unstable. In conjunction with the other dimensions, the attribution can be fleshed out more fully. In terms of the examples we have been using thus far, consistency information would lead us to ask, "Will Ben get joy from the Van Gogh painting the next time he visits the museum?" and "Did Diana's driver use the same type of excessive speed when eluding photographers in the past?"

A Final Example

Before exiting the causal calculus, let us analyze one last example to illustrate how it works (and how it can get complicated). Consider, yet again, President Clinton's affair with Monica Lewinsky. "Why did this happen?" was what most of us at the time were trying to figure out. According to the ANOVA model, what sort of information should we have been gathering? First, we would want distinctiveness information. Did the behavior generalize to other entities? Had Clinton had relationships with other women while married? The answer to this would be yes, as stories of affairs with at least two other women (Gennifer Flowers and Paula Jones) had already surfaced. Thus, unfortunately for Monica Lewinsky (the entity in this example), there was low distinctiveness. The actor's behavior (an extramarital affair) generalized across entities (women other than Monica). Next, we would want to gather consensus information: Did other people in power, especially other Presidents, have extramarital relationships with underlings? Henry Kissinger has said that power is an aphrodisiac. In support of this, the President's scandalous behavior brought to light the fact that many others in politics have behaved similarly. Many of our public officials have had extramarital affairs. Even past Presidents (e.g., John F. Kennedy) have been assumed to have had affairs. Therefore, President Clinton's behavior had high consensus.

Lastly, the model claims that we should have been seeking information about the consistency of the behavior. Did the President continue his relationship with Lewinsky? The answer to this, depending on how we defined consistency, would be either yes or no. On the one hand, the answer would be no, because he eventually broke it off. This was low consistency. But then we may question the termination of the relationship. Did it occur before the scandal broke, or because the scandal was about to break? Perhaps the true question to get at consistency is not whether he eventually broke it off, but whether the behavior occurred more than one or two times. That is, if it happened one or two times, we might attribute the behavior to something unstable—they were drunk, they were working late, and one thing led to another. By this definition, the event had high consistency. It occurred repeatedly, with evidence of multiple meetings between the two.

Thus, what do we conclude in this situation where there was a stable event; where many people have acted similarly; and where this particular person acted as others do, yet he acted in this fashion with lots of different people? Clearly something about the person (the President) caused the behavior, but clearly many other people in his position have acted similarly, suggesting that something about the situation contributed as well. This would be the high-consensus, low-distinctiveness scenario. This scenario is ambiguous and allows the cause to be placed either in the person or in the situation. This would really permit partisan squabbling and naive realism to operate! As you might imagine, similar ambiguity would arise in a case with low consensus but high distinctiveness. In such instances, the low consensus would suggest that something about the disposition of the person caused him/her to act as few others would. Yet the high distinctiveness would reveal that this was not a behavior this person engaged in across a variety of situations or with other people, suggesting that something powerful about the entity might have drawn out this unusual behavior. The attribution is not clear.

A Caveat

You may have noticed that the types of answers to our "why" questions provided by the covariation model are not very satisfying. We can locate cause as internal or external to the person, but we cannot specify reason explanations (Malle, 1999). Take, for example, the story used to illustrate covariation, where cute pictures of cats mysteriously appear on your windshield. The appearance seems to coincide with the presence of another particular person. Even after you have figured out that this covariation exists, you still have no clue as to why this coworker is performing this odd behavior. You just know that the cause can be located in that person. Intentionality is discovered, but specific intentions and reasons have not been. The same is true of many other examples offered, such as Ben, who (like many other people) appreciates Van Gogh paintings, yet does not like the work of too many other artists. The model allows us to see that the cause is probably something about Van Gogh, but this is not likely to be a very satisfying reason for explaining *why* Ben likes Van Gogh. The covariation model has this limitation when it comes to addressing "why" questions: It may point us in a direction so that we may then potentially find those answers, but it does not give us an actual reason.

Evaluating the ANOVA Model

In a direct test of the ANOVA model, McArthur (1972) provided research participants with distinctiveness, consensus, and consistency information relating to a behavior, manipulating the pattern of information that was provided. Overall, there were eight possible patterns or combinations of low and high distinctiveness, consensus, and consistency information. Thus a participant in this research might get a description of a behavior that was said to have high consistency, consensus, and distinctiveness, while another participant would read a behavior described as having low consistency, consensus, and distinctiveness, with each possible pattern being used. The ANOVA model predicts that particular patterns of information lead to specific types of attributions. McArthur found that the actual attributions formed by research participants reflected the use of information in the manner described by the ANOVA model.

For example, when most other people were said to have responded in the same manner as the person whose behavior was described, and the person's behavior was said to be uniquely associated with the entity in question, as well as being consistent over time with that entity (the high, high, high pattern), then research participants judged the cause of that behavior to be located in the entity. However, when a person was described as behaving in a manner that was dissimilar to others, and was described as acting that way with many different entities and consistently over time (the low-consensus, low-distinctiveness, high-consistency pattern), then research participants judged the cause of that behavior to be located in the person.

A Probabilistic Model

The covariation principle implies that causal induction is a normative process. Kelley (1967) described covariation as a process in which people treat causal analysis as a scientist would treat a statistical analysis (ANOVA), making normative, inductive inferences. But the literature suggests that the covariation component in causal induction is not normative. That is, people deviate from normative inductive reasoning when using covariation information in a number of ways. For example, in McArthur's (1972) work, despite evidence supporting the normative predictions of Kelley's model, there was also a marked tendency for people to underutilize consensus information. Furthermore, Cheng and Novick (1992) point out that when people are given a table that crosses the presence and absence of a potential cause with the presence and absence of some effect, people untrained in statistics do not do well in reaching normative and rational conclusions about contingencies between events. Finally, we have already seen a tendency for perceivers to overattribute to disposition, and we will explore that deviation from normative processing as well as a host of others in the next two chapters.

Cheng and Novick (1990) raise an important question regarding causal judgments that deviate from what would be predicted by a normative inductive process. In deductive reasoning, people can use completely rational and logical processes in computing an inference and still arrive at a false conclusion. This can happen when the rules they use are correct, but the information they are given is incorrect. Just as perceivers can arrive at a false conclusion in deductive reasoning through logical information-processing strategies, it may also be possible for inductive reasoning (of the sort people use when applying covariation information to inference formation) to follow rational processing steps and still yield biased or non-normative conclusions, due to the nature of the information that is being used by perceivers to compute their inference. Of course, this does not rule out the possibility that sometimes people use rules of logic incorrectly or make biased inferences. We will discuss this in the next chapter. The point here is that not all deviations from so-called "normative" processes of inference formation are due to irrational/biased processing. Sometimes they result from rational thinking that uses bad information.

Cheng and Novick (1990) propose that deviations from what we would consider normative models of social inference (such as deviations from the Jones & Davis [1965] model of the factors that should, normatively, heighten the occurrence of correspondent inferences) may be produced by perceivers using information in their analysis that observers are not aware of. For example, one problem lies in the type of information that experimenters present to their research participants. In testing the Kelley (1967) model of attribution, researchers typically manipulate the three main factors that Kelley focused on—consistency, consensus, and distinctiveness. Cheng and Novick (1990), however, claim that this is only a limited range of the types of information that perceivers could consider. Therefore, what looks like nonrational processing to the researcher is actually rational processing, with perceivers using information not specified by the experimenters: "Consensus information indicates the amount of agreement between the person in question and other people in their responses to a particular stimulus on a particular occasion, rather than the amount of response agreement between the person and other people with respect to all the stimuli on all occasions" (p. 548).

Cheng and Novick (1992) propose that perceivers, instead of using covariation information irrationally, make probability estimates that go beyond the covariation information provided by the experimenters. To be specific, perceivers are believed to make probability estimates of the likelihood that an effect would have resulted, given the presence or absence of some causal factors that have immediately preceded (that are psychologically prior to) an effect. For example, a person may have an allergy to a cat. This could be something attributable to the cat, the person, or an interaction (a conjunction) between this person and that cat. To test whether the person or cat is responsible, a perceiver might follow the seemingly normative process of computing a probability that the allergy appears in the *presence* of the cat and then computing the probability it appears in the cat's *absence*. The difference between these probabilities is then used to make an inference. However, to test the interaction, or conjunction, hypothesis, the difference just described must be different at different levels of an orthogonal factor. That is, for one cat you would see the difference just described, but for another cat you would not. This is a second-order difference. By using this type of reasoning people perhaps arrive at judgments that appear not to be following logical rules. But they are. They are just using rules not anticipated by the simple use of covariation information. Causal inference is indeed a probabilistic exercise, but it is not simply a deterministic one (did Cause X lead to Event Y?). When we talk about probabilistic causes, we must recognize that these are conjunctive in nature. And this fact can account for why people seemingly do not follow normative rules of induction when using covariation information.

The Abnormal-Conditions (Counterfactual) Model

Hilton and Slugoski (1986) have similarly argued that the logical use of rules, such as those associated with the ANOVA model, does not adequately capture the way in which people actually make attributions. Rather than examining the covariation of consensus, distinctiveness, and consistency information when forming attributions, people may instead rely on "counterfactual and contrastive criteria of causal ascription, as unified in the notion of an abnormal condition" (p. 76). What do these authors mean by this? *Counterfactuals* are alternative realities—those that might have happened if some other path of action or inaction had been chosen. If one chooses to drive home via some alternate route and hits a deer on the way, one might engage in counterfactual thoughts. One would ask, "What if I had acted otherwise?", "If only I took my normal route." Thus a consideration of counterfactuals means that perceivers consider alternative outcomes that might have emerged if a different behavior had been enacted. This is similar to Jones and Davis's (1965) idea that chosen and nonchosen courses of action each have associated effects. The counterfactual (or abnormal-conditions) model assumes that perceivers make attributions by considering such alternative realities. They examine not only the normal conditions, but those usually found when a behavior is absent. For example, when the behavior of driving home a new way is absent, the normal conditions (or those usually found) exist. The model also assumes that attributions are formed by perceivers examining a situation for what is atypical or abnormal. People can assess what caused a behavior to occur not only by looking at what happens when a behavior is absent, but what happens under unique and abnormal conditions, such as when a behavior that is usually absent has occurred. That is, if perceivers want to know why a behavior occurred, they can ask themselves, "What would we expect if the behavior did not occur, and what is unique and unusual about the conditions when the behavior does occur?" By examining what conditions differ between the typical and the counterfactual behavior (what happens if others were to act differently from how they typically do), perceivers can assess the cause for the behavior. They can attribute cause to those factors that are not present when the behavior is absent, but are present when the behavior is also present.

It may very well be that the conditions that are typically present are *necessary* for a given behavior to occur, but without the addition of some atypical factors, the behavior would not have occurred. Thus the typical conditions would not really be considered the cause. Only a consideration of the atypical or counterfactual conditions would allow perceivers to arrive at a reasonable attribution. For example, if a lawnmower catches on fire, it is necessary for a person to have first filled the machine with gasoline and turned on the machine. But these conditions (causes), though necessary for the fire to occur, are also typical of what happens even when a fire does not occur. The fire is dependent not only on the necessary and typical causes, but on the necessary and *atypical* causes as well—such as the engine being excessively dirty. When searching for the cause of a behavior, perceivers are believed to follow a process whereby they contrast the conditions that are typically found (the causes associated with a lawnmower functioning normally) with those abnormal or atypical conditions that are found when the behavior occurs (when the lawnmower catches on fire). An example that Hilton and Slugoski (1986) borrowed from Hart and Honoré (1961) may make this even clearer. When a horrific accident such as a train derailment occurs, people tend to focus immediately on the counterfactual reality: What if this did not occur? Why is it that it did occur now, whereas it has not happened in the past? What atypical or unusual conditions were in place that are not typically in place? These types of questions, which contrast the reality with some more typical alternative reality, are what people seek answers for in order to come to understand the cause of the event. In the case of a train derailment, there are many necessary conditions for the accident (i.e., if those conditions had not been in place, the accident would not have occurred): The freight cars were excessively heavy, the speed of the train was quite high, one of the rails was damaged, and so on. How do perceivers pick from among these necessary causes to determine their attribution? The answer is that perceivers are assumed to engage in a process of contrasting those necessary causes that exist under normal conditions (no behavior) versus abnormal conditions (a behavior has taken place that needs to be explained). Thus, when there is no train wreck (normal conditions), people typically find freight cars of excessive weight and trains traveling at high speeds. Although such conditions were necessary for the wreck to occur, causal weight is instead placed on the necessary cause that is associated with the abnormal event only.

Let us examine one last example, using people instead of lawnmowers and trains. If we want to understand why a behavior has occurred, such as the suicide of Kurt Cobain (the lead singer and songwriter of the band Nirvana, who killed himself with a gunshot to the head), we need to compare the typical versus the atypical conditions. The typical conditions, such as his state of depression, his chronic stomach pain, his addiction to heroin, and his disenchantment with fame, were perhaps all necessary for the suicide to occur. But to determine the cause for his behavior, we need to determine what was unique or abnormal at the time of his suicide—what existed over and above the typical conditions. This process of focusing on the abnormal or counterfactual conditions (those conditions that are different or atypical from what is normally found) and contrasting them with the typical events leads people to place causal weight on the atypical events, even though the typical events may have been necessary.

Finally, an important point relating to this model is that the terms "normal" and "abnormal" are both relative. What is abnormal in one instance may not be considered abnormal if perceivers alter what it is being contrasted against. This is particularly true in attempts to understand the more mundane types of behaviors that are the focus of person perception, such as why a man got angry after a confrontation with a coworker, rather than why a train derailed. The manner in which the comparison or contrast is set up will determine the type of attribution that is formed. For example, the man's psychoanalyst might contrast the man's anger toward the coworker with how other people might have responded in the same situation (thus highlighting consensus information as the relative comparison standard). However, the person's best friend might choose to highlight how the man has responded with other people/entities (thus highlighting distinctiveness information as the relative comparison standard). If the behavior is contrasted against conditions where consensus information is highlighted, a very different attribution may result than if the behavior is contrasted against conditions in which distinctiveness information is highlighted. In our example, if the comparison standard for determining what is typical is how other people would react (the standard established by the psychotherapist), then it might be that other people would not get angry with the coworker, and the man would be seen as at fault for his anger. However, if we ignore what others might do (consensus) and focus instead on how this person has acted with other people under similar circumstances (distinctiveness), we might learn that he has not responded in anger in these other situations. Thus the first contrast for what is typical would lead us to expect that the man is angry by disposition. The second contrast for defining what is typical would reveal that he is not. The act of using what is defined as "normal" and "abnormal" to engage in a process of contrasting alternative realities is what defines this model of attribution. And it is in this manner that the model suggests consensus, distinctiveness, and consistency information to be important. This model holds that such information, rather than being logically and rationally covaried in an ANOVA-like fashion, establishes contrast conditions. If consensus is high, then consensus information is used as a contrast, determining what behavior is normal and abnormal given this contrast condition. But if consensus is low and distinctiveness is high, a different focus for the contrast will exist, and suddenly what behavior seems normal and abnormal (and thus receives causal weight) will be altered.

Goals and Covariation

Sutton and McClure (2001) cycle us back to where this chapter began—to the everyday language (the words "can" and "try") that perceivers use to talk about causes for events. Heider's (1958) discussion of the use of "try" makes it clear that an internal locus often refers to the fact that the observed behavior is *motivated* or *goal-directed*. To say that the cause for a behavior is something internal to the person (such as his/her disposition) is to say that the person has a goal to attain (or is motivated to attain) a certain end state, and that the behavior is enacted to promote the attainment of that goal. Heider's discussion of the use of "can," on the other hand, makes it clear that while some causes for behavior lie in the motives, wants, and goals of the actor, some causes for behavior lie in those factors that *enable* behavior. These include such things as availability of the resources required for the behavior to occur, the actor having the required skills (capabilities), and the situation presenting the appropriate preconditions. Thus Sutton and McClure distinguish between motivating and enabling causes that give rise to behavior. Whereas Kelley's (1967) model can locate a cause as either internal or external to a person, a further analysis of the person's goals and the specifics of the situation that enable the behavior allow for more precise attributions.

Just as there is a tendency to attribute behavior to the person and make dispositional inferences (what has previously been labeled as overattribution to disposition), there is a similar tendency to attribute a behavior to the motives or goals of the actor rather than to the enabling causes. (However, this is merely a tendency; there are instances in which people attribute more to the enabling factors than to the motives [e.g., McClure & Hilton, 1997]. See below.) Perhaps this tendency exists because perceivers see enabling causes as similar to the "normal" conditions described (above) in the abnormal-conditions model (in that even in instances where the behavior does not occur, the person may have resources available for the behavior and may have the capability to enact the behavior). Motivation to act is perhaps seen as more abnormal. Why? Goals can fluctuate across time and situation quite easily. A person may have the ability and resources to act both at Time 1 and at Time 2, but what is distinct about the instance in which the behavior actually occurs (at Time 2) is that the person now has the goal to perform the behavior (whereas he/she did not have that goal at Time 1). The exception to this rule tends to be when the motivating conditions are more typical than the enabling conditions. For example, when a homeless person is seen eating in a high-priced restaurant, we assume that this person always has the goal to eat well. What carries causal weight is the change in the conditions that enable the person to do so. The enabling conditions are abnormal; thus the attribution shifts to reflect this.

Sutton and McClure's (2001) basic point is that whether the attribution a perceiver forms places causal weight on motivating causes or enabling causes is dependent on the perceiver's joint analysis of these causal factors and covariation information. Thus, in an experiment (Study 2), they manipulated the consensus and consistency information for motivating factors and enabling factors to see how attributions were affected. For example, research participants might be told that all people are willing to buy an expensive car (high consensus for the motivating causal factor), but that only the actor they were reading about is able to buy the car (low consensus on the enabling causal factor). In addition, they received consistency information for each causal factor. High consistency for a motivating factor would be that the person is a car enthusiast, meaning that he/she loves cars and is motivated to think about them across a variety of situations (whereas low consistency would be the purchasing of the car on a whim). High consistency for an enabling factor would be that the person can afford to buy the car because of his/her wealth, meaning that the person has the wealth and ability to but a car across many situations (wealth is stable across time). The researchers hypothesized that considering the covariation information along with the motivation information would drastically change the types of attributions they would expect to find. For example, rich people are able to buy more luxury items than middle-class and poor people, yet all people desire to buy luxury items. Thus a rich person buying a big home would be a case of high consistency for both motivation and enabling factors (the rich person always would like to and is always able to buy nice homes), high consensus for the motivating factor (everyone wants a nice home), and low consensus for the enabling factor (few people can buy a large home). This should lead to an attribution to the stable enabling factor (the person's being rich would carry the most causal weight). Such an analysis allowed the researchers to identify situations in which the typical result (that people attribute to motivating factors) was not found. However, when a different pattern of covariation information was provided along with the same enabling and motivating factors, a different attribution would result. For example, when there was low consensus for the motivating factor, the case would be that of a rich person buying an expensive home that few other people want to buy. Rather than the enabling factor being seen as causal, the motivating factor would be seen as causal: The rich person buys the house because he/she wants that house.

CODA

In forming inferences about people and making attributions for the causes of the actions and words they encounter, perceivers use both heuristic and systematic evaluation. Each type of processing can be described as essentially rational, in that perceivers are described as doing the best they can with the information they have (Liberman, 2001). Apparent violations of a normative model (such as Kelley's and Jones and Davis's normative models) are not necessarily indications of bias. The work reviewed in this chapter has illustrated some of the rational processes (e.g., Cheng & Novick, 1990; Jones & Davis, 1965; Kelley, 1967) people use when thinking about the qualities of others. The basic idea is that people act intuitively like scientists, analyzing information in a manner similar to the way in which independent variables are considered as causes for changes to a dependent variable in a statistical procedure like ANOVA. When elaborate processing is blocked, people continue to act rationally, relying on heuristics and inferences about the given information learned through a lifetime of experience with similar people and situations.

This is not meant to imply that people always operate with rationality. They may use faulty heuristics even when they should use systematic analyses. They may use systematic thinking about information relevant to the actions of others, but in a biased way (e.g., Chaiken, Giner-Sorolla, & Chen, 1996)—breaking away from the patterns we would expect to find if people used information provided to them rationally. We turn next to these biases in the attribution process.

7 Correspondence Bias and Spontaneous Trait Inferences

The behavior of the individual is always determined by two groups of factors: by personal factors (attitudes, dispositions, etc.) and by situational factors. The situation plays its part in determining behavior in two ways: as a system of stimuli which provokes reactions, and as a system of opportunities for action (or obstacles to action). We cannot understand the underlying motivation of behavior without taking into account the dynamics of the situation involved . . . the importance of situational factors is often greater than the importance of personal factors: individuals endowed with different traits (attitudes), nevertheless, behave in the same way in identical social situations.

—ICHHEISER (1943, p. 151)

Chapter 6 has detailed the ways people attempt to be rational in making sense of the information they receive about others; they follow rules in analyzing that information, regardless of whether those rules are applied to a heuristic or a systematic analysis of behavior. It has also detailed how apparent deviations from using rules may indicate not that people are nonrational, but that they use information (in a perfectly logical way) experimenters had not anticipated they would use. Now that cool, calculating, rational perceivers have been described, this chapter and the next turn toward the role subjectivity and deviations from "rational" processing play in perceiving others.

We have already touched on one such deviation—the tendency for people to overattribute the cause of another person's behavior to that person's stable qualities (such as his/her disposition), and to (relatively) ignore the role played by the situation in causing the behavior. Consider an example: Ross arranges to meet his friend Clark after they have not seen each other for quite some time. Ross arranges to meet Clark, along with Clark's toddler, at a park, so that the toddler can play while the men are speaking. Clark proceeds to seem distracted, inattentive to Ross, and unable to respond in what Ross considers appropriate detail to Ross's stories of his life situation. Ross concludes that Clark has become rude and is uninterested in his friendship, and departs feeling neglected, hurt, and disrespected. Ross blames Clark's personality and feelings toward him for the action that has occurred, whereas the reality is that the situation dictated that Clark's attention be divided, with his toddler requiring his attention. The fact that Ross specifically chose to meet at a park so that Clark's toddler could accompany them is somehow lost on Ross when he evaluates why Clark has acted as he has. We see a behavior and attribute it to the stable quality of the person, even if a reasonable situational pressure could be pointed to as the cause. A more socially significant example arises from media (and individual) perceptions of the U.S. military personnel who committed socially unacceptable and degrading acts at the Abu Ghraib prison during the occupation of Iraq by U.S. forces in 2004. Their humiliating and offensive treatment of the prisoners may be due to an underlying disposition to be cruel. But virtually ignored are the well-known social pressures that operate in prison settings that drive normal people to cruelty (Zimbardo, 1971; see also Chapter 13, this volume), as well as the social constraint of the military's chain of command. These people may have simply been following orders, as they *must* do in their situation. If so, disposition would have little to do with their acts, despite feeling to the perceiver as if it must.

Heider (1958) identified this tendency as arising from the fact that behavior engulfs the field. Research on this tendency has revealed that there are multiple ways in which information processing can give rise to this tendency, in addition to the one alluded to by Heider. It is perhaps for this reason of being multiply determined that this deviation from objective processing has been so easily identified since the early days of psychological investigation into person perception. Indeed, the robustness of this tendency led Lee Ross (1977) to dub this tendency for overattribution the *fundamental attribution error*. A less dramatic name, *correspondence bias*, arose from the work of Jones and Harris (1967), who discovered this phenomenon while attempting to seek evidence for the Jones and Davis (1965) theory of correspondent inference. Perceivers blame behavior on the person doing the behaving—often at the expense of considering real, external pressure that forces that person to behave in this way. Imagine the impact of such a state of affairs on our evaluations of rape victims, on our ability to evaluate the cause of a crime, or on any plain old interpersonal interaction where the behavior of other people is seen as intended, such that we see more responsibility (and interpersonal consequences) in their actions than is warranted.

EVIDENCE FOR CORRESPONDENCE BIAS

Chapter 1 has asserted that three factors drive perception of others: the situation (broadly defined as in the norms of the culture; more locally defined as in the specific context one is in); the self (motives, goals, expectancies, prior information, and values of the perceiver); and the other person's behavior. The power of the situation alone is often strong enough to determine the behavior of others. This is evidenced by the fact that in some situations, a wide array of people behave identically. Social psychologists recognize this fact and have illustrated it time and again in order to demonstrate the power of the social situation to dictate how people act (e.g., Stanley Milgram's obedience studies, Bibb Latane and John Darley's bystander studies, Solomon Asch's conformity studies). If we recall correspondent inference theory from Chapter 6, Ned Jones was assuming that in this regard people who are in the process of perceiving others are similar to social psychologists; they recognize the power of situations to determine how people act. Social situations can be strong enough that the personality of the individual is not considered a relevant factor for explaining why he/she has acted. Perceivers should notice what Ichheiser (1943) pointed out in the quote above: People with different traits will act identically because the power of situations can determine how they act.

The belief of Jones and Davis (1965) that perceivers understand the power of situations and use this type of information when judging others is evident in examining the factors they claimed promote and inhibit correspondent inference. Jones (1979) stated, "A clear implication of the theory is that behavior under free choice conditions is more diagnostic than behavior under constraint" (p. 108). That is, correspondent inference (the belief that people's traits lead them to act) should decrease as the power of the situation increases (and the belief that a situational press is strong enough to direct behavior emerges). Jones and Harris (1967) sought to test the theory of correspondent inference to see whether people really do follow the rules described by Jones and Davis in forming attributions of others. In doing so, they focused on two factors that were described to affect correspondent inference: the freedom one has to act as one chooses (the lack of situational constraint), and the extent to which one's behavior is unusual (is different from what might be expected, based on knowing what most people do). They expected to find that people use information about obvious situational pressure in deciding how to determine the cause of a person's actions. They were about to discover they were wrong!

The Jones and Harris Attitude Attribution Paradigm

Imagine it is the 1960s. The Cuban missile crisis has brought John F. Kennedy and the United States to the brink of war with the Communist world. Martin Luther King, Jr., is leading nonviolent civil disobedience rallies to change the civil rights laws of the land and bring an end to segregation. Now imagine you are a student at a fairly liberal college during this point in history. It is safe to bet that you expect the average person to be opposed to Castro's political regime in Cuba and opposed to segregationist policies and open racism in the United States. How do you suppose you would react if you learned that a fellow student, Richard, is actually espousing exactly the opposite views— he is pro-Castro and anti-desegregation? According to correspondence inference theory, you should make powerful attributions to Richard, because his behavior is different from how you expect the average person to act (given the social norms at your liberal college). You should assume that he is *extremely* pro-Castro in his political attitudes and racist in his social attitudes.

Let's now throw one more wrinkle into this scenario. Suppose Richard, as it turns out, has been asked to espouse these deviant beliefs by a professor as part of an oral exercise that is required for a course. In this case, the attitudes expressed are no longer freely chosen, but have resulted from a pressure in the situation: If Richard wants to get a good grade, he must attempt to espouse pro-Castro and anti-desegregation beliefs in front of the class as part of the exercise. Now how do you suppose you would react? According to correspondent inference theory, as situational constraint increases, you should be less likely to attribute this set of beliefs to the person. Thus, since Richard has been forced to make the comments (situational constraint is high), you should assume that his beliefs are really no different from the average student's. This sounds like a logical way to test some of the basic tenets of correspondent inference theory. And this was precisely what Jones and Harris (1967) did.

In a now-classic experiment, Jones and Harris (1967) constructed essays that were either pro- or anti-Castro (or pro- or anti-desegregation). Research participants were asked to read an essay, believing either that the person who wrote it was free to write about any position he/she chose, or that the person was asked to write the essay as part of an assignment for a course (such as a final exam question asking the person to make the best possible argument for Castro's regime). The design of this experiment manipulated whether the person had a choice or not and whether a person did something expected or not. The logic of the experiment was that if the writers were not free to choose their actions, then the perceivers should not be forming correspondent inferences. The experiment also applied the idea (derived from the theory of correspondent inference) that the extent to which a correspondent inference is formed will depend on the extent to which the action is different from what one would expect: Correspondence should be high not only when perceived choice is high, but also when the prior probability of the act's occurring is low. For example, if you see a person speak in favor of free elections, and you know that everyone is in favor of free elections, you gain little information about the person from the behavior and should not be likely to make a correspondent inference. How the person differs from others is more informative of personality than how he/she agrees.

In summary, Jones and Harris (1967) asked research participants to read a short essay on Castro's Cuba that supposedly came from another student's political science test. Participants then recorded their estimates of the writer's true opinions on the subject. The essay was either pro- or anti-Castro, and was described as either being written under conditions of free choice or not. Half of the participants were told that the answer was a response to the instructor demanding a particular answer; the other half were told that the answer was written freely. This manipulated the two variables of interest—freedom of choice and normativeness of the behavior. (Recall that in 1965, when this study was conducted, it was highly expected that an essayist freely writing on the topic would be anti-Castro.) Finally, what was being measured was the "pro-Castroness" of the target person's true attitude. The expected and the actual results of this experiment are presented in Table 7.1.

The Importance of Freedom of Choice

It was expected that there should be more correspondent inference when there was choice. And the first finding that jumped out from the data collected was that, indeed, the scores in the choice condition were more extreme. When a pro-Castro essay was believed to be freely written, the person was seen as extremely pro-Castro (59.62), and when an anti-Castro essay was believed to be freely written, the person was seen as

TABLE 7.1. Actual and Expected Results from Jones and Harris's Attitude Attribution Experiment

| | Expected results | | | Actual results | |
| | Essay direction | | | Essay direction | |
	Pro-Castro	Anti-Castro		Pro-Castro	Anti-Castro
Choice	60.00	15.00	Choice	59.62	17.38
No choice	20.00	20.00	No choice	44.10	22.87

Note. Attributed attitude scores ranged from 10 to 70; higher numbers indicated a stronger pro-Castro attitude. From Jones and Harris (1967, Table 1). Copyright 1967 by Elsevier. Adapted by permission.

extremely anti-Castro (17.38). Each response was more extreme than the responses provided by participants who believed the essayist was constrained in what he was to write.

The Importance of the Direction of the Essay, Regardless of Choice

The second finding that jumped out was that the direction of the essay played a huge role, regardless of choice. If the person supported Castro in the essay, participants assumed the person to be pro-Castro. If the person was anti-Castro in the essay, participants assumed the person to be anti-Castro in his/her true attitude. (Thus even the expected position—being anti-Castro—was leading to correspondent inference. Although this seemingly went against the theory, it was also true that because of the political climate at the time, students should have assumed the average person to be anti-Castro.) The clearest test of the model came when people read an essay espousing the unexpected, pro-Castro position. In this case, the essayist was seen as truly holding this opinion and being a Castro supporter.

The Surprising Emergence of Correspondent Inference under Situational Constraint

The theory would predict no effect for essay direction in the no-choice condition. If a person was forced to write an essay, then the perceivers' impression of that person's true attitude should not be influenced by what that person said, because he/she was forced to say it! If a person was forced to say something, the perceivers should just assume that person's true attitude to be the same as everyone else's—if everyone hated Castro, this person should hate Castro too (regardless of what his/her essay might say). Thus the main hypothesis was that the effect of the type of speech given (pro- or anti-Castro) should emerge only in the choice condition (people should only assume that a person was really pro-Castro if he/she freely chose to espouse such beliefs). *This was not found.* Participants rated the essayist's true attitude as corresponding to the essay, regardless of whether there was choice. That is, participants should have adjusted their ratings of the person's true attitudes to account for the fact that he/she was *forced* to write a pro-Castro essay. But they did not. They failed to consider the situation.

Now this is a bit of an overstatement. People were paying *some* attention to the situation. This was hard to see in the anti-Castro condition, because everyone expected the person to be anti-Castro to start with, so forcing him/her to write an essay on this topic should not have affected what participants thought of him/her too much. However, we see from Table 7.1 that it did. Participants were making less extreme judgments (22.87 vs. 17.38), indicating that they were sensitive to the fact that there was some pressure on the person. But still, it is hard to draw conclusions from looking at these cells, since (again) we would expect people at that time to have been anti-Castro. The informative condition about how people handled situational information would be when the essayist was expected to be anti-Castro, but forced to be pro-Castro. People did not seem to take this situation appropriately into account. They took it into account partially, since the score assigned to the essayist's true attitude was markedly lower (44.10) than when the essayist freely chose to write (59.62). But they did not give the situation enough appreciation, and they overattributed, as indicated by how far this rating (44.10) deviated from what the model would have predicted (20; this would have indicated that this person was just like all other people in being anti-Castro, and the only reason the person's essay did not reflect this was that he/she was simply answering an exam question).

Perhaps this finding should not have come as a surprise. Despite the quote from Ichheiser (1943) on the power of situations at the start of this chpater, Ichheiser also believed that people often fail to see the power of situations, while often enhancing the power of disposition:

> [We] interpret in our everyday life the behavior of individuals in terms of specific personal qualities rather than in terms of specific situations. Our whole framework of concepts of "merit" and "blame," "success" and "failure," "responsibility" and "irresponsibility," as accepted in everyday life, is based on the presupposition of personal determination of behavior. (p. 151)

Writing at about the same time, Heider (1944, p. 361) made a similar point regarding a tendency to ascribe changes that occur in the environment to the persons who are in that environment, despite the fact that such changes are often caused by other factors in the environment (either instead of or in concert with factors related to persons): "Changes in the environment are almost always caused by acts of persons in combination with other factors. The tendency exists to ascribe the changes entirely to persons." Heider (1958, p. 79) later reiterated this fundamental belief: "It is an important principle of common-sense psychology . . . that man grasps reality, and can predict and control it, by referring transient and variable behavior and events to relatively unchanging underlying conditions, the so-called dispositional properties of his world."

Our behavior, even if clearly not freely chosen, is believed to be a reflection of our true attitudes and personality. One can imagine (and researchers have already illustrated) the implication this finding has for larger social issues. Consider the implications when a police officer illegally obtains a confession through beating or pressuring a suspect. Please quickly dispel any notion that innocent people never confess to crimes they did not commit. This occurs not merely when people are physically threatened (which Miranda rights ideally prevent). Kassin and Kiechel (1996) found that people can be convinced by authorities that they have committed crimes (when they have not), especially when a defendant's memory for the event is vague and the authorities lie (such as by presenting false evidence). Once the person has been forced to admit to the behavior (via such tactics as misinformation and deprivation of food, sleep, lawyers, etc.), it will now be difficult for a jury to disregard the confession—even when jurors learn that a confession was not freely given (Kassin & Sukel, 1997).

Is Correspondence Bias an Artifact of the Methodology?

Jones (1979) reviewed several criticisms of the attitude attribution paradigm that raise the issue of whether the bias to see disposition as the cause of behavior is indeed something fundamental about how people interpret social behavior, or is instead an artifact of the way scientists have attempted to study this question. Given the implications for social perception, especially as it applies to how the legal system operates, it is important to eliminate doubts regarding the validity and reliability of the findings.

A first, logical criticism of the "Castro" studies is that the research participants were being implicitly told by the experimenter to make correspondent inferences. That is, norms of communication and interaction (Grice, 1975) dictate that people (especially scientists at a university) do not typically provide other people (especially students) with totally irrelevant information. Therefore, if research participants were given an essay to read by an authority figure, were told that it was constructed by a student, and were informed that the task was to determine how well it reflected the true attitude of that student, the implicit communication norm at work would be that the information being provided was probably useful as an indicator of the person's true attitude. If not, the experimenters would not have provided this information (Wright & Wells, 1988).

Another potential artifact concerns the essays themselves. Perhaps the experimenters constructed the essay in such a way as to suggest that the person writing it was truly an expert at these matters. The research participants may have thought, "Who else but an advocate of Castro could construct such clear and expert arguments in favor of his regime?" Thus perhaps the excellence of the essay itself served as an implicit clue to research participants, signaling to them the true attitude of the essay writer as being sympathetic with and corresponding to the position being described (even if the writer was forced to write the essay). Finally, Kelley (1972a) suggested that the research participants may have perceived the so-called "no-choice" condition actually to be one where the essayist had plenty of choice. In Kelley's words, "context factors have not been manipulated as strongly or clearly as has the behavior itself" (p. 18). One approach to dispelling such artifactual explanations for the data would be to run further studies using the attitude attribution paradigm that attempt to control for and address each of these potential methodological flaws. And such work was done. However, rather than review such efforts here, let us turn instead to another approach that addresses this issue—one of convergent validity. That is, can the same basic premise be illustrated with a totally different research design? If the correspondence bias emerges in other contexts, we may begin to conclude that this bias is as real, as robust, and perhaps as fundamental as Ross (1977) described it to be.

The Ross, Amabile, and Steinmetz Quiz Show Paradigm

A primary hypothesis of correspondent inference theory is that as situational constraint increases, people make fewer correspondent inferences. In the attitude attribution procedure, this was tested by manipulating whether people had choice or not. Another type of constraint that limits how people act is the social roles they are asked to play. Consider the roles that teachers and students play. Teachers enjoy the unique advantage of choosing what they will talk about in class and ignoring what they are less confident about. Because of this, their role allows them to appear more intelligent than perhaps they are. A teacher seems to be wiser and to possess vastly more knowledge on a topic than a student does. However, the teacher role also often limits the actions of someone who possesses vast knowledge on a topic. He/she may be forced to ignore the complexities of an issue in order to present it clearly in an undergraduate course, or forced to present material he/she disagrees with because it is a leading theory that students should be taught (yet cannot be critiqued appropriately when the teacher has only 45 minutes to cover a topic). In many ways, this social role dictates what the teacher is able to do, thus constraining behavior.

Ross, Amabile, and Steinmetz (1977) conducted an experiment that provided further support for correspondence bias and took advantage of this type of situational constraint. They manipulated the roles that targets played and observed whether research participants were able to adequately take into account the clear situational constraint imposed by these roles. Participants were asked to take part in a "quiz show." One participant was assigned to be a contestant in the quiz game. The perceiver (another participant) observed the behavior of the contestant as he/she attempted to answer difficult questions. The questions were written by yet another participant playing the role of the "quizmaster" (the person asking questions). Thus the three participants in any given session were randomly assigned to play the role of quizmaster, contestant, and observer, and the behavior of interest was the contestant attempting (and most likely failing) to answer questions. The issue at hand was this: Would the perceiver recognize that the questions in this context were difficult and would be almost impossible for anyone other than the person who composed the questions (and had the role of quizmaster) to answer, or would the perceiver instead assume that the contestant answering the questions (and assigned the disadvantaged role) was not too bright?

To make the test of this issue even more dramatic, the experiment was set up in such a way as to make it quite clear that the situation was one in which the contestant in the quiz show would have relatively little chance at getting the answers correct. The questions were composed by the person assigned to play the role of quizmaster, who was explicitly and clearly instructed to design questions that were in his/her idiosyncratic area of expertise. As a hypothetical example of this, imagine you arrive at an experiment and are asked to be a contestant in a game where some other person is going to ask you questions. Now imagine that this person is an expert on 1960s and 1970s pop/rock music, and is going to be quizzing you on your knowledge of this area by constructing questions to ask you from his/her vast knowledge base surrounding this material. You get questions such as these: At what age did Janis Ian learn "the truth"? Where might the Hollies lead you to expect to find a "long cool woman"? Who sang backup vocals on Lou Reed's "satellite of love"? According to Pete Townshend, where does "nothing ever go as planned"? What is it that Smokey Robinson said would be easy to trace (if you look closely)? From what state does the author of "Mary Queen of Arkansas" hail? Finally, what type of "blues" might one expect to be had by (1) Laura Nyro, (2) Bob Dylan, (3) John Lennon, and (4) Duane Allman and Eric Clapton? The answers are as follows: at 17, in a black dress, David Bowie, by the sea and sand, the tracks of my tears, New Jersey, and (1) wedding bell, (2) tombstone and/or just like Tom Thumb and/or Memphis, (3) yer, and (4) bell bottom. How did you do? Probably not too well. To what do you attribute your failure? It is likely that you see this as a case of being asked hard questions by an expert, and you would not conclude that you know little about pop/rock music of the 1960s and 1970s (or that you are dumb). Unfortunately, this is not the type of attribution formed by people observing your poor performance. The correspondence bias dictates that perceivers will attribute your poor performance not to the situational constraint, but to your own inadequacies.

This was precisely what Ross, Amabile, and Steinmetz (1977) found. Observers in their experiment did not adequately take into account the pressure of the situation when rating either the knowledge of the contestant or the questioner. They rated the person randomly assigned to the role of questioner as generally more knowledgeable than the person assigned to the role of contestant. More dramatically, the person unable to answer the questions specifically drawn from the idiosyncratic knowledge of another person was seen as generally less intelligent, despite the fact that it was clearly the situation that made the person unable to answer the questions. The correspondence bias thus emerged, again, in a totally different research paradigm. Since observers could have been assigned the role of questioner or contestant, they should have been able to imagine what it would be like to be in that role; remarkably, they did not make these considerations when evaluating others.

The Snyder and Frankel Sex Tape Paradigm

Imagine that as part of an exercise for a class, you were asked to discuss extremely private matters about your sex life with a complete stranger. Such an event would be likely to make you feel extremely anxious and nervous. If not, you are an exception to the rule; yet you would probably still be able to guess that if you were watching someone else in that situation, that person would be anxious and nervous. A situation of this type provided for Snyder and Frankel (1976) an excellent way to illustrate the correspondence bias, while controlling for the criticism that Kelley (1972a) had made against the attitude attribution paradigm. If it was the case that the behavioral manipulation in the Jones and Harris (1967) research (strength of the essay) was much stronger than the manipulation of the situation (whether the target was perceived as having free choice), in Snyder and Frankel's case (discussing one's sex life with a stranger) the situational manipulation was obviously stronger. Indeed, there was no behavioral manipulation. The anxiety-provoking situation might lead perceivers to assume that the person was anxious, even though the person did not look anxious. The only rational reason to infer that the person was anxious would be the situation. If perceivers then assumed that the person had an anxious disposition, this would represent a powerful illustration of the correspondence bias. In this instance, having made an inference strictly from the situation would lead perceivers to mistakenly assume that the traits of the person corresponded with the inference that the person must be anxious.

Snyder and Frankel (1976) asked male research participants to watch a videotape (without the sound) of a female target person being interviewed by a strange male. Some were led to think that the interview topic was somewhat bland and uninteresting. Other research participants were told that the woman was being asked to discuss her sex life. The assumption was that the sex tape would be seen as more anxiety-provoking, and that, despite the woman's showing no differences in how anxious she appeared from one tape to the next, the research participants would assume that her level of anxiousness as a person (her trait anxiety levels) would be higher when the topic concerned sex. Results revealed that rather than discounting trait anxiety as a cause for her feelings and behavior (given the power of the situation as a plausible alternate cause), participants instead made correspondent inferences to behaviors that were not observed, but merely implied by the situation. They assumed that the woman on the sex tape was more dispositionally anxious than the woman on the bland tape. Given these various forms of converging evidence, it seems safe to conclude that correspondence bias is a real phenomenon, not an artifact of the methods.

THE ACTOR–OBSERVER DIFFERENCE

Let's return to the example just discussed. To begin with, you were asked to imagine yourself being placed in a situation where you had to discuss your sex life with a stranger, in order to give you a sense of how anxiety-provoking that situation would be. We have then seen how perceivers in the Snyder and Frankel (1976) study reacted when they observed someone who was allegedly in that situation, with the remarkable finding that although they knew the situation was an anxiety-provoking one, they still believed that the person being observed was *dispositionally* anxious. But this example raises an interesting question: What if you were to observe yourself in this situation? Would you be as likely to infer traits (such as being an anxious person) illogically about yourself, based on observing yourself in a particular situation that was known to trigger feelings of anxiety? Although we all somehow exhibit a correspondence bias when examining the causes for the behavior of others, failing to adequately take into account the situation they are in, does a similar shortcoming appear in making inferences about ourselves? Similarly, if you were a contestant in the quiz show experiment, while observers might see you as "stupid" for getting the questions wrong, would you see yourself as stupid (a dispositional attribution), or would you see the questions as unusually hard (a situational attribution)? Jones and Nisbett (1971) illustrated what has come to be known as the *actor–observer difference*. Although as observers of others we have a tendency to underutilize information about the power of the situation and overutilize inferences about the disposition of others, such a bias does not occur when we observers become actors. When we are judging our own actions, correspondence bias disappears.

What is it that others see (when judging themselves) that we don't see (when judging them), even though we may be standing adjacent to them? The answer to this question is multiply determined. Most obvious is the fact that actors are able to "see" their own internal states; they have *self-knowledge and insight*. When judging others, we are forced to infer their intentions, goals, emotions, and so on from their observed behaviors. These behaviors are salient to us and are seen as inextricably linked to the actors. When we are judging ourselves, there is a host of information available to us that we are not privy to when judging others. We need not infer our motives from behavior; we can examine those motives directly. And if they do not provide a sufficient explanation for our behavior, we can seek an explanation elsewhere, in the situation.

Relatedly, *differences in consistency and distinctiveness information exist for actors and observers*. The observers cannot see how the actors behave in different situations with either the same or other entities. Causal data are extended over time and are not available to the observers. Actors' knowledge of their behavior in other situations and at other times should make them potentially excellent judges of the "covariation" between their behavior and the various possible situational and dispositional causes that drive their behavior. If they detect consistency over time, they can infer dispositional causes, and if they detect variability, they can infer situational causes more readily than observers (who don't have access to this information). Consider, as an example, how a person might react after short exposure to his/her family. In many families, it takes relatively little provocation for outbursts of temper and inexplicable (to observers) emotional displays to appear. What appears to an observer as a simple taunt or tease feels, to an actor, like the straw that broke the camel's back. The actor has a history with family members that contributes to his/her responses, and this history is not seen by an observer. Thus, the next time you visit the home of your seemingly rational friend and observe what appears to be an unprovoked meltdown after the friend interacts with his/her parents, consider the actor–observer difference and take into account the situation, as well as consistency and distinctiveness information.

This extra insight into the causes of actors' own behavior might be taken to mean that actors should be more accurate at judging the true causes for their behavior than they are at judging the behaviors of others. However, as we shall soon see, having truckloads of information about themselves available does not necessarily make actors accurate. People can draw on this wealth of information in biased ways, using their increased knowledge to support a particular explanation that they desire and to ward off explanations that are undesirable. From all this information, they can pick and choose among the various options and construct the world in a biased way that suits their needs. We shall return to this issue in the next chapter, when we discuss positive illusions, egocentric biases, and self-esteem motives in attribution.

A final difference between actors and observers concerns the *different aspects of the environment that are salient.* Jones and Nisbett (1971) noted that for actors and observers, different types of information are salient and have an impact on their interpretations of the reason a behavior has been performed. They are attending to different things. For actors, the situation is salient. They are not typically observing themselves when acting, but are focused outward on the environment. This means that if a person is interacting with you so that the person is the actor and you are the observer, the salient factors for the actor are (1) you, and (2) other forces in the situation that he/she is concerned with. The person sees both of these forces that emanate from the situation as powerful causes for his/her own behavior. Observers, in contrast, have actors' behavior as the focal stimulus. To invoke the Gestalt principle of figure and ground, behavior is figural; it is the focus of attention for observers. The situation in which the behavior occurs is ground. Thus actors and observers have divergent perspectives, with attention focused on different things. What is figural to one is ground to another.

We might expect that when the pressure on a person from the situation is excessively clear and obvious, correspondence bias would not be found. People may be bad at perspective taking, but they are not blind. If a criminal holds a gun to my head and I am asked to steal from the man next to me, surely I will not be perceived as the thief in this scenario. Remarkably, we have seen that even people shown blatant situational constraints still exhibit correspondence bias, partially because they hold a different perspective from the actors they are observing. But this fact also presents a possible solution to overcoming the correspondence bias. If actors and observers diverge in their perspective, perhaps getting observers to take the perspective of actors would eliminate the correspondence bias.

Perspective Taking

The previous discussion suggests that a key for removing the tendency to overattribute to disposition is to get observers to notice the situation in the same way an actor notices the situation. Thus, if people are asked to take the perspective of another person, the bias should disappear. As Heider (1958) asserted, successfully taking the perspective of other people is required for accurate attribution to result. If we accept Heider's basic assumption that the "psychological world of the other person" must be analyzed and considered for successful attribution to occur, this requires that as perceivers we must have the ability to consider the world of others. We must be able to stand in the shoes of others, see the world through their eyes, empathize with what they are feeling, and attempt to think and react to the world in the same way that they think and react to the world. Displacing ourselves from our egocentric view of the world and taking the perspective of others is an essential ingredient to accurate attribution. The ability to entertain the perspective of another has long been recognized as a critical ingredient in proper social functioning. Davis (1983) found that perspective taking was positively correlated with both social competence and self-esteem. Piaget (1932) marked the ability to shift perspectives as a major developmental breakthrough in cognitive functioning. Kohlberg (1976) recognized its importance in his classification of moral reasoning. Many empirical studies of perspective taking have focused on the emotional reactions of people who were asked to take the perspective of another individual who was in need. When an individual engages in perspective taking, he/she has an emotional experience that comes to resemble that of the target (e.g., Batson, 1991). Furthermore, this experience of empathy—the consideration of how another person is affected by his/her situation—leads the perspective taker to offer greater assistance to the target. Thus perspective taking can inspire altruism (Batson, 1991, 1998), and its absence can incite aggression (Richardson, Hammock, Smith, Gardner, & Signo, 1994).

However, just because people can take the perspective of others when asked to by an experimenter, this does not mean that perspective taking is something people do naturally. The existence of the correspondence bias suggests that perspective taking is difficult, perhaps not the default approach perceivers take to viewing the social world. Although accurate attribution may depend on it, the natural processes of how people form attributions in reality may not involve adequate perspective taking. But this does not mean that they are incapable of taking the perspective of others. And if it were to occur, what would such a shift in perspective reveal? What do people gain by taking perspective? What they gain is the ability to see that forces exist that might be determining an actor's behavior other than those forces emanating from within the actor (that person's disposition).

Perspective Taking and the Fundamental Attribution Error

An observer's failure to consider the power the situation plays in determining an actor's behavior would presumably be lessened if the observer took the perspective of the actor. This assumption regarding the role of perspective taking in attribution has been examined by both physically taking perspective and psychologically taking perspective. For example, Storms (1973) had observers physically alter their point of view so that they observed the very same physical stimuli that actors observed. Meanwhile, Regan and Totten (1975) asked research participants to psychologically take the perspective of actors (e.g., to imagine what it was like for them, or was like to be them). In each experiment the types of attributions participants formed were then assessed to see if the role of the situation increased (and overattribution to disposition decreased) when perspective taking was introduced.

Storms (1973) claimed that actors and observers have quite literally different points of view. Actors do not normally view their own behavior; observers, on the other hand, are watching the actors. Given these differences in point of view, and the assumption that the actor–observer bias is caused by such differences, Storms asserted that this hypothesis should logically follow: If behavior was videotaped so the observers saw it from the perspective of the actors and the actors watched themselves as if they were observers, the actor–observer difference should be reversed. Actors would make greater amounts of dispositional attributions for their own behavior (with their attention now focused on watching themselves), and observers would take the situation into account (with attention now shifted away from the actor and toward the situation the actor is in). The behavior in this experiment was a conversation between two target actors. Two observers watched the interaction, and each was instructed to observe one of the two actors/targets. Observer 1 watched Actor 1, Observer 2 watched Actor 2, Actor 1 was focused on Actor 2, and Actor 2 was focused on Actor 1. The interaction was videotaped with one camera on Actor 1 and one camera on Actor 2. Participants then watched the videotape of the interaction, and the experimenter manipulated the perspective they saw while watching. One group saw the same perspective they had in the live version of the interaction, so that Observer 1 watched Actor 1, Observer 2 watched

Actor 2, Actor 1 focused on Actor 2, and Actor 2 focused on Actor 1. Another group had the perspective reversed, so that Observer 1 now saw Actor 2 (who had previously served as the situation for Actor 1), and Actor 1 now saw him-/herself (rather than the situation, which he/she had been focused on originally). Similarly, Observer 2 now saw Actor 1 and Actor 2 now saw him-/herself (the method is illustrated in Figure 7.1).

Research participants were then asked to describe either their own behavior (if the participants were actors) or the behavior of the observed person (if they were observers) along several personality dimensions: friendliness, talkativeness, dominance, and nervousness. For each of these dimensions, they had to rate how much they thought each of the following dimensions influenced the behavior: personal characteristics (how important personality, traits, character, and attitudes were in causing the behavior) and characteristics of the situation (how important factors such as being in an experiment, the way the other participant behaved, and the topic of conversation were in causing the behavior).

First, what evidence was found for the original Jones and Nisbett (1971) hypothesis that actors are inclined to attribute to situations and observers to dispositions? Evidence for this was provided by the condition where the perspective of the subjects was the "typical" perspective of actors and observers (i.e., the tape was replayed from the same perspective). In this condition, actors attributed more to situational causes than did observers, supporting the Jones and Nisbett position. However, within each of those conditions, observers should have been attributing more to disposition than to situation, which they did. And actors should have been attributing more to situation than to disposition, but they did not (which, incidentally, was also true in the Ross, Amabile, &

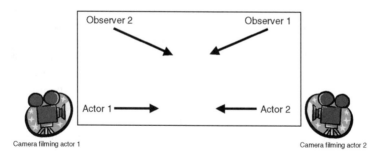

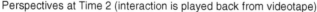

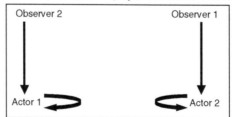

FIGURE 7.1. Perspectives taken in the two phases of the Storms (1973) experiment. Arrows indicate the direction in which attention is focused.

Steinmetz [1977] quiz show experiment). Thus actors attributed more to situation than observers did, but their judgments were not overly situational; they were an even mix of situation and disposition. In summary, this study makes the same general point that the one by Ross, Amabile, and Steinmetz made: Actors pay more attention to situation than observers (who fail to pay adequate attention to the situation), and give it at least equal weight in forming judgments about causality. But what happens when perspective taking occurs, so that actors take the perspective of observers and observers take the perspective of actors? Actors who now are focused on themselves should shift their attributions, so they become more dispositional and less situational. And this was what is found. It was also predicted that observers would become less dispositional and more situational in the types of attributions they form. This too was found: Taking perspective altered actor–observer effects.

Regan and Totten (1975) addressed this same point regarding the shifting of perspectives by focusing on the *psychological* shifting of perspectives. Research participants were not shown information from the perspective of another person; they were simply instructed to take the perspective of that person in some conditions of the experiment. Because people were explicitly asked to take the perspective of others, the dispositional explanations typically formed were turned into situational attributions. Perspective takers made the same attributions for the actors that they would have made had they themselves been the actors in that situation.

In summary, people are capable of taking the perspective of others when that perspective is physically presented to them and when they are explicitly instructed to take the perspective of others. Perspective taking then allows the perceivers to form a more complete and accurate attribution of the causes for behavior. However, the evidence also seems to suggest that although perspective taking is an important ingredient in forming accurate attributions, taking the perspective of others is not something perceivers do quite naturally or spontaneously. It might strike you as odd that even in a situation such as the quiz show paradigm, where the power of the situational force seems so obvious and clear, perspective taking appears not to occur, with the resulting negative consequences (the perceivers form an unwarranted negative, and dispositional, attribution). People still ignore the obvious fact that the quizmaster is making up questions based on his/her own knowledge base, and the contestant is completely at the mercy of being asked difficult questions about something at which the quizmaster is uniquely expert. This might simply suggest that perhaps more is contributing to the tendency to overattribute actors' behavior to their disposition than merely the perspective that perceivers take. This is in fact true, and the factors that contribute to such an overattribution are examined next.

THE CAUSES OF THE CORRESPONDENCE BIAS

1. Situations Lack Salience and Therefore Go Unnoticed by Perceivers

The seeming invisibility of the situation has been mentioned so many times at this point that listing it here seems redundant. Yet let us one last time consider Heider's (1958) influential statement: "[Behavior] has such salient properties [that] it tends to engulf the total field rather than be confined to its proper position as a local stimulus whose interpretation requires the additional data of a surrounding field—the situation in social perception" (p. 54). One implication of this statement might be to conclude that what is salient captures perceivers' attention, and what they attend to is what they assume is the dominant causal factor. An experiment by Taylor and Fiske (1975), reviewed in Chapter 1, illustrated the predominant causal role that a salient individual plays in shaping a perceiver's impressions. When a participant observing a conversation between two confederates was seated facing Confederate 1, that confederate was rated as the more dominant individual—as having set the tone and direction of the conversation. A shift in the perspective of the observer produced totally different findings. When a participant was seated facing Confederate 2, the dominant individual, seen as the cause for what transpired in the interaction, now became Confederate 2. Why would it be that if perceivers attend to a person, they assume that this person's disposition is what causes the effect? According to Gilbert and Malone (1995, p. 30),

> In classical attribution terms, behavior is an effect to be explained, and dispositions and situations are two possible causes of that effect. Why, then, should the salience of the effect facilitate attribution to one of those causes? It is not, after all, the person's dispositions that are salient, but the person's behavior. Indeed, in no other case would reasonable people argue that the salience of an effect 'explains' its attribution: If a physical symptom such as vomiting were particularly salient, this would not explain why physicians attribute that symptom to a virus rather than to a bacterium.

It is not attention to salient behavior per se that causes the correspondence bias. It is the fact that once perceivers have attended to a salient behavior, the role of the situation in causing that behavior goes relatively unnoticed. The explanation offered by Heider (1944) for the fact that the situation seems invisible was that actors and their actions form perceptual units. There is a tendency for perceivers to infer causality by assuming that the cause for a behavior and its consequences lies within the person the behavior is paired with in a perceptual unit: "Origin and the change which occurs to an origin form a unit—the change is seen as belonging to the origin . . . causal effects often play the role of data through which we infer properties of the origin" (Heider, 1944, pp. 358–359). The strength of this perceptual unit, and the relatively complete type of explanation it provides, displace the situation to the perceptual and causal background, where it goes largely unseen. As Heider (1944, p. 361) stated, "Persons, as absolute causal origins, transform irreversible changes into reversible ones. . . . The person can represent the disturbing change in its entirety." But the situation may be more than not figural. Often the situation is not physical, observable, or concrete—literally not seen. One cannot see social pressure. When one person shocked another in the famous Milgram (1963) experiment, observers could not see the pressure the person was feeling from the experimenter. When the Jones and Harris (1967) participants did not realize that a person was forced to write a pro-Castro essay, they assumed that the essay reflected the underlying beliefs of the writer. Situations are often invisible.

2. Underestimating the Impact of the Situation

We have just seen that to avoid the correspondence bias, perceivers must realize that a situation is playing a causal role, and to realize this they must first notice the situation. Yet perceivers may notice the situation and still exhibit correspondence bias, because they have underestimated the role that the situation plays in shaping behavior. There are two distinct ways in which this may occur.

Lacking Awareness of Situational Constraints

The first way in which the situation's impact may be underestimated may occur when a perceiver sees that some situational force covaries with the behavior; yet the perceiver, despite seeing the situation the target actor is in, does not perceive (is not aware) that this situation constrains the individual's freedom to act in any particular way. This is potentially what causes the correspondence bias in the quiz show paradigm. The roles as assigned by the experimenter give a clear advantage to the quizmaster: He/she must know the answers to the questions, since he/she wrote them (the contestant probably will not, since they are specific to a unique area of the quizmaster's expertise). Observers clearly see the situation the contestant is placed in. Where they fail is in their appreciation of the fact that this situation (people being asked to play the roles of contestant and quizmaster) constrains both people in powerful ways. Despite seeing the situation, they cannot see the forces of constraint that this situation (the role playing) is exerting.

Unrealistic Expectations for Behavior

According to Gilbert and Malone (1995), a second manner in which a perceiver may underestimate the role of the situation occurs when the situation is underutilized because the perceiver has an exaggerated sense of how powerful the behavior is and how resistant it would be to the situational force. In this case the situation is not seen as strong enough to deter the behavior, because the behavior is seen as not open to such influences (even though the perceiver has accurately noticed and considered the constraints due to the situation). Thus, if the situation is not perceived as strong enough, and the behavior occurs, it must be caused because the actor desired it to. For example, let us again consider the classic studies of obedience by Milgram (1963). Research participants were asked to administer shocks to another research participant whenever the other answered a question wrong (in reality, no shocks were delivered, but the research participants believed they were). Observers of this situation may have noticed the presence of the experimenter and heard the experimenter saying to the person administering the shocks, "You must proceed." Despite recognizing that the experimenter controlled the freedom of the research participant to some degree, and that the person was being pressured to proceed by an authority, the perceivers may not have expected behavior to be influenced by this situational force. The expectation for behavior would be that people should never shock others and that only extreme pressure from another should ever lead someone to act that way. And the situational pressure the perceivers observed may have led them to conclude that it was insufficient to lead people to shock others. As the experiments by Milgram revealed, such pressure actually is sufficient to get people to act in ways that most people would label as "monstrous." Therefore, perceivers in such cases exaggerate the behavior and its ability to overcome what they perceive to be a situational constraint. We have seen a similar possibility for such an explanation of the Jones and Harris (1967) experiment. Perceivers may have assumed that essayists had some choice—if told to write a pro-Castro essay, they could have refused. If not, they could have at least not have been so enthusiastic or seemingly expert in their position. Thus, even if the situation is not invisible, perceivers may unrealistically expect behavior to be somewhat free of situational constraints and may underestimate its impact on a person. Jones (1979, p. 112) referred to this possible cause of the bias as *underestimated constraints*.

3. Differential Memory Decay for Pallid versus Salient Events

The discussion thus far has been about the invisibility of, and the underestimation of, the situation. But is it possible that situations are retrospectively invisible? Perhaps even when the situation is salient "online" (when information is being received), it becomes relatively less salient as time passes. Thus correspondence bias would be caused by forgetting (as opposed to not seeing) the situation. This is a type of "sleeper effect." The advantage of using disposition to categorize and understand behavior may not be present as the behavior is encoded (especially if the situation is salient during encoding), but its advantage over situational explanations for the behavior increases over time, as the vivid and salient behavior stored in episodic memory has a stronger memory trace than the transient and pallid situation. This explanation for the bias would be particularly useful when people are explaining past behavior, as many times our judgments of others often occur after significant time has elapsed and people are asked to reflect on the others' behavior.

For example, consider how faculty members evaluate graduate students. Graduate students, like faculty members, are attempting to juggle their research interests along with their teaching assignments. However, some graduate students are released from the responsibility of teaching—usually not because of their own work, but because their research advisors have received grants for their (the advisors') research. This allows the students' stipend to be paid by the grants rather than through teaching a course. If some students focus only on their research (without the distractions of teaching), they have a clear advantage in how productive they are in this domain. And it is this domain that typically dictates how well they are evaluated by the faculty. Over the course of a semester, a faculty member may attribute a student's relative lack of research productivity to his/her teaching load (which may be very salient during the semester, especially if the student is helping the faculty member to teach a course). But months later, during the evaluation period, this situational constraint may have waned in its salience. As students are now evaluated side by side for research productivity (which often determines nominations for awards and the quality of letters of recommendation), students who worked for their money are now seen as less successful than those who were assigned (perhaps randomly) to be free of teaching. The power of the situation, though obvious at the time, may lose its power in the future.

4. The Situation Is the Person

Are people randomly assigned to the situations they are in, with their context truly being something distinct from themselves? In many cases, the situations we find people in are perfectly constructed by those people to suit their needs, wants, and disposition. Individuals' homes are likely to be very good extensions of who they are. I knew this intuitively at age 20 when I was looking for a flat in London for the summer. A quick examination of a room (the books, the record collection, the type of furniture, etc.) could tell me much about the person who constructed that situation and whether I would want to share that flat with him/her. People's occupations are other examples where situations may tell us much about disposition. Boxers have a hostile work environment, but would we want to adjust for the hostility of the situation when making a judgment about these persons, or is it safe to assume that people who choose to hit others for a living might construct the hostile situations in which they find themselves?

Such a connection between the disposition of the person and the situation is high-lighted by two lines of social-psychological work. Prentice (1987) examined the relation-ship between a person's possessions and the person's attitudes, disposition, and schemas. The basic conclusion was that the possessions an individual has acquired are consistent in their function for the individual. These possessions are not randomly acquired, but fill the person's context with objects that serve some of his/her underly-ing needs, wants, and beliefs. Prentice noted a similar consistency in the function of the person's attitudes. Attitudes, like material objects, are possessions (of the person's belief system) that serve some function for the individual. And these functions that atti-tudes serve are derived from the same internal source that dictates the possessions mak-ing up the individual's context. A person's possessions (at least the highly valued ones) are signposts for that person's functional and relational schemas. Such self-schemas drive cognition and action across a variety of domains, leading situation to be inextrica-bly linked to personality.

Gosling, Ko, Mannarelli, and Morris (2002) extended this work to making full-blown personality judgments from an examination of people's offices and bedrooms! Their research explicitly linked the individual, the context/environment occupied by the individual, and the impressions formed by observers of the context/environment that the target inhabited. Independent observers of the same social environment came to similar personality judgments of the person who constructed that environment. In one experiment, Gosling and colleagues brought perceivers to 94 offices in five office complexes around the United States (with the permission of the people using those offices) for the purpose of trying to form an impression of the people who inhabited each office, based on an examination of their office space. Each occupant of an office filled out personality scales, as well as nominating two peers who used the same scales to describe the office occupant. The personality ratings made by the target persons (and their peers) were then compared against those made by the people inspecting the office spaces. The two questions of interest were these: (1) How much consensus would there be among the observers, and (2) how accurate would those assessments be? Corre-lations among the ratings of the observers supported the prediction that there would be consensus on personality characteristics as inferred from the "look and feel" of the office. Thus people inferred personality from the rooms that targets inhabited and the possessions that filled them, and there was good consensus across observers. Were these inferences accurate? Yes. There were significant (and positive) correlations between the ratings of the observers (who had no direct contact with the people being judged) and the self/peer ratings. Observers relied on cues in the environment to allow them to develop (what were apparently fairly accurate) impressions of the persons who cluttered their room with the possessions that served as cues to the perceivers. John Steinbeck (1962) captured this idea nicely in the book *Travels with Charley*: "A human occupying a room for one night prints his character, his biography, his recent history, and sometimes his future plans and hopes. I further believe that personality seeps into walls and is slowly released."

Perhaps you are wondering whether this actually is a *bias*. If behavior does seem to correspond with disposition, and if people do construct environments to match their wants and needs, why label the tendency to recognize this a bias? A hippie is unlikely to choose to become a boxer, and an anarchist is unlikely to become a librarian. Indeed, Gilbert and Malone (1995) noted that correspondence bias is not an error when people choose their own situations—such as the person who chooses to become a boxer and the person who chooses to become a librarian. The situation in these examples should not be considered a causal factor. However, this tendency to see people as having caused or constructed their situations may be inappropriately generalized by perceivers to contexts where the individual did not have a hand in constructing the situational constraint. The very fact that situations are often constructed by people may actually be what leads perceivers to become overconfident in the assumption that a situation is just another extension of an individual. Thus, even when the situation should be considered a constraint on the individual, perceivers instead ignore it because it is seen as a construction of the individual. The messy room is seen as a sign of the irresponsible/inconsiderate person, rather than of the stress and time-consuming nature of the person's work that prevented him/her from straightening up.

5. Naive Realism and the False-Consensus Effect

Chapter 1 has discussed naive realism and illustrated one of its manifestations, the false-consensus effect: "[the] tendency to see one's own behavioral choices as relatively common and appropriate to existing circumstances while viewing alternative responses as uncommon, deviant, and inappropriate" (Ross, 1977, p. 188). As a side effect, false consensus can contribute to correspondence bias. If people overestimate the extent to which others agree with them, then they are likely to think that their own beliefs and actions have high consensus. Given this, according to correspondent inference theory, people will be less likely to make dispositional inferences regarding their own behavior. If, however, people observe another person who acts differently from the way they think they would, then they are more likely to think this behavior is unusual or deviant. That is, since they assume most people act as they would, and this person does not, this person's behavior has low consensus and the behavior must reflect something about his/her disposition. Thus the pattern of the actor–observer bias can be produced through a tendency to see false consensus.

6. Anchoring and Insufficient Adjustment

Jones (1979) proposed that correspondence bias might arise from a more global (i.e., not restricted to person perception) deviation from rational processing that was first described by Tversky and Kahneman (1974)–anchoring. *Anchoring* is a phenomenon in which a person's judgment on some task is biased by an initial estimate. When two individuals have different starting points in a judgment task (perhaps because the instructions to each person suggest slightly different points at which work on the problem is initiated), they produce different final estimates, with final judgments biased toward the initial values. Two examples will illustrate the concept of anchoring, at which point we shift toward applying this concept to person perception.

Tversky and Kahneman (1974) provided a classic illustration of the anchoring effect. People were asked to guess how many countries from the African continent were represented in the United Nations—a question to which participants presumably did not know the answer, and which was ambiguous enough that just about any reasonable estimate would be believable. The anchoring manipulation was simple. Prior to guessing the number, people observed the experimenter spin a wheel with numbers on it. People were to estimate whether the number of countries was higher or lower than the number on the wheel, and then provide the estimate. Participants whose spin of the wheel yielded the number 10 reported a substantially lower number of African countries in the United Nations, relative to people who started with the number 65 as an anchor.

Simple judgments of a concrete event were thus altered by trivial, randomly assigned, and irrelevant numbers!

A second example provided by Tversky and Kahneman (1974) came from a different type of task. Research participants were asked to multiply a string of numbers in 5 seconds. The task could not be completed, and the logic of the experiment was that the initial computations would serve as an anchor on which the final judgment was based. The trick was that exactly the same numbers were being multiplied by two groups of participants. What changed was the sequence in which they were presented. The median response of people who saw the string $8 \times 7 \times 6 \times 5 \times 4 \times 3 \times 2 \times 1$ was 2,250; the median response of people who saw $1 \times 2 \times 3 \times 4 \times 5 \times 6 \times 7 \times 8$ was 512. Both these studies illustrate how an initial reference point serves as an anchor against which insufficient adjustments occur.

Applying this concept to person perception, Jones (1979) proposed that if making an inference about a person's disposition and traits is the most available, immediate, or viable hypothesis initially offered to account for the person's behavior, then such a trait inference will act as a starting point, or anchor, which then guides subsequent judgment (see also Park, 1989). Furthermore, corrective inferential work may follow such inferences (meaning that the initial inference is known not to be a final attribution and needs to be adjusted to produce a complete attribution). However, rather than perceivers' starting out at some neutral point and subsequently evaluating causality, they start out with an initial assumption about the person's disposition and attempt to correct or adjust this inference. And as Jones (1979, p. 115; emphasis in original) asserted, "*insufficient adjustment* is a common error in the processing of sequentially presented information." In essence, social perception is vague enough that it is impossible to invalidate a first impression. The work of Asch (1946), reviewed in Chapter 1, where the traits "warm" and "cold" altered the meaning of an entire list of traits, could be seen as another illustration of this point. A first impression can survive to shape final judgments, since it is hard to prove such impressions wrong once they are formed.

7. Cognitive "Busyness" Yields Incomplete Corrections of Dispositional Inference

In the anchoring-and-adjustment explanation of correspondence bias, people notice the situation and are aware it might be constraining behavior, but fail to accurately adjust their initial, dispositional impressions for the impact of the situation. There is a distinction between failing to use the situation because they do not notice it and failing to use the situation even when they notice it and think it might be important. Why would people fail to (or at least insufficiently) use the situation under such circumstances? They may fail to adjust for the role the situation plays in determining behavior because they are unable to do so. Chapter 5 has discussed several reasons why attempts to "correct" first impressions may not occur. One of these is the fact that people lack an adequate theory of the direction and force of the bias that they are correcting for (and this is the logic of the anchoring-and-adjustment explanation of correspondence bias). However, another is that people lack the mental energy or ability to engage in the correction process; correction is effortful, and they may lack the strength of mind to engage in that effort.

Making an adjustment to an initial inference requires people to consider information that is not so salient, and then to engage in either discounting or augmenting of their initial impressions to account for this information. According to Gilbert (1989), this requires mental energy and cognitive effort, and people often simply lack the cognitive resources—the mental capability—to exert the effort needed to adjust and correct an initial inference. The distinction between this explanation of correspondence bias and the anchoring-and-adjustment hypothesis is one of process. In this explanation, people are unable to engage in the correction processes due to the processing resources such processing requires. The anchoring explanation could presumably hold true even if people have the capacity to engage in correction. This explanation draws from the logic of dual-process (and correction) models reviewed in Chapter 5. In this model, trait inference is "automatic" (e.g., Uleman & Moskowitz, 1994), while adjustment is effortful (see Figure 7.2):

> The social inference process seems to be a chain of sequential subprocesses: *Characterization* (or dispositional inference) is followed by *correction* (or situational adjustment) . . . characterization is a relatively automatic process that requires little effort or attention, whereas correction is a deliberate form of conscious reasoning that happens slowly and effortfully . . . when we see others act, we draw dispositional inferences from their actions—even if we 'know' that these actions are coerced and therefore inappropriate grounds for such inferences. And perhaps it is only after we have drawn these erroneous, but effortless, inferences of disposition that we are afforded an opportunity to correct them through the labor of reason. (Gilbert, 1989, pp. 193–194; emphasis in original).

Thus, if correction processes can occur (people are not experiencing cognitive load), the situation will be considered. However, if correction processes cannot occur (they are disabled by making people cognitively busy), correspondent inference should result (Gilbert, 1989). For example, Gilbert, Pelham, and Krull (1988) tested the idea that the correction stage, where more complex attributional reasoning supposedly comes into play, requires more effortful processing, cognitive capacity, and mental energy in order to be carried out. Borrowing the Snyder and Frankel (1976) paradigm, they had participants watch videotapes of someone allegedly discussing either a series of anxiety-provoking topics, such as sexual fantasies, or a series of non-anxiety-producing topics, such as travel. Half the people were under cognitive load, and half were not cognitively busy, at the time they watched the tapes. One potential problem with this design is that the load might make people so distracted that they would not pay attention to the situational information. They might fail to correct because they could not—they might not even see the information they needed to use to do the correc-

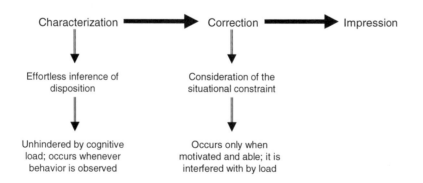

FIGURE 7.2. The Gilbert model of impression formation and correspondence bias.

tion (the fact that the topic was anxiety-provoking). To rule out this possibility, Gilbert and colleagues cleverly manipulated busyness by having participants memorize the discussion topics. So the very thing making them busy and preventing them from correcting was the information they should have been using to make the corrections that they were failing to make!

The videotapes had no sound and depicted a person shifting anxiously in her chair; the topic was displayed on the bottom of the screen. The task was to rate how much trait anxiety the person had (the extent to which she was dispositionally anxious). The prediction was that since all participants observed a person acting anxiously, they should all form effortless trait inferences characterizing the person as anxious. However, the topics should inform people about the reason the person was acting anxiously, and they should correct for this or adjust their initial inference. Participants who thought that the discussion was anxiety-provoking should use the discounting rule and correct the initial inference and not see the person as anxious. Those who thought that the discussion was non-anxiety-provoking should augment and correct their initial inference by really seeing the person as anxious. However, participants who were "cognitively busy" should not be able to perform the correction and should rely on their initial judgment and display a correspondent inference. As Table 7.2 reveals, participants failed to adjust their impressions to account for the situation if they were experiencing a state of cognitive load, even if the cognitive load was the act of thinking about the situation!

8. Prior Information and Context Lead to Inflated Categorizations of Behavior

A perceiver may notice the situation, correctly estimate it to have an influence (to constrain behavior), and be both motivated *and able* to engage in correction processes—and still the correspondence bias may emerge! This can occur because noticing the situation can lead to the paradoxical effect of creating expectancies that then alter the manner in which a person is perceived, inflating the extent to which the person is seen as causal. Why would focusing on the situation actually lead to overweighing a person's personality (rather than, if anything, overweighing the situation)? We will address this question in a moment, but first recall that we have already seen evidence of this fact in the research of Snyder and Frankel (1976). Their participants saw a mildly anxious woman who (they were told) was in the process of discussing extremely anxiety-provoking topics. Even though the woman did not act extremely anxiously, the situation she was in led people to expect that she must have been anxious. Thus noticing the situ-

TABLE 7.2. The Impact of Cognitive Busyness on Correspondent Inferences

	Load	No load
Nonanxious topic	9.3	10.3
Anxious topic	9.0	7.8

Note. Higher scores indicated greater dispositional anxiety ratings on a 13-point scale. Data from Gilbert, Pelham, and Krull (1988).

ation led perceivers to assume that her behavior and emotions were consistent with that situation, even though the woman had not exhibited any signs of this. Once a person acts (even mildly) anxious in a situation that is terribly nerve-wracking, a perceiver, due to the force of the situation, will exaggerate the force of the behavior exhibited and assume that it reflects the power of the situation. The person, despite acting only mildly anxious, will be categorized as being neurotic and a nervous wreck; who wouldn't be in that situation? Trope (1986a) posited that noticing the situation leads a perceiver to assume that behaviors and emotions exhibited within that situation are prepotent, to exaggerate the force of such factors, and thus to develop an inflated sense of what the person is truly feeling and thinking. This leads to an unwarranted dispositional attribution and the fundamental attribution error.

Trope's (1986a) model (see Figure 7.3) begins with a stage of *behavioral categorization* produced through a process of *identification*. This is essentially equivalent to what Gilbert (1989) has called categorization. This is where the perceiver observes behavior and arrives at a label for what sort of behavior is observed; the perceiver characterizes the person's actions, and in so doing establishes an identity for the behavior, or a category into which the behavior fits. For example, suppose you observe a person with tears in his/her eyes, softly sobbing. Before a second has passed, you are likely to have labeled this behavior and made some type of inference about the person. The behavior has been identified (or characterized/categorized). As Gilbert does, Trope assumes that this identification process is capable of occurring preconsciously and spontaneously—it happens within a second and without much (if any) conscious thought. Unlike Gilbert's model, Trope's model specifies what sort of factors determine the initial categorization. This model describes three *types of influences on identification*: the behavior you have observed (crying); the situation in which that behavior occurs (is the person at a funeral or a surprise party in his/her honor?); and prior information (e.g., stereotypes about the groups the person belongs to, and expectancies built-up through past interactions

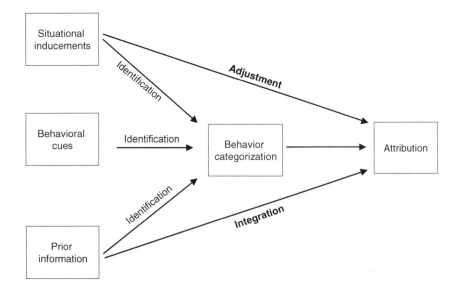

FIGURE 7.3. Trope's (1986a) model of impression formation and attribution. From Trope and Liberman (1993). Copyright 1993 by Sage Publications. Adapted by permission.

with the person). Thus your past knowledge of the person (prior information in the model) will help you make sense of the behavior. Is this someone who is known to cry at the drop of a hat, or someone who is typically stoic and staid? Does your stereotype of this person's gender or ethnicity inform you that people from this group are emotional, or that they are emotionally aloof and inexpressive? This past knowledge is used immediately and without your conscious intent to deploy it, allowing you to label and characterize the behavior. If you know that the person is prone to stoicism, you would label the behavior as tears of extreme sadness. If your stereotypes tell you that people from this group (e.g., men) rarely cry, you might label the behavior as reflecting quite extreme sadness.

Similarly, the context/situation is used in the early moments of interpersonal perception and interaction to help you identify a behavior and make inferences about the character of the person performing that behavior. For example, if the target person is mildly crying, this behavior is ambiguous regarding the person's mental state. People may cry from either joy or grief, and knowledge of this person's situation is used by the perceiver, without conscious intent to engage in such an analysis, to help the perceiver *disambiguate* or identify the behavior. In our example, if the person is at a funeral, you will label the behavior and the person as reflecting sadness. If the person is at a surprise birthday party, you will label the person as happy. Obviously, the way you identify the person's behavior will have an impact on how you treat and react to him/her. If the person is sad, you might console him/her; if the person is happy, you might offer him/her some cake. Without knowing the situation or context in which the behavior occurs, you would be unable to understand the behavior or the person.

To illustrate how context can disambiguate behavior, Trope (1986a) showed research participants faces of people who were displaying real emotions; however, the emotions were ambiguous—for example, they could be interpreted as angry or happy. Participants were then asked to rate the emotions being felt by the person displayed in each picture. An example is provided in Figure 7.4. Is the person happy or sad? This was precisely what research participants were asked to decide. Half of them rated the person as extremely happy, while the other half rated him extremely angry. Why the difference? The half who rated the person angry were told that this was a coach whose team was losing a game (imagine that a bad call had just been made that eliminated his team from the National Collegiate Athletic Association [NCAA] basketball tournament). The half who rated the person as happy were told that this was a coach whose team was winning a game (imagine his team had just won that same tournament). In

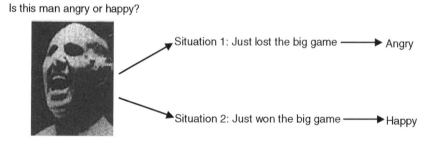

FIGURE 7.4. Situation/context disambiguates behavioral cues and allows for categorization.

see how context was used to identify and make sense of a person's behavior and psychological state, allowing the participants to disambiguate the behavior and categorize the person.

Naturally, perceivers' impressions of other people are not fully formed at the moment the perceivers have categorized them. They can think more deeply about them and alter the initial impressions and snap judgments that are yielded by the original behavioral categorization. Trope's model describes a subsequent, more effortful and deliberate stage of impression formation, where the initial inference is adjusted, modified, and updated to yield a final impression of a person—an attribution for the cause of his/her behavior. In the model, the impact of prior information (expectancies and stereotypes) and of the context in which the behavior has occurred (situational inducements) is felt at *two very distinct points in the judgment process*: first during behavioral categorization, and then again when initial characterizations are being altered and adjusted to form a final impression. Prior knowledge is added to the impression in a process labeled *integration*—a process whereby the conclusions of the initial judgment are bolstered by the prior information. If you have concluded that the person in our earlier example is sad because the person is a man, and you know that men generally don't cry, the further contemplation of the fact that men usually do not cry will only serve to enhance the initial attribution. This man is not only engaging in sad behavior; he must truly be a sad man for him to be crying in sadness. You would infer that only a man dispositionally capable of real grief would sob openly. The prior information is integrated into the final judgment in a way that augments the initial categorization.

However, the model describes an opposing role for the situation at this stage. Rather than augmenting a dispositional attribution, the situation, if considered at this point, leads to discounting of the person's disposition as the cause for the behavior, allowing the impression to be adjusted for the impact of the situation. This man is not sad by disposition; he is at a funeral, and funerals make even men cry. The initial dispositional inference is corrected (adjusted), so consideration of the situation amounts to a subtraction of dispositional forces from being seen as causal. In sum, knowledge of the situation can help you to adjust your impressions of the person accordingly. Once you have concluded that the person is acting sad at Stage 1, the function of Stage 2 is to test hypotheses about the personality of the person. Is he a sad person? The situation is then used here to remind you to adjust the categorization that this person is sad to include the fact that his situation calls for him to be sad.

The final question we must now consider is the one of central concern to this chapter: Why does this model of attribution predict that a fundamental attribution error will emerge where people are unable to adjust their impressions adequately to account for the situation? The logic is that when people use the situation to help them identify the behavior, this can lead them to form an exaggerated sense of how well the behavior illustrates a particular internal disposition. Consider another example: A perceiver observes a football player being mercilessly teased and insulted by his opponent. This intense provocation creates a context in which the perceiver believes the football player must be angry, frustrated, insulted, and hurt. The perceiver expects that in a situation such as this, where a man is insulted, he is likely to lash out in anger. The football player does react, but his behavior is perhaps typical of what the sport calls for: He tackles the opposing player in what might not otherwise be seen as an unusual use of force. However, the context in which the behavior occurs is now more than a football game; it is a context where the player is insulted, angry, and frustrated. Thus the behavior, which is actually a moderate and typical form of football aggression, is not seen as such, but is interpreted as an act of hostility—a severe form of aggression, a retaliation for the insult that the context has created. Trope and Liberman (1993, p. 554) have stated: "[The fact] that a target is aggressive or knowledge of situational provocation (being teased or insulted) may activate the person–situation model for aggression, which may specify a high probability of an aggressive response under such circumstances. This expectancy may lead the target's reaction to be inadvertently identified as aggressive, even when it is not." This exaggerated categorization—one in which the situation actually results in labeling the behavior as having more of a particular trait—is illustrated by the sunburst in Figure 7.5A.

If a perceiver knows a person is in a situation where he/she is being hurt, this knowledge of the situation affects the interpretation of the person's behavior. The person's response of pushing or yelling back may be labeled as highly aggressive behavior, as in the case of the football player above. The situation has led the perceiver to exaggerate the initial categorization. Even when provided with an expectancy that the situation will powerfully constrain and dictate behavior, the perceiver will, ironically, use such situational inducements to augment inferences that identify the behavior as being caused by the person's disposition (e.g., Trope & Alfieri, 1997). However, as the model suggests, the perceiver is able to consider the situation more carefully and elaborately during subsequent stages of information processing. As illustrated in Figure 7.5B, the thick arrow at the top represents the perceiver's attempt to adjust his/her impression to account for the fact that the situation has called for hostility. Perhaps this is not a hostile person, just a situation that calls for hostility.

The individual engaging in this adjustment, however, may still wind up with an attribution that is overly dispositional. Generally the person is not aware that the initial judgment is already extremely exaggerated by the role the situation had played during the categorization stage of processing. Without being aware that the initial identification is augmented, the perceiver is left with a final judgment still weighted toward the side of a dispositional attribution. If the perceiver had accurately categorized the behavior as mildly aggressive, then the adjustment for the context would have produced a judgment that was not an overattribution. But because he/she has unknowingly augmented the degree to which the behavior is seen as aggressive (ironically, because of the detection of the situational inducement), the same amount of adjustment is no longer going to produce a judgment that is evenly balanced. The fundamental attribution error will result, despite the perceiver's having the ability and motivation to correct for and adjust the initial impression for the force of the situational inducement.

This review highlights a distinction between the theories of Gilbert (1989) and Trope (1986a). Trope claims that cognitive load is not needed to produce correspondence bias. Even when a perceiver is perfectly aware of the situation and able to correct for it, the bias can persist. Trope's explanation has to do with the manner in which stages of information processing interact. Even if a person later tries to adjust a judgment for the fact the situation has constrained behavior, the initial inference/anchor is made more dispositional by the force of the situation. The situation gets added to an impression early on (without the perceiver's knowing it), in a manner that augments disposition as cause. Although there is an adequate adjustment for the role the situation may have played after the perceiver has identified the behavior, there is an underadjustment for the role the situation has played in the act of labeling the behavior. Correspondence bias results because context influences attributions at multiple stages.

A. Exaggerated behavior categorization results from considering the situation.

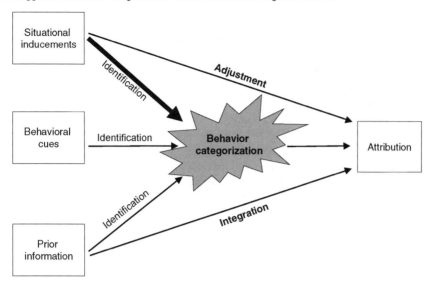

B. Insufficient adjustment results from failure to account for exaggerated categorization.

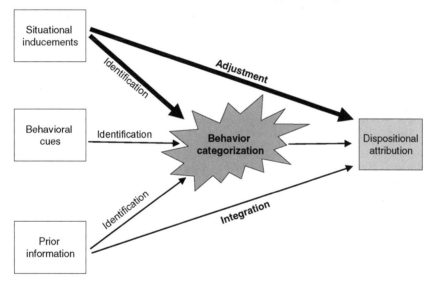

FIGURE 7.5. Fundamental attribution error and the Trope model of impression formation. From Trope and Liberman (1993). Copyright 1993 by Sage Publications. Adapted by permission.

SPONTANEOUS TRAIT INFERENCES

The viability of the anchoring-and-adjustment process as an explanation for correspondence bias, as well as the viability of the processing models of Gilbert (1989) and Trope (1986a), hinges on an important assumption—that a person's most available and immediate hypothesis initially offered to account for an observed behavior (a so-called "snap judgment") is one that suggests *traits* as the cause of that behavior. Each of these explanations for correspondence bias critically relies on a notion that has been dubbed *spontaneous trait inferences* (STIs; Moskowitz & Uleman, 1987).

An STI is said to occur whenever attending to another person's behavior produces a trait inference *without the perceiver's being aware* that such an inference has been formed, and *in the absence of an explicit intention* to infer traits or form an impression (Uleman, Newman, & Moskowitz, 1996). For example, if you observed the person in front of you in the line at the grocery store inform the cashier that he/she had been given too much change, you may have inferred that the person was "honest" without realizing you were even attending to the interaction or forming an impression. Ambady and Rosenthal (1992) find that such short and isolated pieces of information about a person are powerful in impression formation, perhaps as powerful as longer exposure to a person. Winter and Uleman (1984) have proposed that it is possible to judge traits very quickly and accurately (though this may depend on the extent to which the behavioral evidence is infused with meaning; e.g., Heider, 1958; McArthur & Baron, 1983; Moskowitz & Roman, 1992). Indeed, the notion of STIs has been in the field of person perception since its inception:

> We look at a person and immediately a certain impression of his character forms itself in us. A glance, a few spoken words are sufficient to tell us a story about a highly complex matter. We know that such impressions form with remarkable rapidity and great ease. Subsequent observations may enrich or upset our first view, but we can no more prevent its rapid growth than we can avoid perceiving a given visual object or hearing a melody. (Asch, 1946, p. 258)

Although the STI idea was around for a long time, it was also ignored for a long time. Almost all work on attributional reasoning prior to the investigations of Winter and Uleman (1984) had treated impression formation as a process that was consciously intended and monitored. While steps in the process may have been considered to be outside of awareness, the attempt to form a trait inference was always presumed to be consciously intended by the perceiver. This raised an obvious question: Would dispositional inferences be formed at all if experimenters were not asking for them? For example, even Gilbert's (1989) model, which details an explicit role for effortless and unconscious inferences, falls prey to this assumption of conscious intent on the part of the perceiver. In each experiment investigating the model (e.g., Gilbert et al., 1988), the participants were asked to form an impression of a person, and what was found was that trait inferences were formed rather effortlessly, while consideration of situational constraint required mental energy. But would such inferences occur if a person did not have the mindset to form an impression in the first place? And how could researchers examine whether people are forming impressions of others without asking people whether they have formed an impression? Several clever methodologies have emerged (borrowing heavily from cognitive psychology) that allow us to answer this question.

Methods for Illustrating STIs

The Encoding Specificity Paradigm

The first method of investigating whether people form trait inferences spontaneously and implicitly (without being asked to do it or being aware of having done it) relied on the concept of *encoding specificity*, borrowed by Winter and Uleman (1984) from the cognitive psychologists Tulving and Thomson (1973). According to Tulving and Thomson, if two things are stored together in memory, they can serve as cues for each other so that one can be used to help a person remember the other. For example, if two words that are not semantically related—"chair" and "dog"—are paired together in a memory test (i.e., people are asked to memorize a list of pairs like this) then the two should be stored in memory together. If memory for the words is then tested, performance is better when people are provided with some clues or retrieval cues (relative to attempting free recall of the words).Words that are semantically related to the items being recalled should be effective cues (e.g., "table" to help people remember the word "chair"). However, words that have no relationship to the item being recalled, but paired with it earlier, should also be effective, perhaps even more effective because of this link forged between them in memory (e.g., "dog" to help remember the word "chair").

This suggests that if a trait inference was made at the time behavior was observed (when the information was encoded into memory), then that inference and the behavior should be stored together in memory. Rather than asking people whether they formed an inference or asking them to form an impression, researchers can simply test their memory for the behavior. Specifically, researchers want to see how the trait that was supposedly inferred functions as a retrieval cue. Does it help people to recall the behavior? Evidence for STIs is provided if these words operate successfully as retrieval cues. To examine this issue, Winter and Uleman (1984) developed sentences that implied traits (e.g., "The librarian carries the old woman's groceries across the street" would lead to the inference "helpful"). Giving people the word "helpful" later as a cue should bolster recall of the sentence if and only if that trait was inferred at the time the sentence was read. In fact, the trait term should be as useful at aiding recall as words that have a strong semantic link to the sentence—words such as "books," which are related to librarians, or "bags," which are related to groceries. This was precisely what Winter and Uleman found. As an important final note, when participants were questioned about the memory study they had just performed, they denied having any sense that the experiment was about impression formation or having formed any type of judgments about the people whose behavior they were memorizing. Despite participants' denying that such inferences had been formed, and being unable to consciously report engaging in this type of trait inferencing, their recall results clearly indicated that such inferences were being made.

Critics of the encoding specificity paradigm have stated that the STI effect could be an artifact of Winter and Uleman's methodology. It could be that people were not using the recall cues to help them retrieve information stored at encoding, but to generate sample behaviors representing the trait in question, and that these representative behaviors then triggered recall for the actual behavior. "A subject who is given the cue 'clumsy' may think of typical clumsy behaviors, such as 'bumps into people on the dance floor.' . . . These behavioral features may then cue the recall of the stimulus behavior even if the behavior had not been encoded in trait terms" (Wyer & Srull, 1989, p. 146). As Carlston and Skowronski (1994, pp. 840–841) put it, even if people did not form spontaneous inferences, it might look as if they did, because trait terms could still be effective retrieval cues due to "their preexisting links to behavioral prototypes in people's implicit personality theories." However, Winter and Uleman (1984) specifically gave some research participants the trait words and asked them to generate behavioral exemplars in order to see whether a priori links existed between the traits and the behaviors. Fewer than 6% of the responses were behaviors that were even loosely related to the behaviors used in the research reported above. People did not generate "bumps into people" when given the trait "clumsy." This undermines the criticism.

Another way to address the criticism is to manipulate the encoding conditions. If researchers give participants different goals or tasks at encoding, but hold the conditions at recall constant, the alternative explanation (that the inferences are being formed later, at recall) would require that there are no differences in STIs, due to differing conditions happening at the time participants initially encounter the sentences. However, the explanation suggesting that traits are inferred initially (at encoding) would say that goals introduced while the sentences are being presented should influence STI formation. Several studies have found precisely this pattern. Uleman, Newman, and Winter (1992) found that placing participants under cognitive load while they encoded the information reduced the effectiveness of trait cues at recall. Another experiment that manipulated encoding conditions varied the goals of research participants and showed that goals affected recall (Uleman & Moskowitz, 1994). Some participants were provided with goals that facilitate STIs and others with goals that inhibit them. For example, it was posited that trait inferencing would be reduced by giving research participants the goal to detect specific letters in a sentence because it would detract from processing the meanings of words, and the relationship of those words to each other (details provided later in this chapter). It was further posited that trait inferencing could be implicitly increased by making the situation more self-relevant. Some participants were given the goal of imagining how likely they would be to engage in the behaviors described. The logic was that trait inferences might be more likely to occur as an intermediate result in the formation of such a social judgment, but without awareness of the trait inferences. Uleman and Moskowitz (1994) similarly found that manipulating encoding conditions in these ways affected recall. People asked to focus on word features formed fewer STIs than people trying to memorize the sentences, and people making self-relevant judgments formed more STIs than people trying to memorize the sentences. This suggests that the differences in memory were due to inferences formed at encoding, when the sentences were initially being read. However, the best strategy for dispelling criticism that the method is flawed is to provide convergent validity by using a different procedure.

The Relearning Paradigm

As noted above, Carlston and Skowronski (1994) were skeptics regarding the STI phenomenon, believing it to be a product of the methods used. In an attempt to illustrate this, they developed a new method not subject to the criticisms above—one they believed would illustrate that people *do not* form inferences unless explicitly asked to do so. What they ended up discovering (Carlston & Skowronski, 1995) was that despite their efforts to dispel the STI phenomenon, they instead had uncovered a new and powerful method illustrating that such inferences are indeed made! Their method for illustrating that people spontaneously infer traits, even when not explicitly asked to, also borrowed from cognitive psychology. Information that has already been learned, or that is already in memory (even if it cannot be explicitly recalled), is easier to learn again. It takes less time to learn something one already knows. Capitalizing on this fact, they paired both sentences implying traits and sentences not implying traits with photographs (see Figure 7.6, Step 1). If traits are spontaneously inferred from the sentences, then in essence the traits have also been paired with the photographs.

If traits and pictures had already been paired because the trait had been spontaneously inferred, it should now be easier for participants to attempt to learn that these pictures and traits are paired together. It is easier to learn something if one already knows it, even if one cannot consciously recognize that one already knows it. In this procedure, participants were first asked to memorize a list of behaviors that were paired with pictures. Some of the behavior sentences implied traits, and others did not. Participants then were asked to learn a different list. This list once again had pictures (some of which were the same ones seen earlier), but this time the pictures were paired with single words instead of sentences. The words were traits; some of them were implied earlier by the sentences, and were paired with the pictures that the sentences implying the traits had earlier been paired with. Other traits being paired with the pictures were not implied earlier by the sentences, and these were paired with the faces previously paired with the sentences that did not imply traits. If STIs had been made, the implicit association with the faces would make memorizing the pairing of traits and faces easier, and recall would be better than memory for the pairings of faces with irrelevant traits. The results showed that recall was better when a picture had originally been paired with a trait-implying sentence, suggesting that participants had inferred the trait when reading the sentence, and that this STI provided the savings at relearning.

Step 1: Learn sentences (some implying a trait, some not) that are paired with images.

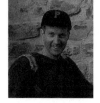   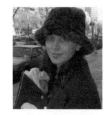

Gordon took the orphans to the circus.   Cindy went for a walk to the store with baby Ben.

Step 2: Learn traits (some implied in Step 1, some not) that are paired with images.

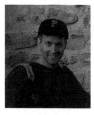   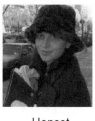

Kind   Honest
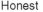

FIGURE 7.6. Carlston and Skowronski's relearning paradigm.

The Reaction Time Paradigm

Given that Carlston and Skowronski (1994, 1995) had set out to undermine the STI concept, Uleman and colleagues had set out to provide supportive evidence for the concept, also attempting to develop a new methodology not subject to the criticism leveled at the encoding specificity paradigm (we never imagined that Carlston and Skowronski's own studies would end up providing supportive evidence as well). We (Uleman, Hon, Roman, & Moskowitz, 1996) borrowed yet another paradigm from cognitive psychology to illustrate how people form STIs. The logic of this experiment was that people are faster at responding to items that are accessible or "primed" (this concept is discussed further in Chapter 9). *Accessible* information is that which is perceptually ready due to its recent or frequent use. Essentially, if you have just thought about snakes, you will be faster at noticing and responding to another snake if it comes along shortly. You are prepared to react to it. If traits are inferred, they too should now be accessible and be responded to faster, even if a person is unaware that an inference has been made! The reaction time procedure of Uleman and colleagues had research participants read sentences that either did or did not imply traits, and then respond to those traits. If a trait had been inferred from reading the sentence, reaction times to the trait would be affected.

Participants read sentences on a computer screen. They then had a word flashed at them and had to decide whether the word was actually in the sentence. The sentences that appeared included some that implied traits. When trait-implying sentences appeared, the word that followed was a trait. When a trait-implying sentence was followed by the trait implied in that sentence, the correct response was "no," since the trait word was not actually in the sentence; it was merely implied by it. If participants had inferred the trait upon reading the sentence, it should take them longer to answer "no" on this task, because they were primed to respond to the trait. Thus, if reaction times were compared between sentences implying the trait and sentences not implying the trait, a slower response to a trait word following sentences implying the trait could only be due to the fact that STIs had happened at encoding and people had inferred the trait, despite not trying to or being aware of having done so. The results were supportive of this prediction.

The False-Recognition Paradigm

Todorov and Uleman (2002) introduced yet another method for examining STIs. The procedure unfolded over several phases. At the first phase, a series of sentences, each of which described a trait-implying behavior, was presented to participants. Each behavior was paired with a picture of a face. The task in this phase (the study phase) was to memorize the material for a memory test that would occur later in the experiment. In the second phase of the experiment (the test phase), the participants were provided with a picture of a face paired with a word. The word was a trait that might, or might not, have been implied by the sentence paired with that given face in the study phase of the experiment. The participants' task was to decide whether the word had actually been included in the sentence that had originally been paired with the face. On critical trials of this experiment, the answer to this question was always "no." The traits were never in the sentence; they were only implied by the sentence.

The logic of this methodology was that if people had inferred the trait upon reading the sentence, then this trait would have been encoded in memory along with the face of the person. Thus, when the face later appeared, it would serve as a cue allowing participants to recall the other events that went on at encoding (that were stored in memory). These would include the inferred trait. However, if this was what is happening, an error would result. Participants would not recall that they inferred the trait stored along with the face, but would assume the reason it was stored with the face was that it was actually in the sentence they read. Thus people would falsely recognize a trait that had been inferred as one that had actually been presented. The familiarity of the trait would be misattributed to its prior presentation (e.g., Jacoby & Whitehouse, 1989; Johnson, Hashtroudi, & Lindsay, 1993).

Two clear consequences were shown by Todorov and Uleman (2002) to have resulted from this state of affairs, thus providing evidence that participants were forming STIs. First, participants showed evidence of false recognition of traits. False recognition was highest when a face that was originally paired with a sentence implying the trait was later paired with the implied trait at the test phase. If the trait being presented at the test phase was paired with some other face—one that was not originally paired with the sentence implying the trait—there would be no reason for people to falsely recognize the trait. It would not have been stored in memory with that face. Thus false recognition was greater when a trait inferred at the study phase was paired at the test phase with a face that at some point had been linked to that trait (through an act of inference) than when the same trait was paired with a different face (and also greater than when the same face was paired with a different trait). The second finding that emerged from this paradigm was that participants were slower to correctly reject an implied trait as having previously been seen, relative to the speed with which they could reject a different trait.

To What Do STIs Refer?

STI research clearly shows that attending to a behavior activates trait concepts associated with the behavior, even when attention is incidental and no conscious intention to infer a trait exists. But what do STIs represent? To Heider, "not the doing only, but the doer" is "susceptible to a value judgment" (1944, p. 365). In essence, it is not just the person's behavior to which we assign a label, but the disposition of the person performing the behavior. For instance, a stupid act is seen as the act of a stupid person. This is why if you tell your friend Larry that he has acted stupidly, he gets insulted! He interprets this to mean that you think him, not his act, stupid. In the English language, traits (such as "stupid") can refer to behaviors and also to the people who perform the behaviors. Research on STIs assumes that these inferences refer to all of the following: (1) a person's behavior, (2) a person's disposition, and (3) a cause of the behavior. But *do* STIs refer to all of these things? Hamilton (1988, p. 377) argued for a distinction between trait inference and attributions:

> If I observe a person's outgoing and gregarious behavior at a party and infer that she is friendly, I am not attempting to explain why she mingled and chatted with others but am simply summarizing a pattern of behavior and inferring a trait characteristic from it. In making the inference I have implicitly assumed that her behavior is at least somewhat representative of her personality.

Although making such distinctions is an important theoretical point for research on trait inferences, the referents of STIs need not affect the consequences of STIs for correspondence bias. Whether (or not) an inferred trait is initially seen as the cause of the person's behavior does not affect the use to which the trait is subsequently put, once it has been inferred. Regardless of its referent, an STI may still operate as an anchor upon which subsequent judgment is based.

Reasons for Forming STIs

The review of STIs thus informs us of one reason why correspondence bias is so fundamental: People have a tendency to infer traits when observing the behavior of other people, and this tendency is something that happens spontaneously and preconsciously. The lingering effect of this "automatic" tendency is for perceivers to be overly reliant on using traits when forming explanations, even when they know the situation needs to be considered. The traits form an anchor for judgment that is hard to adjust away from. But now that we have seen that people form STIs and that STIs are essential to the fundamental attribution error, this does not answer a remaining intriguing and central question: Why is forming such inferences so fundamental? We now know that STIs occur, but why—and why so frequently, easily, and silently?

As reviewed in Chapter 1, a fundamental motive for much of human psychological functioning is the search for meaning, understanding, or certainty in belief. Thus, although people may lack, from moment to moment, an explicit intention or goal to infer meaning, we can conceive of this pursuit as a more permanent and global pursuit (what we might call a *distal goal*). The distal goal of having meaning is one that can be fulfilled by forming trait inferences. Indeed, the more people desire meaning, structure, and closure, the more likely they should be to use trait inferences to categorize the world as a means of delivering such meaning and attaining the distal goal. One study (Moskowitz, 1993a) showed that people who had a high need for structure (a personality variable that establishes one as possessing a chronically high need to attain closure and meaning quickly) were more likely to form STIs. One answer to the question of why this process is so fundamental is that it allows people to resolve a fundamental goal that lies at the heart of the human experience—the need to attain meaning, knowledge, and closure.

We may now wonder why this process, though fundamental, is something that proceeds outside of awareness, in the preconscious. Chapter 2 has illustrated how the intention to act on a goal can be somewhat automatically triggered by the presence of goal-relevant cues in the environment. This "automatization" of goals is said to occur when people routinely practice goal pursuit in the presence of such cues, with such practice allowing the triggering of and the pursuit of the goal to be routinized/habitualized so that it can occur without conscious reflection. Making sense of the world through the use of traits occurs so frequently (is so well practiced) that the process eventually becomes routinized. All that is required for the goal of attaining meaning to be triggered, and for the process of forming trait inferences to be preconsciously initiated in the pursuit of that goal, is the presence of a relevant cue in the environment. In this case, another person's trait-relevant behavior may serve to trigger the STI process. But this explanation for the occurrence of STIs assumes that trait inferences are useful for addressing the goal of attaining understanding/meaning. The notion that trait inferences are useful in this regard is reflected in a variety of attribution models, beginning with Heider (1944) and continuing through Kruglanski's (1990) description of an epistemic process driven by a search for closure/structure.

According to Heider (1944), disposition as an explanation for behavior is both powerful and parsimonious. Other people's actions produce changes—disturbances in the equilibrium that once permitted mastery over events in the environment. Others' behaviors create unexplained occurrences. Behavioral disruptions in a perceiver's understanding of the social environment can be reversed if that behavior is understood and categorized. Heider asserted that traits have the ability to provide complete and sufficient explanations (in a manner unparalleled by other types of causal ascription) that reduce the uncertainty aroused by an observed behavior. A second reason that dispositional inference is pervasive stems from its ability to promote effective interactions with people by allowing the perceiver to develop predictions and expectancies about what others are like and likely to do (Bruner, 1957). In addition, trait inferences help people sustain the belief that the world is a controllable place where things happen because they were willed to happen, and do not result from chance or circumstance (Anderson & Deuser, 1993; Heider, 1958; Jones, 1979; Pittman & Heller, 1987). White (1959) labeled this the *effectance motive*, the goal of which is the maintenance of control over the environment through effective interactions.

However, one important question is still left unanswered by this explanation for the ubiquity of trait-inferencing: Why is it that through the course of their lives, people choose to use traits and dispositions as the best way to explain the behavior of other people? As we have seen, situations are often powerful causes for behavior, so why have we humans not developed the tendency to routinely make sense of the world by using situations as the primary agent of categorization? In answering this, J. G. Miller (1984), as well as Morris and Peng (1994), reminds us of a fact that Sherif (1936) taught us long ago (and that has been touched on in Chapter 3): The culture within which we are raised influences the nature of our cognitive processing. Our cultural heritage not only teaches us the content of the stereotypes that exist within the culture and socializes us to accept the norms that are prominent in the culture, but it infuses our cognitive system with a style for thinking about the world. In explicating this role of culture, Sherif told us:

> Socially established norms are not limited to shaping in us a set of aesthetic standards, or even to prescribing our relationships to other individuals; they have much to do in determining our perception of nature and our attitudes toward it. What we shall notice in the external stimulus field, and what aspects of it will stand out, are largely a function of what we are prepared to see. The socially established norms of a given period create in us lasting expectations and a preparedness to see in the nature that surrounds us much to which another period would be totally blind. (p. 64)

Such modifications to cognition based on culture operate (1) at the perceptual level (e.g., shaping what we notice in the perceptual field, such that, as Sherif [1936, p. 65] says, "the beauty of Lake Constance" would go unnoticed by members of a culture that did not stress an appreciation of nature); (2) at the level of sense making and cognitive organization ("to a person brought up on oriental music, which is built chiefly upon rhythm and melody, the harmony of a musical work coming from a great European orchestra is almost sheer noise" [Sherif, 1936, p. 62]); and (3) at the interpersonal level ("as a consequence of the contacts of individuals, more or less definite 'expectations' of each toward the other appear. Henceforth their reactions to each other are to a large extent regulated with reference to this established 'expectation'" [Sherif, 1936, p. 53]). Thus all levels of experience are filtered through culture.

Morris and Peng (1994) explain how this emphasis on culture can yield a cognitive style that promotes a focus on dispositions as causes for behavior. Their argument is that individuals raised within mainstream Western cultures are taught from birth (indeed, it pervades every level of experience within these cultures) that individuals are autonomous beings, creatures responsible for determining their own destiny through the actions that they perform and the effort that they commit to attaining their various goals. Western civilization is described as a bastion of *individualism,* with the consequence being that individuals are seen as responsible, autonomous, and in possession of free will. Morris and Peng propose that this cultural milieu is what imbues in each perceiver raised within these cultures a tendency to think of the world of other people as organized around behaviors that are freely intended and chosen—behaviors for which these individual persons are responsible. Cognitive processes are by-products of being raised in cultures that teach perceivers to make sense of the behavior of others within the constraint of inferring dispositions first (and asking questions about situations later). Perceivers hold *implicit theories* about the causes for events that are acquired from being socialized within particular cultures: "The person-centered theory that social behavior expresses stable, global, internal dispositions is more widespread in individualist cultures" (Morris & Peng, 1994, p. 952). It is not assumed that what mainstream Western cultures teach are fairly specific sets of relationships between people and actions tied to particular content domains (such as "If one steals, one is a dishonest person"). Instead, it is assumed that these cultures provide a style for thinking about the causes of behavior that influences cognition in a deep and meaningful way. People do not learn that stealing means dishonesty; they learn that behavior is a reflection of an individual's will.

We finally have our answer to why dispositionalism is at the heart of the fundamental attribution error. It is presumably because mainstream Western cultures teach that the way to make sense of the world is to rely on implicit theories about the meaning of events—theories that dictate these cultures' emphasis on autonomy and individualism. Hence, traits drive behavior and are what perceivers see as causal.

THE LIMITS OF CORRESPONDENCE BIAS AND STIs

Although it may be fundamental in some respects, trait inferences are also dependent on the context within which the goals that promote STIs operate. People do not start inferring traits or dispositions about people when the behavior that is observed does not imply a trait! As we have seen in Figure 7.6, the sentence "Cindy took baby Ben for a walk to the store" was not expected to lead to any type of spontaneous inference. The behavior being observed must suggest a trait, and only then will it match the goal of one needing to infer traits to provide control, predictability, and meaning (see the McArthur and Baron [1983] discussion of dynamic stimulus displays, and the Moskowitz and Roman [1992] discussion of stimulus behaviors infused with meaning). One could try to form an impression or form a dispositional inference about almost any behavior if one was asked. Even the sentence "Cindy took baby Ben for a walk to the store" could lead to some type of inference if I asked you to try to form one (perhaps Cindy likes exercise). But it is not functional to draw inferences from such behavior without being asked to do so. Most STI research has simply assumed that in the absence of explicit impression formation goals, STIs occur because distal goals that promote trait inference exist, and behaviors are encountered that readily imply traits.

However, as Krull (1993) has illustrated, trait inferences need not be one's automatic response when explaining a behavior. There are instances in which, rather than forming STIs, people form inferences about *the situation* spontaneously! This suggests there are limits to the occurrence of STIs. Given the appropriate context, situation, not trait, inferences may occur. What other factors limit STIs? Goals disrupt STIs (they are not automatic in the sense that they are uncontrollable, as illustrated by Uleman & Moskowitz, 1994), as does cognitive load (Uleman et al., 1992). However, despite these limitations, the suggestion is (at least in Western cultures) that a fundamental goal for attaining meaning exists, and this leads to a pervasive tendency to infer traits as part of making sense of others. This section of this chapter is dedicated to examining factors— such as culture and goals—that disrupt the so-called "fundamental attribution error."

Culture

The correspondence bias is rooted in the perceiver's basic tendency to think about the world in terms of traits. But perhaps this basic tendency is not so basic, but culture-specific. For example, J. G. Miller (1984) asked research participants of various ages from two different cultures (the United States and India) to form attributions. In the United States, participants showed an increase in dispositional attributions with age, whereas in India no such increase was found. However, Indian participants did reveal an increase in situational attributions with age, whereas American participants did not. Morris and Peng (1994) examining people from the United States versus people from China, found a similar pattern. Americans favored dispositional attributions, while the Chinese favored situational attributions. Shweder and Bourne (1982) found that Hindu participants living in India described the behavior of another person using language that embedded that person's behavior within a particular set of social relationships and contexts. American participants given the same task gave decontextualized descriptions, and instead leaned heavily on dispositions that could be expected to be generalized across situations and relationships.

This difference in how and when (and whether) traits are used to describe the behavior of others is typically attributed to cultural differences in what are called *individualism* and *collectivism* (Triandis, 1989, 1990; see also Markus & Kitayama's [1991] discussion of independence and interdependence). As discussed above, an individualistic culture (such as those derived from Western Europe) is one that emphasizes the uniqueness and autonomy of the individual—one where self-expression and independence are highly valued, if not central to the culture. In contrast, a collectivistic culture (such as those derived from many Asian societies) is one in which the social roles of the individual and the person's ties to the social group are emphasized. The person is seen as interdependent with the collective; rather than being raised to see the self as autonomous and independent, the person views the self as occupying a place in the larger social scheme. These pervasive social forces shape the way the individual is trained to view the world and interpret the actions of others. Members of societies where people are seen as autonomous will use traits to describe the actions of others—individuals control their own actions, so their actions must be derived from their personalities. Members of cultures where individuals are raised to see people as interconnected, and whose actions are dictated by the social roles they are asked to play in society, should be less likely to spontaneously infer traits (or to use traits at all) when describing the actions of others. Rather, people from such cultures should develop the tendency to look to the situation and the constraints of one's social roles to explain behavior. These cultural differences should, therefore, give rise to different attributional tendencies.

Specifically, Morris, Ames, and Knowles (2001) report that when people are judging the behavior of others, there is a greater emphasis on personal traits relative to social situations for members of American (individualistic) relative to East Asian (collectivistic) cultures (Choi & Nisbett, 1998; Morris, Knowles, Chiu, & Hong, 1998; Norenzayan, Choi, & Nisbett, 1998). Morris and Peng (1994) illustrated this with Chinese and American research participants. In one experiment, they showed participants cartoon movies of fish interacting and asked them to rate the cartoons according to internal and external factors. For example, there was a group of fish with one swimming ahead of the group, and participants were asked whether this fish was the leader of the pack (an internal factor being implicated) or being chased by the pack of fish (an external factor being implicated). Americans perceived more internal influence and Chinese people perceived more external influence in accounting for the social behavior (of fish). Morris and Peng took this to be evidence of different implicit theories at work within the two cultures (see Chapter 4 for further experiments by Morris and Peng).

In a similar vein, Newman (1993) found that students from a Hispanic culture (such cultures have also been shown to be more collectivistic) were less likely to make STIs than students from mainstream U.S. culture. Not only were his suburban American students more likely to form STIs than his students from Puerto Rican families, but they were more likely to use traits to predict future behavior. Puerto Rican students "were less likely to assume that behavior would be trait-consistent, and were more sensitive to the effects of situational constraints when predicting the future behavior of other people" (Newman, 1993, p. 249). A similar tendency should be exhibited when explaining one's own behavior. For example, Rhee, Uleman, Lee, and Roman (1995) asked participants to describe themselves by completing the statement "I am ____" 20 times. They found that Asians were less likely to use traits to describe themselves than Americans were. Typical American responses might be "I am hard-working, I am honest," whereas typical Asian responses might be "I am a son, I am a student."

Krull and colleagues (1999), however, provided evidence apparently dispelling the notion that people from collectivistic cultures fail to exhibit the correspondence bias. They used the attitude attribution paradigm and asked participants to read essays arguing either that a person's personality is determined mainly by genetics or that it is determined mostly by environment. The essayist was said to have been required to write the essay. As expected, the U.S. participants rated the person's true attitude as corresponding with the essay position. However, so did participants from Taiwan! Morris and colleagues (1998; see also Choi & Nisbett, 1998) performed a similar study in Hong Kong and the United States, but made the situational factor more salient. They found that for Americans the tendency to attribute to disposition was not changed by the addition of a more salient situational constraint. However, although participants from Hong Kong did display the correspondence bias when this more salient information about the situation was absent, the tendency toward dispositional attributions was dramatically reduced by the addition of a more salient situational constraint. The same pattern of results was obtained when the quiz show paradigm was used.

Finally, one need not look between countries to find these types of differences. Individuals within a country, particularly one as heterogeneous as the United States, can differ in the degree to which they are individualistic. Individualism–collectivism as an individual-difference variable (as assessed using tools like the Idiocentrism Scale; Triandis, Bontempo, Villareal, Asai, & Lucca, 1988) is also known to be able to determine the extent to which people rely on traits in describing the actions of others. For example, Duff and Newman (1997) found that highly idiocentric participants were more likely to make STIs. Participants read sentences (e.g., "On her lunch break, the receptionist steps in front of another person in line") that had both a dispositional interpretation (e.g., "rude") and a situational interpretation (e.g., "in a hurry"). Recall was tested with the aid of either trait or situation cues. Idiocentrism correlated positively with trait-cued recall but negatively with situation-cued recall.

Goals

The correspondence bias is multiply determined. Yet each of the potential causes reflects a failure by perceivers to adequately use information provided for them. They fail to notice situations; they notice situations, but underestimate the impact; they notice situations, but lack accuracy in the type of adjustment they make. What these causes suggest is that perhaps if perceivers try harder to be accurate, or engage in more elaborate and systematic analysis of the behavior observed as well as the context in which the behavior occurs, the bias may disappear. People can perhaps adopt goals when interacting with others that disrupt the bias.

Accountability

Evidence for this role of goals as instigators of more deliberate processing in which initial, more effortless inferences are corrected and adjusted is provided in the work of Tetlock (1983, 1985, 1992; Tetlock & Kim, 1987). Tetlock (1985) examined the impact of making people publicly accountable for their impressions. In Chapter 5, being held accountable is described as a goal state where people feel they need to form justifiable and accurate judgments. This concern with accuracy presumably leads people to be more careful in how they examine the behavior of others, introducing a greater likelihood that they will take note of and account for situational constraint.

Tetlock (1985) led some research participants to expect that they would have to justify their impressions to others. The remaining participants simply performed the judgment task, with no explicit goal provided for them other than that of forming an impression of a person. Research participants who were not accountable showed the classic correspondence bias effect (attributing a speech writer´s position to the true beliefs of the writer, even when they knew the writer was forced to write the speech). However, participants who were being held accountable for their impressions of the speech writer were less likely to attribute the speech to the writer's personal beliefs. Tetlock concluded that this occurred because the goal created more discriminating research participants. High choice clearly signaled a dispositional cause to the careful attributors, whereas forced choice suggested a situational cause. But only the accountable people were discriminating enough to make use of these cues and show attenuation of the effect.

Outcome Dependency

Chapter 5 has defined *outcome dependency* as the goal state where a person is motivated to attain some end with the cooperation of another person. Such motives were posited by Neuberg and Fiske (1987) to be associated with an increase in effortful and accurate processing of information relevant to the partner on whom the person's outcomes are dependent. This occurs because coordination with the partner to attain the desired end depends on the person's being able to accurately assess the skills and qualities of the partner. Thus, as Vonk (1999) states, outcome dependency could lead perceivers "to pay more attention not only to the target's behavior but to everything that is relevant in the person–situation field, as well as to exert cognitive effort in performing a situational correction when necessary" (p. 383). Using (yet again) the Jones and Harris (1967) attitude attribution paradigm, Vonk had participants read an essay they believed was written either under conditions of free choice or forced compliance. However, participants also were made to be dependent either on the person who wrote the essay or on some new person. When the research participant was not dependent on the essay writer, then the experiment was essentially identical to past research on correspondence bias, and the typical results emerged. A person who wrote an essay under conditions of no choice was seen to be just as committed to the attitude expressed in the essay as a person who was able to write freely about the topic in hand. However, outcome dependency alleviated this bias: When the essay writer was said to have no choice, he/she was judged by the participant as having more moderate attitudes than the essay writer who was writing with free choice.

Suspicion of Ulterior Motives

Fein, Hilton, and Miller (1990) point out that in some ways the correspondence bias is counterintuitive. After all, when we observe a person in a commercial pitching a product, such as when Joe DiMaggio attempted to convince us to use "Mr. Coffee" and Phil Rizzuto told us to go to "the Money Store," we somehow knew that the behavior of these former baseball players might not correspond with their true attitudes toward these products. We suspected they might simply have wanted to make a little extra cash after their playing days had long ended. In examples such as this (another good one is when someone compliments you and then asks for a favor), the target person has an ulterior motive. Thus, as perceivers, we face an attributional dilemma: The person's attitude toward the product potentially corresponds with what the person says/does, but the target is potentially simply adopting the observed stance for the purpose of gaining some desired end state. The implication, as Fein and colleagues state, is that "correspondence bias may be less likely to emerge when contextual factors suggest that multiple, plausibly rival motives could underlie the actor's behavior than when contextual factors suggest that the actor's behavior is motivated only by situational constraint" (p. 754).

To investigate this question, Fein and colleagues' (1990) research participants were asked to read an essay and judge the extent to which the essay reflected the true beliefs of the person who wrote it. The essay concerned a rule (Proposition 42) enforced by the NCAA regarding the academic standards that student-athletes must meet. Participants were told that the essay writer was an intern working for a professor. In the no-choice condition, they were further told that the professor had asked the essayist to write the essay for a debate. Thus the position espoused in the essay (pro- or anti-Proposition 42) was determined by the professor. Other research participants were led to believe that the type of essay the person wrote was determined by an ulterior motive. These participants were told that the essay writer was free to write an essay either for or against Proposition 42, but the professor for whom the essay writer was an intern would be reading these essays. The intern knew that the professor had a strong opinion on the topic.

Therefore, although the writer was free to take any position he/she liked, the writer was also dependent on getting a good evaluation from the professor and would probably be motivated to write something the professor would agree with, simply to be ingratiating. The results revealed that in the no-choice condition, the classic overattribution effect was found. If the intern wrote an essay in favor of Proposition 42, perceivers believed he/she truly held attitudes that supported the policy. If the intern wrote an essay opposing it, he/she was judged to be truly against the policy. However, when perceivers believed that the essayist held ulterior motives, this bias disappeared.

The Goal to Shift One's Focus of Attention

Quattrone (1982) demonstrated that sometimes the initial inferences people form are not dispositional, but situational, depending on what their expectancies and mindset are at the time the stimulus information is perceived. Quattrone was able to eliminate overattribution to disposition in the attitude attribution paradigm by changing what information the research participants were led to see as being salient. In fact, the opposite tendency was produced—overattribution to the situation. Quattrone hypothesized that if "behavior engulfs the field," and this leads the traits that describe the behavior to be salient and established as an anchor for further judgment, then altering what "engulfs the field" should alter the extent to which correspondence bias is observed. Asking people to make judgments about someone's personality or attitude should only heighten the extent to which that person's personality or attitude will be seen as salient in explaining the person's behavior. Giving perceivers a goal to make a different type of judgment—one that makes *the situation more salient*—should help to alleviate the correspondence bias.

Research participants were asked to read essays from people whose prior attitudes were known to be congruent with the positions they took in the essays. Furthermore, each essayist was said to have free choice when writing the essay. Yet despite these facts, research participants made an overattribution to the situation. This occurred because of their goals while reading the essay. Rather than having the goal of judging the extent to which an essay reflected a person's true attitude, they were told that their goal was to ascertain the subtle influence of the experimenter on the essayist. Thus, when evaluating the essay, the participants were now focused on the impact of the experimenter (the situation here was another person—the experimenter). Furthermore, rather than judging the true attitude of the essayist, they now had to make judgments of how much the situation had caused the essayist to write the type of essay he/she did. This alteration of participants' mindset influenced whether dispositional inferences or situational inferences were initially formed—a clear illustration that trait inference, while ubiquitous, is subject to being controlled.

Krull (1993) demonstrated a similar effect, due to a perceiver's inferential goal. Krull asserted that the tendency to overattribute to disposition is not a fixed, automatic process (despite being caused by implicit and preconscious cognitive processes), but a strategy that can be controlled. If a perceiver has the goal to learn about a situation (e.g., determine how anxiety-provoking the situation is) rather than to make an inference about the person (e.g., determine how anxious the person is), these goals can exert control over correspondence bias by leading the perceiver to initially draw an inference not about the person's disposition, but about the person's situational constraint (Krull & Dill, 1996). By leading people to form situational inferences, goals defeat the correspondence bias—but not by promoting a stage where effortful correction processes occur to counteract the initial failure to consider the context. Rather, goals prevent trait inferences from occurring at all. In fact, given the appropriate goal, the correspondence bias not only disappears; the effect is reversed, and people overattribute to the situation.

Information-Processing Goals

Krull's (1993) finding is similar to Lupfer, Clark, and Hutcherson's (1990) belief that situational inferences may be formed spontaneously when background information that promotes a situational attribution is present. It is also consistent with our results (Uleman & Moskowitz, 1994) when we asked whether the unconscious trait inferences that contribute to the correspondence bias can be prevented from being formed. Can people control a process when they are not even aware it exists? Uleman and Moskowitz (1994) posited that even implicit inferences can be controlled, despite the fact that these trait inferences are occurring without awareness or conscious intent. This prediction was drawn directly from results found by cognitive psychologists in demonstrating that implicit cognitive processes, such as those that produce the Stroop effect and priming effects, "are not driven by mere stimulus presentation. They are not beyond strategic control" (Logan, 1989, p. 57).

To investigate this regarding STIs, Uleman and Moskowitz (1994) manipulated the types of processing goals participants had while being presented with trait-implying sentences. Some participants were asked to memorize the sentences for a subsequent recall test. Others were asked to analyze the sentences for specific patterns of letters, such as detecting every time an "h" occurred that was not preceded by a "t." Still others were asked to determine whether a set of target words rhymed with any of the words in the sentences. And others were asked to identify whether the pronouns in the sentence referred to men or women, or whether gender could not be determined. What effect did these goals have on the formation of STIs? The results of this study clearly replicated the finding that when participants had the goal of memorizing sentences, STIs were formed. However, when the sentences were processed under alternative processing goals, the extent to which STIs were formed was diminished. Especially when the goals of the experiment competed with meaning being inferred from the sentence (e.g., searching for the letter "h"), the likelihood of STIs' occurring was reduced.

Suppression

As reviewed in detail later in this book, it has been widely illustrated that attempting to prevent oneself from thinking about a topic has an ironic effect: One ends up thinking about the topic even more (Monteith, Sherman, & Devine, 1998; Wegner, 1994). At least initially, suppression appears to work. The unwanted thought is kept out of consciousness and appears to be held at bay. But the mental processes involved in keeping a thought out of consciousness lead to that thought returning with even more force, once the intent to keep it at bay has been released. Yzerbyt, Corneille, Dumont, and Hahn (2001) see this fact as relevant to correspondence bias. They assert that the very correction processes that appear to keep a trait inference from influencing one's judgment too heavily lead to such inferences only returning with even greater force. Thus, when people seem to have successfully removed an overattribution to disposition through adjusting that attribution, they have only temporarily suppressed correspondent bias and have laid the foundation for such overattributions to rebound. Of course, this requires that the correction process must involve more than simply taking the situational constraint into account. It must also include attempts to monitor one's thoughts to prevent premature trait inferences from influencing one's impression.

CODA

It is suggested that trait inferences occur quite passively, effortlessly, and implicitly. Indeed, perceivers have distal goals in place that make such inferences the likely default choice when they are categorizing behavior. This dispositionalist tendency in categorizing the world, arising from a variety of causes, contributes to the tendency (at least in Western cultures) to overattribute the behavior of others to disposition. Detailing the impact of perceivers' implicit theories (derived from culture), mindsets, expectancies, motives, and goals on undermining correspondence bias and STIs is not meant to diminish the importance of trait inferences in everyday psychological functioning. Nor is it meant to underscore the extent to which the correspondence bias is quite a fundamental attributional occurrence. Just because trait inferences are not automatic or inevitable and can be controlled, this does not mean that they do not *usually* occur. And just because they usually occur, this does not mean that perceivers are being overly judgmental or wildly overusing traits in helping them to understand the behavior of others. Trait inferences occur so frequently because they are useful ways to describe behavior; they are functional in that they allow people to understand what they have seen, plan their behavior, and feel as if they have control over the situations that they are placed in (or place themselves in). Traits provide a stable and coherent way of describing the actions of others, and are thus leaned on in initial and preconscious attempts at sense making. But these inferences can be adjusted, overturned, and altered as later thinking deems necessary.

The preceding argument tells us that while correspondent inference may be a "bias," it is a bias born of functionality. It probably evolved out of the important need to make sense of the world and to experience a sense of control (and predictability) over that world. However, contributing to the process of overattribution are a host of factors not necessarily linked to functions—failure to consider the situation adequately, failure even to see the situation, and so on. In the next chapter, we continue discussing processing that occurs in the pursuit of an attribution that we might also consider to be biased. Failing to see or consider the situation may bias perceivers' judgment, but hardly in a way that seems irrational or self-serving. "Bias," in the more typical use of the word, conjures up images of perceivers' steering their thoughts in a self-serving way, serving some quite personal goals. It is to these types of biases in the attribution process that we turn next.

8 Shortcomings and Biases in Person Perception

Since one's idea includes what "ought to be" and "what one would like to be" as well as "what is," attributions and cognitions are influenced by the mere subjective forces of needs and wishes as well as by the more objective evidence presented in the raw material.

—HEIDER (1958, pp. 120–121)

"Exercises for toughening up the nipples!" Anne said in shock as she read the advertisement on the Internet. "I hope I never need to engage in any behavior that requires that sort of an exercise." And so a child-rearing decision had been made. No breast feeding for Anne.

However, imagine that you are a mother who has just spent the better part of 2 years with a child gnawing at your nipples, putting yourself through constant pain (if you had bottle-fed, your nipples would have been touched no more than usual) and sleepless nights (if you had bottle-fed, your partner could have been the one who did not sleep!). What sort of an attitude/impression would you have toward a woman like Anne who chooses not to breast-feed or experience those pains? What sort of impressions would you have of your own behavior and of breast feeding more generally? The most accurate answers to these questions depend on whether there are tangible benefits to breast feeding that you believe you have been providing for your baby, and that those who choose not to breast-feed are denying to theirs. Most people do not engage in painful behavior that has no benefits, so your decision to breast-feed probably reflects your assumption that breast feeding is essential for providing the best care for a child. Armed with such an attitude, it is likely that you might look at those who deny their children such benefits with disdain (at least slightly).

Let's extend our example a bit. Imagine now that you learn that Anne's decision not to breast-feed is based not only on the fact that it hurts, but on the fact that upon examining the best data on the question of whether breast feeding has any tangible benefits, our hypothetical mother (Anne) has deduced that it does not. Anne has discovered an equal number of studies suggesting that here is no reliable difference between breast-fed babies and bottle-fed babies. In fact, she has found that many of the experiments used to convince mothers that there are positive benefits to breast feeding are flawed in their methodology—confounded in ways that make the conclusions tenuous at best—and would suggest to a person trained in the scientific method to disregard the findings.

For example, Anne discovers that most of the research suggesting a benefit for breast feeding was conducted in the period in our medical past when baby formula was simply not as good as it is now, given modern-day advances. Obviously, breast feeding is better than asking children to drink some vitamin-fortified water. But this is not what modern-day alternatives to breast feeding are. As another example, a look at modern research reveals to Anne that studies controlling for factors that could account for alleged differences between bottle-fed and breast-fed babies, such as the IQ of the parents or the socioeconomic status of the family, report no benefit for breast feeding. And of those studies that do provide data in support of the benefits of breast feeding, many ignore obvious problems in the research that would make the conclusion that breast feeding leads to benefits in a child's IQ and health untenable. Anne reads one study published in the *Journal of the American Medical Association* (JAMA) purported to have shown a positive correlation between breast feeding and a child's IQ, while claiming to have controlled for "parental intelligence." Prior studies had been unable to show benefits for breast feeding when controlling for maternal IQ. So this appears to be strong evidence to support breast feeding. Yet Anne's scrutiny of this work reveals that the research *did not* control for maternal IQ. Instead, it controlled for "parental intelligence," defined as "breadwinner's education." This creates three problems with the findings: (1) Since the children studied were born in the 1960s, the "breadwinner" had to have been the father in a vast majority of the cases; (2) education level is not the same thing as IQ or intelligence; and (3) even if we allow education as a suitable substitute for IQ, the research used the education of the parent who spent less time with the child and who was not providing the milk (the father/"breadwinner"). The research defined parental intelligence by virtually ignoring maternal IQ (though it tried to make it sound as if this had been taken into account)—a factor that, if controlled for, is known to eliminate links between breast feeding and a child's intelligence.[1]

Given that people only engage in painful behavior if it has some benefit, and given that our hypothetical mother has found no evidence of such benefits after a careful analysis of the scientific evidence, now how would you (remember to imagine that you are a breast-feeding mom) evaluate Anne's decision to bottle-feed and avoid this pain that you have endured? A rational approach would suggest that you would no longer judge her negatively. Her chosen behavior (bottle feeding) has no proven negative consequences for children, and some studies actually suggest that it is better for children (since it presents fewer problems associated with toxicity). You may not be surprised to learn that people *do not* form such rational impressions of others. If you have just engaged in years of painful behavior, disrupting your life entirely and your sleeping patterns nightly, you are motivated to believe that you have made this sacrifice for a reason. You will not want to think that you have done it because you were following norms and yielding to popular myths. You will want to believe that your suffering is justified by research. If research illustrating no benefits is shown to you, you will have trouble reconciling your pain-inducing decision with the data. Thus many such mothers will not only staunchly defend their decision to breast-feed, but may even *augment* their level of antagonism to those who choose not to—presumably because they are now even more motivated (by the suggestion that some data invalidate their own reasons for choosing to breast-feed) to believe that mothers like Anne are depriving their children of important health and intellectual benefits. Such attributions are *defensive* and *self-serving*, and nicely represent the type of motivated attributional reasoning that is the concern of this chapter.

When an important self-relevant behavior is challenged, we all tend to defend the self and attack the source of doubt. This is particularly interesting in this example, because a bottle feeding mother is making no diatribe against breast feeding. Someone who chooses not to breast-feed has no problem with someone who has decided to; her typical attitude is "More power to them." But it is not uncommon to find breast-feeding women who deride those who do not perform this socially accepted behavior. And attempts to justify the decision to bottle-feed are threatening to people who have chosen the more painful and sacrificing route, almost demanding a self-esteem-enhancing reply through self-serving attributions. Rather than accept scientific data in support of the decision to bottle-feed, such parents can easily point to endless articles in the popular press (*USA Today*, parenting magazines, *CNN.com*) that will provide anecdotal evidence to support their view.[2] The need to justify themselves will steer their attributions so that their own behavior is seen as reasonable, while that of threatening others is seen as negative and unwarranted.

THE POSITIVE SENSE OF SELF

The example above illustrates that we humans do not always follow a rational analysis when forming impressions. Indeed, this fact has already been established in Chapter 7, which has discussed one way we deviate from making "rational" judgments when forming impressions of other people—the correspondence bias (and the related actor–observer difference). This shortcoming in our inferential abilities has been described quite coldly; it is said to occur because the pursuit of accurate assessment is derailed by limitations in cognitive processing abilities. But this is only part of the story. As perceivers, we deal not only with limitations faced by our processing system in the pursuit of accuracy, but with subjective biases inflicted on us by our wants, needs, and desires. We actively twist and fit every piece of information we receive in a way that allows us to meet the needs driving social perception (reviewed in the Introduction to this book) other than attaining accurate meaning—high self-esteem, control, and affiliation.

This chapter starts with an examination of the most discussed form of motivated reasoning: the need to maintain a positive sense of self. Hints of this bias have been seen in Chapter 1, which has shown that we see our own behavior, beliefs, and traits to be consensual—the false-consensus effect. However, we not only see ourselves as having popular beliefs; we also see ourselves as better than most other people (at least in areas that are self-relevant; Tesser, 1988). For example, most of us have a tendency to see themselves as more moral than the average person (Epley & Dunning, 2000; Sedikides & Strube, 1997). Naturally, not all people can be above average in morality. Some of us have to be average, some below average. Despite this relentless fact of life, most of us maintain positive views of their ability, traits, behavior, and attitudes. We have an exaggerated sense of positivity regarding the self. Alicke (1985) found that when asked to judge how self-descriptive various adjectives were, people overwhelmingly chose positive over negative traits. We have not only a tendency to see ourselves positively, but a tendency to rationalize away the negative components of our life. If we are good at something, we see it as important; if we are bad at it, we come to see it as irrelevant. This tendency has gone by many names: *positivity bias, ego-protection, self-esteem enhancement,* and *positive illusions.* The premise is that we are motivated to enhance the positivity of our self-conceptions and to protect the self from negative information. Evaluations are motivated by a need to feel good about the self.

SELF-SERVING BIASES AND POSITIVE ILLUSIONS

Taylor and Brown (1988) argue that *positive illusions,* or unrealistic positive views of the self, are important ingredients of mental health and well-being. It seems that accuracy in self-views is not a panacea; instead, the realism and accuracy of depressive individuals perhaps contribute to poor mental health, while the positive illusions that most people adopt may be adaptive and shelter them. Perhaps when such illusions cross over to the realm of delusions, positivity bias runs awry of adaptiveness. But a healthy dose of unrealistic positive self-regard may be a vital factor for maintaining high self-esteem and well-being. Taylor and Brown classify these illusions into three general categories: unrealistically positive views of the self, unrealistic optimism about the future, and exaggerated perceptions of personal control. The first two of these (plus a related factor, implicit self-esteem) are covered in this section; perceptions of personal control are discussed separately in the next section.

Unrealistically Positive Views of the Self

Attaining and maintaining positive self-esteem can be accomplished if people can assert that they possess mostly positive traits and mostly positive causes for their action. They can do this by using their cognitive apparatus to meet their esteem-promoting needs. People can attend to, interpret, and recall information that is consistent with their predominantly positive self-views. They can also process information in a biased manner, so that negative information is kept at bay.

Self-Serving Bias

People maintain a sense of positivity by selectively processing self-relevant information, so that they attend to and evaluate information with favorable implications for the self and avoid information with negative implications. The tendency to see the self as positive can be discussed as an instance of an "attributional bias," because it is through the manner in which people account for their own behavior and outcomes that they are able to maintain and enhance a positive view of themselves. For example, while we may all like to think of ourselves as moral people, we can also think of times we violated our sense of morality when it was in our best interest to do so. Yet despite sometimes violating what we would consider to be moral behavior, we still manage to find ways to consider ourselves to be fair and moral, even more moral than the average person. How does one manage such feats of mental acrobatics without even realizing one must be an acrobat? This is partly accomplished by our instances of immorality being seen as rare and thus overwhelmed by our supposed frequent instances of obvious morality. (Thus even a lascivious preacher like Jimmy Swaggart can manage the inherent discrepancy between what he practices and what he preaches.) Or, better yet, we may accomplish such feats of positivity bias by using attributions to treat instances of immoral behavior as atypical and resulting from unusual situational constraint.

Attributions come into play in a discussion of positive illusions, because people attribute their own negative outcomes and actions to the *situation*, while positive behaviors are seen as arising from *dispositional and stable causes* (what is known as a *self-serving bias*). The notion of a self-serving attribution suggests a modification to the actor–observer difference discussed in Chapter 7. Instead of actors' being described as focused on the situation and able to use the situation in forming attributions, actors are now also said to be people driven by self-interest and a desire to enhance positive self-regard. We use attributions to defensively protect and enhance a positive self-view. An excellent early review of relevant research on self-serving bias (and criticisms of that research) is provided by Bradley (1978). As Hastorf, Schneider, and Polefka (1970) stated, "we attribute success to our own dispositions and failure to external forces" (p. 73). Thus another difference between actors and observers is that a self-serving attributional pattern emerges for judgments that actors make of themselves, but not for the judgments they make of others (unless they are "significant others" to whom one's identity is linked—spouses/partners, parents, siblings, friends, church members, etc.). (This treatment of significant others similarly to the self is discussed later in this chapter, in connection with the *ultimate attribution error.*)

Stevens and Jones (1976) provided an excellent illustration of the self-defensive nature of attribution. They reasoned that if attribution can be used to protect self-esteem, then the self-protective attribution pattern should be most evident when people's self-esteem is threatened. This may seem like a cruel procedure, but research participants had their self-esteem threatened by giving them false feedback that allowed them to believe that they consistently failed at a task while others consistently succeeded. The task involved matching the length of a line to a set of other lines, one of which was said to be the same length as the target line. Participants were told that they got the vast majority of these judgments either wrong or right. In addition to false feedback, they received consensus information that informed them how other participants had performed. They were told that either most people did the same as they did (84% of others performed equally well or poorly) or most people performed differently than they did (16% had done as poorly or as well).

Attributions were measured in two ways. First, participants were asked to account for their performance on the task by distributing 100 points among four possible causes: ability, effort, difficulty of the task, and luck. Second, attributions were assessed by scales that asked participants to rate (from "very unimportant" to "very important") the importance of each of these factors in contributing to performance. The striking finding was that participants attributed success on the task to personal ability and failure on the task to bad luck. The most threatening case was the one where participants, but few other people, were said to fail on the task. In this case, the smallest percentage of points (18%) was used by people to claim that personal ability had anything to do with their performance, and the greatest percentage of points (40%) was assigned to luck. This was a defensive attribution pattern, because people were ascribing their failure in the face of the success of others to external and unstable factors, and very little to stable, personal qualities.

Miller (1976) extended these findings by also using false feedback to threaten the self-esteem of research participants. Participants were asked to take a test purported to measure their "social perceptiveness." It was expected that participants did not want the test to reveal them to be socially awkward and clueless, so the experimenter could manipulate the potential threat of the feedback by telling people that they scored either poorly (high threat) or well (low threat). Rather than manipulating consensus as Stevens and Jones (1976) had done, Miller delivered this self-esteem threat by telling people either that the test used to measure their social perceptiveness was a well-established one, or that it was a new and unproven measure. It was predicted that the threat to self-esteem would be reduced by the fact the test was unproven, because participants could attribute poor scores to the inadequacy of the test. If they believed the test was valid, the only shelter from negative feedback would be provided by ego-defensive attributions.

The results provided evidence for the self-serving bias. When people received positive feedback, they attributed their test scores to internal factors. Negative feedback, however, was rationalized away through external attributions, and the esteem-protecting bias was greater when the threat was heightened. When participants believed the test was valid and well-established, they were even more likely to attribute their poor scores to luck and their good scores to personal ability.

Sicoly and Ross (1977) obtained similar results. In their study, participants were given false feedback that led them to believe that they either succeeded or failed at a task. They then rated how much personal responsibility they felt they deserved. However, they also then received (false) feedback from an observer (actually another student who worked for the experimenters) that informed the person how much personal responsibility the observer thought the person deserved. Sometimes the observer said that the person was more responsible than the person him-/herself stated; other times the observer reported seeing the person as less responsible. Replicating the results of the other studies, participants made internal attributions for their successes and external attributions for failures. The new twist concerned what people thought about the observers. Here again, there were signs of ego protection and enhancement. When the observer stated that the person was responsible for his/her success, the observer was seen as accurate (ego enhancement). However, when the observer stated that the person was responsible for his/her failure, suddenly the observer was judged to be less accurate than when the person was said to be not responsible for the same failure (ego protection). Thus attributions provide protection and shelter from threatening feedback.

Shelter from the Storm and Motivated Skepticism

Taylor and Brown (1988) describe a variety of ways in which people are sheltered from esteem-damaging feedback. First, because of the norms of interpersonal communication, people do not typically provide each other with scathing (or even mildly negative) feedback. *Feedback is typically positive, and when negative, it is sugar-coated* (Rosen & Tesser, 1970). This is partly what makes the job of a mentor so difficult. A mentor may often need to be critical when others choose not to be; he/she must criticize when people have been accustomed to being praised. Of course, praise is part of the job of mentor as well, but it is less salient than the negative comments, which may come as a shock to a person sheltered behind a wall of positive illusions. Second, *people choose acquaintances and friends with similar views*, thus reinforcing their own opinions and keeping away dissenting views. Third, people promote positive illusions in how they handle negative feedback when it is present. Given that most utterances are somewhat ambiguous, and that most feedback is open to interpretation, *people have a tendency to see ambiguous feed-*

back in the most positive light. If feedback is unambiguous and negative, it is ignored. And even if negative feedback is taken to heart, it has a habit of not planting roots there; its effects are only temporary. Beliefs about the self can change radically in the short term, but tend to drift back to their original state. Finally, if people are unable to ignore the feedback, *they opt to denigrate the source of the negative feedback* by labeling it either as inaccurate ("I need a second opinion") or as coming from a tainted source ("My mentor is a jerk!").

Ditto and Lopez (1992) examined precisely these types of motivated strategies for how people handle positive and negative information. They argue that one way people maintain their positive view of the self (and ward off negativity) is through *motivated skepticism*—a tendency to be skeptical and critically examine information they do not want to receive, yet to readily accept (with fairly little critical examination) information they are happy to receive. For example, the 2000 Presidential election in the United States was so close that at 2:00 A.M. EST on election night, it seemed that the (as yet unknown) results from the state of Florida would yield the overall election winner for the Presidency. When Democrats were eventually told that the Florida vote count revealed extremely (unusually) close results, but that these were not in favor of their candidate, Al Gore, motivated skepticism ensued. Surely there must be some way to critique such a close outcome and perhaps find errors that would overturn it? As it turned out, the skeptical approach did reveal that the state of Florida had prepared for such an eventuality. Given that election returns always have a degree of error, when an election is as close as that particular election was, the law demands an immediate recount using the same techniques. The Democrats did not even need to do anything, because skepticism is built into the way the system operates for election returns that fall within the margin of error. If the margin is still less than 1% of a difference after this initial recount (using the same procedures), the law allows for either of the candidates to be skeptical of the counting procedures and ask for a more thorough counting of the votes using a different procedure. Democrats were motivated to pursue this option and see whether more accurate counting techniques would alter the finding in favor of what they were motivated to see as the result.

However, when Republicans were eventually told that George W. Bush had won the initial count in Florida, but by less than 1%, jubilation ensued. What also followed was an aggressive campaign to resist any recounting of the votes, with Republican officials actually blocking any recount long enough to allow the deadlines for recounting established by the law to be missed. There was motivated skepticism in that they refused to believe the procedure for counting votes could have been faulty (even though the law anticipates that such flaws exist, and allows for recounts). Hence a bizarre scene of motivated skepticism played out on the national stage, with both groups seeking shelter from a storm of negative outcomes. Democrats did all they could to be skeptical of what they labeled an ambiguous result. Republicans did all they could to convince us not to produce for them a negative outcome, and instead to convince us that this ambiguous result was clear and diagnostic—that it had already provided the information and closure we needed. (Keep in mind that skepticism is not always a bias. Sometimes it is correct to be skeptical of a negative outcome. Rather than being biased, it allows for justice to be served and an incorrect decision to be overturned. This is the function of retrials in courts of law, of video replay rulings in football games, and of customer service offices at banks where one's account may have had money incorrectly deducted or service fees incorrectly charged.)

The strategies of motivated skepticism seen in the 2000 Presidential race could have been easily predicted from the findings of Ditto and Lopez (1992). To illustrate that people receiving positive news will uncritically accept it (see it as valid), and that people receiving negative news will challenge it (see it as invalid), they had research participants receive either negative or positive (actually fictitious) news about their health. This may also sound like a cruel procedure, but some participants were led to believe that they lacked an enzyme that would make them susceptible to pancreatic disorders later in life. Others were led to believe that they had sufficient levels of this (actually fictitious) enzyme. The feedback was provided by a "chemically coated" test paper the color of which, upon contact with a person's saliva, would reveal whether the person had the enzyme or not. What were people's cognitive reactions to this information? As predicted, people given the bad news exhibited a defensive pattern of responding. Participants led to believe they had an enzyme deficiency rated this deficiency as a less serious medical disorder than people who believed they had the enzyme. Furthermore, "enzyme-deficient" people saw this deficiency as a fairly common disorder and also saw the saliva test as being inaccurate. However, despite thinking that the test was less accurate, these people were also more likely to engage in the equivalent of "getting a second opinion" by taking the saliva test multiple times to make sure the results were reliable. These people also spent more time before making their decisions about how serious the disease was and how common it was, suggesting that they were analyzing their situation more thoroughly than people who received a clean bill of health. Ditto and Lopez also found that participants who believed they had the enzyme deficiency generated far more alternative explanations for the test results than people who had received a positive test result. Negative feedback triggered motivated skepticism and a more thorough cognitive analysis of the information.

Cognitive Dissonance Reduction

Dealing with negative and aversive thoughts about the self is the primary concern of social psychology's most well-known phenomenon—*cognitive dissonance*. The premise of cognitive dissonance theory (Festinger, 1957) is that when people experience an inconsistency between two cognitions, this causes an aversive drive state (similar to hunger or thirst) that people are motivated to eliminate. To eliminate this state, they must restore consistency between the discrepant cognitions. As an example, receiving negative feedback about the self represents a case of a person having discrepant cognitions: He/she desires a positive view of the self, but has just received negative information about the self. This discrepancy between the two cognitive elements is not ignored or dismissed by the person; instead, it is experienced as aversive and disturbing. It motivates him/her to reconcile these discrepancies and remove the state of dissonance. However, dissonance reduction is *only* motivated when the level of dissonance rises to the point where it is experienced as aversive to the person. What determines the magnitude of the dissonance? One central factor is the importance of the dissonant elements to the self-concept. A person may receive discrepant information, but unless it matters to the person, he/she will not be motivated to reduce the dissonance, because the dissonance will not otherwise be experienced as particularly aversive. This leads to the prediction that people with high self-esteem should experience dissonance more powerfully than people with low self-esteem, due to a greater tendency to expect positive things to happen to the self and for negative consequences to be interpreted as dissonant (e.g., Aronson, 1968; Stone, 2001).

In discussing the reduction of dissonance, Festinger (1957) proposed two general routes toward removing the aversive state. First, one could eliminate the negative behavior that is serving as the source of one of the discrepant cognitions. For example, if one has been receiving negative feedback, one could change one's behavior so that one acts in a way that will result in positive feedback. However, behavior change is not always easy (or possible). If one could act in a way that would result in positive feedback, presumably one would have acted that way initially. Festinger used the example of a person who smokes. Such a person clearly knows that this behavior is bad for health, so there is dissonance: The person engages in a behavior that produces cognitions ("This behavior leads to cancer") that are aversive and dissonant with other cognitions (such as "I want to be healthy"). Does the smoker simply change his/her behavior and stop smoking? No. Behavior change is difficult, and dissonance must be reduced some other way.

The other way one can reduce dissonance and stop experiencing negative and aversive states relating to the self is by justifying or rationalizing the discrepant act and attempting to accommodate the undesirable behavior. Rather than changing what one does, one changes what one thinks about one does! This is a *rationalization*. According to the movie *The Big Chill*, rationalizations are the most important thing people do—even more important than sex! As one character asks, "Ever go a week without a rationalization?" Rationalizing a behavior that causes dissonance with one's sense of self as positive can be accomplished in several ways. First, one can *recruit cognitions that are consistent with the discrepancy*. Rather than thinking about the negative consequences of having failed at a task (as such thoughts are discrepant with other cognitions about the self), the person receiving failure feedback can recruit thoughts about the positive social benefits of having tried a new activity and of having shown an openness to new experiences (as such thoughts are consistent with other cognitions about the self). Second, one can *change one's attitude so that the two cognitions are no longer seen as discrepant*. One may fail at a task, but one can change one's attitude about how one should have performed on the task. If I convince myself that this is a task I should not be good at, then the failure is no longer seen as discrepant with my cognitions. Third, one may shift focus away from a dissonant act and bolster self-esteem through drawing from a vast resource of positive information about the self, *affirming one's sense of self as positive through thoughts in some other, unrelated domain* (distracting attention away from the dissonance and toward one's positive qualities). Finally, one can engage in *trivialization*, in which a dissonant behavior is seen as insignificant and meaningless. Thus one may get negative feedback, but can decide either that the feedback is wrong and stupid, or that the task itself is unimportant and not really relevant to the self. All these styles of rationalizing negative outcomes can bolster and protect self-esteem.

A thorough review of dissonance theory is clearly not the present goal. The objective here is simply to convey how these processes of rationalization and justification are used by people to maintain unrealistically positive views of the self. Dissonance researchers have expended great effort to disentangle when and why one strategy of dissonance reduction is used over another (e.g., Stone, 2001). Let us simply look at one or two illustrations of how rationalization can protect self-esteem and bias the types of attitudes and impressions that we form about the self and others. Consider the first dissonance experiment that was published. Festinger and Carlsmith (1959) asked participants to engage in a mind-numbingly boring task for a long period of time, and paid some of them $20 to do so and some of them $1. They then asked these participants to tell a group of their peers that the experiment was fun and enjoyable. After doing this, the initial participants were asked for their own impressions of the task. One might think that the people paid $20 might have enjoyed the task more, since they received greater reinforcement for having performed the task. But, amazingly, Festinger and Carlsmith found the very opposite: People who had been asked to perform an extremely boring task later provided impressions of the task that indicated it was not boring, but only if they had been paid poorly to do the task! Having created a discrepancy between their initial attitude ("This task is boring") and a behavior that could not be rescinded (telling other people a boring task was fun), *people changed their attitudes.* (But they did so only if they freely chose to perform the act and had no other rationale for having elected to as they had.) Why would they do such a thing? Given no external justification (such as having been handsomely rewarded) for having acted in a discrepant way, they eliminated the dissonance by convincing themselves they liked the boring task. Rather than review hundreds of other studies that illustrate how people change impressions and attitudes to bring them in line with discrepant actions, let us now move toward examining two other illustrations of how unrealistically positive views of the self are maintained that also grow out of the dissonance phenomenon.

One such method, as discussed above, is affirming that one is a good person by focusing on dimensions other than those arousing the dissonance. Steele (1988) proposed that when cognitive dissonance occurs, people are not merely experiencing a specific type of discrepancy between two cognitions in a given domain, but a threat to the integrity of their entire belief system about the self. Steele asserted that the integrity of the self-system can be restored by a change in attitudes (as has been shown in over 100 dissonance experiments, starting with Festinger & Carlsmith's [1959]), but that it can also be restored by calling upon other positive aspects of the self-concept when a person is feeling self-threat or experiencing dissonance—engaging in a process of *self-affirmation*. The person who receives negative feedback can act like the *Saturday Night Live* character Stuart Smalley and think, "I am a good brother, a smart guy, and darn it, I like myself." For example, Steele and Lui (1983) had participants act in a way that violated their attitudes. They found that these people, as dissonance theory would predict, changed their attitudes so that their attitudes became more consistent with the behavior that was performed. However, other participants were allowed to affirm an important component of their self-system before having attitudes measured. They reasoned that this process of self-affirmation would restore the threat to the self-system. If such people then had their attitudes toward the dissonance-arousing behavior measured, they should no longer feel compelled to change these attitudes. This was precisely what was found. Because these participants had handled the threat to the self-concept through self-affirmation, the negative behavior that had been engaged in was now virtually powerless.

Another method for dealing with negative feedback and maintaining a positive self-view that has been mentioned above is the process of trivialization. The purpose of trivialization is to reduce the importance of the dissonant elements, thereby reducing the motivation to engage in dissonance reduction. Simon, Greenberg, and Brehm (1995) reasoned that changing an attitude as a means of dealing with dissonance is going to be hard to do if people are reminded of how important that attitude is to them, or if that attitude is made salient to them. A better strategy for dealing with the threat to a positive self-view is to change people's impression of the feedback—to trivialize the importance of the domain in which they have received negative feedback, or to denigrate the particular person providing the feedback. Simon and colleagues illustrated these self-esteem-protecting functions of trivialization in an experiment. Some students were reminded of their attitudes against a policy proposing that there should be a university-wide comprehensive exam as a requirement for graduation. Other students were not reminded of their attitudes toward this proposed policy (but held them just as forcefully). What was the dissonance manipulation (or threat to the positive sense of self) in the study? Students were asked to write essays that favored implementing the very comprehensive exams that the experimenters knew these students opposed. How did the students deal with the dissonance of having endorsed a policy (the discrepant behavior) that violated their own values? Participants who were not reminded of their attitudes on this issue resolved the discrepancy by altering their attitudes, suddenly indicating that they were actually more in favor of such exams than they had indicated weeks in advance, when their attitudes were previously measured. However, people who had been reminded of their attitudes from weeks before did not currently alter those beliefs. Instead, they chose a trivialization strategy for handling this threat to a positive sense of self. They were more likely to rate the issue of comprehensive exams as less important. Rather than changing their attitude toward the issue, they trivialized the issue and said that it was not so important to them.

Defensive Pessimism and Self-Handicapping

Another global strategy for defending self-esteem is to develop a chronic tendency to prepare for and expect the worst. If people expect bad things to happen, they have a ready-made excuse for failure that they are well prepared to use as a rationalization. People can build walls of negative expectancies that can serve to shelter them from the possibility of negative feedback. Two such strategies that have been explored by social psychologists are reviewed next. The first is called *defensive pessimism*.

Have you ever met a person (maybe you are such a person) who worries after every test that he/she has failed? The person complains before any major event that it will go poorly, proclaiming, "I will not succeed, I am doomed." What usually frustrates others about such people is that they are not doomed. In fact, more often than not, they do better than most people. Their fears were unwarranted. But were these fears useless? Or did the fears motivate them to work extra hard to deal with the eventual task, thus making them well prepared for it and less likely to fail? Many life tasks (goals pursued over a long period of time that are central to a person's motivational system), such as doing well academically, are often confronted with difficulties, frustrations, anxieties, and self-doubts, and the individual's style of appraising these hindrances leads to a typical pattern of goals aimed at overcoming these obstacles (Cantor & Fleeson, 1991, 1994). Take as an example college students like the one described above, who worry about their abilities and the possibility of experiencing failure. Rather than trying to maintain a positive sense of self and ward off the negativity of possible failure by seeking reassurance from others, these students prepare for the possibility of failure by obsessing about the failure itself. They embrace the idea of impending failure so fully that it motivates them to overprepare and, in so doing, to avoid failure. These people try to meet their challenges by mentally enacting worst-case scenarios. Norem and Cantor (1986) called this strategy *defensive pessimism*; being pessimistic about the future keeps negative outcomes at bay and actually serves to defend the self against failure. Indeed, some people turn defensive pessimism into a style of life, imagining the worst-case scenario to every situation so as to protect the self from doom.

Sometimes people do more than imagine the worst-case scenario to defend the sense of self and promote positive illusions. Sometimes people actually put themselves in bad situations to defend the sense of self. That is, we have already seen that external attributions for negative outcomes are able to promote positive illusions. Thus, to the extent that it is easy to form an external attribution for a negative outcome, the easier it will be not to have self-esteem placed at risk. Thus, ironically, people may do things that increase their chance of failure just so they can have a good excuse to account for their failure. *Self-handicapping* is said to occur when people actively try to "arrange the circumstances of their behavior so as to protect their conceptions of themselves as competent, intelligent persons" (Jones & Berglas, 1978, p. 200). Jones and Berglas (1978) claim that this is one reason people turn to alcohol: They use it to create an impediment that removes responsibility for negative outcomes. Imagine the athlete who gets drunk the night before a big game, or the student who claims to be sick before every big presentation (or stays up too late studying so that exhaustion impedes test performance). These people have created external causes for failure, thus protecting themselves from being held personally responsible for that failure if it were to come. For the drunk athlete, the creation of the excuse actually increases the chances of needing an excuse, because it makes the person more likely to fail. In the case of the student who claims to be sick, he/she has created an excuse that will account for potential failure. This is less extreme than performing a behavior that will potentially cause failure, but effective just the same (so long as the student can convince both him-/herself and others that the excuse is legitimate).

Berglas and Jones (1978) provided evidence for the self-handicapping strategy. Research participants were asked to provide answers for extremely difficult questions that they probably had to guess at. However, they then got false feedback informing them that they did wonderfully on the test. After being given feedback that must have seemed miraculous to them, participants were asked again to answer similar types of questions. This created a conundrum: How often could they expect to be lucky and get these difficult questions correct? Having created a context where the individuals must be contemplating failure, the experimenters then introduced a manipulation to detect what types of strategies people would adopt to deal with their fears. Would they attempt to place themselves in the best possible mental state to make their chances for success optimal, or would they create impediments that would allow them to rationalize away any subsequent failure? To examine this, participants were next informed that the researchers were concerned with studying the impact of drugs on intellectual performance. Participants were then offered a choice between two perfectly harmless drugs—one of which would supposedly facilitate intellectual performance, while the other would interfere with it. The results revealed that participants chose the self-handicapping strategy; they preferred to take a drug that would clearly diminish the possibility for success, thus providing an escape route for self-esteem in the event that failure should strike.

Unrealistic Optimism about the Future

People never like to think that negative events will happen to them. It would be dysfunctional to dwell on the probability that people get divorced, develop leukemia, are murdered, personally experience terrorist attacks, suffer from depression, or are victims of rape (yet all of these things have happened to people I know). It would hardly be a bias if people skewed thoughts about their future away from such negative events. But just because people choose to accentuate the positive, this does not mean they can accurately forecast the extent to which their future actually will be positive. There is a difference between being optimistic and being unrealistically positive in predicting what the future holds in store. This unrealistic optimism is first reflected in a bias that is similar to one discussed earlier. We have seen not only that people see themselves as possessing positive traits, but that they believe they possess more of these traits than the average person. Similarly, people see their future as full of positive events; they report four times as many positive things as negative things awaiting them around the corner. We can add to this not only that people accentuate the positive when contemplating their own future, but that this fabulous future is not seen as universal. People estimate their opportunities for positive things (good salary, good job, etc.) as greater than those for their peers (Weinstein, 1980). Meanwhile, the reverse pattern is observed for negative events: People estimate the chances of negative events (car crash, crime victim, heart attack, etc.) as greater for their peers (Taylor & Brown, 1988).

Kunda (1987) has investigated the manner through which people manage to maintain these positive illusions about their future. This unrealistic optimism is said to spring forth from a process labeled *motivated inference*, whereby people (1) generate biased theories about the causes for positive and negative events, and (2) differentially evaluate information that has positive versus negative implications for the self. As Kunda (1987, p. 637) has stated, "the cognitive apparatus is harnessed in the service of motivational ends." Let us focus first on motivated inference in the form of *biased theory generation*—a process whereby people embrace positive causal explanations for their behavior by developing theories in which their personal attributes are seen as responsible for positive outcomes. Kunda has asserted that because these theories allow people to link their personal attributes and traits to the production of positive outcomes, it allows them to expect that their future is likely to be filled with positive events.

Biased Theories about Attributes and Outcomes

If people have theories that their attributes are responsible for positive outcomes, these allow for a feeling that control over future events lies within these personal attributes. And if people control the occurrence of future, positive outcomes, then it stands to reason that they should be optimistic about the future. A good example is that of a man about to marry who convinces himself that his attributes will shelter him from the high divorce rates that will claim the marriages of others. The beauty of this strategy is twofold. First, people are quite gifted at generating just about any theory of self to justify just about any outcome they would like. So the illusion is easy to maintain. Because the man about to marry would like his future to be one of marital bliss, he simply generates a theory that the attributes that produce marital bliss are the very attributes he already possesses. Second, this process allows people not merely to be optimistic about the future, but to feel the much-desired sense of control over their destiny. And with this illusion of control over positive future events comes unrealistic optimism for the future.

To illustrate the impact of causal theories on unrealistic optimism, Kunda (1987) had research participants assess their own attributes, rate how these attributes relate to a future event (marriage), and make predictions about their own success at such an event. Kunda first had participants read about a person who was either divorced or happily married, and who possessed one of two opposing sets of personality characteristics (either he was introverted, independent, nonreligious, and liberal, or he was extraverted, dependent, religious, and conservative). Their task was to decide how much those attributes were involved in producing the outcome of the person's marriage. Next, the participants rated the likelihood that their own future marriages would end in divorce. Finally, they rated the extent to which they possessed the same attributes as the person about whom they had read. The findings revealed that when participants shared an attribute with the person they had read about, then that attribute was seen as one that promoted a good marriage. In addition, information about the outcome of the person's marriage had an impact on the ratings: An attribute was more likely to be rated as good for a marriage if the person was said to have a good marriage (and the attribute was less likely to be linked to marital happiness if the person had been divorced). Thus people seemed to be developing a theory about the cause of a good marriage—namely, that it is caused by people who have certain traits. But, furthermore, people then used these theories to promote an optimistic view of their own future. If people knew that they had certain traits, they were more likely to conclude that those traits promote good marriages. Finally, even though participants were told that the divorce rate at the time was 50%, their estimated likelihood for their own marriages ending in divorce was 20% (thus illustrating the unrealistic optimism produced by the theory about how their own attributes would promote a good marriage).

Warding Off Links between Negative Outcomes and Attributes

According to Kunda's (1987) notion of motivated inference, there are two processes by which people establish unrealistically optimistic expectations for the future. Let us focus now on what Kunda called *differential evaluation of information*—a process whereby people are more critical of information that has negative implications for themselves and more accepting of information that favors them. People ward off negative explanations for their behavior and keep at bay information threatening to their self-concepts. We have already seen one manner in which people accomplish this in the research of Ditto and Lopez (1992) on motivated skepticism. Kunda further examined whether the ways in which people reason about and evaluate information can lead to unrealistically optimistic expectations for the future. Kunda argues that people see positive events as being caused by their own positive attributes. Furthermore, they must be able to believe that their attributes are not the cause of negative events. This creates a problem (which we might also call cognitive dissonance): If people see their positive attributes as the cause for positive events, what do they do when evidence to the contrary erupts in front of them? This should be dissonance-arousing.

Kunda (1987) asked research participants to read a supposed article in *The New York Times* about the negative effects of caffeine consumption and its (fictitious) link to a disease called fibrocystic disease. The disease was said to cause painful lumps in the breast that in the advanced stages were linked to breast cancer; it was described as being brought on by consuming caffeine in amounts equivalent to three or more cups of coffee per day. Caffeine was said to lead to the development of an increased concentration of a substance called cAMP, and this substance was claimed to provide the link among caffeine, fibrocystic disease, and cancer. When participants were asked to evaluate the evidence in the article in support of both a link between caffeine and the disease and a link between caffeine and cAMP, an interesting pattern of defensive processing emerged: Participants were divided into groups based on the amount of caffeine they consumed. Men did not see the disease as threatening, regardless of the amount of caffeine they consumed—because the disease was said to affect women only. As predicted, because they lacked a motive to be biased, the reasoning strategies used and the overall evaluation of the article did not differ for men who had high versus low amounts of caffeine consumption. But for women who consumed a lot of caffeine (relative to women who did not drink beverages high in caffeine content), this article was highly threatening. Such women saw the article as providing unconvincing evidence in support of a connection between caffeine and fibrocystic disease and between caffeine and cAMP. Here we see an interesting twist in positive illusions. Although they may be quite useful at preserving mental health by warding off negative thoughts of disease, death, and pain, these very acts of protecting the self from negative thoughts may lead one to be in greater danger of poor physical health, as signs of disease and scientific data are ignored and dismissed as irrelevant or inconclusive.

Predictions of a Bright Future and Affective Forecasting

Imagine how you would feel if you got the job of your dreams, found the perfect person to date or marry, had a number one single on the pop charts, or received a Nobel Prize (all of these positive events have happened to people I know). Positive events such as these would make you extremely happy and produce a life of joy, right? Just as would winning millions of dollars in a lottery? Yet lottery winners do not report greater happiness, and people with number one songs often find themselves later becoming stars of *Behind the Music*, with tales of loss, depression, and substance abuse. As Wortman and Silver (1989) reported, typical events do not have a lasting impact on well-being, and unusual events (like winning the lottery or losing a friend to cancer) have less of an effect on well-being than people expect. As we have already discussed, people have a tendency to maintain positive self-esteem, and this level of self-esteem, though temporarily altered by day-to-day events, is relatively unchanged over the long haul. When predicting their futures, or at least engaging in *affective forecasting* (forecasting or predicting future affective/emotional states), people seem to be inaccurate at judging the impact of both positive and negative events (Kahneman & Snell, 1992).

In regard to positive events, there is a tendency for people to believe that such events occurring in their future will provide them with far greater, more lasting joy than they actually do. That is, people show a *durability bias* in predicting the power of positive events; *durability* in this context refers to the fact that the positive consequences of such events for emotional well-being are thought to be far more powerful and long-lasting than reality reveals them to be. Although people may be correct in predicting that some event will be positive (e.g., they correctly guess that having a favorite team win the World Series or getting a good job will make them happy), they cannot adequately gauge the duration, power, and impact of such events (Gilbert, Pinel, Wilson, Blumberg, & Wheatley, 1998).

Gilbert and colleagues (1998) discuss a variety of reasons for this overly positive view of the impact of positive events. First, people misconstrue what a positive event will entail. For instance, when we imagine getting a number one song on the charts, we might not predict the ensuing pressure from the record company and fans, a relentless touring schedule that taxes our physical and mental abilities, or a disrupted home life. A second reason for the bias is described by what Schkade and Kahneman (1997) call the *focusing illusion*, whereby people making estimates about their future happiness after an event (such as becoming a pop star) overly focus on the event in question and disregard a myriad of other future events that will also occur. Thus aspects of pop stardom may be positive (e.g., fame, money), but the future will also mix in loss of fame, loss of money, failed romantic relationships, deaths, and breaches of trust by friends. Overall, forecasts of future affect will be skewed by a focus on positive and a neglect of negative events.

Not all forecasts of the future are excessively positive. If people are told that some negative event will happen (such as the death of a parent), and are asked to forecast how lasting (durable) the damage will be, they also display a tendency to exaggerate the impact of the event. Of course, since people have a bias against seeing negative events in their future, the appearance of this bias may depend on their first being forced to confront the inevitability of the negative event. But when they do forecast the impact of negative events, the durability bias is observed. The causes of the durability bias in forecasting the impact of positive events reviewed above would also be causes of this bias in forecasting reactions to negative events. Ironically, one further cause of durability bias in forecasting negative (not positive) events is positive illusions!

How might it be, you may ask, that having positive illusions can lead people to overestimate the impact of a negative event on their future affect and well-being? Gilbert and colleagues (1998) suggest that this occurs because although people use positive illusions to ward off negative feelings, they do not realize they do so. These authors make an analogy between the positivity bias that promotes well-being in mental life and the immune system that promotes well-being in the physical health of the body. Just as the immune system wards off disease, the mental immune system promotes mental health through warding off negative self-views. However, if the mental immune system is to work, Gilbert and coleagues argue that it must work silently and somewhat outside of awareness. If people knew they were engaging in the types of positive illusions reviewed above—selectively ignoring negative information, rationalizing away inconsistencies, attributing their own positive and negative actions and outcomes in grossly divergent ways—the power of the positive illusion would be gone. A good illusion requires sleight of hand, and once the trick can be seen, the illusion is gone. For positive illusions to be successful as a psychological immune system, people must be able to neglect the fact that such an immune system is at work and is propping up psychological well-being. Gilbert and colleagues refer to this as *immune neglect*, and assert that it is a powerful cause of durability bias when the impact of negative events is being forecast.

Gilbert and colleagues (1998) examined this issue by asking assistant professors to forecast their affect if they were to be denied tenure. They then compared these predictions against how people actually felt after being granted or denied tenure (by tracking down former assistant professors who had been granted or denied tenure by the same university as the people doing the forecasting were seeking it from). Forecasters predicted that they would be happier in the 5-year period following getting tenure than in the same 5-year period following being denied tenure. In actuality, people who had attained tenure were no happier in this 5-year period (or at least did not report being any happier) than people who had been denied tenure. Another experiment by Gilbert et al. highlighted the role of immune neglect in producing this bias. If, while forecasting future affect, people fail to consider that their positive illusions will have an impact on their actual affective experiences, then they should predict that their affect will be the same, regardless of whether there is an obvious and easy rationalization for the negative event. Research participants were asked to rate their affect after being rejected by a prospective employer. Some participants gave these ratings by forecasting (imagining) how they would feel; others gave ratings after actually going through a mock interview and being given the negative feedback. In addition, the experiment manipulated how easy or hard it was for positive illusions to be used to rationalize the event. Some participants were told that the decision was being made by one person who was not highly qualified; the other participants were told that the decision was made by a skilled team.

In support of the notion that immune neglect is at work in biasing estimates of future affect, people who forecast their affective reactions believed they would feel equally bad regardless of whether a rejection was caused by an individual or a skilled team, and that this negative affect would persist. Yet people who actually experienced rejection felt better as time progressed. This was especially true when an individual provided the negative feedback, because the person receiving the feedback used positive illusions unknowingly to ward off the negativity by attributing it to the bias of the individual.

Implicit Self-Esteem

For the past 10 (at least) years, fans have been entertained between the innings at Yankee stadium in New York by a subway "race," shown on the monitors at the stadium, with the fictional race being held among the various trains that take people to the stadium. People cheer for the train that they took to the game to win the race, even though they know (or think they know) that they do not really care which train wins. Perhaps one reason they cheer for the train they took to the game is that the train is a small reflection of who they are. Perhaps they live on the East Side, and the 4 train represents this choice. Perhaps they arbitrarily decided to walk west from Fifth Avenue and take the D train; despite being arbitrary, this reflects a decision they made (they could have gone east to take the 4 train), so they cheer for the D train. It seems from this example that positive regard for the self can extend itself even to things that seem loosely (at best) relevant to the self. You would probably not imagine that you would think better of someone just because he/she happened to have the same birthday as you. But research, remarkably, reveals that this is precisely how people react. When research participants were falsely told that Rasputin shared their birthday, Rasputin was rated more favorably than he otherwise was (Finch & Cialdini, 1989). Miller, Downs, and Prentice (1998) found that people were more cooperative with an opponent in a Prisoner's Dilemma game if the opponent shared their birthday. Positive regard for the self can exert itself in ways we never imagined possible, even in cheering for a subway train.

Given the assumption that the need for self-enhancement is fairly ubiquitous, you may have already started to wonder just how conscious and effortful the strategies are that people use to promote positive illusions. Greenwald and Banaji (1995) answer this by proposing that self-esteem has implicit (automatic) influences on how people think. People are so skilled at being self-serving that they are able to promote their positive self-views without trying to do so and without knowing they are doing so. Hetts and Pelham (2001) distinguish between two types of implicit effects of self-esteem. In the first type, the self-esteem itself is explicit (people know they desire positive self-views), but the impact it has is outside conscious awareness. For example, people probably do not realize just how common it is that their positive self-views influence the manner in which they evaluate information (e.g., Ditto & Lopez, 1992; Kunda, 1987). Yet they still may know that they feel positively about themselves. Hetts and Pelham identify a second type of self-esteem, one that is implicit. They argue that people develop automatic, positive evaluative reactions to the self—positive attitudes to the self that unknowingly get triggered any time they come into contact with any feature remotely reminiscent of the self. This implicit positive self-regard then influences how they evaluate others who possess these features (even Rasputin). Thus, *in addition to the implicit influence of explicit self-esteem, there are implicit influences of implicit self-esteem*, such as when people unknowingly favor someone simply because he/she shares their birthday, or cheer for a train line because it is mildly representative of the self.

If implicit self-esteem represents the automatic activation of positive and negative self-relevant affect, it stands to reason that people who have had fewer positive experiences over their lives would have a lowered sense of implicit self-esteem. A person who is born in close proximity to an important cultural event, such as Christmas Day, may suffer from a lifetime of diminished excitement and praise (and presents) on his/her birthday. This should, if the theory is correct, lead these people to have lower implicit self-esteem than people born at other times of the year. And this was exactly what Hetts and Pelham (2001) found in one study: People whose birthdays fell within 1 week of Christmas had lower implicit self-esteem than people in general. And, as we would require of the theory, this lowered implicit self-esteem was not found for people whose families did not celebrate Christmas, such as Jews, Muslims, and atheists.

Hetts and Pelham (2001) review startlingly powerful results of implicit positive self-esteem. People evaluate things associated with the self more positively than things not linked to the self, even if the association to the self is extremely subtle. For example, Koole, Dijksterhuis, and van Knippenberg (2001) found people show a preference for the letters of the alphabet that represent their initials (the "name letter effect"; Nuttin, 1985). In addition, people prefer the numbers in their birthday to other numbers (Kitayama & Karasawa, 1997). Implicit self-esteem even has an impact on life decisions that are not at all trivial. Hetts and Pelham report that people are more likely to marry others with whom they share initials; Pelham, Mirenberg, and Jones (2002) found people to be more likely to settle in places that have a resemblance to their name (such as more Pauls living in St. Paul and more Marys in Maryland). And this is not because people from those places are more likely to give those names to their children. Instead, people are moving to such places. Pelham and colleagues also found a statistically significant relationship between occupations and names (such as more people named Dennis being dentists, more folks named Lawrence being lawyers, and more scientists named Gollwitzer doing research on goals).

THE NEED FOR CONTROL

We have now spent a good amount of time reviewing support for the notion that people process information about themselves (and others) in a self-serving, and a self-enhancing, manner. However, Chapter 1 has outlined several needs that are said to guide the manner in which people process information about the world; a need for self-enhancement (a positive self-view) is only one of these. People also need to feel as if they have control over their social world.

Control and Overattribution

Heider (1944) asserted that traits, as enduring characteristics, provide a complete and stable way of characterizing others—one that affords predictability and control. This need for control and predictability led Heider to believe that there is an unusual contribution from traits in people's impressions of others. This link between the need for control and traits leads to a logical prediction: People particularly concerned with control should be even more prone to using traits as a way of characterizing people than is usually found.

Miller, Norman, and Wright (1978) tested this prediction. Research participants were led to expect to interact with a person about whom they were forming attributions. As hypothesized, when an interaction was anticipated, there was a heightened need to predict what the other person was like, and this promoted the use of traits and attitudes when participants were evaluating the person who would soon become an interaction partner. A later study (Moskowitz, 1993a) used a more subtle manner of examining this issue, rather than creating momentary states of heightened need for control, such states could chronically reside in particular types of people. If such people could be identified, and if traits were used by such people to attain control, then these individuals should be more likely to have developed a cognitive strategy of making sense of the behavior of others through inferring traits. Those who chronically desired structure would presumably be more practiced at, and interested in, inferring traits from behavior than in suspending judgment or forming more complex impressions that would include situational factors. It was found that the extent to which people formed spontaneous trait inferences was determined by their chronic needs for prediction, control, and structure. Given the centrality of control for making predictions and seeing the world as stable, does the need for control lead to pervasive types of perceptual biases?

Exaggerated Perceptions of Personal Control

Since we humans do not wish to feel as if we are subject to random and haphazard forces that are beyond our control, the control need plays an important role in self-assessment as well as in interpersonal perception. This feeling that our destiny is ours to make is promoted by attributions allowing us to feel that what happens to us is a product of what we would like to happen to us. This works somewhat differently when we are judging others, since they are seen as responsible for what happens to them, both the good and the bad. This notion of justice as dictated by the control need recurs below in the discussion of the *just-world hypothesis*. For now, let us focus on establishing the pervasive tendency to desire control and the impact the control need has on self-judgment.

The control need as applied to the self would suggest that since we only want good things to happen to us, anything good that happens must be caused by us. And since negative events are not desired, then accepting responsibility for causing them would reflect that we are not effective at bringing about the consequences we desire; a control need would dictate that negative consequences would be ascribed to powerful external forces that are beyond our control. This illusion produces the same pattern as the self-serving bias, but is not necessarily caused by self-esteem enhancement. An illustration of the control need would be provided by an exaggerated sense of responsibility and internal attribution for events with positive consequences. Langer (1975) labeled this exaggerated perception of personal control the *illusion of control*. For example, Wortman (1975) found that people tended to see themselves as controlling outcomes they actually had no effect on whatsoever. Random outcomes (such as those occurring strictly due to luck) appeared to people as if they were the result of their own skill. In research illustrating this, each participant was told that two marbles were in a can, and that if one of them was picked the participant would receive a desirable prize. The trick was that only some of the participants were told in advance which marble would get them the desired prize. Furthermore, some of the participants were simply handed a marble, and others were allowed to reach into the can and blindly pick one. Despite the fact that there was no control at all in any of these scenarios, people who knew ahead of time that a particular marble represented a good prize, and who were allowed to blindly pick a marble (rather than being handed one), were more likely to see themselves as responsible for a good outcome (getting the marble that represented a prize) than the other participants.

Self-Verification

Swann (1990) has claimed that people are guided in their reasoning about the world by a motive to evaluate the self in a way that verifies and maintains existing self-views. Such a strategy may also be unrealistic and biased, except that rather than individuals' twisting existing information so that it promotes a positive view of the self, they twist it in a manner that promotes a confirmatory and consistent view of the self. Swann states that such *self-verification* emerges as an important strategy in evaluating the self because of its link to people's need to predict what will occur, and in so doing to verify that their own traits are responsible for (control) their outcomes:

> Self-verification theory assumes that people want to confirm their self-views *not* as an end in itself, but as a means of bolstering their perception that the world is predictable and controllable. From this perspective, self-verification processes are "warmed up" by a desire for prediction and control (rather than, e.g., a desire for self-enhancement). ... The desire for prediction and control presumably grows out of interpersonal (pragmatic) considerations as well as intrapsychic (epistemic) ones. From an epistemic perspective, stable self-conceptions act like the rudder of a ship, bolstering people's confidence in their ability to navigate through the sometimes murky seas of everyday life ... events that confirm people's self-conceptions fortify their feelings of security, and events that disconfirm their self-conceptions engender fears that they may not know themselves at all. (pp. 414–415; emphasis in original)

From this summary, we see that the need for control (and self-verification) develops out of people's more general epistemic need to avoid uncertainty and to have consistent and balanced cognitions (Dewey, 1929; Festinger, 1957; Heider, 1958; Osgood & Tannenbaum, 1955). James (1890/1950) described the fact that people attempt to maintain consistent views, even struggling to fit new information so it is seen as consistent with what they already believe, as the most important feature of their mental structure. He referred to this as "the principle of constancy in the mind's meanings" (p. 459). Of course, while keeping old knowledge unaltered, to be utilized time and again, is functional, James (1907/1991) did not believe that people were incapable of breaking from their set knowledge: "You listen to me now with certain prepossessions as to my competency, and these affect your reception of what I say, but were I suddenly to break off lecturing, and begin to sing 'We won't go home till morning' in a rich baritone voice, not only would that new fact be added to your stock, but it would oblige you to define me differently" (p. 74).

Swann (1990) has applied these notions of consistency and control to how people think about and evaluate information concerning the self. Thus, rather than solely being concerned with promoting a positive view, they seek to promote a stable and consistent view of the self. This does not mean that people are incapable of processing information that violates their prevailing self-views, or that they do not seek positive feedback. It simply means that people prefer positive feedback in domains of their life in which they think positively about themselves (e.g., "I am a good lover, so I must accept all information that supports that notion, and must reject any feedback that suggests otherwise as the rantings of a lunatic"). This also means that self-verification predicts that people actually *prefer to receive negative feedback in domains of their life where they know quite well that they have deficiencies* ("I know I am a terrible cook, and anyone who attempts to tell me I have done well must be patronizing me or engaging in ingratiating flattery"). Thus, rather than a bias toward a strictly positive future, the self-verification view proposed by Swann suggests a bias toward a future that people can control and predict, with such control obtained through *preserving* existing knowledge about the self, not promoting an overly positive and false view.

Evidence for self-verification was provided by Swann, Pelham, and Krull (1989). Research participants were first asked to identify their worst attribute—such as "I am unhappily out of shape." They were then informed that two observers had been watching them over the course of the experiment and that these observers had rated them on performance dimensions, such as the attribute they had just listed as their worst attribute. The participants also learn that one of the observers had rated them positively on this bad attribute, while the other observer had rated them negatively. Participants were then asked to pick one of these two observers to interact with in the next phase of the experiment. Rather than choosing the person who would enhance their self-view on the negative dimension, people instead chose the self-verifying person who had rated the person negatively on an attribute for which the person held a negative self-view.

A similar type of evidence for self-verification is attained by taking an individual-difference approach. People with low self-esteem (such as depressed people) should not seek to defend their esteem by bolstering it, but by verifying it. In support of this, Swann (1990) reported that depressed people did not show the defensive pattern observed in nondepressed participants in studies on positive illusions. Highly depressed people preferred to be evaluated by a person who thought poorly of them rather than a person who thought positively of them.

A Conflict among Motives?

We have now examined three different motives that push people in vastly different directions. However, the self-assessment (accuracy), self-verification, and self-enhancement motives need not be seen as adversaries. It is possible that one motive is triggered in some circumstances and in particular types of interpersonal interactions, whereas another motive becomes dominant in a different interpersonal interaction (or even in an interaction with the same person but in a different context). At times, the motives may even work in parallel, such as the situation described earlier where both the control motive and the self-enhancement motive lead people to attribute positive outcomes to the self.

Swann, Bosson, and Pelham (2002) examined the opposite scenario, where motives compete and conflict with each other. For example, imagine you are someone with a negative self-view in the domain of attractiveness. We have just reviewed how Swann and colleagues (1989) illustrated that people who feel as if they are not attractive may prefer not to receive feedback from others telling them that they are attractive. But this self-verification motive can run straight into a conflicting motive. For example, if you want to date or marry, you must hope that, despite your negative sense of personal attractiveness, your partner at least thinks you are attractive. Swann and colleagues (2002) examined how such goals linked to romantic relationships would influence self-verification goals that would typically lead a person who feels ugly to want to be seen as ugly.

Swann and colleagues (2002) hypothesized that such conflicts between goals would be handled by people with low self-esteem by limiting the number of dimensions on which they would allow themselves to be seen in a positive light (such as relationship-relevant domains). People should seek self-confirming evaluations in other dimensions. In addition, the apparent discrepancy between the feedback from a loved one and what a person would expect from the world at large could be handled by recognizing that different relationships require different interaction patterns and feedback. People should know it is important for their loved ones to see them as attractive. In support of this, Swann and colleagues found that participants who thought they were unattractive desired to receive positive evaluations of their attractiveness from dating partners, even though they desired to receive self-confirming evaluations from their dating partners on dimensions not related to attractiveness. And this type of positive feedback in specific domains was limited to specific relationships. Although it was acceptable for dating partners to call such people attractive, this type of positive feedback was not acceptable from partners in other close relationships, like friends and family.

Deserving What They Got: The Just-World Theory

Seeing the world as controllable requires a perception of justice at work in the world, so that people will get what is coming to them (e.g., Lerner & Miller, 1978). Without such a sense, the world would be viewed as in anarchy. In fact, for almost all events, positive or negative, people suppose a justice is at work in the universe, thus making these events seem reasonable and even necessary outcomes, given the behavior and intentions of the people affected. Sadly, a result of this form of the control motive is that people often blame victims. It is not uncommon for perceivers to hold rape victims accountable for being attacked; the perceivers use rationalizations such as "She was dressed suggestively," "She was flirting relentlessly," or "She has a history of promiscuity." Part of this may be due to correspondence bias: Bad acts are assumed to happen to bad people because of their stable bad qualities. But part of this blaming of victims comes from a need for control. Lerner (1965) explained this pattern of making attributions by positing that people have a need to believe in a *just world*. Random acts of violence, innocent people being made to suffer and die, and nasty bastards being rewarded with awards and money are events suggesting that the world is unfair, cruel, and unpredictable—a place where good people cannot be protected from harm and do not benefit from hard work and clean living. So we convince ourselves these outcomes were deserved.

Hafer (2000) argues that the belief in a just world serves an important function. The sense of control that such beliefs engender allow people to invest in long-term goals. Without such a belief, it would be foolish to do anything but act on immediate impulses and live for the moment. Exactly how people define justice in order to determine whether an outcome is just or not is beyond the scope of this chapter. Psychologists who speak of *procedural justice* emphasize the perception of justice in the procedures used by people to attain outcomes (e.g., Tyler, Degoey, & Smith, 1996), while psychologists who speak of *distributive justice* focus on whether outcomes are dispensed fairly and equitably (e.g., Walster, Berscheid, & Walster, 1973). Our concern is not with how people define justice, but with how they use their perceptions of justice (once formed) to maintain their belief in the controllability and predictability of their own futures. Attributions that allow people to perceive the world as just, therefore, allow them to believe in their commitment to and efforts to pursue their long-term goals. The negative side effect of this functional belief is that people blame innocent victims for terrible events that are outside the victims' control. For example, Lerner (1965) found that when research participants had been randomly selected to receive electric shocks, other research participants who learned of this denigrated these individuals. As if receiving shock was not bad enough, they had to suffer the injustice of being seen as responsible for this negative event, simply so that others might maintain the belief that the world is just. This is a sad irony of the control motive.

In order to test whether the belief in a just world is in fact linked to the need to remain future-oriented, and that this requires a belief that future events are controlled by and caused by people's chosen actions, Hafer (2000) posited that the belief in a just world should most strongly affect the types of attributions people make when they are highly concerned with long-term investments. When people's commitment to a long-term goal is weak, there should be little need for them to engage in strategies that promote the belief in a just world. Concern with long-term goals was manipulated in this experiment by having some of the participants write essays about their plans after graduating from the university, while others were simply asked to write a list of their current courses and extracurricular activities. All of the participants then watched a videotape where a student who was said to have contracted a sexually transmitted disease (STD) described to a counselor a variety of symptoms that indicated she was feeling depressed. Half of the participants were informed that the STD was the result of an accident, when a condom broke while the woman was having sex. Half of the participants were informed that the woman had contracted the STD because she had failed to use a condom at all when having sex. The question of interest was whether people would blame an accidental negative event on the innocent victim.

Hafer's (2000) results showed that when participants contemplated their long-term goals prior to seeing the video, the innocent victim was derogated to a greater extent than when goals had not been contemplated. This difference in how much the victim was derogated did not emerge when the woman was clearly responsible for her outcome (failing to use a condom at all). People not only disliked the innocent victim more when contemplating their own long-term goals; they also found her to be more blameworthy and responsible for her fate. Finally, people even dissociated themselves from the innocent victim, being more likely to say, "She is nothing like me." The belief in a just world leads people to a variety of strategies for blaming victims, thereby serving their own sense that their own future goals are attainable and controllable.

Transparency Illusion

On the 1965 Beatles album *Rubber Soul*, John Lennon and Paul McCartney wrote one song entitled "I'm Looking Through You" and another called "You Won't See Me." If you were to accept the proposition put forth by Lennon and McCartney in these songs, then you should believe you can easily see the traits of others, while simultaneously believing that others people do not see your qualities quite so well. In other words, you would exhibit the correspondence bias and think you see right through others (so that other people's behavior is evidence of who those people truly are, suddenly making them seem like totally different persons when they exhibit a wholly new behavior), but you fail to think that others are looking straight through you—in fact, others don't see the real you at all. But what is the evidence for this flip side to the correspondence bias? Should "You Won't See Me" be the flip side to "I'm Looking through You"?

People are likely to be correct in assuming that others are thinking about what they are like. For instance, just as you look at others and believe you can easily see the internal states and traits that have caused the other persons' behavior, you should assume that these others are doing the same to you. The question not yet addressed is whether people assume that when others are looking at them, they believe that the others can truly "see" them. Recent literature disagrees with the "You Won't See Me" proposition. Rather than assuming that others don't see "the real me," people instead have a pervasive tendency to overestimate the extent to which their internal states are easily seen by others. Egocentrism, combined with the need for control, leads to the belief that one's internal states, wants, desires, and goals are obvious to others. In other words, just as I'm looking through you, I tend to believe not that you won't see me, but that you are looking right through me. Thus if you are having a "bad hair" day, you are convinced it is the first thing others will notice. If you are feeling sad, yet have not told others, you will assume that your heart is on your sleeve and that your true self has bubbled to the surface, even though no discernible cues may actually be provided for others.

Vorauer (2001) has labeled this tendency to exaggerate the extent to which the self is believed to be clearly revealed to others as *transparency overestimation*. Vorauer defines this bias as a special case of person perception that involves *metaperceptions*, or people's beliefs about other people's beliefs and impressions about them (which are formed as a function of others' having observed their behavior). Egocentrism is invoked in this bias because people assume that others see and feel what they do, even if they are so focused on the self that they fail to provide the others with any relevant cues to their inner states. Control is invoked in this bias, because beliefs about how others see people are essential for making predictions about how the others will react and how an ensuing interaction with them will unfold. As Swann (1990) has illustrated, people look to others for feedback—especially at times of uncertainty, in order to restore feelings of control and reduce the tension associated with feelings of uncertainty. In addition, for people to make predictions about their own abilities, it is useful to get information from others that allow them to understand where they stand in relation to others. As stated by Vorauer, "this process, whereby people look to another person's reactions to get a sense of their skills and attributes and to develop personal standards, corresponds to the 'looking-glass self' advanced by Cooley (1902/1983)" (p. 261).

Vorauer and Claude (1998) examined the transparency illusion by focusing on people involved in a negotiation, because in a negotiation others must be able to read negotiators' objectives and intentions. The ability to communicate these internal states will be a dominant determinant of whether the negotiation is successful. If negotiators incorrectly assume that these states are clear to others, but this sense of the transparency of their position on an issue is greatly exaggerated, the negotiation will be doomed. For example, you might think that your adversary in a negotiation is being insensitive to your wishes and needs, when the problem actually is that you have not adequately told the adversary what you need. Thus your hostile reaction to your adversary is actually a result of your own miscommunication, born of transparency overestimation.

Vorauer and Claude (1998) examined whether negotiators believe that their adversaries can accurately deduce their goals (such as the goal to be cooperative vs. assertive) in the negotiation when in fact the adversaries are uncertain about what those goals may be. Participants were asked to negotiate a solution to an interpersonal problem that was known to be difficult and to have no easy resolution. The task asked participants to read about an interpersonal problem, offer their solution to the problem, and then read and evaluate the choices made by their partner in the negotiation. In reality, the partner was an experimenter, who carefully controlled the responses that were being provided. In addition, this entire process was being observed by other persons. The negotiators' belief that their goals were transparent to others was assessed by having the participants rate how well the observers were able to identify those goals, based on having perceived how participants responded during the negotiation. The true degree of transparency was calculated by having the observers actually judge the goals they believed were being reflected by the negotiators' responses. The results revealed a large overestimation of transparency. Participants believed that the observers would be able to discern their "true" objectives 60% of the time, yet in actuality the observers only correctly guessed the objective 26% of the time.

Gilovich, Savitsky, and Medvec (1998) explored the transparency illusion by looking at liars, not negotiators. How well are people able to predict whether their lies are transparent to others? People exaggerate their transparency here as well. For example, when participants in this research were asked to lie to others when answering questions (e.g., "What is your favorite type of music?"), their estimates of how well others could detect the fact they were lying was greatly exaggerated. Therefore, observers are not as good at detecting lies as people think they are. This is also true for lies of omission. If people attempt to conceal their emotions from others, failing to tell them how they truly feel about something, they fear that their true emotions will nonetheless become apparent. Savitsky and Gilovich (1998) found that people who were nervous when speaking in public exaggerated how nervous others thought they were. Despite trying to conceal anxiety, people still believe that this anxiety "leaks out" and reveals the hidden insecurity. But this is an illusion, as concealment of an emotional state typically works far better than the transparency illusion will allow people to believe.

Vorauer and Ross (1999) illustrated not only that people believe their opinions, emotions, and lies are transparent to others, but that they overestimate the perceived transparency of their personal attributes as well. These authors further demonstrated that transparency overestimation is exacerbated when people feel self-conscious or have a heightened sense of self-awareness. That is, if people overestimate the extent to which others can see their internal states, then the more accessible those internal states are to them, the more they will think others can see them. Self-awareness is known to heighten the accessibility of self-relevant information (Carver & Scheier, 1978). This has been shown in a variety of ways, and not merely by identifying types of people who have chronic states of heightened self-consciousness (e.g., Fenigstein, Scheier, & Buss, 1975). Even subtle manipulations, such as having people perform a task in front of a mirror or a camera, can heighten self-awareness and lead to the increased accessibility of self-knowledge (Duval & Wicklund, 1972). Vorauer and Ross utilized these facts to demonstrate that increased self-awareness would heighten the accessibility of self-relevant thoughts, and in so doing promote the transparency illusion.

The need for control is not the only motive capable of producing the transparency illusion. (And it should be noted that Vorauer [2001] explicitly states that it is quite possible that the illusion can be produced without any motive whatsoever, but simply from heightened self-awareness and the accessibility of self-relevant information.) As was argued in Chapter 1, the need to belong to social groups and affiliate with others is central to human nature (Baumeister & Leary, 1995), and such belongingness needs may also play a role in the development of illusions of transparency. They certainly create heightened concern with the perceptions of others. For instance, if you want to date someone or get promoted by your boss, you need to know what that person thinks of you in order to make them desire you in the way you wish for them to desire you.

BELONGINGNESS: GROUP-SERVING BIASES AND POSITIVE SOCIAL IDENTITY

The transparency illusion introduces the notion of *metaperception*—people's perceptions about the perceptions of others. This concern with reflecting on the self by looking through the mirror of others is not unique to psychology. Cooley's (1902/1983) notion of the *looking-glass self* and Mead's (1956) concept of the *significant symbol* both reflect the importance of individuals' looking to others to understand the social world. In fact, despite attempts to distinguish the need to attain meaning from the need to belong to social groups and affiliate with others, such social affiliation actually gives rise to meaning. This belief was central to William James's (1907/1991) notion of *pragmatism*: James defined truth as that which can be verified by others, and as knowledge functioning in a manner that allows people to navigate social interaction successfully. Hardin and Conley (2001, p. 1) have summarized this position that belongingness needs have quite an explicit impact on how people perceive the social world:

> Mead emphasized in particular the role of ongoing cooperative social interaction in the creation and maintenance of meaning. Mead's synthesis of self and society was also predicated on the necessity of human relationships for survival, but through a mechanism of organized exchange of social gestures and concomitant perspective taking. . . . Central to Mead's theory is the concept of the *significant symbol*, on which rests the human capacity for language and cognitive representation. The significant symbol is realized when an individual evokes in itself, by its gesture, the functionally identical response the gesture evokes in others. According to Mead, it is only through significant symbols realized in ongoing social interaction that people are able to remember the past, anticipate the future, and experience the present. From this perspective, mind cannot be separated from cooperative social action, but instead arises out of it.

Positive Social Identity

Belonging to social groups and affiliating with other people not only helps us to construct meaning; but reflecting on ourselves through the eyes of others also serves important identity functions. It is only through social comparisons that we may engage in self-evaluation (see Blanton, 2001), and it is through such evaluations that we can develop a positive sense of identity. Let's refer back to an example from Chapter 5. Think about a time when your grades were posted after an exam. Did you simply check to see how you had done, or did you compare your score against others? Why? Because a score is only seen as good or bad in relation to others (even if objectively you know the grade received was an A). But other people may serve as more than points of comparison. Other people may also be internalized to become a part of the self. As we seek groups of others to affiliate with and join for companionship and social bonding, these groups of others come to be seen as part of us. We develop a social component to the sense of self/identity; that is, our self-concept and self-esteem are linked to the social groups (e.g., families, friends, fraternities/sororities, religious organizations, political parties, sports teams) to which we belong (Tajfel & Turner, 1986). Just as we engage in social comparison to evaluate our performance against others, so too do we evaluate and compare the social groups to which we belong against other groups, hoping that these comparisons will reflect positively on our groups.

Thus we look to others for constructing meaning and self-evaluation; yet we also look to others, through the formation of social groups, to provide us with a sense of affiliation and belonging (Baumeister & Leary, 1995). This is basic to human existence. From the earliest moments of life, we enter into social groups—starting with families and religions, and evolving into ethnic and socioeconomic communities, school clubs and other affiliations, work groups, recreational groups, and many others. And by joining groups of others to satisfy the need to belong, we thereby link the self-concept to these groups and develop a complex, layered notion of the self that has the individual at its core, but a sphere of social influences that are essential to it as well. We develop a *social identity* and *collective esteem* to accompany our personal identity and self-esteem. Brewer (1991) sees each of us as in a constant state of juggling the need to assimilate with and join a variety of groups that will contribute to the self-concept, while at the same time attempting to maintain some sense of distinctiveness and uniqueness that defines us as more than just members of groups.

Just as we engage in self-enhancement processes to defend self-esteem and promote positive (and ward off negative) evaluations, the same type of defensiveness is used to enhance the esteem we derive from the groups with which we identify. When these groups are perceived as doing well through positive evaluations against other groups, it reflects positively on us. This creates a positive sense of self through promoting a positive social identity (e.g., Brewer, 1991; Tajfel & Turner, 1986) and what Crocker and Luhtanen (1990) called *high collective self-esteem* (self-esteem derived from the various groups or collectives with which we identify). As an example, when my son Ben was 1 year old, I described to a friend one day that Ben had just been ill and had vomited for the first time. The friend looked at her young daughter sitting next to her and proclaimed, "She is not the vomiting type." As if vomiting when struck by a virus was an attribute one could (or could not) choose to possess! This friend bolstered her own positivity by linking her identity to her child and then distancing that child from the negative attributes that other children (such as mine!) possess. It is in this type of reflexive, unconscious bolstering of and identification with significant others that social identity can promote a positive sense of self—one far more complex than that achieved from simply reflecting on our own accomplishments.

Indeed, when one of the social groups we identify with has succeeded at something, we take extra steps to highlight the fact that we are members of those groups. We use the behavior and status of the group to bolster the self; that is, we *bask in reflective glory* (BIRG) of the successes achieved by others with whom we identify. In support of this idea, Cialdini and colleagues (1976) found that university students altered the manner in which they dressed on the day following a victory by their football team in an intercollegiate game. Presumably fans can bolster a positive sense of self by wearing the hats and jerseys of their favorite sports teams after a victory, because this links the self to the social group and allows for the positivity associated with the achievement to extend from the group to the self. Just as BIRGing may occur after positive group events, downplaying a link to a group may occur after negative events.

Group Enhancement

> They take the Christians to be the cause of every disaster to the state, of every misfortune to the people. If the Tiber reaches the wall, if the Nile does not reach the fields, if the sky does not move or if the earth does, if there is a famine, or if there is a plague, the cry is at once, "The Christians to the Lions." Tertullian (Third century A.D.) . . .
>
> —ALLPORT (1954, p. 243)

This quote from an early Christian writer in Allport's (1954) *The Nature of Prejudice* highlights an essential ingredient in the study of how, why, and when social identity and group membership influence the types of attributions people form. To promote positive social identity, one's own group must appear in a positive light following a social comparison. This can be accomplished both by enhancing one's own group (in a manner similar to that described when discussing positive illusions) and by denigrating other groups (especially disliked or stereotyped outgroups). For example, attributions formed toward an outgroup may be negative and dispositional, even when the same behaviors performed by a member of the majority group are seen as externally caused (because of one's goal to be self-promoting). Outgroups get blamed for negative events, even events having nothing to do with them (see Allport's discussion of scapegoating), whereas one's own group is not seen as responsible for negative events. Heider (1958, p. 361) referred to this point in stating that "attribution depends on the value of the other person in the life-space. If we are inclined to disparage him we shall attribute his failures to his own person, his successes to his good luck or unfair practices. When Nietzsche says 'Success is the greatest liar,' he refers to this error in attribution." One's own positive behavior (and that of other ingroup members) is seen as a reflection of a positive disposition, while in disliked others it is seen as a fluke. Such an attributional style ensures that one's own group identity is not threatened by failures or shortcomings within the ranks, or by merit and virtue within the ranks of other groups.

Research in the area of stereotyping and prejudice has found support for this attributional bias, where the types of causal explanations people use to explain their own group's negative and positive outcomes are drastically different from the manner in which they assign responsibility to other groups. Taylor and Jaggi (1974) suggested that people would account for negative acts by their own group and positive acts by members of a disliked outgroup by using situational attributions to explain away the behavior. Similarly, they predicted that people would use dispositional attributions to account for positive behaviors performed by their own group and negative behaviors performed by members of other groups. This attribution style would allow them to preserve positive identity while helping to maintain negative stereotypes about disliked groups. Taylor and Jaggi's research was conducted in southern India with Hindu research participants. Participants read a series of stories that described positive and negative acts performed by Hindu (ingroup) or Muslim (outgroup) individuals, and then gave the causes for these events by completing attribution ratings. Hindus were found to make internal attributions for socially desirable behaviors performed by Hindus, but external attributions for undesirable behaviors. The reverse pattern was found when these Hindus were judging Muslims. Pettigrew (1979) dubbed this group-level version of what Ross (1977) had called the fundamental attribution error the *ultimate attribution error*. The bottom line is that motivation to see the self in a positive light can cause one to attribute the behavior of significant others to dispositional causes when those behaviors are positive (and to external causes when they are negative). Members of outgroups do not benefit from this attributional bias, and may in fact suffer from a similar bias that explains away their positive behavior (and blames them for negative behavior).

If defensive attribution, in which one is motivated to enhance esteem, is actually what causes such differential responding, then a pattern of outgroup-denigrating and ingroup-enhancing attributions should be heightened under conditions that facilitate and enhance the motive for self-esteem bolstering. In order to test this, Dunning, Leuenberger, and Sherman (1995) manipulated the extent to which esteem was threat-

ened by having participants either succeed or fail at a task just prior to making evaluations of others. In some cases, the other people who were being evaluated were similar
to the research participants, thus making evaluations of these "others" relevant to the
participants' own esteem. In other cases, the people being evaluated were dissimilar to
the participants. In this sense, the evaluations being formed were similar to the ingroup
and outgroup evaluations in Taylor and Jaggi's (1974) experiment. What Dunning and
colleagues found was that when self-esteem was threatened, participants restored their
positive sense of self through the types of attributions they made. As predicted, they
made more positive evaluations of the similar others than of the dissimilar others, but
only after failure (when esteem motives were high), not after a personal success. Fein
and Spencer (1997; see also Spencer, Fein, Wolfe, Fong, & Dunn, 1998) have made a
similar point in research examining implicit (automatic) responses. Essentially, their
argument is that the response of denigrating others when experiencing lowered self-
esteem is learned through experience and repetition, and eventually it comes to operate
automatically. In this research, thinking about the stereotypes of other groups was
shown to be a form of automatic self-affirmation. When research participants had experienced a threat to their identity, they were more likely to have the goal of repairing the
threatened self-image triggered. Their lowered state of self-esteem was repaired by stereotyping others and contemplating the others' negative characteristics.

Finally, Crocker, Thompson, McGraw, and Ingerman (1987) illustrated that the
ability for self-esteem threat to trigger defensive attributions was qualified by participants' chronic level of self-esteem. They examined individuals with low versus high
chronic levels of self-esteem who belonged to either high-status or low-status sororities.
The logic was that belonging to a low-status sorority would cause negative social comparisons and low collective esteem, and that this should trigger a defensive attribution
pattern. Members of low-status sororities should be more likely to try to bolster their
group's image and denigrate other groups, whereas members of high-status groups
should not. What the researchers found was that this defensive attribution pattern was
exactly how people with high self-esteem responded. If participants both had high self-
esteem and belonged to a high-status group, there was no threat, and they had no reason to bolster their identity. If they had high self-esteem and belonged to a low-status
group, such bolstering occurred. However, people with low self-esteem did not react
this way. They bolstered self-esteem regardless of the status of their group. People with
low self-esteem evaluated their sorority more favorably than another sorority, regardless
of whether their self-esteem had been threatened or whether their sorority was low-
status.

Ingratiation

Group enhancement is an interesting mix of self-enhancement needs and belongingness
needs. When we attempt to belong to social groups and feel a sense of connectedness
with others, these groups contribute to our identity and lead us to enhance our sense of
self through our connections with the groups. However, we do not only evaluate groups,
and other individuals with whom we wish to affiliate and whose approval we seek to
gain, in order to promote a positive sense of self. We also evaluate them positively in
hope that our praise, loyalty, and positive regard will lead them to accept us and grant
us the right to affiliate that we crave. Thus the need to belong may initiate *ingratiation
goals*, which contribute to our positive evaluations of the desired group and negative
evaluations of their enemies. An ingratiation goal is the wish to be liked by and
accepted by others, and to attain this goal, we often implement a strategy that we hope

will get others to like us. But this strategy, according to Jones (1990), is an implicit one. We do not want others to know that we are being strategic in an attempt to be accepted, as that would violate most people's norms of how social exchanges operate. According to Jones, "Ingratiation exploits the logic of social exchange while subverting it. The goal of being liked merely because one has made an effort to be liked can best be attained only if it is concealed. It is not, in other words, contained in the implicit contract underlying social interaction" (p. 177).

It is paradoxical how illicit and negative (if our ulterior motive is discovered) ingratiation is taken to be, given that it arises out of a basic human need to be liked and accepted by others. Indeed, when research participants are asked how they could go about getting others to like them, there is fairly good consensus about what should be done (engaging in a little flattery, showing interest in and agreement with what someone is saying, making eye contact, and smiling; Godfrey, Jones, & Lord, 1986). Yet, somehow, trying to get others to like us renders these positive actions to the domain of falsehoods, misrepresentations, and ulterior motives. The negativity associated with ingratiation probably evolves from the sycophantic possibilities linked to these ulterior motives. When the persons or groups by whom we want to be accepted are intensely popular, high in status, high in power, wealthy, or famous, the incentive value for being linked to such persons or groups is high, and the reason for seeking their acceptance is less likely to be perceived as genuine (Jones, 1964). Thus the behavior aimed at ingratiating ourselves with a group will not necessarily be objectively evaluated, but evaluated in terms of the benefits the group might bestow upon us. The movie star is more likely to trust the flattery of a friend whom he has known prior to stardom than a stranger he has met at a party. The high-status sorority member is more likely to see as genuine the friendship and help of a person with no interest in either gaining sorority membership or dating one of her sorority sisters.

The preceding discussion suggests that ingratiation is only perceived as negative if a person or group being flattered is able to recognize that we are being ingratiating because we have some ulterior motive. Ingratiation should be more likely to work as a strategy for getting group members to like us if they perceive our flattery (or whatever strategy we have chosen) in a self-serving manner. To the extent that they want to be liked, praised, and viewed in a positive light, the more willing they will be to accept our ingratiating remarks as not the products of an ulterior motive (Vonk, 2002). Therefore, ingratiation dovetails nicely with positive illusions. People want to hear others agree with them and view them positively, and they are critical of information that opposes this self-view. This should lead to a propensity to accept ingratiating comments (unless they are given a reason to be suspicious; Fein, Hilton, & Miller, 1990). Vonk has shown that because of positive illusions, the target of ingratiation is more likely than a neutral person who has observed the interaction to accept ingratiating comments as genuine. An observer must decide whether to attribute ingratiating comments to the ulterior motives of the ingratiator or to the wonderfulness of the ingratiatee. In such a case, the motives of the ingratiating person are likely to be called into question.

EGOCENTRIC PERCEPTION

Chapter 7 has noted that perceivers often fail at taking the perspective of others. Rather than seeing the world as it affects others, they see the world only as it affects them, neglecting the fact that the environmental forces that have an impact on others are different from those that influence them (or at times even failing to see those forces at all). Indeed, often people are so caught up in their view of the world and their pursuit of their own goals that they act as if others do not even exist. An example of this type of self-centeredness that you can easily draw from your own experience happens whenever you drive your car. Inevitably, a few other drivers will fail to use their signals when making a turn. They fail to realize that those signals are not a nuisance that authorities have instituted to make all drivers' lives miserable, but a form of communication with others. Without the use of a turn signal, other people on the road do not know where a driver is going and must wait at the intersection to learn, only at the last second (when the driver in question turns without signaling), that an opportunity to enter a busy intersection has now passed. The purpose of a turn signal is solely to alert other drivers (and pedestrians) about where a driver is going, so that these others can act. Using the signal for this purpose requires drivers to realize that they are interacting with other people, even as they are "alone" driving their vehicles. However, the fact that others are waiting in a busy intersection, and have few opportunities to enter this highly trafficked road, escapes many drivers. They fail to consider the perspective of other people, and may prevent others from moving on because they fail to signal.

This example illustrates that it is difficult for actors (drivers) to see the world like observers (other drivers waiting to continue their travel) because of the differing visual perspectives actors and observers hold. However, a differing visual perspective is not the only reason people fail to take perspective; they fail at taking the perspective of others when vision is not even relevant. For example, even if people are reading or hearing about information, they have a tendency to process that information from their own point of view, seeing the world through blinders. There is a type of self-relevant tunnel vision that leads people to cling quite closely to that which is important and relevant to them—to see the world in an egocentric way while ignoring the perspective of others. This type of perception, in which the self is all-important and the world is filtered through the lens of "self," is referred to as *egocentric perception*.

Metacognition and the Child's Theory of Mind

Egocentrism in the form of failed perspective taking is quite common in children. Why? Because they lack the mental tools that taking the perspective of others requires. In particular, such a task requires engaging in *metacognition*, which means being able to think about mental states. In the case of perspective taking, one must be able to think about the mental states of others. One reason why children exhibit egocentrism is that cognitive development has not yet progressed far enough to allow them to *think about what others are thinking about*. In addition, children, through the course of development, have a constantly shifting sense of how the world operates. Like scientists with a theory about some phenomenon, children are said to possess a *theory of mind* (Carey, 1985; Wellman, 1990) that allows them to make sense of their world. Wellman (1990) believed that even in early childhood, children's theory of mind allows them to make distinctions between mental things (such as wishes and wants) and physical things (such as balls and cars). Yet these theories are still incomplete, and evolve throughout childhood. In early childhood, it is just not possible to think about the wishes and wants of others.

One characteristic by-product of early, immature theories of mind is a child's inability to distinguish between the mental representations that others hold about the physical world and those that the child holds. The child, though capable of understanding mental states such as wants and beliefs exist, still believes that others see and know only what the child sees and knows. A classic illustration of this is derived from a task where a child has some information that others do not have (Wimmer & Perner, 1983). Will the child think that the others will act as if they know what the child knows, failing to make the distinction between their two perspectives? In this task, the child learns about a boy named Maxi who loves chocolate. Maxi places some chocolate his mother gave him in a cupboard and goes outside to play. The child, observing this, then sees the mother move the chocolate from one cupboard to another while straightening up. Maxi later returns to the kitchen to retrieve his chocolate. The child is then asked where Maxi will look. Children under the age of 4 incorrectly guess that Maxi will look for the chocolate in the place to which it has been moved, rather than in the place where Maxi left it. There is an inability to distinguish self- from other-knowledge (though see Wellman & Bartsch, 1990, for an account of these findings that does not require the assumption of limitations in a child's reasoning ability).

Egocentric Communication

Egocentrism, though it diminishes with age and the development of metacognitive abilities and more complex theories of mind, does not disappear altogether. Keysar, Barr, Balin, and Paek (1998) have proposed that everyday types of miscommunication in adults often arises from a type of egocentrism similar to that in children, in which others' perspective is simply not (initially) taken into account. A prominent example is people's failure to realize that others do not know what they are thinking! One reason why people have difficulty explaining concepts to others is that they fail to realize that others lack basic information and assumptions that the "teachers" possess. For instance, if you have ever tried to teach your grandmother about using a computer, you may have attempted to be clear by being extremely simple, saying something like "Move the mouse so the cursor is on the little picture of the globe, and click twice." However, despite your attempt to take her perspective, your egocentrism may have prevented you from realizing that even words like "mouse," "cursor," and "click" are meaningless and confusing (perhaps threatening) to one who has never used a computer before. We all often fail to adjust what we say to take into account the difference between information that is in our minds alone and information that is shared knowledge between us and those we are speaking with.

Egocentrism in communication is not limited to the domain of explaining things to others. Even everyday conversation is marred by the fact that people speak about ideas that pop into their heads, yet fail to realize that they have not informed their conversation partners about the shift in topic. For example, you may be driving with a friend, talking about the author of a book you have just read, when a song comes on the radio that leads your friend to think about the lead singer. Your friend then remarks, "Isn't she from New York?" This requires you to know that the friend is now referring to the lead singer and not the author. This is obvious to your friend, since it is the clear topic of his/her current thoughts. Yet to you the statement is ambiguous. Keysar and colleagues (1998) argue that when people communicate with others, most of the utterances exchanged are ambiguous in that they have multiple meanings. For example, the statement "one has to wonder about Hillary Clinton" could mean just about anything—positive or negative. It clearly means one specific thing to the person who said it, but this is not necessarily what will be "heard" by the person it is said to. Egocentrism can lead two such communicators to fail to detect their differing perspectives. A perceiver, in attempting to make sense of an utterance, may not even realize that an utterance has more than one meaning or that the other person has intended something other than what was interpreted. Instead, an utterance is automatically interpreted in terms of the perceiver's own egocentric point of view, using his/her own accessible knowledge.

Keysar and colleagues (1998) have tested this by examining whether people misunderstand a definite reference made by another person. They propose that meanings that could not be implied by a speaker (because they are outside the speaker's realm of knowledge, for instance) are used by a perceiver in attempts to understand what the speaker has said. They refer to this as a failure to consider "common ground," or what might better be known as shared information between two people. The example they provide is of a man who is watching his daughter while his wife is out for the evening. The child falls asleep, and the man considers calling the woman he is having an affair with. But he realizes that his illicit lover is also likely to be asleep, so he does not call. Just then his wife returns and asks, "Is she asleep?" The wife clearly is referring to the daughter, but the perceiver feels anxiety and guilt at his momentary assumption that the wife is referring to the lover, whom she does not even know exists. Keysar and colleagues conducted an experiment to see whether people would make these types of confusions regarding the referents of a pronoun (thus illustrating failed perspective taking). They found that research participants acted just like the children who had privileged information about where Maxi's chocolate had been moved. Perceivers who had privileged information (that a communication partner did not have) failed to take the perspective of the other person into account and responded as if the pronouns used by the other person referred to things the person could not have intended them to refer to. Regardless of what the communication partner intended to say, his/her perspective was not (at least initially) taken into account. It was only after miscommunication and confusion entered the picture that perceivers might shake free of their egocentric perception and understand their communication partners.

It is not only the perceiver who fails to take the perspective of the communicator into account. Keysar and colleagues (1998) report that when a speaker plans an utterance, he/she does not always take into account whether the conversation partner has shared knowledge that will allow him/her to know to what the speaker is referring. For instance, I might just say, "Peter sure likes to be in control," without regard for whether you know to which Peter I am referring, or to whether you know Peter at all. Only your exasperated "What are you talking about?" brings the conversation to normality. (Though speakers do attempt some monitoring of their utterances before they let them leap from their mouths, the initial planning of an utterance typically does not include a perceiver's perspective, which means the monitoring process does not always catch the reference that will be misunderstood by the perceiver.) Egocentrism gets in the way and trips us both up.

Perspective Taking and Egocentrism

Since failing to take the perspective of others is one sign that people have egocentric biases, this might suggest that the cure for egocentric perception is somehow to get people to take the perspective of others. But there is no guarantee that this cure will work. In fact, Robins and John (1997) argue that perspective taking can make an individual (or at least some individuals) even more egocentric. They relate the tale of Narcissus from Greek myths, who when looking upon his own image, and seeing himself from the perspective of others, fell in love with that image! The tragedy of the tale is that this enhanced egocentrism led Narcissus to be so captivated with his own image that he was unable to stop looking at himself long enough to care for the simple needs of his physical body. His self-love was enhanced by perspective taking rather than diminished by it, and this led to his death.

Robins and John (1997) found that individuals they identified as being highly narcissistic did in fact choose to observe themselves on a videotape during an experiment rather than choosing to observe others. And this type of perspective taking (viewing the self as others do, with one's focus not outward on others but on the self) had a different impact on these individuals than on individuals who were not narcissistic. As reviewed in Chapter 7, when most (non-narcissistic) people take the perspective of others, the actor–observer bias in perception tends to disappear. But perspective taking did not alleviate this bias for the narcissistic participants in this study. When Robins and John had the narcissistic persons view (on videotape) and evaluate their own performance in a group task, they actually showed a heightened actor–observer bias. They were even more positively self-biased in the perspective-taking condition than when they were focused on others.

Even when perspective taking does allow one to overcome a bias in person perception (such as when actor–observer bias is attenuated), it perhaps does so by simply imposing one's egocentric view on others, rather than eliminating the egocentricism. That is, ironically, one's very egocentrism is still in operation during perspective taking and interferes with some bias of interpersonal perception! Galinsky and Moskowitz (2000b) considered this point in more detail. The findings illustrated that although perceivers tended to use stereotypes when responding to members of stereotyped groups, people asked to take the perspective of those individuals failed to show a reliance on stereotypes; the bias toward stereotyping was eliminated. When asked to write an essay about a day in the life of an elderly individual, people who took the perspective of the elderly person did not use stereotypes in their essays. In addition, when measures were taken to see whether the stereotype of an elderly person was even being contemplated by the research participants, the results suggested that they were not. But in the Galinsky and Moskowitz (2000b) research, the impact of perspective taking on stereotyping did not guarantee that people were no longer being egocentric. Instead, it may have been their egocentrism that disrupted stereotyping (see also Galinsky & Ku, 2004). To illustrate this, we asked the following question: If perspective takers were not thinking about the stereotype, what were they thinking about? Apparently they were thinking about themselves, extending their egocentrism to others. The characteristics associated with the self were being used to describe the group they were judging, creating a merging of the self and the other. Similarly, Davis, Conklin, Smith, and Luce (1996) have found that after perspective taking, a perceiver sees greater overlap between ratings of the self and the target whose perspective the perceiver has taken; that is, the perceiver sees an increased number of self-descriptive traits in the target. Taking perspective allows perceivers to see how others are like them.

EMBRACING NEGATIVE INFORMATION

The discussion of positive illusions has (ideally) created the impression that people prefer to think positive thoughts about themselves. But this preference to cling to positive illusions does not mean that people fail to process negative information. In fact, results reviewed above, such as those of Ditto and Lopez (1992), suggest that people will more thoroughly analyze negative information (perhaps in an effort to ward it off; rationalization requires effort, whereas accepting something positive about the self or consistent with one's beliefs is rather easy). Despite being displeasing and presenting a challenge to positive illusions, negative information must be processed, and perhaps processed even faster than positive information. At first glance, such a statement may seem inconsistent with the robust positivity bias we have been discussing. But this bias in favor of noticing negative information, and processing it in a more thorough manner, is actually quite consistent with the positivity bias. If people are to maintain a conscious focus on positive information and ward off negative information, then a system for processing negative and unwanted information must be in place that will allow that information to be recognized, dealt with, and rationalized away.

Hansen and Hansen (1988) reasoned that one manner through which people discern whether another person poses a threat is through a quick and implicit evaluation of the other person's facial features. Facial expressions are a form of nonverbal communication that Darwin (1872/1998) believed to hold survival value for a species (particularly if verbal communication does not exist). If detection of facial features has survival value, then presumably such detection processes will have become routinized so that they happen efficiently, perhaps automatically. And by this logic, detecting negative expressions should have a superiority, as they should warn the individual of danger. The experiments conducted by Hansen and Hansen revealed an asymmetry in how people detected positive versus negative faces. Participants examined a crowd filled with faces that all shared the same affective expression, save for one (e.g., a group of all smiling faces with one negative face buried in the crowd). The threatening faces seemed to pop out of the crowd and capture attention more readily than a positive face. The researchers suggested that this phenomenon occurs through a preconscious process in which an individual searches for a signal that a threat exists.

Cacioppo and Berntson (1994; see also Cacioppo, Gardner, & Berntson, 1997) have even argued for the likelihood of *distinct and separate neurophysiological substrates for handling positive and negative information*. The valence of a stimulus, rather than being seen as ranging from highly negative to highly positive on a bipolar scale, is instead presumed to be detected by separate systems that record the degree of negativity and degree of positivity. An implication of this is that a highly negative stimulus need not be seen as low in positivity. And this can explain the existence of ambivalent attitudes, in which people have both positive and negative affect for a person simultaneously (e.g., in the area of racial attitudes, people have both positive and negative feelings toward members of stereotyped groups; Thompson, Zanna, & Griffin, 1995). Another, more relevant implication is that a system that serves the function of quickly scanning the environment for threats and other forms of aversive stimuli is potentially in place, making attention to and detection of negative information not only necessary, but perhaps primary. Zajonc (1980b) claimed that such a neurological system would allow people to deal with threats to well-being. This functional perspective suggests that people have the capability to detect the valence of stimuli automatically, so that harmful objects may be detected early enough to be avoided, and people can react to such stimuli before the stimuli reach consciousness.

Automatic Affect and the Detection of and Attention to Negative Stimuli

Zajonc (1980b) laid the groundwork for the possibility that affective appraisal can occur automatically by asserting that affect is activated separately from and prior to cognitive responses. This meant that cognitive and evaluative responses are the products of separate processing systems. Affective reactions, rather than being the results of a cognitive appraisal of a stimulus, were believed to be capable of being generated prior to cognitive analysis of the stimulus. *Preferences need no inferences.* It is not a great leap from Zajonc's notion of early affective appraisal to the notion that evaluation can be automatically activated (e.g., Bargh, Chaiken, Govender, & Pratto, 1992; Fazio, Sanbonmotsu, Powell, & Kardes, 1986). From this perspective, the inherent properties of the stimulus trigger an evaluation; affect is produced by the mere presence of the stimulus. And if the purpose of this perceptual system is to protect the individual from harm, it is only logical that negative stimuli (e.g., those with potential for harm) are more likely to be automatically attended to than positive stimuli (those that are appetitive), due to their ability to address more pressing (because they require immediate action) needs.

To demonstrate the attention-directing power of an activated negative evaluation toward undesirable and disliked objects, Pratto and John (1991) used a Stroop-like color interference paradigm. Participants were instructed to name the color of the ink in which each word was written. But rather than the words that were to be named spelling out the names of opposing colors (e.g., the word "blue" written in red ink), the words were traits. Trait words that were either positive or negative (and ranging from either extremely positive or negative, on down to mildly so) were presented in different-colored inks, and the task was to name the color in each case (and ignore the word). The prediction was that negative items would cause a slowdown in the task relative to positive items, because negative items would be more likely to capture attention and keep attention lingering on them. This misdirected attention should distract people from the focal task (naming the color) and slow them down. Pratto and John found (Experiment 1) that undesirable traits produced greater interference with the color-naming task than desirable traits. In Experiment 2, they showed it was not that both positive and negative information were attended to equally and the negative information was then deliberately blocked from consciousness. Rather, automatic vigilance—a heightened, preconscious attentional focus (on negative stimuli)—led to the interference effect.

Negativity Bias

Not only has it been posited that positive and negative affect have evolved separate evaluative systems that operate preconsciously to provide information as to whether a stimulus is aversive or appetitive (e.g., Cacioppo et al., 1997); we also need not assume that positive and negative evaluation are weighed equally in terms of their ability to direct processing. For example, Kahneman and Tversky (1984) reviewed robust findings that people place greater weight on those aspects of a situation that suggest risk, loss, and negative consequences. People show a greater concern for avoiding losses than approaching gains; they are *risk-averse.* (An exception occurs when a decision is framed in terms of potential losses, at which time people actually seek risks, presumably feeling that taking risks is the only way to avoid a loss. This can be seen in sports, such as when an excellent golfer such as Phil Mickelson must play a risky style of golf to avoid losing to Tiger Woods. Perhaps if Woods did not lead others to fear losing, but allowed opponents to frame a tournament in terms of a win—gain—they would be less inclined to take risks that lead to both increased birdies, but also increased bogeys.)

Kanouse and Hansen (1972) examined "the idea that people are generally cost oriented in forming overall evaluations—they weigh negative aspects of an object more heavily than positive ones" (p. 47). Early evidence for this negativity bias emerged from research examining how people combine information about others into a coherent impression. Asch (1946) had given people lists of traits and asked them to integrate them. But how do people do this, especially when some of the information is negative and some of it is positive? Anderson (1965a) described two methods people might use—an *averaging model* and an *additive model*. In an averaging model, people presumably average the positivity–negativity of each trait in the list, thus producing an overall evaluation that is somehow the mean overall affect for the person. If a target person is extremely hostile, mildly annoying, and somewhat generous, a perceiver takes the average of these three traits to produce an overall negative evaluation of the person. The additive model should by now be quite predictable: Rather than averaging the observed traits together, people instead are posited to add the valence of each trait in producing an overall evaluation. To test these models, Anderson gave people lists of four adjectives that described a person and asked them for an overall evaluation. In some cases, the adjectives were all extremely positive; in other cases, they were a mix of extremely and mildly positive traits; and in still other cases, they were all mildly positive traits. The same patterns of combinations were also constructed for negative traits. The pattern found was not predicted by either the averaging or adding models: When people judged negative traits, they tended to rate the overall evaluation as farther from the neutral point in the negative direction than the ratings of people evaluating positive traits were in the positive direction. The negative adjectives thus had more power in determining the overall evaluation.

Skowronski and Carlston (1989) propose that negative information is unusually influential in guiding one's impression of the person performing the negative behavior because of the *diagnosticity* of such information. *Diagnosticity* essentially means that a piece of information allows observers to make distinctions readily among various possible alternatives. For example, if you are told that a person likes to drink beer, this is not highly diagnostic for determining the person's more general eating habits. But if you are told that the person refuses to eat beef, this is more diagnostic for classifying and categorizing the person among various alternatives. He/she is likely to be a vegan or a vegetarian. More information, such as that the person refuses to eat cheese, would be needed to allow you to diagnose further whether the person is a vegan (who does not eat cheese) or a vegetarian (who may).

Skowronski and Carlston's argument is that negative information, rather than being powerful in guiding impression formation simply because it violates expectancies, has a powerful impact on impression formation because *it is more useful for distinguishing between possible alternative interpretations for a behavior—it is more diagnostic of a specific category than positive information*. For example, if we are trying to diagnose whether a person is honest, then positive behavior, such as revealing all earned income on his/her tax return, is less informative than negative information, such as failing to list all income earned through tips and untraceable cash payments. As Skowronski and Carlston (1989, p. 137) put it,

> a good person must act good most of the time to retain that categorization, whereas a bad person need act bad only some of the time. A person who both robs banks (a dishonest act) and reports income to the Internal Revenue Service (an honest act) will generally be perceived as dishonest. As a consequence of such perceptions, negative behaviors should be

perceived as more diagnostic of negative traits than positive behavior is of positive traits. Therefore, subjects confronted with two equal but opposite cues should generally assign the negative cue more weight, producing a negativity bias.

Consistent with this logic, Birnbaum (1973) found that a person who was described with several moral behaviors and just one immoral act was, nonetheless, rated as more immoral than moral: "Bad deeds have an overriding impact on the overall judgment. A person may be judged mostly by his worst bad deed." Similarly, Birnbaum (1972) found that if people had pairs of immoral acts described to them (e.g., stealing a waitress's tip money from her table and killing a neighbor's dog because the incessant barking is annoying you), the more severely negative act was given greater weight in determining the overall evaluation of the person.

Reeder and Brewer (1979) claim that this unusual diagnosticity for negative information arises from the use of *implicational schemas* by perceivers. The term *implicational schema* is meant to capture the idea that people have theories, or schemas, about the implications of traits for behavior. If we conceive of an individual as possessing a trait to a specific degree (e.g., we conceptualize a trait like intelligence on a scale from "very unintelligent" to "extremely intelligent," and assume that each person we meet falls somewhere on this unipolar scale), then possessing a trait to that degree informs us of a range of behaviors likely to be seen as a function of having that specific trait to that specific degree. These define several types of implicational schemas that direct attributional processing and can lead to non-normative responding. The *hierarchically restrictive schema* is the one that is believed to give rise to the form of negativity bias just described. This form of the implicational schema is one in which an attribute rating that falls at the extreme high end of the scale (e.g., very intelligent) is believed to have fairly unrestricted implications for behavior. A very intelligent person can act in an extremely intelligent way (scoring the highest in a class on an exam), but can also act in an extremely unintelligent way (failing an exam, locking his/her car keys in the car, using the wrong word in a speech). However, our schema tells us that if a person's perceived attribute level falls at the low end of the scale (e.g., very unintelligent), the range of behaviors that can be committed is extremely restricted. Whereas the intelligent person can act in either an intelligent or a stupid fashion, dependent on the circumstances, the unintelligent person simply does not have the means to act in a highly intelligent fashion. How does this schema relate to the negativity bias?

When a negative behavior is observed, such as acting in an immoral fashion, what type of attribute could have produced it? According to the schema, an immoral person (a person high in the attribute of immorality) can produce both moral and immoral behaviors (as his/her behavior is unrestricted). But the person low in immorality has highly restricted behavioral possibilities. A person low in immorality cannot act in an immoral fashion. Thus, if one immoral behavior is observed, it must indicate that the person is high in immorality. Therefore, even though multiple positive behaviors can be observed, a confident attribution cannot be made. But with one negative behavior, the implicational schema leads the attribution to be sealed. Reeder and Brewer (1979, p. 76) have summarized the logic in this negativity bias well: "A single highly immoral behavior will imply the presence of an immoral disposition in the actor. A single highly moral act, however, may (depending upon the situation) imply a range of dispositional classifications." In the language of Skowronski and Carlston (1989), a negative act is more diagnostic of a trait.

ACCURACY IN SOCIAL PERCEPTION

Let us end this chapter with a brief review of accuracy in social cognition. Are people any good at judging the personality of others, even given the biases reviewed throughout this chapter? One problem in answering this question (and perhaps the reason why asking it has been reserved until now) is that accuracy is a tricky thing to define. Gage and Cronbach (1955) argued that defining *accuracy* as the mathematical difference between one person's estimates of another's personality and some psychological test that measures the other person's personality is inherently flawed. However, Kenny (1994) argues that the factors that might be conflated via such a technique can, through the use of recent advances in statistical analyses, be teased apart; this allows us to assess accuracy and define it as the match between a perceiver's predictions about what a person is like (and likely to do) and the measurement of what someone is actually like (and does). Funder (1999) argues that accuracy in person perception is substantially higher than what might be predicted, based on the current review of subjective biases in attributional reasoning. But being able to detect such accuracy in perceivers requires identifying moderating factors that have the power to shape whether a perceiver will be accurate or not in a given interpersonal judgment.

Positive Evidence for Accuracy

To end on an optimistic note, research has revealed that people are at times quite good at using their inferential powers to infer the properties of other people with some accuracy. For example, Kenny, Horner, Kashy, and Chu (1992) took strangers and had them meet in person briefly before making personality judgments of one another. Two findings emerged: First, there was consensus among participants regarding a given individual, so that perceivers seemed to make the same personality inferences. Consensus among perceivers has been found even when personality judgments of others are based on photographs (Berry, 1990). Second, these impressions were predictive of a given target's ratings of him-/herself (see also Funder & Colvin, 1988). We have seen similar evidence in Chapter 2, where the work on *thin slices of behavior* is reviewed and in Chapter 7 where personality was inferred from examining a person's office. Berry (1991) extended these findings to illustrate that accuracy could be attained even without having met the target of one's personality judgment. Research participants were asked to examine either a photograph of a target person or a recording of the person's voice as he/she simply recited the alphabet in a neutral voice. The participants then rated the targets for warmth and power. Finally, the people whose faces and voices were being used to make inferences about personality were asked to make self-perceptions of their own warmth and power. To what extent did the targets' self-ratings correspond with the inferences made by perceivers (i.e., to what extent were perceivers accurate)? First, perceivers seemed to be using cues such as the babyishness of the face and voice to make inferences about the targets' warmth and power. Thus, even in such limited conditions, there are cues available for people to use. More importantly, the impressions formed by perceivers based on these cues did remarkably coincide with the self-views of the people being judged. Therefore, accuracy can exist even at zero acquaintance.

It might naturally be expected that accuracy has an even greater chance of appearing when judgments of other people are not made at zero acquaintance or based on thin slices of behavior, but based on more extended contacts. Kenny, Kiefer, Smith, Ceplenski, and Culo (1996) examined the impressions of people who knew each other well—fraternity brothers. The average ratings of several fraternity brothers regarding the behavior of one specific brother turned out to be quite predictive of that "target brother's" behavior across a host of situations. Interestingly, the brothers were not very good at predicting how that same brother might act in a one-on-one interaction with any given one of them. As an aggregate, they could predict behavior in the group and in group settings, but they did not have particularly accurate judgments in the individual context. This finding might seem counterintuitive, but given the nature of the types of interactions such people share, it is likely that they are quite accurate when making predictions about the types of interactions that are common (hanging out in a group) and less accurate when asked to make predictions about contexts that are not experienced much between the individuals in question. This finding might even suggest that accuracy is perhaps best achieved by (and perhaps even best defined as) the ability to make predictions about others when the goals of the interaction context are taken into account and when relationship-specific factors are considered. We turn to this next.

Pragmatic Accuracy

Gill and Swann (2004) propose that understanding the person perception process requires first understanding what the people being perceived are trying to do within their social exchange. As is the case with fraternity brothers, most social interactions are fairly specific in terms of the goals and contexts they occur within—they are limited in scope. Gill and Swann argue that accuracy is not really a matter of knowing what a person is "objectively" like across a host of contexts, but is a pragmatic matter; it is an issue of predicting what a person is like and likely to do within the confines of a given situation and the goals that are adopted within the borders of a specific relationship. These authors refer to this as *pragmatic accuracy*. In essence, it is a form of accuracy that matters to people because it serves an important function: It has utility within their important relationships and interactions. Groups often need to coordinate social activities and maintain cohesion among actions, as do relationship partners of various sorts, making it necessary (pragmatic) to know one's partners accurately and well. If accuracy is defined this way, we might expect it to be found much more often than the biases reviewed in this chapter would lead us to believe, because it is measured within relationships that have meaning to individuals and have goals to guide the nature of their impressions ("the accuracy of social beliefs is . . . determined by how well they serve the goals of perceivers"; Swann, 1984, p. 461). If accuracy is measured in contexts that have little utility to the perceivers, we might expect it to be low.

Gill and Swann (2004) illustrated pragmatic accuracy in two separate domains—important social groups (families and fraternities) and romantic relationships. To investigate whether people would make accurate assessment of others on relationship-relevant traits (but not on relationship-irrelevant traits), they investigated dating couples and had members of the couples predict the responses of their partners on items that were either relevant or irrelevant to the dating relationship. Accuracy was measured by how well the perceivers (one member of each couple was randomly assigned to be the perceiver of the partner) predicted their partners' self-views. They found that accuracy increased as the relevance of the trait being judged to the relationship context increased. And this was not because relevant traits were more positive and people were assuming that their partners had positive traits (and the partners were assuming they had positive traits as well); the effect emerged even when the researchers controlled for the valence of the traits. It is thus illustrating something different from positive illusions: People are accurate predictors when the persons being predicted are confined to important relationships and the qualities being judged are relevant to those relationships. As Chapter 5 has indicated, accuracy can be promoted when the judgment at hand matters to people.

The work on the pragmatic nature of accuracy fits well with work on what has been called *empathic accuracy*—which is defined as the extent to which partners in a relationship can accurately infer each other's thoughts and feelings during an interaction (Ickes, 2003). Findings support the idea that partners who solve conflicts in a direct fashion rather than avoiding them develop more accurate understandings of each other's thoughts and emotional responses as the interactions unfold. In addition, perceivers tend to be more accurate at judging emotionally negative behaviors displayed by their partners than at judging positive or neutral behaviors; this probably reflects the greater salience of negative information in dyadic interactions. Empathic accuracy is a double-edged sword. It can cut through the relatively trivial misunderstandings that occur in every relationship; yet it can cut right to the core of pain and dissatisfaction in a relationship, because it can trigger intensely negative feelings when it is used to ascertain or uncover differences that threaten the relationship. This accounts for the fact that accuracy is in some studies found to be positively associated with relationship satisfaction, while in other studies a negative correlation between accuracy and relationship satisfaction is found (Simpson, Blackstone, & Ickes, 1995).

CODA

To some extent, this chapter has read like a laundry list of all the sorts of nonrational things that perceivers do when making sense of themselves and others. The motives and goals that perceivers possess can bias the types of inferences they form, with often dramatic effects for how interpersonal interaction unfolds and consequences for the self. For example, the desire to maintain positive illusions and enhance self-esteem can lead people to engage in motivated skepticism, motivated reasoning, self-serving biases, and unrealistic predictions about the future. In sum, people avoid negative information about the self; they attribute negative outcomes to sources external to them; they predict that the future will be positive because they see positive self-attributes as the cause for positive things' currently happening; and they accept positive news all too readily. This may have many positive consequences for mental health, especially so long as these tendencies stay on the side of illusions and do not slip into the realm of delusions. However, even positive illusions can present dangers to individuals. For example, it may cause people to avoid visiting a doctor in order to shelter themselves from receiving negative feedback—an act that will not have any benefit whatsoever. Many women avoid the simple act of breast self-examination (as a means for early breast cancer detection) specifically for fear of shattering their positive illusions. As a second example, it may cause people to make decisions based on predictions about the future that are distorted by the durability bias. One might decide to move to Florida because one focuses on the wonderful feeling of having warm weather almost continually, failing to realize that this positive feeling is fairly short-lived (with the possible exception of the case where one's hobbies, a major source of life satisfaction, all require extensive time in the outdoors).

The motive to protect self-esteem is ubiquitous and multifaceted. Indeed, the menagerie of self-protective mechanisms is so broad and varied that it has even been refereed to as the "self zoo" (Tesser & Martin, 1996). However, it is not the only motive that drives self- and other-perception. The need to control can create distortions to the attribution process that have severe consequences. The transparency illusion can lead people to believe that others are being insensitive to what they perceive to be clear signals they are sending to these others. This can lead negotiators to walk away from the table and lovers to develop feelings of resentment and being misunderstood. The belief in a just world can lead people to hold innocent victims responsible (partly or wholly) for the crimes that have been committed against them.

Similarly, the need to belong to a group of others can have deleterious consequences that might seem impossible to predict from such a positive-sounding motive. However, the desire to belong can lead one to denigrate others, if those others are perceived as threatening to the group that one wishes to identify with. From such positive motives, prejudice can spring forth. On the more personal level, striving to join other groups can lead one to act in sycophantic and ingratiating ways in order to garner favor with the group. These are the ugly sides of the need to bond with others. However, such needs to belong serve a purpose, and the ugliness is an unintended consequence of the main function that belonging to social groups serves: they provide group members with a sense of connectedness and a positive reflection on themselves. Through processes associated with basking in reflected glory and social identity, individuals attain a positive sense of self through a connection with social groups.

In summary, people affirm, verify, enhance, and assess. How do they do it all? When is one motive likely to rear its head versus another? How do people reconcile instances of motives in conflict? These issues are beyond the scope of this chapter. Our goal has been simply to illustrate the various sources of influences on person perception, and to discuss a mere handful of the ways in which attribution is influenced by these sources (motives). Trope and Neter (1994) assert that the manner in which people evaluate information about themselves and others is not uniformly driven by any one motive, but involves essentially balancing their various goals in an effort to provide the long-term attainment of a sense of self-worth. This means that they are willing to think negatively about the self at times if it means some benefit in the long run. Thus people actually seek out negative information about the self if it confirms their identity, but also if such negative information is useful and will allow them to grow and develop. But seeking accurate, negative information about the self is typically only done when people feel good about themselves. When people are in a bad mood, or are feeling bad about their abilities, they typically do not choose those moments to seek constructive criticism. Trope and Neter asserted that when people feel poorly about themselves, they do not wish to get negative feedback about their abilities, but instead prefer information that is self-enhancing. But self-enhancement is discarded in favor of gaining more accurate information about the self, even if negative, when people are feeling good (see also Trope & Pomerantz, 1998). For each person, the self zoo is under the watch of a very careful keeper.

NOTES

1. Making matters worse is that supposedly unbiased sources, such as medical journals, admit to publishing articles with potentially biased findings. On June 5, 2002, CNN.com reported a statement released by JAMA that studies financed by pharmaceutical companies were getting pushed through the review process in that journal without receiving proper scrutiny. Essentially, not all data published in JAMA have been scrutinized according to accepted scientific standards.

2. Studies published in academic journals rarely make such statements as, "It has been determined conclusively that . . . " Instead, they tend to use language like "The data suggest that . . . " However, the popular press invariably alters the language in such a way that the average reader can make sense of the findings and not have to worry about the subtleties of the findings. They give the impression that the case is closed (e.g., the layperson may conclude that breast feeding "will" make a child smarter because a CNN bullet point scrolled across the bottom of the screen and said so). And this does not even touch on the cases in which the media are biased in what they present, deliberately distorting rather than poorly simplifying. To continue with the current example, a recent study found that both day care and bottle feeding do not have the previously believed (slightly negative) impact on health issues such as asthma. However, reports in the media pursued this issue by talking about day care exclusively, ignoring that the study had just found one of the few traditionally believed benefits of breast feeding to be nonexistent. Thus people can expose themselves to biased data quite easily if their goal is to support a prior belief.

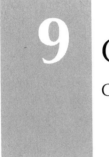

9 On Perceptual Readiness

CHRONIC SOURCES OF JUDGMENTAL INFLUENCE

CAIRO—It was a picture of Arab grief and rage. A teenage boy glared from the rubble of a bombed building as a veiled woman wept over the body of a relative. In fact, it was two pictures: one from the American-led war in Iraq and the other from the Palestinian territories, blended into one image this week on the Web site of the popular Saudi daily newspaper Al Watan. The meaning would be clear to any Arab reader: what is happening in Iraq is part of one continuous brutal assault by America and its allies on defenseless Arabs. . . . the daily message to the public from much of the media is that American troops are callous killers, that only resistance to the United States can redeem Arab pride and that the Iraqis are fighting a pan-Arab battle for self-respect . . . images, however, are not presented as fragmentary evidence of the evils of war but as illustrations of a definitive black-and-white view of the war and the United States. The way they are presented, and the language that accompanies them, amplifies their impact. President Bush, in one Egyptian weekly newspaper, is shown on each page of war coverage in a Nazi uniform. American and British forces are called "allies of the devil." Civilian casualties are frequently reported as "massacres" or, as another Egyptian paper said, an "American Holocaust."

—SACHS (2003)

In the spring of 2003, the United States invaded Iraq, with American media outlets revealing time and again the U.S. name for the war: "Operation Iraqi Freedom." Most Americans, even many opposed to the war, were willing to assume that the reason for the invasion was to rid the world of a dangerous madman—one who posed a threat to the lives of both Americans and Iraqis, because of his stockpile of chemical and biological weapons. As the media declared, the troops were going to free the people of Iraq from tyranny (while freeing the rest of the world from the tyranny of the chemical and biological weapons believed to be in the possession of the Iraqi leader). Americans, prepared to think of their country as a force of freedom and good will, viewed the attack as one intended to topple a tyrannical force. Even most Americans opposed to the war were opposed because they felt it was not America's place to engage in preemptive strikes (for fear of what Iraq might do should it not be proactively disarmed), or to impose its values on Iraq without prior provocation (or at least with more provocation than Iraq's violation of U.N. resolutions relating to weapons). Though they disapproved of instigating war to attain the stated desired ends of the Bush administration, few doubted that those ends would preserve freedom at home and deliver it abroad.

What shocked and awed many Americans was that their troops were not widely greeted in Iraq as liberators. The Iraqi press, and the media across the Arab world, saw the invasion as an act of American aggression. It would be more likely for the Arab media to use a phrase like "Operation Evil-Doer Colonialism" or "Operation Greed: Grab the Oil" to describe the American war effort. An article in the op-ed section of *The New York Times* (Sachs, 2003; quoted above) nicely illustrated the gulf between Arab and American perceptions of the war as portrayed in the respective media outlets. Reporting the same day in *The New York Times*, Rami Khouri (2003) asserted not only that the horrific images were singled out for Arab media attention, but that "sometimes, an image that would get an innocuous description in an American newspaper is given a more sinister interpretation in the Arab press." Ranging from the broad goals of the war to the meaning of specific interactions between U.S. troops and Iraqi civilians, the two groups saw and described two different sets of events.

This is similar to a form of naive realism described in Chapter 1: *seeing information in the opposite way from a competitor's view*. The media, as well as the partisans to whom the media broadcast their messages, are ready to see the world through a specific lens. Americans are raised in an environment where freedom and liberty are central concepts. These values are frequently encountered and endorsed, and have come to have a sort of favored status over other concepts that are less frequently encountered and endorsed. This relative state of readiness to view the world through the lens of these concepts makes Americans especially likely to use the concepts when they encounter a person (or people) to whom those concepts might be relevant. Thus, for Americans, the most reasonable explanation for American actions in relation to foreign peoples is that Americans are attempting to spread freedom and liberty. These concepts are ready to be used even before the government and press attempt to convey the reasons for American intervention (this is why it is so easy for many Americans to trust the government in these matters—they are ready to believe and see those concepts). Iraq in spring 2003, however, was not a society that stressed freedom, independence, and personal liberty. It was a country ruled by an iron fist, whose people were raised under an anti-Western dogma easily associated with British colonialism and American cultural imperialism (and its associated immorality, as defined by the powerful force of local religious teaching). Their readiness to see the world through a lens of Western aggression and colonialism made them especially likely to use those concepts when they encountered people to whom those concepts were relevant. Thus, for Iraqis, the most reasonable explanations for American intervention in their country were aggression, greed, and colonialism.

This is not meant to be a political analysis. Obviously, a complex set of forces will contribute to American intervention in any region of the world, as well as to the perception of that intervention by the vastly diverse peoples of the world. What is meant to be illustrated is that one powerful force contributing to that perception is what a given person is *ready* to see and believe. Readiness to perceive others in certain ways is determined itself by many factors—attitudes toward the groups that a person belongs to, culturally transmitted beliefs about those groups, exposure to information about these groups (from the government and media), what significant others think about a group (peer pressure), and so on. Our concern in this chapter is with a specific source of influ-

ence on impressions and judgments: the influence of perceptual readiness in the form
of available concepts that have a chronic and stable level of accessibility in the mind.

AVAILABILITY VERSUS ACCESSIBILITY

Knowledge Availability

We must begin by making a distinction between knowledge that is available and knowledge that is accessible. *Availability of knowledge* means that some piece of knowledge is known by an individual, stored in long-term memory. When you say, "Yeah, I know that," what you are saying is "Yes, that information is available in my long-term memory." But just because you know something (or have it stored in memory), this does not mean that it is very accessible to you. And here you can use the term *accessible* in the traditional sense. When you have some old clothes in storage, they may not be very accessible to you, as they may be stored in a place that is difficult to get to. Perhaps they are in an attic that is hard to climb into, or buried under dozens of other boxes. This is a useful metaphor. You have lots of information available in memory (a lifetime's worth of acquired knowledge), but some of it is easier to retrieve than others; it is more accessible.

If knowledge can be accessed, it obviously must be available. However, the fact that information is not easily accessed does not mean that it is not available. With the help of a cue or mental clue (e.g., Tulving & Pearlstone, 1966), you may be able to suddenly recall information that had previously been buried in your mind's attic. Take a concrete example to distinguish what is available to you from what you can easily access. You may know stereotypes of Polish people, yet you may be fairly confident you do not know any "Polish jokes." However, if pressed, or if provided with a mental cue/clue (such as "Do you know the one involving the light bulb?"), you could probably suddenly remember a Polish joke learned as a child. Memory researchers use examples like this to make a distinction between free recall and cued recall. Here it is used to illustrate that information available in memory is not always accessed. This begs the questions: What does it mean for information to be accessible, and what determines accessibility?

Knowledge Accessibility

Bruner (1957) introduced the concept of *category accessibility*, distinguishing a concept's status as lying dormant in long-term memory from its status of having a heightened readiness or state of activation. The dormant concept, construct, or category is still available; it can be, but as yet has not been, retrieved from memory. The activated concept, however, is in a state where *it is not dormant, but has the potential to influence thought processes*. It is more than merely available, but has a heightened state of potential use. Higgins (1996) defined *accessibility* as "the activation potential of available knowledge. The term *potential* nicely captures several characteristics of accessibility ... that it is capable of being activated (and then used) but exists in a latent rather than in an active state" (p. 134). In this sense, accessibility of a concept means that because of the concept's heightened activation, a person who has encountered a stimulus relevant to the accessible concept can access the category/concept in question with greater speed and ease, making that category more easily retrieved from memory (see Chapter 3). The more easily a concept is retrieved from memory, the more likely it is to be used in noticing, attending to, and interpreting a stimulus. It has *perceptual readiness.*

Higgins, Bargh, and Lombardi (1985) used the metaphor of an energy cell or battery to describe what is meant by accessibility. Each of the concepts stored in long-term memory can be thought of as being a chargeable unit, like a battery, and each exists at any point in time in various levels of power. Some are out of energy, but can momentarily be charged and attain enough energy to be retrieved from the long-term store and attain a state of perceptual readiness. Such is the case with our Polish joke that we could not retrieve. It initially has too little charge to be accessed and used. But the appropriate stimulus in the environment can trigger or activate the unit and provide it with a momentary charge. Its accessibility, once attained, now makes the concept ready to be used, whereas it had previously been dormant/inaccessible. Other concepts exist at varying levels of charge or degree of accessibility. Thus the concepts of freedom and democracy are fairly charged for the average American, as these concepts are triggered (and momentarily charged) fairly often. Concepts that have a fairly constant level of charge are ones that have been frequently and consistently encountered and used. These concepts need not await a cue or stimulus from the environment to trigger them (or provide them with a momentary charge); they are in a state of permanent charge or *chronic accessibility,* making them relatively more accessible than other concepts, and therefore more pervasive tools in guiding how a person sees the world.

Chronic Accessibility

Kelly (1955) argued that people's fairly routine and habitual experiences in life make specific sets of social situations frequent and result in the repetition of specific types of social behavior. People are repeatedly in situations that call for kindness, helpfulness, intelligence, and so on, depending on the types of daily routines they repeatedly enact. This personal history creates a unique set of constructs that are typically encountered, through habit and repetition, and become chronically accessible to an individual. Chronic accessibility thus creates a permanent screen or filter through which the person's world is experienced. According to Kelly, constructs that are chronically accessible serve as a "scanning pattern which a person continually projects upon his world. As he sweeps back and forth across his perceptual field he picks up blips of meaning" (p. 145). Bargh (1990) has similarly argued that goals and motives can also attain a chronic state of accessibility. Each person has sets of goals he/she pursues across a variety of situations and that are fairly stable across the life span (e.g., goals to be egalitarian, tolerant, successful, independent, etc.). Given the frequent and habitual pursuit of these goals over time, these concepts come to have a chronic state of accessibility. For instance, a person does not need to plan consciously to act in an egalitarian fashion if he/she has chronic egalitarian goals. Instead, egalitarian goals are constantly "charged," making the individual ready to take advantage of situations that present an opportunity to act in an egalitarian way (e.g., Moskowitz, Salomon, & Taylor, 2000).

Preconscious Perception

The concept of chronic accessibility poses an interesting problem. It suggests that dormant concepts, of which we humans are not consciously aware and which have not yet been retrieved from long-term memory, have an impact on how we perceive the world. It suggests that we scan the environment through a filter outside our conscious control, under the direction of concepts that have some heightened state of activation. In addition, this heightened state of activation has not been attained because of some current, conscious decision to think about those concepts or to pursue momentary goals related to those concepts. Rather, there are permanent states of activation that, because they are linked with dormant concepts that we do not consciously reflect on, exert a silent influence on our judgment and behavior. The discussion of automatic processing in Chapter 2 has raised the concern that automatic processing may mean that we have no control at all, with "free will" reduced to a "ghost in the machine." Here we see the opposite paradox: Our free will is operating, but at a silent level, due to the fact that the concepts with a heightened state of activation are lying in perceptual wait below the threshold of conscious awareness. These dormant, charged concepts direct social cognition and perception without our awareness, but in accord with our goals and prior interaction history with stimuli. Thus, rather than the concern expressed regarding automatic processing that stimuli dictate our responses with the absence of free will, free will is instead posited to dictate what stimuli we respond to and detect (in the absence of consciousness).

Thus, even without our deliberating from moment to moment about the concepts that we find to be important, chronically accessible concepts run on automatic pilot, freeing us from needing to scan the environment consciously for things that matter to us. Chronic concepts can pick and select such information from the environment without our needing to ask them to do the job. Much like breathing, the process occurs without conscious monitoring. Think of the so-called "cocktail party effect." You have probably experienced your own ability to detect your name being spoken in a loud and crowded room when you were engaged in a conversation with someone and not paying attention to what people engaged in other conversations were saying. Yet somehow when they speak your name, it turns out that you were, at some level, attending to what others were saying in the din.

Why has this ability been referred to above as a paradox? The paradox resides in our intuitive sense that it is impossible to react to a stimulus if we have not yet discriminated that stimulus from among the multitude of stimuli that bombard our senses. It is seemingly not possible to attend to a stimulus when we have not allocated conscious attention to it, or to perceive things we report being unable to consciously detect/see (*subliminal perception*). The paradox is resolved only by accepting that much of our perceptual experience takes place in the preconscious and prior to our conscious awareness getting involved. Our minds see things before it reports to us (and sometimes without ever reporting to us) that these things have been seen! This ability is linked to a differentiation between short-term and iconic memory. Due to the huge amount of information that bombards our senses at any given moment, we have developed the ability to momentarily store large amounts of information, for very brief periods, without our consciousness necessarily getting involved. The vast sensory storehouse of visual information is known as *iconic memory* (*echoic memory* is said to exist for auditory stimuli). Information does not stay in the iconic storehouse very long, but within this brief period, vast amounts of information from our environment are represented by the perceptual system. Once information enters this storehouse, we are able to "decide" what information, from this bombardment, passes through a metaphorical filter and enters consciousness, capturing our focus of attention, and being represented in short-term memory. These "decisions" about what information to keep and what to filter out occur prior to our being aware that any information has even been internally represented (and are thus made without conscious reflection or awareness). Thus, although you may not have been consciously attending to another conversation in the crowded party room, the contents of other conversations were being preconsciously scanned and placed in your iconic storehouse. When that content is deemed relevant, attention shifts and alters what is consciously attended and perceived. Chronically accessible concepts help the filter operate.

> The perceiver can scan or examine the contents of the icon and, on the basis of at least partial analysis of its contents, exercise control over what to encode—and therefore what to reject—for further processing. The rejected material would be lost to the perceiver beyond a fraction of a second. . . . It may be assumed that encoding selectivity is not restricted to laboratory-produced sets . . . presumably a host of "chronic sets" (personality predispositions) are built in through years of experience. (Erdelyi, 1974, p. 17)

CHRONICALLY ACCESSIBLE NEEDS, GOALS, AND VALUES: THE "NEW LOOK"

Recall that Chapter 1, in reviewing the notion of naive realism, has discussed several ways in which the perception of stimuli from the environment is thought to be altered and twisted in the perceptual process, without conscious awareness of these twists. One of these is that the context in which the behavior occurs alters the meaning of the behavior. Another is that the perceptual system attempts to make sense of a stimulus (via Gestalt perceptual principles of holism, closure, etc.). Finally, Chapter 1 has reviewed the so-called "New Look" in perception that emerged in the 1940s. What was new about this approach to perception was the argument that perception is more than a mere transcription of the environment by the senses, but instead involves subjective twists of the data bombarding the perceptual system. In addition, it proposed that the subjective twists arise from the needs and states of perceptual readiness of the person doing the perceiving; these serve to manipulate what is perceived and attended to.

People's habitually pursued needs, values, and goals were described as making them chronically ready to detect and perceive certain stimuli from the environment. The chronic accessibility of certain concepts was said to be attained because of the relevance of these concepts to the individuals' important needs and values. And this heightened state of accessibility was believed to imbue the perceptual process with the power to detect stimuli relevant to these important needs and values. The term *perceptual readiness* refers to this power to facilitate the detection of information relevant to accessible concepts. Thus the New Look introduced both the notion of accessibility and its main consequence for social cognition—perceptual readiness.

Seen, but Not Seen: Chronically Accessible Goals/Needs/Values and Perception

Postman, Bruner, and McGinnies (1948) conducted an experiment that nicely illustrates the impact of chronically accessible concepts on fundamental and basic processes of perception. In the experiment, words were presented to people on a screen. Postman and colleagues varied the speed at which the words were presented, with presentation speed starting subliminally (the words were presented so quickly that they were not consciously registered) and gradually slowed until a word could be consciously identified. The research participants were instructed to watch the screen and report when they could actually see something. The subliminally presented words were carefully selected so that they were values that participants could embrace to varying degrees. For example, from the category of "political" values were words such as "politics," "dominate," and "govern"; from the category of "social" values were words such as "loving," "kindly," and "friendly." The experimenters first assessed the extent to which participants valued each of these constructs, and then observed whether there were differences in how quickly participants could consciously perceive these words as a function of whether the words were of central importance to them or not. They found that words describing values that participants had listed as being of central importance to them were perceived at a faster rate than less valued words. This finding of lower thresholds of recognition for desired words suggests that participants were responding favorably to stimuli prior to conscious recognition. Their subjectivity was operating prior to consciousness!

Bruner and Goodman (1947) similarly proposed that the need associated with a stimulus leads to the perception of the stimulus to be altered in line with the need state. If the object is something people value, they will accentuate it in their perception, so that its perceived size grows as the value of the object grows. Perhaps an admired person seems taller in stature (so that the perceived size of the person grows with the admiration), and a loved one appears to have a giant intellect. The degree of the effect was predicted to increase as the need of an individual increases. The more the individual wants something, the more the perception should be distorted. To demonstrate this, Bruner and Goodman used a quite simple paradigm. Research participants were asked to hold an object in their palm and draw it, using a variable circular patch of light controlled by a knob. The object was either a coin or a disc the size of a coin. The researchers found drawings of coins to be distorted relative to drawings of discs of the same size, so that money (something valued) was seen as larger than an object of the same size. This occurred despite the fact that the object participants were asked to draw was being held in the palm of their hand as they were drawing it. The object could not have been any more concrete and open to inspection, yet the perception was still subjectively distorted by need and value states. Even more dramatically, this distortion did not vary directly with the size of the coin, but with the value of the coin. A nickel is larger than a dime, but the relative distortion of size (of a nickel compared to a nickel-sized circle and a dime relative to a dime-sized circle) was greater for a dime than for a nickel (and was greatest for a quarter). As one final illustration of this subjective influence on perception, distortions in drawings of coins were greater for poor participants (who presumably needed money more) than for rich participants.

Auto-Motives

The concept of perceptual readiness took some time to take root in social psychology, being revived and moving to the mainstream of the field only in the late 1970s and early 1980s, some 20 years after Bruner's (1957) review of over a decade of research. By the time it had taken root, its form had changed somewhat. It referred to the accessibility of information stored in memory (such as schemas, traits, stereotypes, and exemplars), not to the accessibility of goals, needs, motivation, and values (this is reviewed later in this chapter and in the next). These newer forms of perceptual readiness were described as functioning in much the same way as the goals and values described by the "New Look": Accessible knowledge structures serve an important processing function that guides attention, encoding, and retrieval of information.

Bargh (1990) finally connected more modern research on perceptual readiness to its origins in the "New Look" by proposing that much of human interpersonal behavior is directed by what he called *auto-motives*. These were defined as chronically accessible goals, motives, and needs that have the power to exert an influence on attention, judgment, and behavior across a wide array of interpersonal situations. The pursuit of these goals is automatically initiated. The feeling of conscious willing is not needed to trigger goal pursuit; the only things needed are cues embedded in the context signaling that this context affords one the opportunity to pursue chronically accessible goals. "Chronic goals and intents, and the procedures and plans associated with them, may become directly and automatically linked in memory with representations of environmental features to which they are frequently and consistently associated" (Bargh, 1990, p. 100). Thus chronic goals lie in wait, and when appropriate contexts appear, these contexts trigger the goals and the pursuit of the goals. The goals' chronic state of accessibility allows them to function, once an appropriate context is entered, automatically. Since Bargh's review, a literature has been building that more directly provides evidence of the impact of chronically accessible goals on person perception. Let us sample from this ever-growing list to illustrate the impact of chronic goals on (1) what people attend to, (2) how they judge others, and (3) how they behave in interpersonal interaction. The first example is drawn from my colleagues' and my own research, because it bears theoretical similarity to the research of Postman and colleagues (1948) reviewed above.

Auto-Motives and Perception

When people have chronic goals (such as chronic egalitarian goals), these will be triggered by appropriate cues in the environment. Given the presence of such cues, two things should happen. First, the goals will be made even more accessible and will direct attention to stimuli compatible with the goals (i.e., ones that present an opportunity to pursue the goals). Second, the goals' activation will disrupt incompatible processing from occurring, what is known as *goal shielding* (Moskowitz et al., 2000). Let us focus here on the first point. Does the presence of cues in the environment that signal the presence of an opportunity to be egalitarian lead to the increased accessibility of chronic egalitarian goals and the subsequent ability for those goals to direct what people holding them attend to? To be even more specific, the interpersonal cue that was used in this research was whether or not the face of a member of a minority group (one that has historically been treated in a nonegalitarian fashion) was present. Such people represent opportunities to act in an egalitarian way, because they are often the targets of injustice. The measure of whether such goals would have an impact on attention was whether participants were able to detect stimuli relevant to egalitarian goals in their environment more quickly than other types of stimuli following exposure to these cues. Thus, for a person with chronic egalitarian goals, the presence of a Black man should trigger these goals, whereas the same man, encountered by a person without chronic egalitarian goals, would trigger only the culture's stereotype of that group. Once chronic goals were triggered, they should alter what was seen, how quickly it was seen, and the types of impressions formed.

In one experiment (Moskowitz et al., 2000) people were identified who were *chronic egalitarians*. These were individuals who habitually pursued goals of fairness and equality to such a degree that these had attained a state of heightened accessibility. Once these chronic egalitarians had been identified (vs. plain old nonchronic people, who very well might value egalitarianism, but not enough for it to be the dominant theme in their life strivings), such people were asked to engage in a perception task where they had to identify words that flashed on a computer monitor. Some words were relevant to the goals of egalitarianism ("equity," "tolerance," "fairness," etc.); some were not ("humility," "courteous," "responsible," etc.). In addition, each word was preceded by a face—a yearbook picture of either a White or a Black man. It was predicted that seeing faces of Black men (a group that has historically been discriminated against) would trigger egalitarian goals in chronic egalitarians but not in nonchronic participants. Pictures of White men would afford no opportunity to think or act in an egalitarian way and would not trigger egalitarian goals. The triggering of the goals would be evidenced in the speed of responding to the words. This was what was found. People labeled as having chronic egalitarian goals had these goals automatically triggered by the mere presence of a goal-relevant stimulus (a Black man). These goals, once triggered, had an impact on perception: Such individuals were faster to perceive words relevant to the goals of egalitarianism in their environment, but showed no increased speed to perceiving words irrelevant to these goals. Chronic egalitarians only showed this effect when the words were preceded by pictures of Black men, not White men. Consistent with the auto-motive model, the chronic goals were triggered by specific contexts with which they were associated. Once triggered, the goals passively guided what people were prepared to see.

Auto-Motives and Judging People

What is perceptually ready not only determines what we humans attend to and perceive. Once a goal, need, motive, or value is activated, it arms us with tools for judgment. The way we interpret the behavior we see, the types of attributions we form for the people performing those behaviors, and the opinions we are ready to express are all filtered through our perceptual readiness. There has been such a large collection of literature illustrating how differences in chronic goal orientations, motives, values, and needs influence how we judge others that it would be impossible to review it all here. Among the chronic forces known to influence how we judge other people are locus of control (Lefcourt, 1976; Rotter, 1966), attributional style (Anderson, Horowitz, & French, 1983), need for cognition (Cacioppo & Petty, 1982), control motivation (Pittman & D'Agostino, 1989; Pittman & Pittman, 1980), need to evaluate (Jarvis & Petty, 1996), motivation to respond without prejudice (Plant & Devine, 1998), modern racism (McConahay, Hardee, & Batts, 1981), and uncertainty orientation (Sorrentino & Short, 1986). And the list goes on. Instead of reviewing all of these, let us focus on some chronic orientations that could be added to this list, while ignoring others. The goal here is not to be comprehensive, but to provide converging illustrations of the role auto-motives may play in how we judge others.

Values

Rokeach (1973) argued that values are chronic preferences for specific modes of conduct (*instrumental values*) and end states (*terminal values*). Thus values are like needs in that they specify movement toward a preferred (and important) state of being, but are different from needs in that "values are the cognitive representations and transformations of needs, and man is the only animal capable of such representations and transformations" (whereas all animals have needs; Rokeach, 1973, p. 20). As an example, a terminal value is a need to attain a state of being that has a particular set of characteristics. At the personal level, a terminal value might include the need to attain "peace of mind," a desired end state that serves one's personal being. Terminal values can also have a more interpersonal flavor, such as the need to attain "world peace" or "brotherhood." These end states, held as enduring preferences of the individual, are preferences that describe relationships between people in society, rather than simply one's own state of being. Finally, in describing a value as a preference for one specific end state, Rokeach meant that "a person prefers a particular mode or end-state not only when he compares it with its opposite but also when he compares it with other values within his value system" (1973, p. 10). Thus there is a hierarchy of values, and the higher a value is in the hierarchy, the more enduring and important that value. It is the enduring nature of values (their chronic quality) that gives them the power to guide action and judgment across a wide variety of domains. Rokeach saw values as standards that serve as a frame of reference both for interpreting the social world (as in shaping impressions of people) and in making comparisons (as in ascertaining the relative standing between people on some dimension). Values that are higher in one's value hierarchy will be more likely to be automatically triggered and guide one's impressions.

Rokeach (1973, pp. 98–99) described an experiment that illustrates how values, as chronic states, guide how people interpret the meaning of events in their social world. A national survey conducted in 1968 asked Americans to offer their reactions to the assassination of Martin Luther King, Jr. People were asked to choose from among the following reactions the one that best characterized their own reaction: sadness, anger, shame, fear, and "he brought it on himself." Clear patterns emerged in the reactions people offered for this event that were determined by their value systems. People who possessed the terminal value of "equality" (i.e., ones we might call chronic egalitarians) were the least likely people to have characterized their response to this event as one marked by fear and the feeling that King got what he deserved. What values were possessed by people most likely to characterize the event in this way? These people had the terminal values of obedience, salvation, and materialism. A survey that assessed people's overall level of racism toward Black Americans revealed similar findings: People who had a chronic commitment to the value of equality were among the least racist type of people. That is, their responses to a whole host of race-related questions came out on the racist end relatively infrequently (relative to people with other chronic values) and on the anti-racist end very frequently. Rokeach reviewed a litany of such attitudes and interpersonal opinions that had been examined up to the early 1970s, with the results being similar. The chronic states of an individual—in this case, values—direct how the person interprets the world, sees other people, and forms impressions of the events that occur in his/her social world. People with different value hierarchies interpret the events of their day in drastically different ways as filtered through their value systems.

The Authoritarian Personality

Maslow (1943) identified what he called a certain type of personality structure, associated with the chronic motives of power, cruelty, and superpatriotism. This set of chronic motives was said to serve as a means of providing for an individual a framework for judging and interpreting the world. It was believed to evolve from childhood experiences that teach a child to bury any immoral impulses. Harsh parenting styles lead the child to desire protection from the punishment associated with giving in to basic impulses. The evolving chronic motives that allow this protection to occur emphasize extreme punishment for any type of violation of societal norms, mores, and values. They also create the desire to become subservient to leaders who will protect the individual from the immorality that exists, leaders who will exert strong control. Such a hierarchical view of the world (punishers lording over the wicked) creates a need to dominate and be dominated, which leads to sadistic or masochistic tendencies, depending on which position one is in (the dominator or the dominated). Such a person comes to see power, order, definiteness, strictness, morality, power, and nationalism as affording the best protection from others, but in reality these chronic motives are smoke screens used to protect the person from his/her own "undesirable" impulses.

Simple desires to be good and moral in an overly simplistic way, which serves an overdeveloped and feared superego that is harsh and punishing, lead people to form impressions of others who look different from them as threats that need to be harshly dealt with (Adorno, Frenkel-Brunswik, Levinson, & Sanford, 1950). Thus they have a need to alleviate the guilt associated with the repression of their own basic instincts or repressed impulses. Since the fear of punishment from society, parental figures, and the harsh and punishing superego that has internalized these impulses is so great, such individuals need to express these impulses by projecting them onto others. Rather than admit their own failures, they create a world that is filled with evil and with villains, against which they need power and structure to protect them. Minority group members and foreigners are seen as threats to their way of life—to their stable, secure world—and to the values these authoritarians hold dear. In response to this pressure to preserve values, these people become highly ethnocentric, closed-minded, and in need of certainty; they dislike ambiguity and anything that is not clear-cut or black-and-white (Block & Block, 1951; Frenkel-Brunswik, 1949). This leads to prejudice and the dislike of people who are "different." The chronic motive pervades social judgment.

Early research created personality scales to attempt to measure the prevalence of this personality type. One such scale focused on the motive of feeling superior to others; it was labeled as a measure of *ethnocentrism*, or the need to see one's ethnic group as better than other groups. Another was called a measure of *intolerance of ambiguity*, or the extent to which a person needed to have clarity, certainty, and black-and-white solutions to questions. One scale measured anti-Semitism, or the degree to which an individual was motivated to dislike a specific group of people—Jews. Each of these personality scales was shown to have a relationship to prejudice, so that people who were chronically ethnocentric or chronically motivated to rid their environment of ambiguity were more likely to be prejudiced. As Frenkel-Brunswik (1949) stated, we should "expect prejudice to be associated with perceptual rigidity, inability to change set, and tendencies to primitive and rigid structuring of ambiguous perceptual fields" (p. 122). Adorno and colleagues (1950) developed a measure to assess one's chronic levels of authoritarianism that used this earlier work as its model. They called this measure a *fascism* (F) scale.

These chronic motivational states that characterize the authoritarian personality structure are matched by some cognitive consequences that have an impact on person perception. The most important and well-researched of these consequences—the relationship between authoritarianism and prejudice—has already been mentioned. An even more basic form of influence on impression formation, one more subtle and easily overlooked, is the impact of such chronic motives on the very early stages of impression formation that occur preconsciously. Uleman, Winborne, Winter, and Shechter (1986) predicted that the very meaning assigned to the behaviors people observe should differ between two people, dependent on their chronic levels of authoritarianism. Just as the Arabs and Americans described in the quote at the start of this chapter came to see the very same event in different ways, people high and low in authoritarianism (F) should come to see the very same behavior in different ways. What is most significant about this particular form of chronic influence on judgment is that this influence not only comes from a source that people do not know is biasing them, but affects judgments that they do not know they are making. Uleman and colleagues relied on the cued-recall procedure, reviewed in Chapter 7, for studying spontaneous trait inferences. Participants read sentences pretested to be ambiguous regarding the traits that they implied, and then had to remember those sentences when prompted with cues (such as traits implied by the sentences). They found that the inferences spontaneously formed by people high in authoritarianism were different from those low in authoritarianism. For example, the sentence "The secretary invited the man she had just met at the party to come home with her" led to the impression that the secretary was a "promiscuous slut" for people high in F, but "friendly and assertive" for people low in F. The sentence "The pilot reported his neighbor to the police for smoking marijuana" was predicted to lead to the impression that the pilot was "an honest citizen" for people scoring high on the F scale, but to the impression that he was "nosey" for people scoring low.

Need for Structure/Closure

Frenkel-Brunswik (1949) illustrated that people with an intolerance of ambiguity are more likely to be prejudiced. However, this need to structure judgments and attain closure (removing ambiguity) is a useful skill for navigating through the social world, and need not be linked to the prejudiced/authoritarian personality. Thompson, Naccarato, and Parker (1989) proposed separating this important element of social cognition from its link to prejudice and the emotional/repression-laden theory from which it emerged; thus was born the concept of *personal need for structure*. That is, a person may require structure not to satisfy buried urges, but to satisfy the cognitive system's need to categorize and simplify the environment in order for the person to function effectively in a complex stimulus environment.

Thompson and colleagues (1989; Thompson, Naccarato, Parker, & Moskowitz, 2001) proposed that imposing meaning on the environment is a pervasive goal for all individuals. How to expend time and cognitive effort toward accomplishing this end (how long people are willing to tolerate ambiguity) is determined in part by chronic tendencies. High personal need for structure is characterized by decisiveness and confidence, with discomfort experienced if the environment lacks clarity. Individuals with a high chronic need for structure prefer structure and clarity in most situations, with ambiguity and "grey areas" proving troublesome and annoying. They dislike and are disturbed by people who vacillate and who express opinions that lack coherence.

To examine the impact of a chronic need for structure on social judgment, Neuberg and Newsom (1993) examined how narrow or comprehensive a person's thoughts about other people were as a function of the perceiver's chronic need for structure. The idea was that high need for structure should be associated with structured and narrow thought, less ambiguity, and cleaner definitions of what it means to be a particular type of person. If asked to describe an introvert (or an honest person, or a successful person, etc.), people with a high need for structure might use fewer types of traits and a more narrow characterization of what such a person would look like, compared to people without a chronic need for structure (or low in this tendency). Research participants were given a set of index cards with information printed on them. They were told that the experiment was examining organizational style, and that they were to sort the cards into piles or groups, organized according to whether information fit together. Each participant received cards that contained one of four types of information: pictures of furniture; colors; traits they were to sort on the basis of how well they described old people; and traits they were to sort on the basis of well they described the self. The researchers then examined the relationship between the participants' need for structure and the complexity of the "sorts" that were created, and found the predicted relationship—a negative correlation. People who were high in need for structure created groupings of traits and images that were less complex. Neuberg and Newsom concluded: "Given that the nature of cognitive categories has crucial implications for the ways in which we perceive ourselves and others, for the ways in which we search our environment for new information . . . differences in the preference for simple structure may be quite important" (p. 123).

Indeed, to drive this point home, Neuberg and Newsom (1993) conducted an experiment to illustrate directly how need for structure influences the types of judgments made of other people. Participants were asked to read a story describing the actions of a person and were told that they would soon need to answer some questions about this person. The person was described as a student having difficulties both with tasks involving math and with a romantic relationship. The story also was somewhat ambiguous in describing the qualities of this person on some traits that are relevant to the stereotype of women, such as being overly emotional and irrational. The most important ingredient of the study came next, when half of the participants were led to expect that the person described in the story was a woman, and the other half were led to expect the person described was a man. The researchers predicted that people high in need for structure would be more likely to try to use stereotypes when judging other people, because stereotypes provide a fast and convenient way to explain another person—one that is simple and easily attained (see Chapter 11 for a detailed review of this idea). When the person in the story was described as a man, there would be no relevant stereotype to match the behavior described. However, when the person was described as a woman, the behavior would suddenly be relevant to the stereotype of women, and a person inclined to use stereotypes should now see this as an opportunity to do so. People high in need for structure should have just that inclination. This was exactly what was found. When the person in the story was a man, participants high and low in need for structure did not differ in their ratings. When it was a woman described in the story, the people high in need for structure rated her as more emotional and irrational (a stereotypic judgment) than the people low in need for structure did.

A further illustration of how impression formation is influenced by chronic levels of need for structure was provided by Webster and Kruglanski's (1994) examination of primacy effects (discussed in Chapter 1). A *primacy effect* is the disproportionate use of information one learns fairly early about a person (relative to information learned later) in forming an impression. Webster and Kruglanski reasoned that using the first bits of knowledge one learns about a person represents a tendency to form a structure quickly and then cling to that structure, avoiding ambiguity or uncertainty, and keeping the initial impression in place. If a primacy effect is essentially a case of quickly structuring another person's qualities into a coherent impression, then people high in the need for structure should be particularly likely to engage in this type of processing. To examine this issue, Webster and Kruglanski focused on an important interpersonal domain—job interviews. One would hope that in this situation, the interviewer would be sensitive enough not to allow stereotypes or first impressions to overly influence his/her conclusions about one's qualifications. Unfortunately, if an interviewer has a high need for structure, it may be particularly difficult to avoid relying on first impressions and on information revealed early in the interview process. This was precisely what was found. Research participants asked to play the role of the person doing the hiring in a job interview listened to a recorded interview that described the qualities of a job applicant. What was manipulated was the type of information they heard first. Ratings of participants low in need for structure did not change as a function of whether the information heard first was positive or negative. However, participants with high need for structure showed a primacy effect: When positive information was heard first, they liked the applicant, but when negative information was heard first, they disliked the candidate.

Social Dominance Orientation

Most societies have a hierarchical nature, with some groups superior to others (even if not officially designated as such). And in the structure of most societies are built-in institutions and social roles that allow for the maintenance of a status quo, in which the hierarchy is preserved and a few groups of people are permitted to remain superior over others. The social dominance of these few groups is contributed to not only by societal structures that keep the hierarchy in place, but by individuals who possess chronic motives to have the hierarchical structure of society maintained. Pratto, Sidanius, Stallworth, and Malle (1994) have identified what they called an implicit value that is relevant to intergroup relations, or a chronic motive to have the hierarchical placement of groups maintained. They refer to this as *social dominance orientation* (SDO)—"the extent to which one desires that one's in-group dominate and be superior to out-groups" (p. 742).

SDO manifests itself through what these authors call *hierarchy-legitimizing myths*. These are cultural beliefs and ideologies present in the society that serve to make discrimination legitimate. "They minimize conflict among groups by indicating how individuals and social institutions should allocate things of positive or negative social value, such as jobs, gold, blankets, government appointments, prison terms, and disease" (Pratto et al., 1994, p. 741). There are two paths through which SDO exerts itself and helps to sustain hierarchy-legitimizing myths. The first is by influencing the social structures that determine the opportunities and penalties facing people from different social groups. The second is by determining the attitudes of individual people toward things such as race relations and social policy, and by determining the types of jobs that individuals feel are appropriate for people from particular groups to pursue. Given that the concern in this book is with a given individual's social cognition, let us ignore the impact of SDO on cultural institutions (but see Sidanius & Pratto, 1999, for a discussion of a link among SDO and discrepancies among social groups in job pay, hiring, housing approval, mortgage approval, and bias at every stage of the legal/criminal justice system, from incarceration rates to severity of punishment).

Let us focus instead on the individual level—on how impressions of an individual, and even impressions of the self, are guided by this chronic motive. Pratto and colleagues (1994) argued that one's impressions about the types of jobs that are appropriate for one to pursue—something as fundamental as one's career choice—is determined by one's SDO. People who have high levels of SDO should form the impression that careers best suited for them are those that have a hierarchy-enhancing function—ones that keep the status quo in place. These would include careers as prosecuting attorneys, government officials, military personnel, and police officers. Similarly, people with low levels of SDO should form the impression that the careers best suited for them are those that have a hierarchy-attenuating function—ones that challenge the status quo and seek change to the social order. These would include careers as defense attorneys, social workers, and counselors. To test this prediction, Pratto and colleagues engaged in a massive data collection effort in which close to 2,000 college-age people were asked to answer a battery of questionnaires. Included among these was a measure of SDO, as well as questions pertaining to what sorts of careers the individuals felt were appropriate and that they intended to pursue. Responses to the question concerning career intentions were coded so that a person was labeled as intending to pursue either a hierarchy-enhancing career or a hierarchy-attenuating career. The results supported the notion that people's impressions about what careers were best suited for them would be determined by their motivation to see their ingroup as dominant. The people selecting hierarchy-attenuating careers were found to have reliably lower levels of SDO than the people selecting hierarchy-enhancing careers.

One final illustration of SDO's impact on impressions can be seen in the domains of racism and sexism. SDO determines whether people view others in prejudiced ways. In the Pratto and colleagues (1994) research, people high in SDO were more likely to express anti-Black sentiment and anti-female sentiment when answering surveys about these groups than were people low in SDO. The conclusion drawn from this finding is that such impressions help to rationalize the reasons for the lower-standing of these groups in the societal hierarchy. Thus, independent of cultural institutions that help to maintain the hierarchy, individual impressions of people from these groups help to justify and rationalize the status of these groups, making the boundaries unlikely to change. People chronically motivated to see these boundaries kept in place have developed a hierarchy-legitimizing style of impression formation, which allows people from stigmatized groups to be held accountable for their negative status.

Interpretation versus Comparison Goals

Interpretation and comparison are two of the primary ways in which people produce impressions (Stapel & Koomen, 2001). *Interpretation* occurs when people are attempting to encode behavior and understand/identify the behavior they have observed. *Comparison* occurs when people are forming a judgment and need to make relative assessments of the degree to which a person exhibits a given trait or behavior relative to a standard of comparison (some example against which the current act is judged). Comparison goals are a primary tool of pursuing self-esteem needs. In order to feel a positive sense of self-worth, one must engage in comparisons of the self against others along relevant dimensions (e.g., Festinger, 1954b). Because of the fundamental nature of comparison processes for human well-being, these goals are presumed to be chronic, triggered automatically by situations that present opportunities for engaging in social comparison (Stapel & Tesser, 2001). Interpretation, on the other hand, is linked to epistemic needs. To attain closure and meaning, to understand the world, requires people to pursue the goal of identifying and interpreting the events and behavior they observe. These goals are also chronically pursued, and would be triggered by environments that present opportunities for making valid interpretations. Given the central role these goals play in impression formation, and given the assumed chronic pursuit of these goals, it should be the case that cues in the environment relevant to these goals should trigger them automatically. Which of these goals is triggered will determine the degree to which a person engages in social comparison versus interpretation processes when interacting with others.

Stapel and Koomen (2001) examined this auto-motive hypothesis by implicitly triggering either an interpretation goal or a comparison goal in research participants. They then looked to see how social cognition was affected. To trigger the goal, participants performed a task that had words associated with the goal embedded in the materials. Half the people incidentally read words relating to interpretation (e.g., "understand," "comprehend," "interpret," and "meaning"), while the other half read words relating to making comparisons (such as "distinguish," "opposition," "contrast," and "difference"). Without realizing that this had triggered any goals, participants then engaged in an impression formation task supposedly unrelated to the former task. Their judgments were clearly affected by the chronic goals triggered in the current setting. When comparison goals were triggered, people formed impressions by making contrasts—looking at how the person they were forming an impression of compared to relevant standards of comparison that were present in the immediate environment. These comparison/ contrast processes led the person to be judged as not at all like the relevant standards that were present. However, when interpretation goals were triggered, the opposite pattern emerged. Rather than contrasting the person with relevant standards that were present in the environment, the perceivers used the traits of the "standards" as an interpretive frame that provided a way to make sense of the target person's behavior. As an example, if Gandhi had been recently mentioned in the participants' environment, then people with a comparison goal used Gandhi as a standard of comparison against which the new person was judged. Gandhi was extremely benevolent, so the new person was seen in the opposite manner—as not benevolent at all, given the behavioral standard established by Gandhi. However, when an interpretation goal was triggered, the benevolence of Gandhi was seen as a framework for making sense of the behavior of the new person, and thus he/she was seen as benevolent too. Clearly, the chronic goals triggered by our environment can play a central role in determining the types of judgments and impressions we form.

Auto-Motives and Behavior in Interpersonal Interaction

As noted in several places throughout this book, thinking is in the service of action (e.g., Allport, 1954; James, 1890/1950). So too are goals and motives, which are merely mental states seeking to deliver our desired ends. If goals and cognition help us to prepare and select appropriate behavior, we should naturally expect behavior to be influenced by implicit cognition and implicit goals. In this section, we explore several ways in which chronically pursued goals have an impact on behavior. Fitzsimons and Bargh (2003) have proposed that most of our important relationships with other people can be characterized by some set of goals—whether it be the goal to make our mothers proud or the goal to be supportive and helpful to our friends. Because these goals are chronically associated with these specific relationship partners, the presence of these people triggers these goals and influences our behavior, regardless of whether we are consciously aware of the goal being triggered. When with friends, we nonconsciously start acting helpful; when with our mothers, we begin to act in situation-appropriate ways that might make her proud. In fact, we do not even need these relationship partners to be physically present to trigger these goals automatically and to start us behaving in ways consistent with these goals. Any cues in the environment that might remind us of our mothers would trigger the chronic goals we have associated with our mothers and lead to behavior consistent with that goal. Thus cues in the context that are associated with any of our significant relationships can trigger whatever goal is associated with those relationships and lead to behavior aimed at delivering that specific goal.

Fitzsimons and Bargh (2003) provide several illustrations of how the mental representations of specific relationship partners, including the chronic goals associated with those relationship partners, can be triggered by the cues in the current environment. Once these chronic goals are triggered, they influence actions. In one experiment, these authors relied on the fact that people seem to have chronic helping goals associated with close friendships. Therefore, they had people simply think about their friends and then measured whether such people were subsequently more likely to help others (thus indicating that thinking about the friends triggered the goal to help, and this influenced how the participants chose to act). As predicted, people who thought about friends actually chose to help a stranger to a greater degree than when they had previously been asked to think about coworkers.

Another experiment illustrated the powerful motivating influence of mothers. Fitzsimons and Bargh (2003) first classified research participants as being people who either possessed the chronic goal of making their mothers proud or people who did not have this chronic goal associated with their relationship with their mother. Participants then had thoughts about their mothers triggered (or not) by asking half of them to describe their mother's appearance. Following this, they worked on a task aimed at detecting whether there were behavioral differences between the groups. The task involved generating as many words as possible from a series of scrambled letters. People not asked to think about their mothers did not perform differently on this task as a function of whether their relationships with their mothers were marked by thoughts of making them proud. However, participants asked to think about their mothers showed a difference in how well they performed on the task as a function of their relationship with their mothers. Those who had the goal of "making Mom proud" included in their mental representation of "mother" had these chronic goals triggered, whereas people who did not have this goal associated with their mothers did not. Once this goal was triggered, these participants outperformed all the other people in the experiment on the word generation task. They implicitly made their mothers proud by trying harder and doing better. In these examples, an automatically triggered goal influenced a consciously chosen behavior. However, goals can influence how people act even when they do not realize they are acting. Let's illustrate what is meant by this next.

The Chameleon Effect

Al Gore was a Senator and Vice-President of the United States, and the son of another Senator. He had lived in Washington, D.C., most of his life, but when he ran for President in the year 2000, we got to see him in a variety of new contexts. Interestingly, it seemed as if whenever he made an appearance in the American South (especially his home state of Tennessee), his accent seemed to change, and a Southern drawl appeared. Some people saw this as evidence that he was disingenuous, willing to morph his very speech patterns to try to please the locals. "That man would stop at nothing to try to get a vote," they charged. However, there are several other possible explanations for Gore's Southern accent. Let us concern ourselves with one specific possibility here, mimicry. Chartrand and Bargh (1999) have proposed that the mere perception of other people's behavior will increase the likelihood that the perceiver will begin to enact that behavior. This mimicry of others is believed to be a passive and nonconscious process. "One may notice using the idiosyncratic verbal expressions or speech inflections of a friend. Or one may notice crossing one's arms while talking with someone else who has his or her arms crossed. Common to all such cases is that one typically does not notice doing these things—if at all—until after the fact" (Chartrand & Bargh, 1999, p. 893). This act of nonconsciously taking on the accent, speech patterns, and behaviors/mannerisms of an interaction partner has been dubbed *the chameleon effect*. With no intended insult to Al Gore, a familiar and applicable saying is "Monkey see, monkey do."

Nonconscious mimicry is not a new phenomenon. Berkowitz (1984) used this idea to explain why violence seen on television is so readily imitated by children. Adopting the posture and body movement of an interaction partner has been repeatedly illustrated, especially when the interactants have a rapport of some sort (La France & Ickes, 1981). It is even seen in neonates, who are known to mimic the facial expressions of adults (Meltzoff & Moore, 1977). The question we are concerned with here is this: Why do people so readily mimic? Is there some chronic goal that drives them to imitate the behavior of others? Chartrand and Bargh (1999) assert that "the consensus position appears to be that behavioral coordination is in some way related to empathy, rapport, and liking . . . mimicry and behavioral coordination are said to serve the adaptive function of facilitating social interaction interpersonal bonding" (p. 896). Thus, if goals associated with the need to belong are associated with mimicry, then the chameleon effect should be especially pronounced in people who have chronic goals associated with empathy and liking. Specifically, people who have chronic goals to take the perspective of others should be especially likely to illustrate the chameleon effect. To get along with others and to act in a coordinated manner requires being able to empathize with others and take their perspective. Thus people particularly motivated to engage in perspective taking should be particularly likely to reveal the behavioral manifestations associated with this chronic goal. Chartrand and Bargh identified research participants who scored either high or low on a measure of chronic levels of perspective taking. They then measured whether these groups differed in how much they nonconsciously mimicked others. Each participant was brought to the lab and asked to work with a partner on a task. This "partner" was actually a confederate working for the experimenters who was trained to display two nonverbal behaviors while interacting with the participant—rubbing the face and shaking a foot. The measure of mimicry was simple: Did the participant also rub the face and shake a foot? Remarkably, most of them did, and this was more pronounced for chronic perspective takers.

Intimacy Goals versus Identity Goals

Let's move from mimicry to dating. What determines how people behave in intimate relationships? Obviously, the answer to this question is complex and multiply determined. However, among the important ingredients are the chronic goals that each individual brings to the dating relationship—the things each one hopes to attain in a romantic relationship. Does one seek companionship, dependence, emotional support, physical contact, a partnership that allows one to pursue independent activities, financial security? Which of these goals is most important will dictate whether one enters a relationship and how one behaves within that relationship. Sanderson and Cantor (1995) identified people with chronic *intimacy goals*—goals aimed at using interpersonal relationships for attaining interdependence, relying on others, and communicativeness. These can be contrasted with *identity goals*—chronic states of seeking to use interpersonal relationships for exploring the self and establishing one's unique identity. It may be that intimacy goals, which represent a more advanced stage of emotional and social development, are not ready to be pursued by individuals who have not yet established a secure and stable identity (one must be secure in the self before turning one's goals toward emotional intimacy and interdependence with others; Erikson, 1959). Thus behavior in interpersonal relationships should be influenced by the chronic goals of the dating partners (Cantor & Malley, 1991; Sanderson & Cantor, 1995; Zirkel, 1992). As an example, people with chronic intimacy goals have fewer sexual partners, have longer-lasting relationships, spend more time with their partners while in their relationships (day-to-day time spent together), and have greater satisfaction with their relationships than people with identity goals do. For the latter group, their goals are better served by exploring their personality within the context of many different relationships.

The relationship between how one acts and whether the context triggers one's chronic goals was illustrated in the domain of sex. Sanderson and Cantor (1995) predicted that whether people practiced safe sex (such as using condoms) would be dependent on whether the relationship context was associated with their chronic goals. That is, they predicted that the context in which individuals with such goals found themselves would determine whether these goals were triggered, and whether these goals could be carried out with goal-relevant behavior. As a hypothetical example, consider Jane, a woman with chronic identity goals. Jane's chronic goals are best served in relationships that provide an appropriate context for pursuing her chronic goals. Thus sexual relationships characterized by a lack of emotional intimacy and casual sexual encounters will trigger her identity goals, and will promote behavior that helps to promote the successful completion of those goals. In such relationships, one must be careful not to contract a sexual disease, and this would mean that practicing safe sex would be a behavior well matched to one's goals. Thus, if the dating context triggers Jane's goals, then she should practice safe sex. However, if Jane enters a relationship with a person who desires emotional intimacy and a long-term commitment, she may now be in a context that does not trigger her own chronic goals and leads her to abandon the behaviors that are associated with those goals, such as practicing safe sex. It is not that people with one type of goal are more likely to use condoms than the other, but that the match between goals and relationship partners can determine this behavior.

Now you may be saying to yourself that this logic is confounded: A person in a long-term relationship would always be less likely to use condoms, because the partner is not a stranger and there is less of a need to be defensive. However, Sanderson and Cantor (1995) were not predicting that people in committed relationships would be less likely to use condoms. They were predicting that people would be likely (or unlikely) to use condoms when doing so met their chronic goals. Thus, in a dating context allowing for chronic goals to be pursued, then the compatibility of condom use with those goals would be the determining factor governing whether safe sex was practiced. Thus, perhaps counterintuitively, Sanderson and Cantor found that people with chronic intimacy goals were actually more likely to use condoms when they were in intimate and committed relationships, and were less likely to do so when in casual sexual encounters! For such people, their chronic goals involved communication and interdependence, and when they were with partners who fostered these goals (committed relationships), they were more likely to feel comfortable enough to discuss and use sexual protection. A context not triggering these chronic goals (such as casual dating) would make it less likely for such people to see an opportunity to pursue their goals and less likely to act in ways compatible with their goals; this would place them in substantial risk simply because of their auto-motives.

Learning versus Performance Goals

One last illustration of how auto-motives influence behavior is focused on how people form impressions and react to their own behavior, especially when people discover they have failed at some task. Chapter 8 has discussed how failure is threatening to the self and leads people to try to protect self-esteem through a variety of possible mechanisms. How people respond to negative feedback is in part determined by what chronic motives they have, and whether the context in which the failure occurs can trigger a relevant chronic motive. Dweck (1991, 1996; Elliott & Dweck, 1988) identified two chronic goals that are pertinent to the achievement domain and can help predict how people respond to failure. *Performance goals* are those that lead individuals to strive toward evaluating, measuring, and judging the relative degrees to which they possess a particular ability or trait—that is, their efficacy in a given domain. In the achievement domain, this would mean having goals of understanding how well they perform. This chronic goal orientation is marked by *the assumption or theory that ability, efficacy, and traits are fixed and stable qualities* and can be measured. Performance goals can be contrasted with *learning goals*, which are goals that lead individuals to strive toward developing their aptitude in a given domain. Rather than being marked by an assumption that ability is fixed and need only be measured, learning goals are associated with *an implicit theory that ability is malleable, dynamic, and open to change*. It is the goal orientation of cultivating skills in a particular domain rather than assessing them.

These goals are conceived of as having opposing consequences for impression formation and behavior. Chronic learning goals will be associated with a belief in change and growth, and will lead individuals to approach contexts with the task of using information attained in that context as feedback to promote an ever-changing level of efficacy and skill in a given domain. They want to know where and why they are making mistakes in order to learn how to improve. Chronic performance goals will be associated with a belief that attributes are fixed, and will lead individuals to enter situations for the purpose of diagnosing efficacy—to find out, via task performance, how capable they are. Feedback situations, therefore, should trigger different chronic goals for different people. For individuals with chronic performance goals (who hold *entity theories*, or theories that specify ability as a fixed entity), negative outcomes or negative feedback should trigger these goals. With these chronic goals triggered, the negative feedback being received should lead them to form impressions about themselves that characterize the cause for the failure (or negative feedback) as being a lack of intelligence or ability on their part. With their goals guiding these impressions, the behavioral response initiated as a function of these auto-motives will be one of disengagement and withdrawal; the individuals, convinced that they simply lack aptitude, will display a helpless reactions (e.g., low persistence). People with learning goals, on the other hand, will have these goals triggered in feedback situations. When feedback is negative, these individuals will form impressions about the feedback that are guided by their goals, and come to see the feedback not as reflecting a stable quality or attribute, but as a relevant source of information about their current standing in an evolving skill domain. Thus they are not lacking in intelligence or ability; they are in need of harder work or more practice. Very different behavior should now be evidenced as a function of the auto-motive that has been triggered. These persons should view setbacks as cues that alert them to focus on new behavioral strategies. Their behavior should be oriented toward mastering the causes of the setback. Rather than helplessness, they should display persistence.

CHRONIC GOALS AND PERCEPTUAL DEFENSE

The likelihood that subjective discriminations among and reactions to stimuli occur prior to consciousness suggests not only that we humans can use chronically accessible goals to help us detect the presence of things in our environment compatible with those goals, but that we may be able to establish a preconscious defense system to ward off stimuli that are threatening to our chronically accessible goals. As Postman and colleagues (1948) stated, "value orientation not only contributes to the selection and accentuation of certain percepts in preference to others, it also erects barriers against percepts and hypotheses incongruent with or threatening to the individual's values" (p. 152). This type of preconscious defense system, in which we prevent ourselves from consciously seeing concepts that are displeasing and threatening (or at least delay the recognition of such concepts), is known as *perceptual defense*.

Perceptual Defense

In order to illustrate that we preconsciously detect undesirable stimuli and then prevent ourselves from consciously noting these, McGinnies (1949) conducted an experiment in which people were asked to make verbal responses to the presentation of threatening and disliked word stimuli (i.e., to report when they could see each word). In addition to assessing at what point in time people were consciously detecting each stimulus, physiological arousal was simultaneously measured as an index of people's reactions to the stimulus not guided by consciousness. Such words should not only affect verbal reports, but cause autonomic arousal. Verbal reports should be pushed in the opposite pattern of the valued words in the Postman and colleagues (1948) study: They should take longer to identify (have higher thresholds of recognition), leading to a preconscious avoidance.

McGinnies (1949) assessed reactions to "taboo" words (emotionally charged words that research participants desired to avoid, such as "whore" and "penis") in a manner similar to Postman and colleagues (1948)—by measuring the time it took to consciously recognize a word as its presentation speed was gradually slowed from being initially flashed so quickly that it could only be subliminally detected. In addition, reactions to the words were assessed through the use of galvanic skin responses. It was found that it took people longer to recognize the taboo words than to identify control words such as "broom" and "clear." Furthermore, and most significantly, it was found that emotional reactions to taboo words were being registered by galvanic skin responses when such words were not yet being consciously detected. That is, people were having autonomic responses to subliminally presented, despised words before they were able to issue verbal responses signaling conscious perception of them. The preconscious was apparently detecting these words and defending the conscious mind from them, delaying recognition (raising the perceptual threshold). McGinnies assumed that perceptual defense "serves, in many instances, to protect the observer as long as possible from an awareness of objects which have unpleasant emotional significance" (p. 244). Chronically accessible concepts play a role at the preconscious level, determining what will pass through the iconic storehouse and into conscious attention. Although alternative explanations for these early studies can be generated (and perhaps you are rushing them to mind now—e.g., participants effortfully suppressed speaking words they did not wish to speak, even if they really could see them; or perhaps the effort involved in suppressing the speaking of such words caused the changes in galvanic skin responses). However, subsequent, more thorough research, with compatible findings, helps us to keep hold of the idea that there is preconscious analysis of environmental stimuli, and that this analysis is guided by such things as perceptual readiness (for a review, see Erdelyi, 1974).

The Homunculus Paradox

A new paradox becomes evident when we consider perceptual defense. Earlier in this chapter, we have settled the so-called paradox of subliminal perception by allowing for the possibility that information processing can be broken down into several steps (including iconic and echoic perception), some of which are preconscious and provide outputs that feed into consciousness. The new paradox, however, revolves around how the decision is made to allow some stimuli to pass through the iconic/echoic filter and ultimately become consciously detected and attended. Given that these "decisions" are made without conscious awareness, the process, paradoxically, seems to involve "the will" without the will's being phenomenologically involved. It appears as if there is a "little man in the head" (a *homunculus*) making decisions for each of us. Of course, psychologists do not think a homunculus is the solution. This might be how Homer Simpson's brain works, but not yours and mine.

The Threshold Metaphor

Deutsch and Deutsch (1963) have explained our ability to decide what to allow through the preconscious filter by using the analogy of signal detection theory. Although our conscious will may not be involved from moment to moment in terms of deciding what to allow through the filter, the will can be involved at setting the threshold for determining what stimuli will pass through such a filter. If we conceive of concepts (such as goals) as having certain levels of charge or accessibility, we can have a filter in place that allows stimuli to pass into consciousness only if they have a certain degree of fit to concepts with a certain level of accessibility. Thus, if each stimulus entering the storehouse is conceived of as a signal, for the signal to be detected it may need to have a certain level of strength/fit relative to the parameters defined by the filter. Thus each of us has a unique set of chronic goals that perhaps define what stimuli will have the "right fit," and because which chronic goals are in greater relative states of accessibility shift from situation to situation, which stimuli will have the appropriate "signal" will also shift. The threshold defined by the filter may be constantly shifting along with our passive, chronic goals, altering the point at which a signal will be strong enough to pass through the filter (as our needs and goals shift from context to context, the filter may adjust itself with the activation of goals and concepts relevant to that new context). Such a threshold metaphor (e.g., Treisman & Geffen, 1967) posits that all information is first perceived and analyzed preconsciously, but that only certain elements with a required level of excitation are allowed through the threshold to be consciously recognized, responded to, and remembered. Information important to our concerns will have a level of excitation associated with it, and our goals and concerns specify for us, even if we are not aware of it, the level of excitation that a percept needs to be charged with in order to pass through the filter.

Interference and Inhibition

The preconscious filtering of information is not the only way that perceptual defense could occur. A second explanation has less to do with the simple blocking of information from passing through a filter and more to do with a preconscious suppression or inhibition resulting from a competition between two or more concepts that each desire to enter consciousness and capture a stimulus. More than one response may be associated with a stimulus, and each may rush to be made. Consider again the Moskowitz and colleagues (2000) study, where an image of a Black man triggered egalitarian goals in chronically egalitarian persons, but stereotypic thoughts in people who were not chronic egalitarians. Importantly, even a chronic egalitarian knows the stereotypes of Black men; such a person simply finds it distasteful and wrong. Given that such knowledge is available, how does one prevent it from becoming accessible? Shouldn't all information associated with the category be triggered, as the notion of spreading activation suggests? Or is some information triggered because of its increased accessibility, and other information (especially that incompatible with the triggered information) inhibited? That is, if two concepts are associated with a category and are incompatible with each other, one may actually serve to lower the accessibility of the other, making it less perceptually ready. Rather than simply being not selected to enter consciousness, it is actually given a lowered likelihood of being used. This is what is meant by saying that *inhibition* of a concept has occurred.

In order to understand the concept of inhibition, we must first be certain to understand what is meant by a *preconscious competition* between concepts. For example, in the Stroop (1935) effect (see Chapter 2), people are asked to name the color of the ink of a printed word. But if the word itself is the word "blue" yet is written in the color green, there are two responses that compete: The correct answer is "green" (the color of the ink), but the automatic processing of the semantic meaning of the word makes a person want to respond by saying "blue." These different responses can have different points at which the threshold for allowing the response to be made is set, and the thresholds for each of the responses may interact with each other, either facilitating or inhibiting a particular response. Thus, if color naming is one response, and the automatic occurrence of detecting semantic meaning is the other, when these two responses produce conflicting reactions to the stimulus (saying "blue" vs. "green"), a competition between the responses can be observed. Given that reading words is an automatic process, and detecting ink colors is a temporary goal, the more well-practiced and efficient response wins the metaphorical race. Therefore, people begin to read aloud the word listed ("blue") before correcting themselves to say the correct response ("green"). It is for this reason that people are slow to name the ink color; their initial response is incorrect, and it needs to be quickly inhibited before the correct response can be offered. To return to the example of perceptual defense as seen in the research of McGinnies (1949), if one response is the chronic avoidance of sexually explicit and embarrassing stimuli, and the other is the iconic recognition of all words (including sexual words), the former response may compete with and interfere with the further processing of the latter. As Bruner (1957, p. 145) states, failure to perceive is most often not a lack of perceiving but a matter of interference with perceiving. Whence the interference? I would propose that the interference comes from categorizations in highly accessible categories that serve to block alternative categorizations in less accessible categories. As a highly speculative suggestion, the mechanism that seems most likely to mediate such interference is probably the broadening of category acceptance limits when a high state of readiness to perceive prevails.

Inhibition in Social Cognition

Let us now illustrate how these ideas are important for the interpretation of other people. The first example is from the domain of stereotyping. A person who wishes to see the world in nonprejudiced ways faces a dilemma (reviewed in detail in Chapter 11): Even if the person denounces stereotypes, he/she knows the various stereotypes of social groups in the culture, and these come to mind quite easily. The nonprejudiced person is faced with the dilemma of not wanting to think about stereotypes, but having these thoughts triggered easily and frequently. What is the person to do? The best the average person can do is to try to recognize when these stereotypes come to mind and to try not to let them influence judgment (and to reject them when appropriate). But the person who is chronically egalitarian—who has habitually pursued the goals of being fair, tolerant, and nonstereotypic—has a different strategy available. For this person, a lifetime of detecting stereotypes, rejecting stereotypes, and being committed to this process has made doing these things a chronic state of affairs. This should lead him/her to have egalitarianism chronically accessible and manning the gate at the threshold to consciousness. The filter is ready to detect stimuli relevant to egalitarianism and antagonistic to egalitarianism.

Chronic egalitarians, should, therefore, be more likely to detect information relevant to this chronically accessible construct (as reviewed earlier in this chapter), but they should also be more likely to *inhibit* incompatible information, making information relevant to stereotypes harder to detect and be brought to consciousness. Why? Practice at associating goals (in this case, egalitarian goals) with stimuli (in this case, members of stereotyped groups) can lead to the implicit activation of the goals in the presence of the stimuli (Bargh, 1990). What happens when a person has *practiced a goal of suppressing a construct in the presence of a stimulus*? If attempts at stereotype suppression can be routinized through practice (or through contextual conditions that create a strong enough commitment to the goal), perhaps the presence of a relevant cue will trigger inhibition of a stereotype. Fox (1995) suggests that a process perhaps better labeled as *spreading inhibition* can be produced if attention is repeatedly focused on ignoring a stimulus and the semantic content associated with it. Practice at avoiding a construct can result in that construct being implicitly inhibited, rather than facilitated. Tipper (1985) has labeled this inhibition effect associated with ignored stimuli *negative priming*. Neill, Valdes, and Terry (1995) describe spreading inhibition from negative priming as represented by a "slowdown" rather than a facilitation to words linked to the to-be-ignored category.

Exactly this type of preconscious inhibition in egalitarian individuals has been illustrated (Moskowitz, Gollwitzer, Wasel, & Schaal, 1999). Male research participants with chronic egalitarian goals (in this case, regarding the treatment of women) had attributes and thoughts associated with the stereotype of women actually inhibited (or less accessible) after they saw a woman, relative to people without chronic goals of this type (who, instead, had stereotypic traits and attributes more accessible). Participants were asked to perform a task in which words either relevant or irrelevant to the stereotype of women were presented on the screen. Participants had to speak the words aloud into a microphone, with the computer recording their pronunciation speeds. Half of the time these words were preceded by faces of women, and half of the time by faces of men. Participants were asked to ignore the image, or essentially to inhibit thinking about the image. The logic was that a picture of a woman (but not a picture of a man) would trigger goals to be fair to women in chronic egalitarians (but not in nonchronic participants), and that the goal of ignoring an image of a woman would trigger automated inhibition processes associated with that group. If a chronic egalitarian habitually ignores thinking about stereotypes when thinking about women, then the goal of ignoring this group should automatically trigger these automatic inhibition tendencies. The face of a woman should trigger the goal and establish a preconscious defense system, warding off responses incompatible with the chronic goals, such as thinking of the person in a stereotypic way. This was exactly what was found. People with chronic egalitarian goals were slower to pronounce words relevant to the stereotype of women, but only when the word was preceded by a picture of a woman that they were trying to ignore. This did not occur when the words were preceded by pictures of men; this did not occur when words irrelevant to the stereotype were preceded by pictures of women; and it did not occur at all for people without chronic egalitarian goals. The semantic content linked to a cultural stereotype may thus be inhibited as a function of categorization, rather than activated.

Inhibition is not always caused by chronic goals. Stereotypes, for example, not only are incompatible with goals of being egalitarian, but may be incompatible with other stereotypes. For example, the stereotype of African Americans involves the traits "aggressive" and "hostile," while the stereotype of women involves the traits "dependent" and "weak." African American women clearly cannot be both weak and aggressive, and it stands to reason that because of this incompatibility, the triggering of one stereotype could inhibit the triggering of the other. When we meet people, there are multiple ways to categorize them (TV host, Black man, athlete, celebrity, killer, etc.). All these categories could be used to describe the same man (O. J. Simpson). Which stereotype is activated (if any) will depend on which category is used.

This type of evidence for inhibition between incompatible constructs was provided by Macrae, Bodenhausen, and Milne (1995, reviewed briefly in Chapter 1). They showed a competition between activated constructs and a preconscious inhibition process by examining two opposing stereotypes relevant to the same stimulus. Participants observed a Chinese woman in one of two possible contexts: one that triggered stereotypes of women, and one that triggered stereotypes of Chinese people. They found that when gender stereotypes were made accessible (by showing a videotape of a Chinese woman applying makeup), people were likely to have gender stereotypes accessible, but not stereotypes of the Chinese (which instead were now inhibited by the presence of the woman, rather than made accessible). However, if the Chinese stereotype had been activated (by showing a videotape of a Chinese woman using chopsticks to eat noodles), the stereotypes of the Chinese were most accessible, and gender stereotypes were no longer accessible, but inhibited. Macrae and MacLeod (1999) examined similar types of interference and inhibition between competing constructs in the domain of memory and forgetting. The inability to remember information may be caused by interference from a competing representation that blocks the desired information from reaching consciousness. Macrae and MacLeod extended the research of Anderson, Bjork, and Bjork (1994) by positing that the retrieval of social information is regulated by implicit processes that lead to the temporary forgetting (suppression) of competing constructs. For example, when one wants to remember the name of a date one is meeting at a restaurant, this goal is served if the names of past dates taken to the same restaurant can be automatically suppressed. Retrieving a specific item from memory leads to the suppression (rather than the increased accessibility) of relevant, but competing items.

Whereas the Moskowitz and colleagues (1999) and Macrae and colleagues (1995) studies illustrated how a preconscious inhibition can be produced by a competition between two incompatible concepts (a goal and a stereotype in one case, two competing stereotypes in the other), Dijksterhuis and van Knippenberg (1996) found that such inhibition can occur even when the need for a competing category or goal is not currently present. The inhibition process is already triggered by adopting one goal or by having one stereotype triggered, so that information incompatible with that goal or stereotype is simply inhibited, tuning the cognitive system toward relevant information and defending it against irrelevant information. Dijksterhuis and van Knippenberg (1996) illustrated that priming a stereotype facilitated access to stereotype-consistent traits and inhibited access to stereotype-inconsistent traits. Research participants in the Netherlands were first asked to imagine a typical "soccer hooligan" and to spend 5 minutes writing down the behaviors, lifestyle choices, and attributes of such a person (the stereotype of this group includes notions of such people as aggressive, fanatical, violent, and insolent). Later in the experiment, the participants were asked to work on a separate and "unrelated" task in which they were to try to recognize whether a string of letters was a word or not. On the key trials of the experiment, the letters did form words, and these words were either consistent or inconsistent with the image of a soccer hooligan. The results showed that after having thought about a soccer hooligan, people were slower to recognize words inconsistent with the category (e.g., "friendly," "intelligent," "understanding") than control words (and words consistent with the category, which were recognized faster). There was inhibited access to incompatible words.

Rothbart, Sriram, and Davis-Stitt (1996) obtained similar results by looking at how stereotypes would facilitate or inhibit the ability to think about types of people instead of stereotypical traits. They found that stereotypes, rather than promoting access to stereotypic traits and inhibiting access to incompatible ones, increased the ability to retrieve typical category members while limiting access to atypical members. The more counterstereotypic a category member was, the lower the probability that this member would be activated and retrieved when the stereotype was accessible. The role of typicality in exemplar retrieval was further explored in a field study involving rival fraternities; typical members of the rival fraternities were more likely to be recalled, and atypical examples (specific individuals who disconfirmed the stereotype) were inhibited and less likely to be recalled. The Rothbart et al. experiments are important because the ascription of traits to a person is often determined by the exemplars that come to mind (Smith & Zarate, 1992), and the findings suggest that counterstereotypic traits and exemplars are being inhibited when stereotypes are accessible.

We have been using stereotypes as examples of this interference and inhibition process, because the domain of stereotypes is simply an interesting one in which to illustrate this point. However, inhibition should occur whenever a chronic goal is in place and incompatible stimuli are present in the environment (Moskowitz, Li, & Kirk, 2004). Kunda and Thagard (1996) offer what they call the *parallel-constraint-satisfaction model* to account for such inhibition. This model asserts that not everything in the lexicon associated with a category/stereotype is triggered upon encountering a member of that category, or a behavior that falls within a particular category. Instead, chronic goals, expectancies, and context bolster the activation of some information while simultaneously (in parallel) inhibiting or constraining the activation of other information. Kunda, Sinclair, and Griffin (1997, p. 721) offer a nice example that moves us out of the domain of stereotyping: "*Aggressive* may activate both *punch* and *argue*. The context in which *aggressive* is activated may serve to narrow its meaning. Thus, *courtroom* may activate *argue* while deactivating *punch* . . . a given trait may have a rich and diverse network of associates; only a subset of these is activated on any occasion." This model holds that not all information associated with a category is triggered. In fact, the goals of the perceiver and the context the perceiver is in inhibit some associations, making them less (rather than more) likely to be accessible and used. (In a courtroom, for instance, notions of punching are not activated, but notions of being argumentative are.)

CHRONIC ACCESSIBILITY AND SCHEMATICS

Bruner (1957) focused his discussion of perceptual readiness on motives, needs, and values that are chronic states of the perceiver. However, when the notion of chronic accessibility was gaining widespread interest in the field some 20–30 years later (e.g., Bargh, Lombardi, & Higgins, 1988; Bargh & Pratto, 1986; Bargh & Thein, 1985; Higgins, King, & Mavin, 1982; Markus, 1977), the emerging research was predominantly void of motivational concepts, and was focused instead on the chronicity of cognitive structures—a chronic style of thinking, such as a habitual focus on a particular set of traits (such as those constituting the self-schema). This was similar to Kelly's (1955) assertion that habitual experiences serve as a scanning pattern that sweeps the environment, and Heider's (1958) notion of perceptual styles as chronic states of readiness that guide impression formation from situation to situation. Bargh (1982) summarized this well:

> People possess a variety of long-term, or chronic expectancies that have evolved out of frequent and consistent experience within specific environmental domains (Broadbent, 1977; Logan, 1979; Shiffrin & Dumais, 1981; Shiffrin & Schneider, 1977). Considerable experience in a domain results in associations between its constituent elements forming and strengthening in long term memory (e.g., Hayes-Roth, 1977; Hebb, 1949). Because chronic expectancies are relatively permanent characteristics of the perceptual system itself (Broadbent, 1977), one's active direction is not necessary for them to influence the interpretation of stimuli. (p. 426)

Chronically Accessible Knowledge and Judgment

Higgins and colleagues (1982) reasoned that people whose routines frequently place them in contact with the same stimuli will have those concepts in a permanent state of excitation. "To the extent that people's social experiences vary in respect to which constructs are frequently activated (e.g., long-term differences in socialization experiences, goals, etc.), one would expect there to be individual differences in construct accessibility" (p. 36). A teenager who spends an inordinate amount of time with friends who focus almost exclusively on doing schoolwork and commenting on other people's intelligence will come to have notions of intelligence chronically ready to be used to interpret other people. Another person, who is immersed in a culture of friends consumed by people's physical appearance, may, upon hearing a prominent lecturer, only comment about the color of the lecturer's shirt or the style of his/her haircut. Higgins and colleagues sought to illustrate that such stability in accessible constructs exists as a chronic state, and that such stable levels of excitation influence impression formation, so that the same information should be interpreted differently by different individuals as a function of what traits, concepts, and beliefs they have chronically accessible.

Higgins et al. first assessed what concepts were chronically accessible to their research participants. They asked people to list up to 10 traits describing a type of person that they (1) liked, (2) disliked, (3) sought out, (4) avoided, and (5) frequently encountered. These questions were used to ascertain the types of traits each partici-pant had chronically accessible. From these traits, an essay was constructed (tailored to each participant) that described a person in the following manner: Half of the per-son's behaviors implied traits consistent with the participant's accessible concepts, and half implied traits not chronically accessible to the participant. Participants did not know that their task of reading the essay, forming impressions of the person, and reproducing the essay from memory had any link at all to the earlier task. The find-ings suggested to the researchers that "the effects of construct individuality on impressions and reproductions were found a week after subjects' accessible trait con-structs were elicited . . . an individual's accessible constructs remain fairly consistent over time" (p. 42).

Chronically Accessible Knowledge and Attention

Bargh (1982) illustrated that chronically accessible knowledge has an impact not only on the types of impressions people form, but on the more primitive processes of atten-tion and perception—what information in the environment automatically captures attention. Bargh identified people who had the trait "independence" central to their self-conception. People with a particular chronically accessible trait were labeled as *sche-matic* for that trait (meaning that this chronically accessible trait played a central role in their self-schemas). Thus participants in the experiment were either schematic or aschematic (i.e., the trait was not chronically accessible to them) for the trait "indepen-dence." It was predicted that schematics would detect and attend to words relevant to their chronically accessible knowledge more easily in the environment, and that such words would even distract attention if it was focused elsewhere. Schematics were identi-fied by asking people to fill out a personality questionnaire (2 weeks before the next phase of the experiment) on which they had to rate the extent to which each of 25 traits was self-descriptive.

To test the hypothesis relating chronicity to attention, Bargh (1982) used a para-digm reviewed in Chapter 2, called a *dichotic listening task* (e.g., Kahneman, 1973). In such a task, people wear headphones and have separate streams of information pre-sented to each ear. They are asked to ignore the information presented in one ear and attend to the information in the other (repeating the information in the attended ear out loud—a task known as *shadowing*). Bargh manipulated the type of information being presented in the ear participants were to ignore. Half of the participants heard adjec-tives that were both relevant and irrelevant to the chronically accessible concept "inde-pendence" (and in the ear they were attending to, they heard nouns irrelevant to inde-pendence). For the other half of the participants, the adjectives relevant and irrelevant to independence were presented in the ear that participants were attending to, and were therefore being shadowed. The information to be ignored (in the unattended ear) consisted of nouns that had nothing to do with independence. Could participants ignore, or would their attention automatically be drawn to, information relevant to their chronically accessible constructs?

To see whether attention was being uncontrollably drawn to the ear that had the self-relevant information, people were asked to perform a task simultaneously with the dichotic listening task—turning off a light whenever it came on. The light was rigged so that it sometimes came on precisely at the moment when information relevant to the self was being presented. If people were automatically drawn to that self-relevant information, this should have an impact on both the shadowing task and the task of turning off the light. According to Kahneman (1973), attentional resources (the number of things one can attend to at any point in time) are limited, so that the reaction to the light is related to the amount of attention one is giving to the shadowing task. If attention to the shadowing task is distracted and interfered with, one has fewer attentional resources to dedicate to turning off the light, and response time will be slowed. If attention to the shadowing task is focused and facilitated, one has greater attentional resources to dedicate to other tasks and responses to the light will be faster and more efficient. Thus Bargh could determine whether his participants' attention was focused on the shadowing task or distracted away from it by measuring whether their response times to the light were slowed or quickened. If chronically accessible information was automatically directing attention, it should affect people's performance and attention on the shadowing task. Adjectives relevant to "independence" should automatically direct attention, so that when presented (intermittently) in either the ear being ignored or the ear not being ignored, it would nonetheless not be ignored, but have the power to capture attention. When presented in the ear people were attending to as part of the shadowing task, it should facilitate performance on the shadowing task, and in turn increase the speed with which people could turn off the light. If presented to the ear people should be ignoring, a reduction in the response speeds to the light task would indicate that people were not ignoring these words, but having attention automatically drawn to them. This was what was found: "Automatic processing of the self-relevant information facilitated the shadowing task when part of the attended channel, and inhibited performance when on the rejected channel . . . schematics apparently made automatic attention responses to the self-relevant adjectives" (Bargh, 1982, p. 433).

Bargh and Pratto (1986) performed a conceptual replication of this finding, using a Stroop-like paradigm (Warren, 1972). Rather than looking to see whether words participants were supposed to ignore interfered with how quickly they could turn off a light (if and only if those words were relevant to their chronically accessible constructs), they looked to see whether such words would distract attention when people were to ignore the word meaning and simply pronounce the color of the ink in which the words were written. Words pretested to be part of a participant's self-concept were presented in colored inks, and participants were to name the color of the ink. The reaction times to naming ink colors were reliably slower when the word content (which should be ignored to do the task efficiently) was consistent with the participants' self-concept. Attention was automatically distracted by word content that was relevant to the participants' chronically accessible constructs. This slowed down performance of the focal task (color naming).

Depression as Chronic Accessibility of Negative Beliefs: The Depressive Self-Schema

Chronic perceptual and explanatory styles—modes of thinking—have become increasingly popular in explaining the cause of depression. Aaron T. Beck (1967, 1976) proposed a cognitive model of depression in which a *depressive schema* develops—one that guides the types of beliefs a person holds, the types of explanations the person gener-ates for positive and negative outcomes, and the types of interpretations he/she forms for the behavior of others. The depressed individual has developed a chronic style of perseverating on negative beliefs and explanations for events, and this style leads to negative affect, depressed mood, and feelings of helplessness. The depressive self-schema becomes so strong in the depressed individual that it pervades all levels of psy-chological functioning. As with perceptual readiness more generally, the more accessi-ble the schema becomes, the wider the range of events seen in the light of this schema, and the wider the range of behaviors seen as validating and supporting the negative self-views that have come to characterize the self-concept. Beck (1976) argued that this depressive schema spins its negative web over perception and interpretation without the individual's awareness; he/she concludes that the world is a negative and threaten-ing place where failure predominates. The ability to control such thoughts is the focus of cognitive theories of depression, and if such control is possible, we would not want to label the process as wholly automatic. But, nonetheless, it is a pervasive and silent pro-cess of seeing the world through the lens of a negative self-concept that constitutes a chronic belief system and perceptual style. Martin Seligman (1975, 1991) and his col-leagues have taken Beck's cognitive formulation of depression and investigated the impact of these schemas on explanatory styles—the types of attributions depressed peo-ple arrive at for negative events.

Explanatory Styles

Attributions have been described in Chapter 6 as explanations people make for events in their world. People experience some new event, and they engage in a causal calculus to determine whether the cause of the event is internal or external, stable or unstable, and so on. Seligman (1975, 1991), along with his colleagues, developed the idea that people do not always evaluate new events from some fresh perspective, using the causal calculus to help them determine causation. Instead, people have particular *explanatory styles* for seeing the world—chronic tendencies to rely excessively on some dimensions of the causal calculus (rather than weighing each of them on each occasion). Seligman's (1991) argument is that people develop automatic tendencies to explain events in par-ticular ways. What sorts of "styles" develop? Seligman identified two broad styles: the *optimistic* and *pessimistic* styles of explaining behavior. These styles determine not only people's attributions for the behavior of others, but their attributions for their own behavior and one's own consequences. The optimistic style is one in which positive events are seen as stable, dispositional, and global. It is a chronic way of seeing the world in which people perceive good events as caused by them, as pervading everything they do, and as doing so across situations and over time. The pessimistic style is just the opposite. It is the tendency to make the same types of attributions, but for negative events. People see bad things as caused by them, as pervading everything they do, and as stable across time and situations. Seligman's concern has been with how these attributional or explanatory styles affect mental and physical health; he has arrived at the conclusion that they have long-term effects for well-being across a wide variety of domains. Most centrally, Seligman (along with Albert Ellis and Beck) has suggested that depression is caused by the pessimistic explanatory style.

How do we assess attributional styles? Seligman proposes that three dimensions must be assessed. The first he calls *personalization*, and this means the extent to which the cause for an event is seen as internal versus external. When evaluating the self, does one have a tendency to explain behavior with an internal or an external cause? This component of the explanatory style is essentially identical to what Heider (1958) earlier called *locus of causality*. The second dimension that Seligman claims is important in determining attributional style is called *permanence*. This is the extent to which one thinks an event is permanent versus transient and temporary. The pessimistic style is associated with seeing negative events and outcomes as permanent, while positive events and outcomes are seen as temporary and fleeting. Negatives are described with words like "always," while positives are described with words like "sometimes." The optimistic style has the opposite pattern. This component of the explanatory style is essentially identical to what was earlier called the *stability* dimension. Finally, the third dimension Seligman believes contributes to explanatory style is called *pervasiveness*. This refers to the extent to which an explanation is fairly global in nature versus fairly specific. Does a positive or negative explanation get put in a box so that it is seen as linked only to the event at hand, or is it seen as pervading one's very existence? Is the attribution made to something quite specific or to something more general? A pessimistic explanatory style is one in which negative events are ascribed to global and universal forces, whereas positive events are ascribed to very specific causes. For example, a person with a pessimistic style who fails on an exam will say, "I always do poorly on exams," or "I'm just not that smart." However, the person with the optimistic tendency will do the opposite, making global attributions for positive outcomes and specific attributions for negative ones (thus containing them within limits).

Seligman (1991) has marshaled two general types of evidence to support the idea that chronic attribution styles lead to depression. The first is correlational in nature and involves measuring (1) how depressed people are and (2) what type of attributional style people have. Such research has consistently revealed that depression and the pessimistic attribution style are correlated. People who attribute negative events to internal, stable, and pervasive causes are more likely to be depressed. Of course, it could well be that this attributional style does not cause depression, but that depression causes people to adopt this style. If we want to establish that people's styles are what determine their mental health, we need to examine their styles ahead of time and see how well people protect themselves from depression when life eventually beats down their doors. Such evidence has also been gathered, and reveals that people with the pessimistic style are more prone to depression following failure and negative life events than people with an optimistic style. One compelling example comes from the Princeton–Penn longitudinal study—an experiment that followed children for 5 years, starting in the third grade, to examine how their attributional styles related to the development of depression as childhood progressed. Children with a pessimistic style were more likely to develop depression and in turn to do poorly in school. A style of seeing negative events in a pervasive, personal, and persistent (permanent) way leads to depression (Nolen-Hoeksema, Girgus, & Seligman, 1992).

The implications of these findings range from the pragmatic to the therapeutic. For example, if depression is caused by pervasive, automatic thoughts that assign negative events to the permanent and global nature of the self, treatment for depression would involve (1) training people to identify these thoughts; (2) trying to marshal contrary evidence to the conclusions suggested by such thoughts; (3) teaching people new styles of explaining negative events that can replace the automatic ones currently springing to mind; (4) developing automatic strategies for recognizing when pessimistic explanations are likely to be made; and (5) developing new automatic associations that move people toward more self-affirming explanations. A practical use of these ideas can come in the form of improving job performance. Seligman (1991) has noted that salespeople suffer rejection daily; in fact, they suffer from volumes of rejection daily. The cumulative effect of this incessant rejection is that salespeople often quit their jobs. Seligman recounts a discussion with a life insurance executive who told him:

> Every year we hire five thousand new agents. We select them carefully out of the sixty thousand who apply. We test them, we screen them, we interview them, we give them extensive training. But half of them quit anyway in the first year. . . . By the end of the fourth year eighty percent are gone. It costs us more than thirty thousand dollars to hire a single agent. So we lose more than seventy-five million dollars every year in hiring costs alone.

Aside from money, imagine working in a place where 50% of your colleagues leave each year. This is not a happy work environment. Seligman's research informs us that despite the time and money being exerted and spent on tests and interviews to detect people who like sales and who are good at sales, the workforce is still not able to perform this job. He posits that this is because an important component to success and longevity on such a job will be attributional style. People who can attribute repeated failure to external causes will be more likely to deal with the rejection, and less likely to quit. If Seligman's optimistic view of his own work is true, then attribution theory can save the insurance industry millions of dollars, lower all our premiums, and create happier lives for the workforce more generally.

Indeed, we need not focus only on the pessimists who become depressed. We can also examine the health benefits of the opposing explanatory style—attributing positive events to internal and stable events. Seligman (1991) has proposed that such benefits include the possibility of defeating cancerous tumors and generating a will to live. We have all heard anecdotes of elderly persons who die shortly after their spouses of many, many years have died, or of people who seemingly through sheer force of optimism defeat incredible odds to survive a fatal illness. One classic study from the 1970s helped pave the way for exploring the benefits of attributional styles. Langer and Rodin (1976) explored how having a sense of personal control could affect physical health, using life and death as their measure of interest. A *sense of personal control* means the belief that there are stable and internal causes for life events. People without this sense attribute life events to external or unstable causes. Seligman (1975) famously described the phenomenon of *learned helplessness*, in which people develop such a strong perceived sense of lacking control that they withdraw altogether. They learn that any action is futile, so they just stop trying; they stop attempting to change their surroundings or engaging in proactive behavior. Langer and Rodin reasoned that if the externalizing style associated with pessimism has negative health benefits, positive health benefits should be associated with an internalized style that places control firmly within the individual. To examine this question, they chose an environment where people are known to lack control and to develop a chronic expectation that they lack control—a nursing home. When people move to a nursing home, they move from an environment where they care, feed, clothe, and plan for themselves to one where much of their daily activity is structured and planned for them. Indeed, one study found that patients who came to a nursing home from their own homes died sooner than patients who had come from other hospitals where control had already been relinquished. It seemed possible that loss of control (learned helplessness) could cause death. Can the feeling of having control hold back death?

Langer and Rodin (1976) posited that differences in feelings of control would have an impact on mortality! The attributions made for events could alter feelings of control and optimism, and this could affect life expectancy. In this research, patients living on the fourth floor of a nursing home repeatedly interacted with a worker who stressed how much control and choice they had in their daily lives, whereas the patients on the second floor interacted with a worker who reminded them that many positive things were available to them at the home that the staff of the home provided for them. The fourth-floor patients were told that they could pick their meals, room arrangements, and films; the second-floor patients were told that their rooms, films, and meals were exquisitely prepared for them by the staff. On the fourth floor, patients were given the option of selecting plants for their rooms and taking care of them. Patients on the second floor were given plants and had them cared for by the staff. Thus two groups of people, equal in all respects except the amount of control they perceived themselves to have, lived in a nursing home. What became of them? After 3 weeks, 71% of the people on the second floor were rated as having a condition that worsened, whereas 93% of those on the fourth floor had improved. And after a year and a half, the mortality rates reflected this trend: 15% of the residents of the fourth floor had died, compared to 30% of the residents of the second floor. Therefore, attributions not only pervade our lives from the moment we are born; the pattern of attributions we make may be an important factor in determining when we die. (See also Taylor, Lichtman, & Wood, 1984, for a discussion of how attributions for the cause of disease, as well as beliefs about controllability of disease, affect physical health and adjustment to disease.)

Automatic Processing and the Depressive Schema

Spielman and Bargh (1990) have argued that not only explanatory styles, but the constructs that are chronically accessible, differentiate depressed from nondepressed people. Depressed people are said to be people who have chronic accessibility for negative information, and this increased accessibility is thought to be what gives rise to differences in explanatory style and depressed affect. Spielman and Bargh explain that "once [an] event is recognized as a negative one, other negative events may also become accessible in memory, thus leading to the globality, or over-generalization, that is characteristic of depression" (p. 119). There is a triggering of negative beliefs, concepts, and traits, and this spreads through the associative network, providing a web of negativity for interpreting the meaning of events.

Bargh and Tota (1988) suggest that Beck's notion of the depressive self-schema is tied to automatic triggering of negative thoughts linked to the self-concept. However, research (such as that of Higgins et al., 1982) on chronic accessibility suggests that information chronically linked to the self-concept has an impact not only on self-judgments, but on social judgments more broadly, including the perception of other people. Is self-reference necessary to trigger these chronic negative thoughts in depressed persons? Bargh and Tota claim that "depressed individuals appear to differ from nondepressed individuals mainly in the content of their self-referential thought and not so much in the content of their more general social-perceptual constructs. The greater accessibility of negative concepts in depression seems to be conditional on the activation of the self-concept" (p. 926). Thus negative thinking should be automatically triggered in a depressed individual whenever the self is relevant to a context, but not when judging others.

CODA

If a stimulus is ambiguous or somehow impoverished (such as when it is dark, faraway, blurry, or otherwise hard to see), people have accessible categories—ones that are perceptually ready to be used—to help in perceiving and making sense of the stimulus. Postman and colleagues (1948) found that how quickly people could notice a stimulus was determined by what values were accessible; McGinnies (1949) found that people even had physiological reactions (galvanic skin response) to words they could not report seeing if the words were related to accessible concepts. Higgins and colleagues (1982), as well as Bargh (1982; Bargh & Pratto, 1986), found that chronic accessibility is not limited to goals and values, but can exist for semantic knowledge that is routinely used. Bruner (1957, pp. 129–130) summarized the impact of accessibility as follows:

> The greater the accessibility of a category, (a) the less the input necessary for a categorization to occur in terms of this category, (b) the wider the range of characteristics that will be "accepted" as fitting the category in question, (c) the more likely that categories that provide a better or equally good fit for the input will be masked. To put it in more ordinary language: apples will be more easily and swiftly recognized, a wider range of things will be identified or misidentified as apples, and in consequence the correct or best fitting identity of these other inputs will be masked. This is what is intended by accessibility.

Bruner (1957) thus identified three general effects of accessibility on perception of a stimulus. First, the greater the accessibility, the lesser the input necessary for a categorization to occur; we will be able to categorize a person or identify an object based on fewer features. Readiness leads the accessible item to be seen when there is degraded stimuli, when there is little evidence, and when there is ambiguity. If we have been raised on an apple orchard, we are quicker and better able to identify a tree in the distance as an apple tree. If the trait "hostility" is chronically accessible, we will be quicker to label a behavior as hostile, even if the behavior is ambiguous. Second, a wide range of characteristics will be accepted as fitting the category; we are ready to accept something that resembles the accessible item as an instance of it (although this can lead to misidentifying ambiguous stimuli, due to applying the construct too broadly). For example, a broader range of behavior is subsequently interpreted as being a hostile act if the trait "hostility" is accessible. Third, competing explanations that provide an equally good fit for the input will be masked. Once we are ready to categorize something as an apple tree, alternative categories (e.g., pear tree) are more difficult to see eventually if they are in fact the reality.

In sum, the notion of accessibility flows naturally out of the discussion of naive realism in Chapter 1 of this book. An external object does not present itself and define itself for the perceiver; the perception of, and the meaning attached to, an object are constructed. The perceiver sees not merely what is there, but what the accessible constructs in the mind make that person perceptually ready to see. As Bruner (1957, p. 132) put it,

> In short, the accessibility of categories I employ for identifying the objects of the world around me must not only reflect the environmental probabilities of objects that fit these categories, but also reflect the search requirements imposed by my needs, my ongoing activities, my defenses, etc. . . . the likelihood that a sensory input will be categorized in terms of a given category is not only a matter of fit between sensory input and category specifications.

It depends also on the accessibility of a category. To put the matter in an oversimplified way, given a sensory input with equally good fit to two nonoverlapping categories, the more accessible of the two categories would "capture" the input.

And as noted in Chapter 1, once extrastimulus information is being used to interpret the stimulus, features never observed in the stimulus will be linked to it if those features are suggested by the accessible category. Accessible categories allow perceivers to "go beyond the information given" (Bruner, 1957) and to construct a fuller reality than the actual stimulus may have suggested by itself. Accessible information not only colors what is seen, but fills in the gaps and extends what is seen to features not even present.

The accessibility of goals or any type of semantic knowledge, like a stereotype or trait, is not dependent on having an auto-motive or chronic accessibility. Goals and knowledge can be momentarily triggered and attain a heightened state of activation, with many of the same consequences as those reviewed by Bruner (1957). The current contexts can create perceptual readiness, just as can habitual routines and goal pursuits: "When we have just finished reading Melville's *Moby Dick* and ruminations about dangerous and enigmatic huge sea mammals are foremost on our minds, we are more likely to identify 'a speck on the horizon' as a whale rather than a ship or a drilling platform" (Stapel & Koomen, 2001, p. 230). It is to the silent and preconscious influence of these temporary states of accessibility that we turn next.

10 Temporary Accessibility/ Priming Effects

ASSIMILATION AND CONTRAST IN IMPRESSION FORMATION

A GOP commercial that subtly flashes the word "RATS" across the screen is coming off the air amid allegations the Republicans were trying to send a subliminal message about Al Gore. George W. Bush called the notion "bizarre and weird," and his campaign made light of it all. The GOP admaker said he was just trying to make the spot visually interesting. But Gore's campaign and experts in political advertising said the word choice—as an announcer was denouncing Gore's Medicare plan—could hardly have been an accident. . . . Bush noted that the word appears only fleetingly—for a tiny fraction of a second. Played at full speed, it's barely noticeable, particularly if the viewer isn't looking for the word. "One frame out of 900 hardly in my judgment makes a conspiracy."

—MECKLER (2000)

When individuals are asked to judge themselves or another person, they are unlikely to perform an exhaustive search of memory for all cognitions that have implications for this judgment. Rather, they are likely to base their judgment on some subset of these cognitions that is most readily accessible.

—SRULL AND WYER (1979, p. 1660)

In the 1970s, a poster of the television star Farrah Fawcett (wearing a one-piece bathing suit) was ubiquitous. It sold in such large numbers that a new sex symbol was declared born. Teenagers across the land debated as to why the poster of the scantily clad star had been hung on seemingly every boy's wall in America. One camp proclaimed that the sexy star herself, with her nipple prominently displayed through her bathing suit, was obviously the cause. What the boys saw was titillating enough to warrant the attention. However, another camp claimed that nipples are a dime a dozen, and that what really drove the boys into a frenzy was the unseen, but still subconsciously noticed, placement of the word "sex" in the star's curly hair, with the letters formed by her curls. Subliminally, the word "sex" was being processed, with thoughts of sex being triggered in the mind of those who saw the poster, and this unconscious detection of the concept of sex was what gave the poster its unusual selling power (as they say, "Sex sells").

388

A similar public debate emerged 25 years later, not involving a sex symbol (hardly!), but a political candidate. A commercial favoring George W. Bush over Al Gore for President in 2000 flashed images of the Democrat, Gore, superimposed with subtitles and an announcer calling for citizens to cast their votes for the Republican, Bush. As images flashed on the screen, the word "BUREAUCRATS" (included among the images) did something odd that only very few people could see with the naked eye (and thus it was subliminal to most people). The letters "R," "A," "T", and "S" jumped out very quickly from the word "BUREAUCRATS" so that "RATS" was exposed to viewers, but so swiftly that it was barely (if even) detectable, just as an image of Gore appeared. Democrats claimed that Bush used subliminal messages—in this case, triggering the concept "rats"—to try to make people form negative impressions of Gore. Bush, comically, declared that this was not a case of "subliminable" advertising. He pressed Americans to see that the flashing of the word "RATS" was an honest mistake that could have no effect on a voter's evaluations. What was comical was not merely the fact that a man running for President could not pronounce the word "subliminal," or that letters do not mistakenly appear to leap off film, but must be artfully made to do so by a professional. Rather, the most comical piece was the denial that subliminal information has any impact on judgment or behavior—a fact that the National Science Foundation, which Bush sought to control as President, has spent millions of dollars to establish. But does it have an effect in the examples described above? Can concepts be made accessible if they do not have chronic states of accessibility? Do they have an impact on us? Does it matter if they are subliminally presented or not (and in actuality the case described above is not, since the word "RATS" was detectable if viewers looked for it)?

Consider a quick example. Most likely you would describe the last symbol in the following string as a letter: "A a; C c; L l." However, here is the very same stimulus presented in a different string: "4; 3; 2; l." How would you describe it now? The same stimulus gets interpreted differently because it fits equally well into two, nonoverlapping categories. The way in which it is categorized is determined by what we are ready to see and what concepts have been made accessible (numbers or letters). Many of the behaviors we observe in ourselves and in others are similar in this regard; they too can be placed into more than one nonoverlapping category. The person who helps another person can be seen as kind, ingratiating, or even manipulative. The Senator who opposes changes to the Pledge of Allegiance can be seen as God-fearing, patriotic, or sycophantic. The person who runs in to save a turtle from a burning house can be seen as heroic or moronic. The President who invades a foreign country can be seen as a forward-thinking liberator (stopping a despot before he engages in genocide), or as aggressive, cynical, and manipulative (ignoring peaceful solutions to problems while distorting the potential effectiveness of other solutions to justify the chosen path, instigated for reasons that are never truly revealed). Many of the social behaviors we observe are open to such multiple interpretations; they can be categorized in alternative ways with equal likelihood. And often these potential interpretations are quite distinct and lead to drastically different implications (Kanouse, 1971). *The interpretation that is chosen can be determined simply by whatever applicable concept happens to be accessible at the moment.*

One way in which the interpretation of behavior is determined by accessible constructs is that the behavior is drawn toward, or *assimilated* into, a perceptually ready interpretation. If for some reason we are feeling cynical, the Pledge-promoting Senator will be seen as pandering to an audience that he/she believes wants to keep the Pledge of Allegiance intact. If patriotic themes are accessible (such as in times of war or national strife), the same behavior may be seen as praiseworthy devotion to the country. A second manner in which the interpretation of behavior is determined by accessible constructs is that the behavior is pushed away from, or *contrasted* with, a perceptually ready interpretation. Thus, if we have in mind an extremely patriotic American, such as Thomas Jefferson, the Senator whose best form of patriotism is to espouse attitudes in favor of the Pledge of Allegiance may pale in comparison to the type of patriotism evidenced by Jefferson. Rather than being seen as more patriotic, the Senator is seen as less so (with Jefferson as a standard).

The current chapter explores the relationship between concepts triggered in the mind and the impact of activated concepts on our judgment of others. Chapter 9 has focused on how chronically accessible information influences how we think about people. The current chapter is concerned with the impact of information that is momentarily brought to mind—that is temporarily (rather than chronically) accessible—on our behavior toward and evaluation of others. The chapter details (1) the circumstances in which accessible constructs have an impact on judgment and behavior, (2) the type of impact accessible constructs have, and (3) the processing mechanisms responsible for bringing about this subtle impact. An impact can be exerted on perception and judgment, even if one does not realize a concept has been triggered, does not see the actual triggering event (e.g., it is presented subliminally), or does not realize there is any bias/impact on one's judgments and evaluations. This use of a triggered concept is what we refer to when we talk about *priming effects* or *accessibility effects*. George W. Bush was incorrect in assuming that subliminal concepts can have no impact. We should not necessarily ignore a small number of "frames" embedded within thousands on film, nor should we ignore the power of that which we do not see. But the issue we must be concerned with is when, how, and why such forces, which feel as if they should be random and meaningless, have an impact (and thus allow us to know whether subliminal words in a political commercial can have an influence).

PRIMING: THE TEMPORARY ACCESSIBILITY OF MENTAL CONSTRUCTS

What do we mean when we say that a concept is "triggered in the mind," or that there can be "unconscious detection of a concept" (such as the word "sex" being seen, but not seen)? Chapter 4 has stated that the mind stores many types of constructs and concepts, ranging from exemplars to stereotypes to schemas to implicit personality theories to prototypes to goals to traits. What the current chapter explores is how the retrieval of such concepts from memory activates them in the mind. This retrieval of a concept from memory, even if a person is not aware that the concept is being retrieved, brings to the concept a heightened state of accessibility or perceptual readiness (Bruner, 1957). That is, a concept held in the mind can be triggered by a stimulus in the environment, and once triggered it is now ready to be used by the mind to help to categorize and interpret the stimuli that greet the perceiver. Just as with chronically accessible constructs, the idea is that a mental construct can be "charged" or made accessible so that it has a relatively favored status in comparison to other concepts. Unlike the charge associated with a chronically accessible construct, however, the momentary charge attained by a concept being triggered in memory is not permanent. The strength of the charge is dependent on how recently the concept in question has been encountered, how frequently the concept in question has been encountered, and how strongly the activating stimulus is able to trigger the category/concept in question. If the charge is strong enough, the concept has attained a sufficient level of activation/accessibility that it can be said to have reached a *response threshold*. The concept is now ready to be used and to have an impact on perception and judgment. However, even if the charge has not accumulated to the point where it has reached the response threshold, this does not mean that the charge is unimportant. Rather, the charge is accumulating below the threshold, so that it will take less and less additional stimulus input for the concept to be triggered. If a certain degree of charge is needed for full-blown activation, that charge may not be attained the first time a stimulus is encountered, but it will be reached on a second (or subsequent) encounter with the same stimulus. The charge has been slowly accumulating so that it finally rises above the threshold.

This triggering of a concept in the moment—with the concept being accessed by the mind's attempt to make sense of an external stimulus (thus charging the concept above a specified threshold), and being temporarily pulled from long-term memory—is known as *priming*, and the stimulus that causes the concept to be triggered (or to rise above threshold) is known as the *prime*. The idea that one's context primes concepts and this perceptual readiness determines to what one attends was eloquently stated by James (1890/1950, p. 442):

> When watching for the distant clock to strike, our mind is so filled with its image that at every moment we think we hear the longed for or dreaded sound. So of an awaited footstep. Every stir in the wood is for the hunter his game; for the fugitive his pursuers . . . the image in the mind is the attention.

The Priming of a Construct: Producing Temporary Accessibility

By now, you may be convincing yourself that there is no chance that your perception and judgment are so capriciously determined as to be guided by fleeting thoughts, primed constructs, and accessible information you cannot even detect. However, if I ask you to play a few simple word association games, you may begin to see how such forces can determine what comes to your mind. If I ask you for the first thing that comes to mind when you think "bread," you are likely to say "butter." And if I ask you first to name a nut that comes in a shell, and now ask you to think of an animal, you probably generate an elephant as the animal of choice. And can you deny that you have found yourself at times whistling or humming a song, only to wonder whether that song was actually playing in the shop that you just left? How can you not even be sure that you heard a tune, yet find yourself singing it nonetheless? It is because the song has been primed without your realizing it, and has influenced your own responses despite your being unaware of its influence (or the fact that you even encountered the song). What is accessible in your mind is partly determined by what you have been exposed to in your environment. Not only is the concept that you have seen or heard (whether supraliminally or subliminally) triggered (primed), but the activation spreads to related concepts, making these concepts accessible as well. Accessibility is evidenced by how quickly these concepts come to mind, so that "butter" springs to the tongue after thinking about bread because the concept of "butter" has attained heightened accessibility (Meyer & Schvandeveldt, 1971).

Srull and Wyer (1980) presented a clear illustration that exposure to a stimulus primes a category in the mind that represents the stimulus in long-term memory. However, for the concept truly to be activated, the strength of the charge associated with the concept needs to rise above the response threshold. Once that threshold is attained, the concept is ready to influence how people respond (so long as it stays above threshold or maintains its charge). To illustrate that activation strength accumulates until it eventually reaches a threshold strong enough to make the concept perceptually ready, Srull and Wyer manipulated how frequently research participants were exposed to a particular concept. Participants were exposed to stimuli meant to eventually prime the concept "hostility" (this was accomplished by having them form sentences from jumbled words, with the solution requiring that sentences be formed that described hostile acts—such as breaking someone's legs). Some of the participants were exposed to 15 such stimuli, while others were exposed to 35. The logic was that encountering the concept 35 times would lead to a larger/stronger accumulation of charge and a greater likelihood of the concept "hostility" being made accessible (and staying accessible for a longer period of time—a point we turn to shortly). The test of whether the concept was accessible was a particular form of perceptual readiness that will be described in more detail shortly: Participants were asked to read about the behavior of a person (unrelated to the sentences read as part of the priming task) and make a judgment about the person. If the concept of "hostility" had been primed, then people should be ready to use the concept in describing the behavior of this new person. Such an illustration of accessibility was found—especially in the case where participants had been exposed to the prime 35 times, where there was a clear use of the concept of "hostility" in the descriptions of the subsequently encountered behavior.

Spreading Activation

The accessibility of a concept is determined by exposure not only to that specific concept, but to words or events associated with that concept (e.g., semantically related concepts). You do not need to see the word "hostility" or read about explicitly hostile acts for the concept of "hostility" to be made accessible. As one concept is charged, that charge spreads along the associative network—triggering the related concepts to which it is linked, and thus priming these associated concepts as well. That is, through priming, and *spreading activation along an associative network*, information available in memory has now attained a heightened state of accessibility even if it has not been directly primed by a stimulus in the environment (see Chapter 3). For example, Neely (1977) asked research participants to decide whether a string of letters was actually a word (a lexical decision task). The trick was that the letter strings were preceded by words. The logic was that the presentation of the first word would prime that concept and make it, as well as related concepts, accessible. The more accessible the first concept, the easier and faster it would be to respond to the second concept if it was related to (associated with) the "prime." Thus, if exposure to a concept increased its accessibility as well as the accessibility of related concepts, response times to the lexical decision task would be faster for words that were related to the primed construct. Thus a participant might see "bread" followed by "butter," or "body" followed by "leg." Other participants, however, saw the same initial words, but had these words followed by some new, nonassociated concept—for example, "body" followed by "bird," or "bread" followed by "professor." When responses to the lexical decision task were called for at very fast speeds, where people did not have time to think about their responses, what Neely found was that participants were faster to respond to the related concepts than to the unrelated concepts. This illustrates that when people are exposed to a concept, this concept (and associated ones) become accessible, allowing them to interpret and categorize new, related stimuli more efficiently.

This finding suggests that the thoughts that come to mind when we see a person should include a whole host of behaviors and traits that are linked to that person (or to our impression of that person). For example, if you meet someone who you categorize as an introvert, triggering of the concept "introvert" should trigger associated behaviors and concepts, which should then be perceptually ready to be used in thinking about that person (and other people). This is precisely the point made in Chapter 4 about the consequences of schemas (e.g., Cantor & Mischel, 1977). This process is illustrated in Figure 10.1, where encountering an athlete (Derek Jeter, at bat in the final game of the 1999 World Series, helping to deliver a championship to his team) is shown to trigger the concept "athletic." Activation then spreads from the notion of "athlete" to other related concepts (those linked to "athletic" in an associative network, with activation spreading along the network).

Priming in Everyday Life

Perhaps by now you are becoming convinced that the triggering of concepts can bias what you think you see or hear and what concepts come to mind, without your being aware of the influence these concepts have or their heightened accessibility. But you may still be skeptical about whether this process has any impact on real interpersonal interaction or your moment-to-moment judgments of the people you meet. After all, the procedures this chapter has been describing for making concepts sufficiently charged so as to be perceptually ready are fairly artificial-sounding. They have included (1) commercials flashing words at viewers subliminally, (2) people repeatedly reading sentences that describe hostile acts, and (3) experimenters explicitly asking people to read words that represent a concept (such as the word "bread"). Can people help having

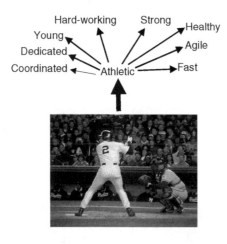

FIGURE 10.1. Spreading activation.

concepts (and associated concepts) triggered when such tasks are performed? Probably not. And perhaps merely incidentally encountering the concept (e.g., seeing a piece of bread or observing person act in an hostile way) is insufficient to trigger or prime these concepts, thus rendering priming fairly irrelevant to everyday life. Do people typically think of others in spontaneous ways that will lead to priming of concepts and, in turn, have an impact on thinking and action?

The research reviewed thus far in this chapter has used mostly artificial means of triggering concepts, with the goal being to show that accessibility can have an impact on how people think about other people. It should not matter *how* the concept is made accessible, so long as it attains a heightened state of activation relative to other concepts. But it is certainly reasonable to ask whether these artificial means of priming a concept actually approximate how concepts actually become triggered in the course of everyday life. As Gilbert and Hixon (1991, p. 516) stated, "The Sufis teach that if a pickpocket meets a holyman he sees only his pockets . . . we offer a revision of the Sufi teaching: When a pickpocket reads the word holyman, he will probably think of a great deal more than pockets—and in so doing he will reveal little about how pickpockets construe holymen in their day-to-day lives." Reading "holyman" may necessarily mean that this concept is activated, whereas in real life it does not get triggered on meeting such a person. Does the fact that flashing the words "quiet," "reads," "books," "shy," and "woman" may activate the concept "librarian" mean that seeing a librarian will activate this concept and its associated qualities?

In one experiment, Moskowitz and Roman (1992) proposed that day-to-day inferences about others operate as primes. That is, the snap judgments people make—the spontaneous trait inferences (STIs) they form in quickly and effortlessly describing others—serve to activate or make accessible the very concepts that have been inferred. This provides one answer to these questions: How can it be that in day-to-day life people have concepts primed outside of awareness? Where does a concept get triggered without conscious awareness, if not by an experimenter (or advertiser) subliminally flashing it? The answer is through the spontaneous inferential processes that people use every day. By definition, an STI is an inference formed without a perceiver's awareness or intent—one that explains behavior in terms of traits (see Chapter 7). Given that these traits are held outside of awareness, they should be equivalent to the subliminal and artificial "flashes" of traits in a priming experiment. Essentially, STIs are self-generated primes, ones produced via the natural course of making sense of the world. In a study (Moskowitz & Roman, 1992, Experiment 1) similar in form to Srull and Wyer's (1980, described above) it was illustrated that self-generated primes function in a manner equivalent to primes provided by an experimenter. In one task participants were "primed," and in an "unrelated" task their evaluations of a new person were assessed. Here the priming was done by manipulating the inferences participants formed spontaneously. Some participants read a sentence that implied the trait "persistent," whereas others read a sentence implying the trait "stubborn." All participants then read and evaluated information about a new person. Although participants did not know that inferences had been made while reading the sentences, evidence for such inferences, and their ability to function as self-generated primes, was found. People primed with (read sentences implying) "persistent" described the new person as persistent, whereas those who spontaneously inferred "stubborn" saw the new person as stubborn.

Perhaps an even more obvious way to test the ecological validity of priming research is simply to examine whether concepts become accessible through seeing images of people who suggest the concept, or imagining meeting such people (as opposed to reading about them). For a White person, does meeting a Black man trigger the concept of "Black man"? For most people, does imagining a supermodel trigger concepts associated with that category? Many experiments have illustrated that seeing images of people (either still photographs or moving pictures) and actually (or imagining) meeting people from a particular group can lead the concepts associated with that group to attain heightened accessibility, and that these concepts can influence what people subsequently attend to and what types of judgments they form (e.g., Bargh, Chen, & Burrows, 1996; Chen & Bargh, 1997; Correll, Park, Judd, & Wittenbrink, 2002; Dijksterhuis et al., 1998; Fazio, Jackson, Dunton, & Williams, 1995; Fein & Spencer, 1997; Gilbert & Hixon, 1991; Kawakami, Dovidio, Moll, Hermsen, & Russin, 2000; Livingston & Brewer, 2002; Macrae, Bodenhausen, Milne, Thorne, & Castelli, 1997; Moskowitz, Salomon, & Taylor, 2000; Spencer, Fein, Wolfe, Fong, & Dunn, 1998). For example, Fitzsimons, Chartrand, and Fitzsimons (2003) illustrated the power of images as primes, showing that pictures of pets trigger the concepts associated with a given animal. Participants shown pictures of cats and dogs had the concepts associated with these pets made accessible. Dogs are associated with the concept of loyalty, and people primed by seeing a dog were more likely to respond in a loyal manner in a subsequent situation. Although it may not be true of every concept that seeing an image triggers it, at least there is evidence that sometimes concepts may be triggered in everyday life by categorizing a person (or pet) according to his/her (or its) group membership.

One less obvious way in which a concept becomes accessible in life outside the lab is, ironically, the result of trying not to think about that concept. An example from the movie *Austin Powers III* helps to illustrate the temporary accessibility that arises from trying not to think about something. In this case, Austin desperately tries not to think about the hideous mole on the face of a double agent. Trying not to think about it makes it so accessible that it is all he can think about. Thus, hysterically, all he can manage to utter in the person's presence is "mole." Less ridiculous examples can be culled from day-to-day life. The decision to diet often brings seemingly unending thoughts about food, even as one deliberately attempts to suppress such thoughts. A failed relationship often produces countless hours of thought mired in the accessibility of one's "ex." No matter how much one tries not to think about the person, the person seems to seep into conscious thought more and more. Wegner and Erber (1992) suggested that attempting not to think about a concept—which they call *thought suppression*—requires one actually to hold the unwanted thought in the unconscious mind, in order to prevent the thought from entering consciousness. If Austin does not want to think about moles, at some level he needs to be constantly but preconsciously reminding himself, "Do not think about moles." Thus, in the movie, he fails miserably at this. Why is it that unsuccessful suppression seems so common? That is, why does it seem that the more one tries not to think about something, the more one thinks about it? We will discuss the cognitive processes underpinning thought suppression in Chapter 12, when relating this notion to political correctness and the attempt not to think about stereotypes.

There are many ways in which concepts are triggered in our minds in the course of our day-to-day lives. The point here is simply to illustrate that often it matters not how the concepts are made accessible, so long as they attain a heightened state of activation, and that heightened state of activation makes the concept perceptually ready. Artificial procedures for making a concept accessible illustrate this point just as powerfully as more naturalistic priming methods.

Retrieval and Accessibility

Why does exposure to a concept lead to its accessibility? The prevailing explanation is that when we perceive or think about a concept/person/object, the act of focusing attention requires that we understand, label, and categorize what we have focused on. To do this requires retrieving relevant information from memory. If I see a round object with a sugar glaze, I must retrieve my concept of "donut" from memory in order to label the object. If I attempt to think about the concept of "rudeness," I must be able to first retrieve my notion of "rudeness" from memory to accomplish this task. Logan (1989, p. 65) assumes that "retrieval from memory is an obligatory consequence of attention; whatever is related to the current focus of attention is retrieved." Thus exposure to a concept—either through its contemplation in the mind or through a physical encounter—leads automatically to the retrieval of the concept, and associated concepts, from memory. This creates the accessibility of a concept.

Many concepts are quite complex. If I ask you to think of your mother, perhaps no clear, single association immediately comes to mind, but many, complex associations do. Thus multiple concepts and meanings may be associated with a single stimulus, and not all of them need to be retrieved when attention gets focused on the stimulus (Logan, 1989). The natural question that follows is this: What gets activated when many associations exist? This has been addressed in Chapter 9 in reviewing the notion of inhibition, and the discussion will turn again to this issue in Chapter 11's review of stereotyping. However, an answer has already been provided by Logan's assertion, reviewed in Chapter 3, that retrieval of any association to a concept takes time, and that each association to a cue has its own retrieval distribution. What concept becomes accessible, and what response is elicited, are essentially determined by a race between associations. Whichever construct or association is retrieved more quickly will be what becomes accessible and determines the response a person elicits.

In summary, we interpret the behavior of others (and ourselves), as well as produce social behavior, with the aid of what is most accessible to us. What is most accessible will vary from person to person, and within the same person from situation to situation. When we retrieve a concept from memory through having recently been exposed to a stimulus associated with that concept, the concept is said to have *temporary accessibility*. What is temporarily accessible will change as we move from one situation to another and encounter different stimuli that retrieve different concepts from memory.

Types of Temporary Accessibility

Recent research has suggested that a wide range of concepts and constructs, not merely semantic knowledge, can be primed. Let us now sample a few of the types of concepts/cognitive processes that can be made accessible: attitudes, emotions, goals, and mindsets. The accessibility of stereotypes is discussed in Chapter 11.

Attitudes

The affect or evaluation associated with an object can be automatically activated (Fazio, Sanbonmatsu, Kardes, & Powell, 1986). The *automatic activation of affect* (also called *attitude accessibility*) occurs when the presence of an object leads to the activation of positive or negative evaluative responses that are linked to that object. For example, whenever a snake is seen, the attitude associated with snakes (negative, in my case) is unconditionally triggered, along with the perception of the snake. This makes that attitude accessible. The corresponding consequence, given the discussion thus far of these matters, is that one should now be perceptually ready to respond to objects to which one has similar affect. That is, if an attitude is accessible, one should be faster to respond to (notice, attend to, make a judgment about) a new target that has similar valence. Having just seen a snake, for instance, I should be faster to respond to a spider.

A clear illustration of the increased accessibility of an attitude is provided by Chen and Bargh (1999). They posited that if the valence of an object is automatically activated (i.e., attitude accessibility) by the presence of the object, then this should make people faster to respond in a manner consistent with the attitude. If a positive attitude is triggered, then people should be faster to move toward or approach a positive stimulus, and if negative attitudes are made accessible, they should be faster to move away from or avoid a new negative stimulus. The attitude, if accessible, should make the responses associated with it easier. Chen and Bargh reasoned that pulling something toward the self is associated with liking things, and pushing something away is associated with disliking. Therefore, the response they used that was believed to be compatible with a positive attitude was arm flexion (pulling an object toward the self); the compatible response for negative attitudes was arm extension (pushing the object away from the self). They asked research participants to move a lever when a word appeared, with half the participants moving the lever toward themselves and half moving the lever away. Participants responded faster to positive (vs. negative) words when asked to flex the arm (to move the lever toward them when a word appeared), but responded faster to negative words when asked to move the lever through arm extension (to move the lever away from them when a word appeared). The words triggered the associated affect, and the evidence for the increased accessibility of the attitude was its impact on responses, such as how quickly participants moved a lever.

There has been some disagreement in the literature as to how pervasive this effect may be. Fazio and colleagues (1986) argued that weak feelings and attitudes (ones that are not strongly held) are not triggered by the mere presence of an object. If I have ill-formed and weak attitudes toward goats, for example, there is little reason to predict that an evaluation will be triggered that is part and parcel of my perception of a goat. Roskos-Ewoldsen and Fazio (1992) provided support for this by illustrating that the stronger an attitude toward an object, the more likely that object was to capture attention when briefly flashed at people as part of a larger stimulus display. Attitude strength thus seemed to have an impact on degree of accessibility when the target item was present. However, Bargh, Chaiken, Govender, and Pratto (1992) asserted that any object triggers an evaluation, regardless of the strength of the attitude. Thus even a goat will trigger an affective response, regardless of whether my attitude toward goats is weak and ill-formed.

Emotions

Emotions can also be made accessible, and the accessibility of these emotions can have an unrecognized impact on impression formation. It is easy to imagine everyday experiences where your current emotions affect how you interpret a stimulus. I recently had a friend visiting me at my new home in the woods of Pennsylvania, and because I had just moved there from New York City, my reaction to every noise in the night was comical to him, a country boy. These same noises encountered during the day were not interpreted

by me as dangerous or scary. But when I was frightened by my environment, each stimulus was encoded in light of that emotion.

Niedenthal, Halberstadt, and Setterlund (1997) illustrated this impact of accessible
emotions by exposing participants to word lists that made emotions such as happiness,
sadness, anger, and love accessible. People's reaction time in determining whether a letter string was a word was faster when the word was compatible with the emotion that
had been primed. Happy people were faster to recognize words related to happiness,
and people with the concept of anger made accessible were faster to recognize words
related to being angry. Niedenthal and colleagues reasoned that the increased accessibility of an emotion spreads to concepts associated with these emotions, thus increasing
the speed with which such concepts can be recognized. When people are angry, experiences and concepts linked to anger more readily come to mind, and ambiguous stimuli
are now ready to be perceived in a manner consistent with the accessible emotion.

Goals

Chapter 9 has reviewed several examples illustrating that chronically accessibile goals
operate in the preconscious. But are temporary goals, those not chronically held, capable of being triggered or primed by the current context? The tip-of-the-tongue effect,
reviewed in Chapter 2, suggests that this is indeed possible. A goal, once triggered (e.g.,
to figure out who was the most valuable player of a particular championship game),
remains accessible even after people stop consciously trying to regulate the goal. As
reviewed in Chapter 2, I (Moskowitz, 2002) found that explicitly asking people to pursue a goal had primed that goal, allowing people to respond faster to goal-relevant
words on a reaction time task that they did not even know contained words, let alone
words related to their goal. However, in each of these examples an individual is explicitly asked to adopt the goal at some point, and the research illustrates that at some later
time the goal is still accessible. The question still remains as to whether cues in the environment can trigger goals even when the individual is at no point in time consciously
deciding to pursue the goal. For example, can a goal be subliminally primed and then
influence what people desire and strive to do? Can subtle cues in the environment
silently prime goals?

Chartrand and Bargh (1996) posited that goals can be implicitly activated and are
capable of directing cognition. The test of this proposition relied on the assumption
that activated goals exert the same effects regardless of the manner in which they are
triggered. Explicitly being asked to do something, or consciously adopting a goal to act
a certain way, should lead to the same responses as when those same goals are primed
without a person's knowing it! If a pattern of cognitive responding on a task is known
to be an effect of having an explicit goal, then the same goal triggered implicitly should
have the same effects on cognitive responding. For example, as reviewed in Chapter 4,
Hamilton, Katz, and Leirer (1980a) found that impression formation goals (asking people to form an impression of a person based on some information they read) versus
memorization goals (asking people to memorize some information about a person) differentially affected how the information about that person was organized in memory.
And as reviewed in Chapter 3, Hastie and Park (1986) found that impression versus
memorization goals affected the relationship between participants' impressions and the
recall for the information: What participants recalled about a person and the impression they formed about the person were much more similar when they had a memory
goal as opposed to an impression formation goal. Chartrand and Bargh argued that if

these impression formation and memorization goals were activated *implicitly* (even if they were presented subliminally), exactly the same pattern of cognitive responding would be observed as that found in the experiments of Hamilton and colleagues and Hastie and Park, where goals were explicit. This would suggest that the goals were in fact primed implicitly.

Chartrand and Bargh (1996, Experiment 1) examined this hypothesis by priming goals through a sentence completion task similar to that of Srull and Wyer (1980, reviewed above). They then examined the effect of having been subtly exposed to goal-relevant words in the priming task on people's subsequent information-processing strategies. To do so, they used the methods of Hamilton and colleagues (1980). The behavior of a person was presented to research participants in the form of a list, and later in the experiment there was a surprise recall test that assessed both memory for the behaviors and the amount of clustering in the participants' free recall of those behaviors (an index of how the information was organized in the participants' memories). Hamilton and colleagues found that recall for the information was better when participants were asked to form an impression than when they were explicitly asked to remember the behaviors. In addition, these two goals led to differences in how information was organized in memory. Consistent with the findings of Hamilton and colleagues, Chartrand and Bargh's participants with primed impression formation goals had higher clustering scores and recalled a greater number of behaviors during the recall test. The very same pattern of responding was found when people were merely exposed to goal-relevant words as when people were explicitly asked to adopt a goal.

A similar illustration of goal priming was presented by Bargh and Barndollar (1996). In these studies, goals were activated through a word puzzle containing words related to either achievement or affiliation goals. The effects of the primed goals were assessed by examining the participants' behavior with a partner with whom they were asked to work on a new task. The partner was actually a confederate of the experimenters who was instructed to perform poorly on the task. To examine whether the goal was primed, Bargh and Barndollar examined whether participants chose to be affiliative-oriented toward the confederate (taking time to console and help the partner) or achievement-oriented (trying to attain the highest individual score on the task). They found support for the notion that goals can be primed: Participants exposed to achievement goals during the initial task were more achievement-oriented (and performed better) on the task performed with the partner than those primed with affiliation goals (who apparently diverted time they could have spent achieving on the task to helping the other person).

Higgins, Roney, Crowe, and Hymes (1994) argued not merely that goals are activated preconsciously, but that a strategy ("regulatory focus") for pursuing a goal can also be triggered. A strategy that regulates goal pursuit through a focus on approaching a desired state is called *promotion focus*, while a strategy focused on avoiding an undesired state is called *prevention focus*. For example, the same goal can be framed through either a promotion or a prevention focus. The goal of not allowing stereotypes to influence you in how you think about people could be framed through a promotion focus by asking yourself to approach a state that is not compatible with stereotyping, such as asking yourself to try to be fair or egalitarian. However, the same goal could be framed through a prevention focus by asking yourself to avoid a state that is compatible with using stereotypes, such as by asking yourself to try to avoid thinking in a stereotypic way. In these two examples, you have the same goal; it is just framed in terms of either approach or avoidance. Higgins and colleagues argue that whether a goal is framed with an approach or an avoidance regulatory focus will actually alter how you go about pursuing the goal (and whether you are successful at attaining it). We will examine this specific example more closely in Chapter 11 when we discuss how and when people's goals influence the degree to which they stereotype others. For now, let us stay focused on the question of whether general strategies of goal pursuit can be accessible and have an impact on goal pursuit (e.g., Förster, Higgins, & Idson, 1998; Förster, Higgins, & Strack, 2000; Higgins et al., 1994; Shah, Higgins, & Friedman, 1998).

To examine this question, Förster and colleagues (1998, Experiment 2) used a priming procedure to temporarily trigger either promotion focus or prevention focus. Though participants were not aware that a particular regulatory focus was more accessible than another, this preconsciously triggered strategy for goal pursuit influenced subsequent behavior, facilitating responses that were compatible with their regulatory focus. Förster and colleagues had research participants pursue a very easy goal—they were asked to press a button. But they were asked to press the button either by pushing an arm forward toward a button that was in front of them and away from their own bodies (arm extension), or by using an arm movement in which they moved their arm toward their own bodies in order to press the button, thus flexing their arm in a drawing-toward motion (arm flexion). The logic was identical to that of Chen and Bargh (1999), described earlier: Arm flexion is compatible with the goal of approach, because to approach something means to bring it closer to one's body. Meanwhile, arm extension is compatible with avoidance goals, because to extend one's arm is to engage in a pushing away motion, consistent with what one does when trying to avoid something. This very subtle test of whether a regulatory focus could be primed and have an impact on behavior was successful. People with a promotion focus pressed the button with greater force when they were flexing an arm, while people with a prevention focus pressed harder when they had to extend an arm. Participants not only lacked awareness that a regulatory focus was primed; they were not aware of how this interacted with their arm position in determining the strength of their button pressing.

Mindsets

The concept of *mindset* was introduced by the Würzburg school (Külpe, 1904) to explain the fact that asking people to solve a specific task created a related cognitive orientation (i.e., a set) that facilitated solving the task at hand (as well as related tasks), but hampered solving unrelated tasks. Relevant cognitive procedures become activated when people are working on a task, and these procedures themselves, rather than any specific semantic content, become more accessible. Gollwitzer (1990) posited that different mindsets should be endowed with those cognitive features that facilitate the respective tasks and are thus functional to task completion.

Higgins and Chaires (1980) provided a first test of the idea that instead of specific semantic content, mindsets or general cognitive orientations can be made accessible and influence subsequent information processing. The general cognitive orientation they made accessible was the use of what they called *interrelational constructs*, with the idea being that once such a construct was made accessible, the cognitive orientation described by this concept would now be accessible and be more likely to be used in the future when new stimuli are encountered. By *interrelational constructs*, they simply meant the types of relationships between objects/people that are created when we use words such as "or" versus "and." That is, when you say "cake and pie," it suggests a wholly different relationship between these two things than if you say "cake or pie." Higgins and

Chaires were positing that even a mindset as abstract as thinking about things as belonging together can be made accessible, so that people are ready to "see" future events as things that can belong together. To make these orientations accessible, they presented participants with a list of objects and their containers as part of a memory task (e.g., "cherries, jar"; "vegetables, bag"). The object and its container was described with either the conjunction "and" or the preposition "of"; half of the participants saw a list with such phrases as "carton *of* eggs," and the other half saw such phrases as "carton *and* eggs." After these orientations were primed, participants were then asked to perform a separate and ostensibly unrelated task—the Duncker candle problem.

In the Duncker candle problem, people are shown some objects—a box of thumbtacks, a book of matches, and a candle. They are told to affix the candle to a wall in such a way that the candle burns properly yet does not drip wax on the table or floor. The correct solution requires participants to realize that the box can be used not just as a container for tacks, but also as a flat surface that can be tacked to the wall and support the candle. The priming of the different mindsets facilitates performance on the task by promoting the ability to see the tacks and box as separate entities. In their experiment, people primed with "and" as a grammatical connective were more likely to solve the Duncker candle problem than people primed with "of," because priming "and" created a mindset that promoted thinking about objects as separate entities.

Gollwitzer, Heckhausen, and Steller (1990) found that there are unique mindsets associated with *how* people go about pursuing goals, and that these mindsets, as orientations for how goals are pursued, can be primed just as easily as goal content. One mindset they discuss in relation to pursuing a goal is the *deliberative mindset*, a cognitive orientation in which people are evaluating and selecting a goal from among many alternative goals that could possibly be pursued at a given point in time. In contrast, a separate cognitive orientation associated with pursuing a goal is the *implemental mindset*, where people are concerned with specific planning on how to pursue or implement a chosen goal. In Gollwitzer and colleagues' experiment, participants were given either a deliberative or an implemental mindset as part of an initial task. The deliberative mindset was primed by asking people to weigh the pros and cons of initiating action regarding an unresolved personal problem; the implementational mindset was primed by asking people to plan the implementation of a chosen personal project. The participants were then asked to perform a "second experiment" in which they were presented with half-finished fairy tales, and were asked to complete the stories. The impact of the mindset was gauged by the degree to which the participants' cognitive orientation was used to describe the actions of the characters in the story. Were the characters described as being deliberate and lost in thought like Hamlet, or quick to act like Indiana Jones? Deliberative mindset participants ascribed deliberative actions to the main character, from contemplating courses of action to seeking advice. On the other hand, implemental mindset participants had their characters plunge into action.

Many experiments have illustrated the impact of various mindsets on how people form judgments, including an *accuracy motivation mindset* (Chen, Shechter, & Chaiken, 1996), a *comparison mindset* (Stapel & Koomen, 2001), *imitative mindsets* (Li & Moskowitz, 2004b), and a *counterfactual-thinking mindset* (Galinsky, Moskowitz, & Skurnik, 2000).

The Decay of Temporary Accessibility

How long-lasting is the "temporary" impact of having been incidentally, randomly, unknowingly, and unintentionally exposed to a concept? We have examined evidence that concepts can be made accessible, and that this accessibility spreads to associated concepts; we will soon discuss in detail how such accessibility influences judgments. But you may not yet be willing to accept the idea that this influence is one that will last for very long. For example, if the concept "reckless" gets primed because I have witnessed someone driving past me in a reckless manner (and have thus spontaneously inferred the concept "reckless"), how long does this concept remain accessible? Is a broker who witnesses such an act on the way to work likely to arrive at work and make a reckless decision regarding a stock portfolio because earlier in the day he/she saw someone acting recklessly? Neely (1977) showed that accessible constructs have an impact on how fast people notice related words a quarter of a second later. This is important for illustrating that concepts can indeed be made accessible. But the next questions are these: What does accessibility do (what impact does it have on judgment), and for how long does it do it (what determines when a concept that is primed will cease to be accessible)?

Higgins, Bargh, and Lombardi (1985) proposed that accessibility is not a binary affair, with a concept either being triggered or not. Instead, their *excitation transmission model* proposes that the accessibility of a construct is like an energy cell that can be charged to various degrees. Just as the battery on a laptop computer can last longer if it is charged more fully, the length of time over which accessible constructs can be expected to have an impact on judgment will depend on how strongly activated the concept is. Just as a concept accumulates charge until it reaches a threshold, once it passes that threshold it continues to accumulate charge, becoming not only activated, but strongly activated. Higgins (1996, p. 147) states that "excitation transmission models account for priming effects in terms of the heightening and the dissipation of excitation (or energy levels) from stimulation and decay." Thus the dissipation of accessibility effects depends on how strongly activated the construct is. Note the connection here to the model proposed by Logan (1989). Not only is the duration of the accessibility of a construct linked to its strength of activation, but so too is the likelihood that one construct will win the metaphorical "race" against other competing constructs to "capture" a stimulus. That is, the time it takes to retrieve a concept from memory and thus be able to apply it to judging some stimulus is directly linked to how strongly activated that concept is, or, in the language of the model, how strong the excitation level for the concept being retrieved happens to be. If one has recently been exposed to a concept, its excitation level will be high; it will be strongly accessible; and it will win the race to capture the stimulus against other potential constructs that could also fit.[1]

Thus far we have asserted that the length of time accessible constructs can be expected to influence a perceiver is tied to the energy level or the amount of excitation associated with the priming of the construct. A stronger prime will result in a larger degree of excitation, and therefore a longer-lasting influence. But we are still only speaking in relative terms. What do we mean by a "larger degree of excitation," and to answer our original question, just how long in real time do these effects typically last? The construct is, after all, only *temporarily* accessible. The answers to such questions are examined next.

Recency of Concept Activation

Srull and Wyer (1979) offer an initial answer to the question of what determines the amount of excitation or accessibility of a concept. It is partly determined by how much time has elapsed since the priming event was encountered (how recently the concept was activated). Concepts recently primed are more accessible (all else held equal) than those primed earlier. As time elapses from the encounter, new concepts become activated momentarily, and the activation of the initial concept fades. Even in the absence of new priming (such as when people are in a lab and prevented from thinking about new events or encountering new stimuli), activation fades as the stimulus that triggered the concept is no longer a "recent" event.

For example, Srull and Wyer (1979) made concepts accessible by having participants read sets of four words that did not form a grammatically correct sentence. The task was to take three of the four words from a given set and use them to form a correct sentence. The priming occurred through the concepts implied by the sentences. For example, one set included the words "the hug boy kiss," and any use of three words to form a correct sentence must imply the concept of "kindness." Participants completed 30 such sentences, 20% of which were related to kindness. To measure how long the accessibility lasted, participants were asked to make a judgment of a person whose behavior was known to be ambiguous with regard to kindness. If the concept of kindness was accessible, it would influence the judgment formed of the person, and he/she would be seen as kind. The time interval for making this judgment was varied from making an immediate judgment, to waiting 1 hour, to waiting 1 day (24 hours). Srull and Wyer found that the accessibility only seemed to be strong enough to influence judgment when the judgment was made immediately—when the prime had been recently encountered. An hour later, accessibility had faded.

Frequency of Concept Activation

Extending this finding, both Higgins and colleagues (1985) and Srull and Wyer (1979, 1980) proposed that the amount of excitation (or the strength of accessibility) and the duration of the accessibility are connected not only with what concept has recently been encountered, but with how often that concept is encountered. The more frequently one encounters (or contemplates) the primed concept (such as when 80% vs. 20% of the stimuli prime the same concept), the stronger the accessibility, and the longer the duration of its heightened accessibility. As an example, the experiment of Srull and Wyer (1979) that was described above was in reality more complex. Participants not only had concepts primed by seeing 30 items, 20% of which were related to the concept "kind"; the researchers also manipulated the frequency with which the prime was encountered. Thus, some participants read 30 items, 80% of which were related to kindness. They also had some participants read 60 items, with either 20% or 80% of the items related to kindness. Obviously, the persons who saw 60 items, 80% of which were related to kindness, encountered the concept of kindness more frequently than the persons who saw 30 items, 20% of which were related to kindness. Each group had recently seen this concept, but one group had been exposed to it far more frequently. What impact did frequency of priming have on the durability of the concept's accessibility? Accessibility was greatest when measured immediately, and when a concept had been activated numerous times in the past (such as 60 sentences that had 80% of the items related to the prime). Frequent priming led to effects that persisted through an hour, and beyond: "[The effects] are sometimes detectable even after 24 hours" (Srull & Wyer, 1979, p. 1670). Whereas the recent prime faded quite quickly, the frequently primed concept had strong initial effects, and these survived an hour and at times a day.

The Interaction of Recency and Frequency

What happens when two concepts are activated—one made accessible because you have recently been exposed to it, but the other made accessible because you have frequently been exposed to it? For example, let's say you have been listening to Eminem music all day, and the concept "hostile" has been frequently primed. Yet moments ago you were watching television reruns and saw an episode of *Seinfeld* where the character Elaine playfully shoves someone. You have recently been exposed to "playful," but have frequently been exposed to "hostile." How will you then interpret the behavior of a person who you then see shoving another person? Will this individual be seen as playing around or as hostile?

You could predict that whichever concept is more highly accessible when the priming of concepts stops is the one that will be used. Thus, even though you have frequently heard hostile music, "hostile" may be less accessible than "playful" after you have recently seen someone being playful, and therefore "playful" will be what you use to help you interpret the shove. However, you could also argue that it is not the accessibility *at the time priming stops*, but the accessibility *at the time the judgment is made* that matters. That is, if accessibility decays over time, and if decay rates are not uniform, it could be that even though the frequently primed construct "hostile" is less accessible than "playful" immediately after you have seen the playful behavior on TV, the decay rate associated with a frequently primed construct may be slower than the decay rate of the recently primed construct. Therefore, you may be more likely to interpret a shove as consistent with the recently activated construct if the shove happens very soon after the priming event. However, this effect may flip-flop as more time elapses between the judgment being made and the end of the priming episode. If the frequently primed construct has a slower decay rate, it may end up initially having less of an impact on your judgment than a recently primed construct, but subsequently have more of an impact as time elapses. In essence, recent priming may be like a burst of hot flame, which has intense heat initially but burns out quickly, whereas frequent priming may be like a slow burn—the heat may never be as great as the initial burst from a flare-up, but it maintains its heat longer and fades slowly, allowing the accessibility to linger.

To examine whether accessibility effects depend on the rate at which accessibility decays, Higgins and colleagues (1985) conducted an experiment similar to the example above. Participants were primed with one concept repeatedly ("independent"), but were primed with another concept more recently ("aloof"). They therefore had two constructs primed, each of which was potentially useful for describing a behavior they then had to judge—a person acting in a standoffish manner. Was this person seen as independent or aloof? The answer was that *it depended on the length of the delay between when a construct was primed and when the judgment was made*. When the delay was brief (15 seconds), the recently primed concept was more accessible and guided judgment. When the delay was of a longer duration (2 minutes), the frequently primed concept was now more accessible and guided judgment. Higgins and colleagues concluded that "after a sufficient delay, the frequent construct will be at a higher level of action potential than the recent construct given its slower rate of dissipation" (p. 66). The excitation level of a construct decreases over time since the last encounter with the priming stimulus, but *the decay function is not uniform* because the level of excitation is not merely tied to how long since the priming event has been encountered, but how often it has been encountered. Thus frequency and recency of activation both influence the duration of accessibility effects—sometimes in ways that are compatible, but potentially in ways that are incompatible.

Closing the Construct's Activation (Use It and Lose It)

Thus far we have discussed dissipation of excitation over time as the manner in which a temporarily accessible construct loses its readiness. But decay is perhaps not the only factor that determines how long an accessible construct remains in a state of perceptual readiness. Liberman and Förster (2000) propose that concept accessibility declines after the concept has been used. We might think that using a concept results in even greater accessibility of the concept, as the individual has greater exposure to the concept while using it. But rather than being seen as an instance of increased frequency of exposure to the stimulus (and heightened accessibility), use of the concept seems to deactivate the concept's accessibility, closing it down. This issue, however, is tied to the nature of the activated concept. Chapter 2 has discussed how *goals* can be primed. The claim being made here is that when a goal is primed, it stays primed until one has had a chance to attain the goal. In fact, the accessibility will only increase in strength as time passes (e.g., Bargh, Gollwitzer, Lee-Chai, Barndollar, & Trötschel, 2001). This is in contrast to what occurs when semantic information is primed. Rather than the typical effect that semantic concepts decrease in accessibility as time passes, an accessible goal increases in accessibility until it is used. But once one has had the chance to pursue and attain the goal, the accessibility of the construct is released: If one uses the construct (attains the goal), one loses the accessibility.

To investigate this, Liberman and Förster (2000) relied on the fact that the goal of trying to suppress a thought leads to that thought's accessibility. Thus concepts were activated by giving people the goal of *not* thinking about them. In a first experiment, the concept that people had the goal to suppress were colors. Participants were asked to describe a colorful painting, but were instructed to do so without using color-related words. Other participants were simply asked to describe the painting, with no restriction on their descriptions. The logic was that the goal to suppress thoughts of colors should give rise to the feeling of heightened accessibility linked to those concepts. Liberman and Förster posited that the difficulty of suppressing a thought (e.g., Wegner, 1994) would imply to the participants that they had the goal to think about that thought. In this phenomenon, the goal would be inferred from the sensations being experienced as a consequence of thought suppression. Thus a goal to use the suppressed concept would arise, regardless of whether that goal really existed or was mistakenly inferred from the sensations associated with suppression.

Following the first task of describing a painting, half of the participants should now feel they had the goal of using color words and half should not. In a second task, half of the people were given another picture to describe, without any mention of restrictions regarding word use. Thus half of the people who had been previously asked to suppress now had this restriction lifted; they had the opportunity to use color concepts. The review of semantic priming would suggest that if participants had concepts accessible from having suppressed them, and if the opportunity to use them in the second picture-describing task was a case of frequently priming the same concepts, then color concepts should be extremely accessible. However, if these were goals that were accessible, then as soon as the goal was fulfilled, the accessibility should die out. People who had suppressed the use of color words and then had the chance to express those thoughts should show a decrease in accessibility rather than an increase. (The remaining half of the participants did not describe a second painting and moved immediately to the next task.)

Participants next performed a task that provided a measure of concept accessibility. People were asked to provide descriptions of their homes, with the experimenters coding the material to see how often people used color terms in their descriptions. The more accessible the concept, the more colors that should be listed in the description of the home. The results showed that rather than leading to increased accessibility, describing colors in a second painting (i.e., using the concept) led to decreased accessibility—but only for some people. This happened only for the people who suppressed the use of colors on the first task and then had the chance to use colors on the second task. Giving expression to their unwanted thoughts (being allowed to use color concepts) satisfied the goal of using those thoughts, and accessibility was reduced. People who had been denied the opportunity to satisfy the goal persisted in having these concepts accessible.

Accessibility Effects

You may now be convinced that concepts in our minds can be triggered by events in our environment to which we have been incidentally exposed. Having recently thought about or seen a particular concept—whether it be a type of person (e.g., Saddam Hussein), a trait (hostile), a goal (to have power), or a stereotype (e.g., a dictator)—will trigger that concept and make it perceptually ready. The focus now turns to the impact such accessible information has on how we interpret other people. Is it possible that we are influenced by concepts in our minds of which we are not aware? Do we start to see people as being similar to or matching these concepts, simply because they are ready to be used in interpreting others? And do they continue to have an influence on us even if we become aware of their influence? Or are we able to control our impression formation processes so that we can "factor out" or "correct for" the influence of an accessible construct, should we become aware of its potential influence?

As an example, in the days before the invasion of Iraq in spring 2003, President Bush repeatedly spoke of Saddam Hussein as an evil tyrant. He made references in speeches to how Hussein had killed and tortured Iraqi citizens without remorse. How would citizens of the United States—mainly those who knew little about Iraq and its leader—think about the invasion and the need to overthrow Hussein, as a result of recent exposure to such information? One possibility was that having been recently exposed to President Bush's use of the concepts "evil" and "tyrant" would make these concepts accessible, and that the perceivers, with such concepts accessible, would be more likely to interpret Hussein in such a fashion, even in the absence of real information about him. Without being aware that they were simply agreeing with the President, or using these descriptions because they readily came to mind, they might form a fairly firm impression of Hussein as a tyrant. Even more interestingly, they might use this accessible information to describe a totally different person. Just because it was talk of Hussein that made these concepts accessible, the use of the concepts, once accessible, might not be limited to just describing the person who triggered the concept in the first place. These concepts might be used to describe any person whose behavior might be relevant. Thus, if asked to form an impression of the leader of China, these perceivers might also be disposed to lean toward the concept "tyrant." The point here is not whether such impressions were accurate or not. (Hussein probably was a tyrant, and

China's President, Jiang Zemin, may or may not be one.) It is that the basis for the impression was a reliance on whatever concepts just happened to be sitting in wait at the top of the perceivers' heads, without their realizing that this was the basis for the impression.

Finally, it was also possible for these perceivers to realize that their impressions were not based on an analysis of the information, but on fairly effortless processes. They might detect that the reason they were thinking so extremely negatively of China's leader was that the President had just been using the term "tyrant" in describing Saddam Hussein. Thus they might try to adjust their impression so that the concept of "tyrant" played less of a role in their impression of Jiang Zemin. But this would not guarantee that they were not influenced, even as they tried to remove the impact of this influence. In doing so, they might go too far in the other direction and see him as less of a tyrant than they otherwise would have had they not become worried about being influenced to start with (see the discussion of correction processes in Chapter 5). These two forms of influence on judgment—assimilation and contrast—are discussed next.

ASSIMILATION

Assimilation is said to occur when people lean on activated knowledge about a construct, using it as an interpretive frame for subsequent information (i.e., interpreting new information consistently with the activated construct). The interpretation of some behavior or person is drawn toward, or seen in the light of, the accessible concept. Heider (1944, p. 365) described assimilation as follows: When an actor is performing an act, one of these two ingredients (act and actor) colors the interpretation of the other, making the two ingredients seem similar. When the knowledge we have about an actor's behavior (observed actions) is used to interpret the actor and make inferences about the actor's personality (what Heider called "influences of effects on origins"), the traits implied by the behavior are used as "data through which we learn to know about the origins" (and one can trace attribution theory's origins to this notion). When the knowledge we have about an actor is used to interpret his/her behavior (what Heider called "the influence of the origin on the effect"), a perceptually ready construct (such as a trait or expectancy we associate with a person) provides the meaning that is ascribed to the behavior. Accessibility effects can be linked to this idea.

However, assimilation is not dependent on knowing that a relationship exists between the act/person being judged and the concept to which it is seen as similar. Accessible constructs (1) can be used to interpret behavior without awareness of its influence, and (2) can have an impact on the impressions of people other than the people whose traits served to make the concept accessible (i.e., the priming event can be different from the judgmental target). Perhaps most cases of assimilation can be described as cases of *misattribution*. One attributes an accessible concept (or the feeling of perceptual readiness—perhaps a feeling one cannot even consciously detect or define) to some person who is not responsible for the concept's heightened "charge." For instance, contemplating Bill Clinton might make the concept "liar" perceptually ready; however, one would not be limited to using that perceptually ready concept in describing Clinton only. Although the correct attribution for the perceptual readiness would be to Clinton, if one were to encounter some new person (such as George W. Bush), one might attribute the feeling of the concept's accessibility and perceptual

readiness to the new person. Bush's behavior would be assimilated to the accessible concept and be seen as the cause for the concept's ease of retrieval from memory and
readiness to be used (see Figure 10.2). One might ask (unconsciously), "Why do I see
Bush as a liar?" And one might answer (also unconsciously), "It is because his behavior
seems to suggest lying." And in so doing, one would fail to recognize that the true cause
for accessibility was a discrete priming event unrelated to the target of judgment to
whom the accessibility of the concept was now being attributed.

The Experimental Paradigm: Priming Task and Judgment Task

Despite Heider's (1944) discussion of assimilation and Bruner's (1957) discussion of
accessibility, links to modern-day accessibility theory are usually drawn through Higgins, Rholes, and Jones (1977). In this research, a classic procedure used in many priming studies was implemented. A typical priming study is divided into two parts: a *priming task* and a *judgment task*. In the priming task, people are incidentally exposed to
information—such as a stereotype, trait, exemplar, or goal—in order to make associated
concepts accessible. For example, seeing "reckless" as part of a list of words to be
remembered in a "memory experiment" increases the accessibility of the associated
knowledge structures (such as notions of recklessness and related constructs). After the
memory task, an ostensibly separate judgment task occurs, where people learn about
and report impressions of a person described as having performed an ambiguous
behavior that could be characterized in at least two, nonoverlapping ways (e.g., driving
a jet-powered boat without knowing much about such devices could be characterized as
"reckless" or as "adventurous" behavior). The concepts made accessible in the first task
are relevant to the possible nonoverlapping impressions that might be reached. This
allows researchers to examine whether having the concept primed in the first task
influences judgments on the second task.

For example, Higgins and colleagues (1977) exposed participants to trait words,
along with some filler words, as part of a so-called "perception task." The content of
these words was supposedly not important, and in no way did participants think that

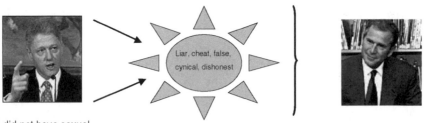

"I did not have sexual
relations with that woman."

"I am convinced this is not intentional;
we don't need to play cute politics."

FIGURE 10.2. Assimilation as a misattribution of fluency: Accessibility carried to a novel target. Exposure to Bill Clinton with his finger wagging might trigger the concepts "liar," "cheat,"
"false," and so on. The concept, once activated, would be used in framing a new event relevant to the concept. If one next saw President Bush denying that the subliminal message in his
TV commercial was intended, one might now attribute the reason for the accessibility of the
concept "liar" to Bush, assimilating one's judgment of him to the accessible construct. Had the
concept not been primed, Bush might not have been seen in this way.

these concepts would be used other than for the perception task. The perception task was actually being used, unbeknownst to participants, to prime specific traits. Participants were shown a series of slides that contained words printed on backgrounds of different colors, and they were asked to name the color of the background in each case. However, prior to each slide they also received a separate "memory" word that they were to repeat 8–10 seconds later, after they had noted the color of the slide. These memory words were carefully selected so that four of them were used to prime four separate traits. Some participants, for example, saw the words "reckless," "conceited," "aloof," and "stubborn." Others saw the words "adventurous," "confident," "independent," and "persistent." Later, as part of an ostensibly separate experiment on reading comprehension, participants were asked to read a passage in which the main character, named Donald, was acting ambiguously. Importantly, Donald's ambiguous behavior was along the trait dimensions previously primed. That is, he acted in a way that could be characterized as reckless or adventurous, as confident or conceited, as independent or aloof, and as persistent or stubborn.

Finally, after having been primed and having read about Donald, participants then made judgments (formed impressions) of Donald. What the research showed was that having been exposed to traits (e.g., reckless) in "Study 1" affected which of the two, nonoverlapping ways the ambiguous behavior was interpreted. If participants had been exposed to the words "reckless," "conceited," and so on in the first task, they would see Donald (some person whose behavior had nothing to do with the perception task just performed) as more reckless than adventurous, more conceited than confident, and so on. Of course, if they had been incidentally exposed to the words "adventurous," "confident," and so on in the first task, an opposite impression of Donald would be formed. Trivial exposure to these concepts determined how people reacted to Donald, without their realizing that their judgment was being influenced at all; instead, they probably believed that Donald's behavior alone dictated how he was being judged (see Figure 10.3).

Higgins and colleagues (1977) thus illustrated that perceivers assimilate judgments of people they observe to match accessible constructs. But they also importantly introduced some limitations and qualifiers to this influence that are quite important. As Stapel and Koomen (2001) noted, having thoughts about Chinese food is not going to have an impact on what you think about your friend's baby sister. And as George W. Bush claimed, being exposed to the word "RATS" would not have an impact on anyone's impressions of Al Gore. Or would it? We turn next toward examining four factors that determine when people will, and when they will not, assimilate judgments to primed concepts.

The Four A's of Assimilation: Applicability, Ambiguity, Assertibility, and Awareness

Applicability

The applicability of the primed concept to the stimulus/target/person that is being categorized and judged is a question of how relevant the accessible information in the mind is relative to the information we are attempting to understand. As perceivers, we do not attempt to foist whatever concepts that have been brought to mind upon each and every person we encounter. When notions of shyness are brought to mind, increasing the accessibility of this concept, and we then come across "Donald," who acts in a

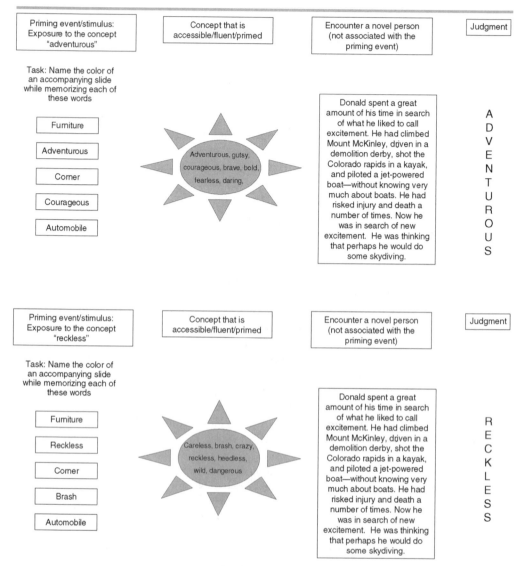

FIGURE 10.3. Assimilation as illustrated by the "unrelated studies" paradigm (e.g., Higgins et al., 1977).

manner that fits equally well into several alternative, nonoverlapping categories, how is he judged? The answer is that accessible information exerts an impact on our judgment only if the person we are judging is behaving in a fashion that is relevant/applicable. Although certain concepts are "perceptually ready," this should not be interpreted to mean that they are perceptual "givens." Bruner (1957) noted that as accessibility increases, less stimulus input is needed for that category to be used, and a wider range of stimuli will be captured by the accessible category. While this is true, it occurs within the confines of the fact that the stimuli being judged must first be identified as having features that at least make the item relevant to the category. The wide range of stimuli/

behavior that may be captured by the accessible construct is not so wide that it extends to all behavior.

Higgins and colleagues (1977) thought this point central to understanding accessibility effects. To illustrate the role of applicability in determining when accessible information is used, they manipulated whether the behavior that was observed was applicable to the accessible category. We have already discussed the behavior being judged in their experiment: A person named Donald acted in a way that could be seen as reckless or adventurous, as confident or conceited, as independent or aloof, and as persistent or stubborn. And we have already discussed how the interpretation perceivers arrived at was determined by what was accessible, so the behavior of Donald was assimilated into the accessible information. What has not yet been mentioned was that in addition to the experiment's priming either the positive or negative versions of the possible interpretations for the behavior (e.g., confident vs. conceited), it manipulated whether the concepts being primed were applicable to the behavior being judged. Therefore, some participants were exposed to trait words in the initial "perception task" that were relevant to the behavior of Donald that would soon be judged, and some saw trait words that were not applicable. This resulted in four types of primes: positive and applicable ("adventurous," "confident," "independent," and "persistent"), negative and applicable ("reckless," "conceited," "aloof," and "stubborn"), positive and nonapplicable ("neat," "satirical," "grateful"), and negative and nonapplicable ("disrespectful," "listless," "clumsy," "shy").

Higgins and colleagues (1977) found that, as noted already, applicable primes shaded the type of judgment made regarding Donald's behavior. This difference in judgments of Donald did not emerge when nonapplicable concepts were primed. What these results suggest is that people do not "see" the concepts that are accessible to them in all places they look; they only see them in the relevant places. But if the target person behaves in a way that is perhaps even remotely relevant, given that perceivers are perceptually ready to see that behavior, their accessible category may assimilate the behavior into it. The results also mean that accessibility effects are truly linked to the specific constructs that are primed. It is not the case that the findings of Higgins and colleagues are due to perceivers' simply being ready to see others positively when they are primed with positive concepts. The behavior must be relevant and applicable to the accessible concepts not in their affective tone, but in the meaning they suggest. Research participants primed with shyness did not see Donald as shy if his behavior did not fit it, nor did they come to see him as negative in a general sense.

Just how wide can the gap between the behavior and the concept be in order for it to still be seen as relevant and applicable? Donald's behavior in the Higgins and colleagues (1977) study was clearly not shy or satirical, and hence he was not seen as such. Yet it was clearly either adventurous or reckless, and as such was seen in such a fashion, with the direction of the judgment assimilated in the direction of the prime's valence. Although it may be the case that the range of stimuli/behavior captured by a prime does not extend to all behavior, it is also the case that the stronger the accessibility, the wider the range of behaviors and stimuli that will be captured and be deemed as relevant. Higgins and Brendl (1995) examined this component of the notion of applicability—namely, that *applicability* is a relative term, and what is deemed as applicable can vary along with the strength of the accessible concept. Thus, on the one hand, applicability is in some sense an absolute thing; reckless/adventurous behavior will never be seen as applicable to the concepts of "shy," "satirical," "grateful," or "disrespectful." On the other hand, there are perhaps numerous behaviors that might be seen as relevant to the concept of shyness, dependent upon just how ready one is to see that trait in others. The judgment of applicability is not solely based on the features of the stimulus, but on the strength of the excitation of the accessible construct.

Higgins and Brendl (1995) examined this by manipulating the behavioral information. For some participants the behavior was said to be vaguely related to the trait of "conceited," and for others the behavior was more clearly applicable to one of the two, nonoverlapping trait categories of "conceited" and "confident." The participants who read about these behaviors and judged the person performing them were primed so that they had varying degrees of accessibility of the trait "conceited." The most important finding emerging from this research was that when a stimulus was, as the researchers labeled it, "extremely vague," the strength of the activation compensated for the weakness of the stimulus. The more accessible the construct ("conceited"), the more likely the vague behavior was assimilated into the construct (the person was more likely to have been judged as having acted in a conceited way). Higgins and Brendl concluded that accessibility and applicability determine whether assimilation occurs.

Ambiguity

Thus far we have assumed that an accessible construct will work only when the person being judged behaves in a manner that is somewhat unclear. That is, the person's behavior must be either ambiguous (equally relevant to at least two, alternative, nonoverlapping constructs) or vague. When we observe a person acting in a highly diagnostic, unwaveringly clear fashion, there is little room left for our implicit biases as perceivers to work their magic. If someone is acting in an unambiguously kind way, being primed with "hostility" will not lead us to the judgment of "hostility." If someone acts in a clearly counterstereotypic way, an accessible stereotype will not be used in our impression (e.g., Locksley, Borgida, Brekke, & Hepburn, 1980; see Chapter 5).

Thus accessibility effects are dependent on the stimulus information being somewhat open to interpretation. When we are forming impressions of people whose traits are so evident in their behavior that their behavior impels one and only one interpretation, then accessibility of a construct will not matter much at all. But if, as is the case with much social behavior, the acts observed remotely lend themselves to subjective twists and spins, then we perceivers will interpret the actions in line with what is suggested by our accessible concepts.

Assertibility

Often we feel we simply are not allowed to assert a particular opinion. A sense that our expectancies, stereotypes, and accessible constructs should not be asserted (whether due to conformity pressures, political correctness, or our own sense of values informing us that to do so is unjust) can limit the degree to which assimilation effects occur. As just noted in the discussion of ambiguity, one factor that determines what we will assert about a person whose behavior we have observed is the quality of the stimulus information. Information about another person's behavior may stray too far from being ambiguous to allow accessible constructs to have an impact on our impressions. However, we have examined the case where the information strays from ambiguity in the direction of *increased clarity* (diagnostic information suggests one clear interpretation). There is another way in which information may travel away from being ambiguous, and that is when, rather than being ambiguous, information is just plain *uninformative*. Ambiguous information is information that suggests multiple possible alternative interpretations—but at least it has possible interpretations. Uninformative information does not suggest any particular interpretation. If the behavior of a person we observe is uninformative, then we may feel a constraint on our willingness to assert an impression that is consistent with an accessible construct. As with diagnostic stimuli, uninformative stimuli leave an accessible construct no room to work its magic, this time because we perceivers do not feel licensed to assert any impression whatsoever. We are unwilling to assert an impression that will be assimilated toward the accessible construct, because the stimulus information does not provide an opportunity to formulate what could be considered a valid and justifiable impression.

An uninformative stimulus is not the only factor that determines whether a feeling of assertibility exists. Another factor is whether we perceive a social constraint that does not allow us to express a particular thought or feeling. Many thoughts may cross our minds that we know are not appropriate, allowable, or acceptable to utter or to use in our judgments of others; they are not socially sanctioned thoughts. Thus, even if a behavior is ambiguous and relevant to one of our accessible thoughts, we may still prevent ourselves from using such thoughts because of the social constraint. In essence, we need a license to speak our minds, and some situations clearly revoke that license. Classic demonstrations of this lack of assertibility (a removal of the license to judge) were provided by Darley and Gross (1983) and Yzerbyt, Schadron, Leyens, and Rocher (1994); these are reviewed in Chapter 11. A more recent illustration of the notion of assertibility, and its impact on impression formation, has been provided by Monin and Miller (2001). These authors argue that in order for accessible information, such as a stereotype or an expectancy, to influence people's social judgments, they must feel that it is warranted to use such information—that they have a license to do so. The condition of assertibility must be in place. Concerns over licensing can initially constrain the impact accessible constructs have on judgment. Without a license, accessible constructs are not free to drive impression formation, and people keep them locked up, unexpressed. However, once the license is returned, their accessible constructs now drive their impressions. That is, a feeling that the use of accessible constructs is warranted and people can assert whatever they wish may subsequently free these accessible constructs and allow assimilation to occur.

The logic of Monin and Miller's (2001) research hinges on the belief that people sometimes become so comfortable in the public perception that they are fair and just, they soon feel as if they no longer need to guard against what they say and do. The public perception of them is so strong that they need not be concerned about damaging it. Thus, once people become convinced others see them as fair, or they become secure in their own sense of themselves as fair, they now feel no obligation to censor their biases and stereotypes from influencing their judgments. Whereas concerns about what people may or may not assert—what is socially licensed and allowable—may initially constrain accessibility effects, these constraints are eventually lifted if they feel sufficient credentials of fairness have been established that will not be damaged by what they say. Once this social constraint is lifted, they are licensed to react according to whatever is perceptually ready.

Monin and Miller (2001) illustrated that people make judgments consistent with accessible concepts only after they have first established credentials that would seemingly allow them to get away with a behavior, secure in the knowledge that they have a license to judge and act. In their research, the accessible concepts being examined were stereotypes, and the logic was that social norms should prohibit using stereotypes to judge someone in a stereotypic way. However, if people had the opportunity to illustrate that they were nonprejudiced, to establish their credentials as fair persons, such persons would now, ironically, feel free to stereotype others! Their credentials as fair persons would make them feel immune to the social constraints, because their public image as being nonprejudiced persons would protect them from being seen as biased if they said something politically incorrect. For example, participants were asked to make a choice between candidates for a job. The job was stereotypically male, and the job candidates included both men and women. Monin and Miller hypothesized that the accessibility of the stereotype should lead people to see the male candidate as fitting the job better if they were assimilating the job to the male stereotype. However, using stereotypes to make a hiring decision, rather than actual information about a person, is not licensed by our society. In the absence of any information that people could use to justify their decision, relying on the stereotype alone would be a blatantly bad thing to do. Thus, in the absence of either diagnostic information about the candidates or ambiguous information about them, participants should be unable to assert any preference, regardless of whether the stereotype was accessible. However, this constraint should disappear if participants felt they had the moral credentials, the license, to speak freely and use whatever perceptually ready impression they have. This was precisely what was found. Assimilation was more likely to occur after participants first had the opportunity to establish their credentials as nonsexist persons. These credentials were established by first allowing some of the participants to express their disagreement with blatantly sexist statements. This disagreement then, ironically, licensed them to go ahead and act in a sexist fashion, free of the social scrutiny, because they were secure in their sense of themselves as nonsexist. Without the buildup of credentials, people did not feel allowed to assert a judgment that aligned their judgment (who was the best candidate for the job) with the accessible stereotype.

Social pressure is another force that determines what we feel licensed to assert as perceivers. What we are willing to assert in private is often different from what we will assert in public, because social forces censor us. Thus social forces may inhibit our sense of feeling licensed to say what we think. It can even alter the very type of judgment that is formed. Whether we use an accessible construct, and whether a judgment is assimilated to an accessible construct, may be limited by what we are willing to assert in the face of a particular social pressure. If a judgment is made anonymously, perhaps social pressures regarding what it is acceptable to assert are not so central. However, if we are forming impressions we need to justify to others, or that will be publicly expressed, then the confidence with which we feel we can assert our judgment will impact on whether we feel free to allow our internal states to guide judgment.

One such social pressure comes from needing to justify decisions and impressions to others. Being held publicly *accountable* in this way motivates people to be more accurate in how they evaluate information and more deliberate in considering what types of factors should influence one's judgment. Accountability leads people to think through issues in a careful and thorough fashion in order to form a position that is defensible (Tetlock, 1985). It motivates people to contemplate the arguments on both sides of an issue to prepare for the criticisms of others and have a well-articulated and carefully constructed point of view. Accountability to social forces has been shown to influence people's susceptibility to the correspondence bias by making people more likely to consider all possible influences on impressions, including situational pressures, that are typically not fully considered (see Chapter 8).

Just as Tetlock (1985) showed that the correspondence bias was eliminated by accountability—people failed to make overattributions to disposition under conditions of low choice when accountable, but did so, as is usually found, when unaccountable—we (Thompson, Roman, Moskowitz, Chaiken, & Bargh, 1994) predicted that accessibility effects would be eliminated when people were accountable. Rather than relying on what is most accessible to shape judgment, a person concerned with justifying judgments will draw conclusions from a precise evaluation of the data, rather than a quick and effortless application of whatever interpretation is perceptually ready. Accountability will alter what people feel licensed to assert, and this sense of what they are licensed to assert will determine whether accessible constructs are used in forming an impression. We (Thompson et al., 1994) primed people with concepts such as "reckless" or "adventurous" and "persistent" or "stubborn," and then looked to see whether people assimilated their judgment of an ambiguous target to fit with the accessible information. Half the participants were accountable to others for the judgments being formed, half were not. As predicted, when participants were not accountable, priming effects emerged (as usual); when accountable, the assimilation of targets to accessible traits did not occur. When people were carefully, elaborately, and accurately processing the information about Donald, they no longer asserted that the target resembled whatever perceptually ready information that had been made accessible.

Awareness

For assimilation to occur, people must not be aware that an influence is being exerted on their impressions. If they become concerned that some force is biasing what we think, and this force is one they do not want as an influence, they will take steps to remove its impact on judgment. Given that most people would not like to think their impressions are determined by something as trivial as whatever happens to be accessible, or that what influences them could be caused by unintentional exposure to a concept, they will probably take steps to account for the effects of an accessible construct if they are aware of them (i.e., correction processes; see Chapter 5). Assimilation is a form of naive realism; thus people must remain naive to the influence for assimilation to occur. With this said, at this point you may be suspicious as to whether participants in the experiments discussed in this chapter truly were not aware of an influence on their judgment. After all, the words that were used to make a concept accessible (e.g., "reckless" as part of a perception task) were consciously presented to the participants. Was it possible that people did not really notice any link between seeing such words in one task and then reading about a person whose behavior was relevant to those words? It could be that participants knew the experimenters expected them to use those words in their later judgments, and they were merely obliging the experimenters rather than illustrating assimilation.

To rule out this possibility and demonstrate that temporary constructs really exert an unconscious influence, Bargh and Pietromonaco (1982) subliminally primed people. If one is never aware of having seen a word it would be impossible for one to be aware of any impact that word might have on one's later judgments and impressions. This would rule out the possibility that being conscious of the priming episode at some point could influence the effects of the priming. Bargh and Pietromonaco used the same basic paradigm we have been reviewing: They exposed participants to trait words and then gave them a passage to read about a person named Donald as part of a supposedly unrelated, second experiment. This time, however, the words were subliminally presented (below the threshold of conscious awareness). The traits that were subliminally primed were related to the concept "hostility." Next, in the supposedly unrelated experiment, people read a description of Donald who was ambiguously hostile, and were asked to form an impression of him. They rated Donald on a series of scales, some related to and some unrelated to hostility. If the concept was made accessible by the subliminal presentation, then Donald should be seen as increasingly hostile as that concept is made more and more accessible. Given this prediction that strength of accessibility should have an impact on assimilation, the experiment manipulated how strongly the subliminally presented concepts would be activated. Either 20% or 80% of the words subliminally presented were related to hostility (e.g., "hostile," "unkind," "punch," "hate," "hurt," "rude," "stab"). Were people primed to see the world in terms of the construct "hostility"? The results showed that Donald was judged more hostile in the 80% than in the 20% condition on the related traits, but there was no difference in ratings of Donald on the unrelated traits. Subliminal primes shape impressions.

Thus assimilation occurs even if people never consciously see the trait words. However, this should not be taken to mean that a concept must be subliminal for it to exert an influence on judgment. Rather, all that is needed is for people to remain naive about the influence being exerted. It is not whether or not they are aware that a concept was ever exposed to them that matters; it is whether they are aware that having been exposed to those concepts has any impact on their later thoughts and actions (Bargh, 1992). In most experiments, people are vividly aware of the primes themselves. The trick is for the experimenters to introduce the judgment task in a manner that does not allow the perceivers to realize that the words they were just exposed to will be related in any way to the judgment task. Subliminal presentation of words is one way to ensure that, but it is not required. For assimilation to occur after priming, people must not be aware of an influence on their judgment. It does not matter that they have seen the actual stimulus serving as the prime.

What happens when people do become aware of an influence on their judgment from an accessible construct? For example, what happens to the judgment of Mr. Vance, the teacher described in Chapter 5 who worries that he will be too easy on his own child (who happens to be in the class), because his accessible "pro-child" feelings may bias his judgment? What about a Jewish admissions officer who worries that she may be using more lenient criteria for admitting Jewish students to her college? Or take as an example the worry that driving in speeding traffic will make you also drive at excessive speeds, without realizing it. In many instances, people not only see the event that primes a construct; they develop a theory that this accessible concept is in fact influencing them by assimilating their judgment and action toward it. Once people develop such theories, they dictate a response that will allow them to counteract the influence. Mr. Vance tries not to be too positive in assessing his own child's work; the Jewish admissions officer tries to use the same criteria in evaluating all students.

Essentially, people engage in a process very similar to that discussed in Chapter 5. The perceivers detect a possible bias on their impressions/judgments, and attempt to *correct* for that bias or remove the unwanted influence. This process of perceivers using some theory of how they are being biased to make adjustments to their impressions/ judgments has been called a process of *correction* (e.g., Gilbert, 1989; Wegener & Petty, 1995), *dissociation* (Devine, 1989), and *debiasing* (e.g., Thompson et al., 1994). Unfortunately for the perceivers, the theories they have about what might be influencing them may be incorrect (e.g., Nisbett & Wilson, 1977). And even if they are correct in identifying what is influencing them, they may still incorrectly gauge how it is influencing them (e.g., Wegener & Petty, 1995; Wilson & Brekke, 1994) or how much it is influencing them (e.g., Martin, Seta, & Crelia, 1990; Moskowitz & Skurnik, 1999). For example, the admissions officer may have an incorrect theory that she is biased in favor of Jewish students, and any attempt to correct for this bias (which doesn't really exist) would end up creating a new bias against Jewish students. Mr. Vance may correctly think that he is biased in favor of his child, and then try to correct for this bias (which really does exist), but in so doing he incorrectly gauges the strength of his bias. Thus, he ends up being harsher on his child than he needs to be.

We will explore this question more fully in the next section when we discuss contrast effects. When judgment is pushed away from, or in the opposite direction from, an accessible concept (rather than assimilated toward it), it represents a form of judgmental *contrast*.

CONTRAST

Perhaps the focus to this point on assimilation has given the impression that our "natural" response to a construct's heightened accessibility is to use that construct as an *interpretive frame* through which later stimuli are seen; new information is assimilated to match what we are perceptually ready to see. However, this need not be the case. First, attempting to interpret new information need not be our goal. For example, as reviewed in Chapter 9, sometimes we have the goal of evaluating, not interpreting others. Second, even if we are interpreting others, the interpretation need not be produced through a process of assimilation. Contrast and assimilation are types of accessibility effects; the discussion here does not attempt to claim that one is more basic or primary than the other. Indeed, both types of effects were introduced by Heider (1944, pp. 363–368) in discussing influences on social perception. What is *contrast*? Just as coherent meaning can be assigned to a stimulus by drawing it into an accessible concept, sometimes clean and simple meaning can be produced by pushing information away from an accessible construct. Moving a stimulus away from an accessible concept while categorizing the stimulus is a *contrast effect*. The Ebbinghaus illusion reviewed in Chapter 1 is a fine example of contrast in perception. In Figure 1.3, the circle surrounded by smaller circles appears larger than the same-sized circle surrounded by larger circles. The perception of a circle is shaped by what is accessible (the circles in its immediate context), leading the target circle to seem less like the comparison circles.

Heider (1944) similarly described contrast in person perception as a case of *dissimilation*—a process whereby an actor performs an act, and the qualities of the actor color the interpretation of the act by making the act and actor seem "as much unlike each other as possible" (p. 363). Like assimilation, contrast is a type of accessibility effect where activated knowledge is used in interpreting a given stimulus; it is simply used to illuminate the stimulus in a manner that makes it seem *opposite* to the accessible information. For instance, Heider gave several classic literary examples to illustrate the meaning of contrast. In *Othello*, Shakespeare develops the title character in a manner that leads us to be certain he is not the type of person who is prone to jealousy. When Othello then exhibits jealous behavior, the behavior acquires dramatic force when contrasted against the accessible expectancy. Thus the jealous behavior is seen as extremely jealous in light of the character's nonjealous nature. As a second example, Heider stated, "Sophocles' Philoktetes offers a similar example. Philoktetes is presented as possessing a high degree of self-control. That such a man cries out loud in pain is very impressive" (p. 364).

It should be noted here that a contrast effect is "an effect," and in this section several cognitive processes that may be able to bring about this effect are reviewed. The use of the Ebbinghaus illusion as an illustration here is not meant to imply that a specific type of perceptual process is the only way in which contrast is produced in person perception. Two prominent explanations have been put forth to explain how contrast effects occur. The first is the *standard-of-comparison* model, and the second is the *correction* model. In the latter, contrast is produced in the manner discussed at the end of the preceding section: In attempting to remove a bias on one's judgment that one has become aware of, one engages in a correction or debiasing process that ends up producing contrast. In the standard-of-comparison model, contrast occurs through a process of comparing stimuli (people) against accessible constructs, such as traits and exemplars—producing a perceived difference between the two, whether one is aware of the accessible standard or not. This is akin to the perceptual contrast in the Ebbinghaus illusion. We next examine each model in turn.

The Standard-of-Comparison Model of Contrast

The standard-of-comparison model proposes that when a concept is primed, it is then used as a standard of comparison against which new and applicable stimuli are evaluated and judged (e.g., Herr, 1986; Herr, Sherman, & Fazio, 1983). For example, if one is primed with an exemplar that represents extreme hostility, such as "Hitler," "Dracula," or "Osama bin Laden," subsequent people who are behaving in an ambiguous way that is relevant to hostility will have that behavior evaluated in the context of the accessible exemplar. Hitler was evil, so Donald, seen through Hitler-colored glasses, does not seem hostile at all. The perception of Donald is pushed away from the accessible construct, rather than drawn toward it. For instance, Herr (1986) found that increasing the accessibility of the construct "hostility" through exposing participants to hostile primes, such as "Dracula," led to subsequent impressions that a target person was less hostile.

Latitudes of Acceptance and Rejection

This model has its roots in social judgment theory and the concepts of *latitudes of acceptance and rejection* (Sherif & Hovland, 1961). Sherif and Hovland (1961) examined how contrast effects in perceptual stimuli, such as those in the Ebbinghaus illusion, could be applied to social perception. Social judgment theory asserts that attitudes are evaluative in nature, and that these evaluations are represented in the mind in terms of an internal reference scale. The manner in which this internal reference scale is constructed is said to be according to latitudes of acceptance and rejection. A *latitude of acceptance* is the range of the scale where the beliefs one person finds acceptable are contained; a *latitude of rejection* is where beliefs one finds unacceptable are contained. Sherif and Hovland argued that one's existing attitudes determine latitudes of acceptance and rejection, and therefore establish reference points or standards that subsequent information is judged against. Just as the perception of a circle's size is determined by the size of other circles around it, one's view of a person, or the positions espoused by that person, are influenced by one's relevant attitudes. These authors reasoned that one's prior attitude on a particular issue serves as a standard against which information relevant to it is judged.

When one is receiving information relevant to one's existing attitudes, and this information falls within the latitude of rejection, the reaction to it gets polarized and contrast occurs: "The statement or position is perceived to be farther from the person's own attitude than it truly is. Within this contrast range true discrepancy is overestimated, and the magnitude of overestimation grows larger as true discrepancy increases" (Eagly & Chaiken, 1993, p. 367). For example, if one has a very strong attitude about an issue, such as when one is a pro-environment activist, this attitude will serve as a standard (and a relatively extreme standard at that) against which new information about the environment is judged. If one receives information from another person that is neutral toward, or even moderately in favor of, protecting the environment, one's own extreme attitudes on this issue will, by comparison, make the positions offered by the other person seem almost anti-environment. We have noted such effects in Chapter 1 when discussing how extremists view the "neutral" media as actually biased against them and how negotiators see their opposition as having more extreme positions than is actually the case. We can see this in religious life, too, where extremists see more moderate worshipers of their own faith as heretics. These nonextreme views fall within the extreme persons' latitude of rejection.

The Extremity Hypothesis

Moving away from contrast in the domain of attitude evaluation and into the domain of impression formation, the standard-of-comparison model asserts that people do not or cannot typically bring all relevant information out of memory when forming an impression of a person. Instead, they rely on a subset of accessible knowledge. If specific examples of the judgment category are at hand, people will employ them as standards of comparison against which new information is evaluated. For example, Herr and colleagues (1983) found that accessible exemplars led to contrast effects when nonhuman stimuli (exemplars of animals) were used as primes. The construct "hostile" was made accessible by exposing participants to ferocious (e.g., "grizzly bear," "shark") and nonferocious (e.g., "dove," "kitten") animal names. They then were asked to judge the ferocity of some new, ambiguous animals (ambiguous in that they did not really exist, so participants could not know how ferocious they were). It was found that accessible exemplars led to contrast. If the concept of "shark" was accessible, the ambiguous animal was seen as not very fierce; if "dove" was accessible, the animal was judged as fierce.

Herr (1986) posited that the extremity of the prime has an impact on the type of judgment formed. Extreme primes should lead to greater contrast in one's impressions than more moderate primes, because an extreme construct shares few features with other targets. If an extreme exemplar is accessible in memory, the target being evaluated against this standard will seem less extreme on the quality in question, resulting in contrast. In the language of social judgment theory, the extreme prime is more likely to set a judgment standard in which the moderate behavior of others will fall into the latitude of rejection. On the other hand, if an accessible construct is a moderate instance of the category in question, the construct will now share many features with the target stimulus. If a person is seen as sharing many features with the accessible construct, the behavior will be assimilated into the accessible construct. The more moderate standard of comparison will allow for the moderate behavior of others to fall within the latitude of acceptance (see Figure 10.4).

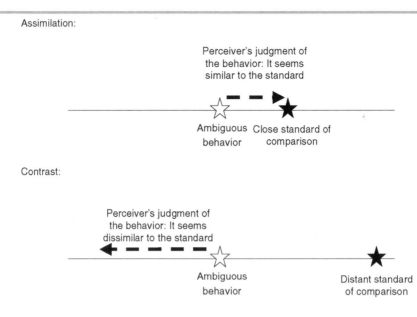

Assimilation:

Perceiver's judgment of
the behavior: It seems
similar to the standard

Ambiguous Close standard of
behavior   comparison

Contrast:

Perceiver's judgment of
the behavior: It seems
dissimilar to the standard

Ambiguous   Distant standard
behavior   of comparison

FIGURE 10.4. Standards of comparison and a case of judgmental contrast.

Herr (1986) examined this extremity hypothesis derived from the standard-of-comparison model. Participants were exposed to an extremely hostile prime, like "Dracula," and an extremely nonhostile prime, like "Gandhi," in an initial experiment. They then performed a supposedly separate, unrelated experiment where they had to form impressions of a person (Donald) whose behavior was ambiguously hostile. Herr found that Donald was judged as more hostile if people had been initially exposed to the name of Gandhi in the earlier experiment. Poor Donald paled in comparison to Gandhi, and his ambiguous behavior was now seen as hostile by the perceivers. But if Dracula had been seen earlier, Donald was now rated as friendly, not hostile, despite performing exactly the same behavior. All that changed was the context that served as an evaluative frame for the behavior. However, Herr also found that whereas extremely hostile exemplars led to contrast, moderately hostile primes such as "Alice Cooper," "Robin Hood,"and "Joe Frazier" led to judgments of greater hostility, or an assimilation effect. In sum, contrast increases as primes increase in extremity, since more extreme primes share fewer features with the target and serve as more distant judgmental anchors.

What about the Four A's?

The issues of applicability, ambiguity, assertibility, and awareness of the prime are as relevant to contrast effects as they are to assimilation effects. For example, ambiguity was addressed by Herr and colleagues (1983). They primed the names of extremely ferocious ("shark") and moderately ferocious ("rhinoceros") animals and examined the impact on judgments of an ambiguous target's (a novel animal's) ferocity. However, they also had people rate the ferocity of unambiguous targets, such as goats and pigs. With ambiguous targets, they found that extremity of the prime mattered; the more extreme the prime, the greater the contrast. But this was not the pattern found with unambiguous targets. Here, prime extremity did not matter. Contrast effects resulted regardless of whether the prime was extreme or not. To put this a slightly different way, if the primes were extreme enough, ambiguity did not appear to matter. Contrast occurred with both ambiguous and unambiguous targets. But if the primes were not very extreme, then the ambiguity of the stimulus was very important. As Herr and colleagues stated, "Clearly, the ambiguity of the target to be judged plays a critical role. In the case of prior activation of moderately extreme categories, it is the ambiguity of the target that determines whether assimilation or contrast effects emerge" (p. 334).

Applicability is also important for determining whether accessibility effects occur when the standard-of-comparison model is examined. The behavior of the person being judged must be relevant to the concept being primed. Earlier it has been noted that when traits are accessible, but are not relevant to a behavior, then no accessibility effects are found. Research on the standard-of-comparison model has examined a related question regarding applicability: What happens if the concept implied by the accessible construct (such as "hostile") is relevant to the behavior being judged (Donald's ambiguous behavior), but the manner in which the concept is made accessible is by priming an exemplar that is not relevant or applicable? This may sound confusing, so let's use an example. Suppose "hostile" is primed by exposing people to an exemplar of a hostile animal, such as a tiger. If you are then asked to evaluate the ambiguous behavior of a person, will a contrast effect occur, or will the animal fail to be used as a standard of comparison because the concept "tiger" is not applicable to evaluating human behavior? Stapel and Koomen (2001) predict that "*animal* exemplars like 'Shark' and 'Tiger' are not very likely to be used as a comparison standard when judging the hostility or friendliness of a *person* named Donald. These exemplars are not similar, do not belong to the target category (persons), and thus lack comparison relevance which makes contrast unlikely to emerge" (p. 241; emphasis in original).

The role of applicability in determining whether contrast effects occur was examined by Stapel, Koomen, and van der Pligt (1997). Participants in this experiment were exposed to names of either extremely hostile persons (e.g., "Hitler") or extremely hostile animals (e.g., "shark"). Stapel et al. had their participants perform an ostensibly separate experiment after being primed: They read about a person named Donald whose behavior was ambiguously hostile–friendly. The task was to form an impression of him, rating his friendliness–hostility. The researchers found that when a person's name was used as a prime, the typical contrast effect emerged; people rated Donald as more friendly after they had been exposed to the name "Hitler." However, contrast effects were not found in the animal-priming conditions. As noted above, animals are not relevant comparison targets for judging people, so in this sense the prime is not an applicable standard of comparison.

Although assertibilty has not been examined regarding contrast effects, presumably the same principles that determine whether one will assert an opinion about a person or topic by using accessible constructs will govern contrast as well as assimilation. If there is no license to express an opinion, the lack of feeling that rendering a judgment is socially acceptable and warranted should prevent one from expressing an opinion, and thus should keep contrast from occurring.

Finally, whether one is aware of a prime is not a strong factor in determining whether contrast occurs when a standard-of-comparison process is responsible for contrast. Like perceptual contrast in Gestalt psychology, contrast in person perception results from exemplars' being used as anchors that provide the context for perceiving and interpreting the meaning of a behavior. The process is believed to be a fairly automatic one. What would happen if one was aware of the construct's accessibility and that it was being used as a comparison standard? Presumably it would still be used as a standard and contrast would result (so long as the prime was applicable and relevant to the judgment). If one is conscious of the fact that Hitler is one's standard for hostility, Donald's behavior will still pale in comparison. In fact, being aware of the prime might exaggerate contrast effects if it served to strengthen the likelihood of the prime being used as a standard. But this is not to say that awareness of the prime is not an important factor in producing contrast. In fact, the second model of contrast effects—the correction model—hinges entirely on whether one is aware of the prime. Thus awareness is relevant to whether contrast effects occur, but this relevance depends on the manner in which contrast is produced via standard of comparison or via correction processes.

The Correction Model of Contrast

A standard-of-comparison process in which a target is evaluated against a standard is one possible way contrast is produced. But there is another mechanism capable of producing contrast—a correction process. According to the correction model (also called the set–reset model), contrast depends on people's attempting to interpret a stimulus and judge it in some way. In doing so, if they are aware of being biased and have a theory about how that bias is affecting them (L. L. Martin, 1986; Martin, Seta, & Crelia, 1990), contrast can result. In an attempt to remove a potential source of bias from their judgment, people correct the judgment by subtracting the biasing influence. Contrast arises from people's difficulty in determining whether their judgment has been shaped by the behavior of the target (what seems a reasonable basis for judgment) or the primed construct (what seems a biased basis for judgment). How is it that the inability to differentiate between a genuine reaction to a target and the contributions of irrelevant forces, such as primes, can lead to contrast effects?

Contrast is dependent on one's first associating the accessibility of information with one's reaction to the target. Accessible information is initially assumed to be accessible because the target person's behavior has made it accessible. Thus judgment is "set" in place by merging the observed behavior with the primed construct. This is the availability heuristic: A concept's accessibility is assumed to reflect the fact that the ease with which a particular thought comes to mind is an indication of its relevance to the target of judgment. However, if one becomes aware of the possibility that the "feeling of accessibility" may be due to some other source, and may not really be associated with the observed behavior, then an unwanted influence is being exerted on one's judgment. In such cases, one does not wish for judgment to be "set" in a manner that links the accessibility to the current target of judgment, since one suspects that the accessibility is due to some other source. One will then engage in "resetting" of judgment to correct for the prime's unwanted influence. One attempts to exclude information related to the prime from one's judgment. But in doing so, one may extract part of one's genuine reaction to the target—an overcorrection. Certainly, it is possible that when judgment is being adjusted for a potential biasing influence, one can be accurate and correctly partial out *only* those contributions to judgment uniquely contributed by the biasing force. However, people "may not make a perfect discrimination between their reaction to the priming task and their reaction to the target" (Martin et al., 1990, p. 28).

An Illustration

Let us illustrate this process with a concrete example. You observe a person acting in an ambiguous manner that has elements both of boldness/bravery and of recklessness/craziness. Think of Donald from Figure 10.3. Is he excessively brave? Is he suicidal? These concepts, and those related to them, are all related to his behavior. Your mind is full of positive thoughts, such as "bold," gutsy," "dauntless," fearless," and "daring." But your mind is also full of negative thoughts, such as "reckless," "dangerous," "crazy," "rash," and "suicidal." Now imagine you begin to worry about a potential influence on your judgment. You remember that just before encountering Donald, you had read a story on the Internet about the suicide of Kurt Cobain. You now worry that the concept "suicidal" may be tainting your interpretation of Donald's behavior—not because he really is acting that way, but because the concept was accessible to you. Finally, you attempt to remove the unwanted influence and judge the action based only on what you see. But the problem is that the behavior you see *is* partially crazy, reckless, and suicidal. By preventing yourself from including these concepts in your impression, you have gone too far in the reverse direction, now removing elements from your perception of the behavior that actually should not be removed if you want to form an unbiased judgment. Thus, rather than seeing Donald as reckless and suicidal as the "prime" suggested, you now see him in the opposite manner—as brave and bold.

In more technical language, an ambiguously reckless or bold target contributes both positive and negative elements to one's reaction (Figure 10.5A). If the concept "reckless" has been primed by some event not related to the behavior, this concept, and its related negative elements, now have increased accessibility (Figure 10.5B). Next, if this construct is not only accessible, but is being used to help one interpret a stimulus, features of both the construct and the stimulus are merged together in one's perception (Figure 10.5C). Finally, if one becomes aware of the influence and wants to remove it from judgment, one must "reset" one's judgment and eliminate this unwanted influence. But since the two sources of influence (one's real reaction to the person untainted by the prime, and the elements contributed by the accessible construct) have been merged, separating them is difficult and imprecise. In the process of adjusting judgment for the unwanted influence (resetting), one may overadjust. By *overadjust* is meant that one removes part of one's real reaction to the person, untainted by the prime. The result is that one's reaction to the target is left without some elements that were consistent with the prime that should have remained as part of the unbiased evaluation. This is a contrast effect. Rather than a judgment's being drawn toward the prime, a judgment is produced that has fewer elements of the prime.

Evidence for the Correction Process

Initial support for the correction model of contrast effects came from experiments where the researchers attempted to make the primes extremely obvious to the perceivers, presumably heightening the probability that the perceivers would be aware of the prime's impact on judgment. L. L. Martin (1986) and Martin and colleagues (1990) created construct accessibility by blatantly presenting prime words to participants. Presenting prime words blatantly (rather than subtly) did in fact lead to contrast effects, presumably because awareness of a potential biasing influence (the blatant primes) motivated attempts to remove the bias from judgment. Further evidence for

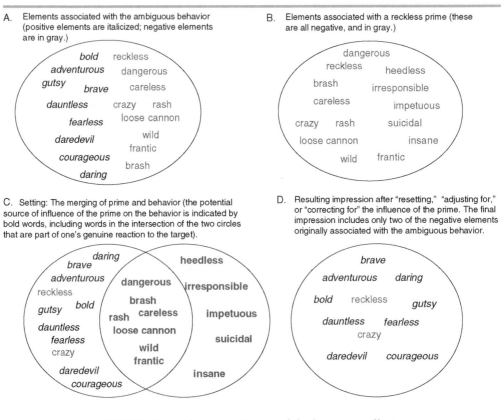

A. Elements associated with the ambiguous behavior (positive elements are italicized; negative elements are in gray.)

B. Elements associated with a reckless prime (these are all negative, and in gray.)

C. Setting: The merging of prime and behavior (the potential source of influence of the prime on the behavior is indicated by bold words, including words in the intersection of the two circles that are part of one's genuine reaction to the target).

D. Resulting impression after "resetting," "adjusting for," or "correcting for" the influence of the prime. The final impression includes only two of the negative elements originally associated with the ambiguous behavior.

FIGURE 10.5. The correction model of contrast effects.

the role of awareness in producing contrast came from experiments in which research participants were able to consciously report remembering the primes. The ability to remember the prime words at the end of the experiment was correlated with a tendency to exhibit contrast effects. Both Lombardi, Higgins, and Bargh (1987) and Newman and Uleman (1990) included in their experiments measures that assessed recall for the primes, and found that recall for prime words was correlated with contrast in judgment. These findings suggest that memory for the primes indicated a heightened awareness of the primes and their presence in consciousness. Awareness of the primes led perceivers to believe that their judgments were influenced by the primes. Attempts to correct for this influence led to contrast effects.

The first direct test of whether awareness of a primed trait (and thus correction for an influence on judgment) led to contrast was conducted by Moskowitz and Roman (1992). It was reasoned that if an activated construct was conscious to perceivers, then they would be less likely to use it to interpret the behavior of a target person. Ironically, in attempting not to use the construct, people would end up using it nonetheless, but not in the manner they had expected. Rather than interpret the person's behavior in a fashion consistent with the primed trait, they should show a contrast effect caused by overcorrection. To examine whether awareness of the prime triggered a correction process, research participants' awareness of the primed words was manipulated by having them read trait-implying sentences. Half the participants were instructed to form an impression of the people described in the sentences, thus making conscious trait inferences. The other half of the participants were instructed to memorize the sentences, and traits would thus be activated only through spontaneous processes of trait inference. If people spontaneously generated traits that made that trait accessible, but this activation and its potential influence were outside of awareness, then assimilation should be found. However, contrast should be exhibited for those who formed conscious inferences. They would be attempting not to allow inferences formed on the first task to influence judgments of a separate person on the next task.

Participants next read a passage about a person behaving in an ambiguous manner that was relevant to the traits that had just been primed. The participants' task on this second, "unrelated" experiment was to form an impression of the person being described (once again, named Donald). As predicted, it was found that when the sentence task promoted traits' being inferred spontaneously (the equivalent of trait constructs' being activated outside of awareness), assimilation effects emerged. However, when traits were consciously inferred, participants were aware of the source of their trait inferences (and their potential biasing influence), and showed contrast effects in subsequent judgments. If they had first read a sentence that implied a person was reckless, they later judged a new person, Donald, not as reckless but as bold.

In a conceptual replication of the finding that awareness of the prime produces contrast, Strack, Schwarz, Bless, Kübler, and Wänke (1993) primed people and asked half of the participants to remember the priming episode (reminding them of the primes) just prior to reading about a target. Thus, rather than measuring recall for the primes after the experiment and correlating it with contrast effects (as had been done in earlier research), they directly manipulated whether people were aware of the primes by reminding some of the people of the priming phase of the experiment. Participants who were not reminded of the priming part of the experiment showed assimilation; reminded participants showed contrast in their judgments.

Comparing the Two Contrast Processes

We have been discussing two supposedly separate ways in which one's judgment of a person can be contrasted away from an accessible construct. One difference between the two processes concerns the types of accessible constructs that appear to trigger them. One process is triggered when accessible constructs are created by people being exposed to exemplars ("Hitler" and "Gandhi"), while the other process is triggered by people being blatantly exposed to (or reminded of) traits ("conceited" and "reckless"). Another difference is that one process is said to be fairly automatic and occurs essentially as part of perception, while the other is dependent on people becoming consciously aware of the accessible construct and making an attempt not to be influenced by it (and, in so doing, being influenced in the opposite manner). Finally, and perhaps least obvious, the two processes suggest that different judgments should be expected when primes are extreme versus moderate. The standard-of-comparison model predicts that extreme standards should lead to contrast. However, the correction model predicts that extreme primes should lead to less contrast (because people would be less likely to see something so extreme as a source of bias; it instead seems so different from the target behavior as to be irrelevant). These three differences between the models suggest that contrast effects truly are produced through at least two very different mechanisms.

Before any research on this issue had accumulated, Heider (1944) essentially described the standard-of-comparison and correction processes as two distinct ways through which contrast could be produced. Heider explicitly stated that a *perceptual* contrast effect, in the manner described by Gestalt psychology and social judgment research, may be produced in person perception through exemplars serving as standards of comparison:

> Contrast does not seem to occur as influence of act on person. The unit of origin and effect is a hierarchical unit: the origin is a superordinate part, the effect a subordinate one. Therefore, the effect can be seen with the origin as background and the latter can provide a standard according to which the meaning of the effect appears, but the reciprocal relation (origin with effect as background) is impossible. (p. 365)

To Heider, the origin of an effect (a person) provides a background against which the effect (the behavior and its consequences) is judged. People (exemplars) can be used to ascribe meaning to behaviors, since exemplars can assume the role of "ground" (in Gestalt terms) or a standard of comparison, against which the context of the action is determined and its meaning derived.

Heider (1944) also stated that an effect very similar to perceptual contrast can be produced even when exemplars are not being used: "[Behavior] can be evaluated in reference to an environmental 'press,' and thereby something like a contrast phenomenon can arise. If we perceive that a person stays moderately calm under extremely exciting circumstances we shall judge him as very quiet" (p. 368). By *environmental press*, Heider meant that one becomes aware of some biasing influence in one's environment that exerts pressure on the type of judgment one forms. Awareness of these pressures allows one to take those constraints into account when assigning meaning to the behavior. For example, a person who is observed crying at a funeral will not be seen as sad by disposition. The perceivers are aware of the sad context, and this will allow them to adjust their perception of the target to account for the influence of the contextual features. However, perceivers do not excel at this (hence the correspondence bias) and often make imprecise adjustments. For example, if the perceivers are made aware of a biasing influence (such as realizing that the sad context of a funeral will have an impact on the person behavior and should be accounted for when forming an impression of the person), Heider explains that *too much adjustment* may result. This would produce a judgment that takes the biasing influence too much into account. Rather than the person being seen as sad, the attempt to adjust for the influence makes the perceivers see the person as not a particularly sad person at all. This "something like a contrast" phenomenon is exactly what person perception researchers have labeled as a correction process.

Let us next examine the evidence in support of Heider's (1944) theorizing that contrast in person perception can be produced by two distinct cognitive processes. As reviewed above, the evidence has accumulated around the fact that there are three observed differences between the research on the correction process and that on the standard-of-comparison process. First, one process relies on exemplars as primes to produce contrast, the other on traits. Second, if a construct is being used as a standard of comparison then the more extreme the concept, the greater the resulting contrast should be. Thus, we can examine whether different processes are being used by examining whether extreme traits versus extreme exemplars both lead to more contrast. If not, it suggests they are not working via the same cognitive processes. Third, if correction processes are not used, then the process through which contrast is produced should not be the effortful and deliberate one described by the correction model, but the rather effortless and automatic one described by the standard-of-comparison model. That is, the correction process requires cognitive capacity and should be disabled by cognitive load; the standard-of-comparison process should not.

Traits versus Exemplars as Primes

What determines whether people use an accessible construct to assimilate new information or use it as a standard against which they can compare the new information? Perhaps quite accidentally, it turns out that all of the initial research providing evidence for contrast effects created a concept's heightened accessibility by using exemplars (e.g., "Hitler," "Gandhi," "Dracula," "Robin Hood," "shark," "tiger") as primes, while that in support of assimilation used traits (e.g., "daring," "reckless," "aloof," "conceited," "hostile") as primes. Thus it is quite possible that *whether assimilation or contrast occurs is dependent on the features of the accessible construct*.[2] It may depend on whether the accessibility of the concept is triggered by an exemplar (e.g., "Hitler") or a trait (e.g., "evil"). Exemplars and traits are different from each other in a variety of ways. Stapel and Koomen (2001) point out that they differ in terms of how distinctive they are, how abstract/narrow they are, and in how exclusive they are (there are many ways to be evil, but only one way to be Hitler). Stapel and colleagues (Stapel & Koomen, 1997, 1998, 2001; Stapel, Koomen, & van der Pligt, 1996, 1997) assert that the narrower, more exclusive, and more distinctive a primed category is, the more likely it is that contrast will occur. This is why extreme exemplars are so likely to lead to contrast—they possess all of these features. But Stapel and colleagues (1996) point out that traits—such as "evil," "hostile," "daring," and "rude"—possess none of these features. Traits, instead, are abstract concepts. This is why when traits are primed, they are used to draw the behavior of the person they describe inward and assimilate it.

This idea that the features of the prime dictate whether assimilation or contrast is the type of accessibility effect that results suggests that if a prime is made to be narrower, less abstract, and more exclusive, then contrast should be more likely to occur. In fact, Stapel and colleagues (1996) suggest that if a trait prime could be made less abstract and more distinctive, then it suddenly should lead to contrast rather than assimilation, even if the prime is subtle and not aware to the person. In support of this, they replicated the Moskowitz and Roman (1992) research, but added pictures to accompany the sentences. They hypothesized that the pictures would promote exemplars' being held in mind when participants were making judgments. The results showed that participants who were asked to memorize sentences, and who would therefore have traits passively primed, showed assimilation if no picture was provided (replicating the Moskowitz and Roman results). However, if a picture of the target was provided, a contrast effect was now found instead of assimilation. Stapel and colleagues explained this finding by saying that the picture encouraged participants to use an exemplar, and thus triggered the standard-of-comparison process. This seems a plausible account for promoting contrast where assimilation would otherwise occur by altering the features of the prime so it is more narrow, exclusive, and distinct.

Extremity of Primes and Contrast Effects

However, whether the prime is an exemplar or a trait is not the only feature of the prime that determines what type of processing is triggered. If that was the case, concepts triggered by inferring traits would never produce contrast effects, only assimilation. However, contrast effects via overcorrection for a prime's influence also occur— and this process is most likely to occur, as reviewed above, when one perceives a biasing influence on one's judgment. It has been further proposed that not simply whether the prime is an exemplar or a trait, but its *extremity*, can determine whether correction processes are initiated or not (Moskowitz & Skurnik, 1999). When a concept is triggered by a *moderate* trait prime (e.g., "troublesome"), contrast in judgment is more likely to result than when the concept is triggered by an *extreme* trait prime (e.g., "malevolent"). However, the opposite pattern emerges with exemplar primes: Increased extremity produces an even greater likelihood of contrast. The fact that extremity leads to different types of outcomes in judgment for different types of primes suggests that there may well be very different cognitive processes at play in producing each type of judgment. Let us explore this more closely.

Moderate primes, more so than extreme primes, will be seen as sharing some features with ambiguous target behaviors. A moderate prime, such as "troublesome," will be perceived as a more appropriate characterization of ambiguously hostile behavior (such as arguing with a store clerk) than an extreme prime, such as "malevolent." The consequence is that once one becomes aware of a prime's increased accessibility, moderate primes will be more likely to be seen as having potentially contaminated one's reaction to the target and less likely to be seen as irrelevant to the ambiguous behaviors of the target. The more likely the prime is to be seen as having contaminated one's reaction, the more one will adjust one's initial reaction to the target to correct for the prime's influence, and the more likely it is that one will remove part of one's genuine reaction. In essence, one plays out a process whereby one thinks, "I was just thinking about a hostile person; I better be careful not to let that influence me." The closer the prime words come to resembling the target's vaguely hostile behaviors (the less extreme the primes), the more likely that an influence will be deemed possible and contrast will emerge. For example, if one reasons, "I was just thinking about a malevolent person; I better be careful not to let that influence me," then no cause for concern is likely to emerge. Malevolence hardly seems applicable to the behavior observed, so becoming aware of the possibility for its influence does not make one likely to conclude that it actually did have an influence. One can discount the possibility that one was being biased and trust one's judgment. A more moderate prime is a more worthy contender for having an influence, and thus is more likely to trigger correction.

If you think back to the earlier review of the standard-of-comparison model of contrast, exactly the opposite prediction has been made there. It has been earlier asserted that extreme primes will be more likely than moderate primes to be perceived as occupying categories of behavior that are separate and distinct from ambiguous behaviors located along the same semantic dimension. The more extreme the prime being used as a standard of comparison is, the greater the perceived dissimilarity between the standard and the target, and the greater the contrast. In essence, one plays out a process whereby one thinks, "Relative to Hitler, this person isn't hostile." The more Hitleresque the exemplar, the greater the contrast. This pattern of contrast is suggestive of a standard-of-comparison process, because a target's behavior should fall outside the latitude of acceptance when evaluated against an extreme exemplar. This would result in seeing the target and the prime (standard) as sharing few features, and consequently in the target seeming unlike the standard.

One way to illustrate that contrast effects may occur through two different processes is to simultaneously manipulate prime type (exemplar vs. trait) and prime extremity (moderate vs. extreme). If there are two different processes involved, judgments should be influenced differently when people have previously seen extreme versus moderate traits versus exemplars. This is precisely what we (Moskowitz & Skurnik, 1999) did. We primed concepts by exposing research participants to either extreme traits (e.g., "malicious," "malevolent"), moderate traits (e.g., "unfair," "troublesome"), extreme exemplars (e.g., "Mike Tyson," "Dracula"), or moderate exemplars (e.g., "Bart Simpson," "Kurt Cobain") relevant to the concept "hostility." We then had participants read about a person acting in an ambiguously hostile manner. We found that extreme exemplars were more likely to produce contrast effects than moderate exemplars. Yet a different pattern of findings emerged for trait primes: When traits were used as primes, greater contrast was seen with moderate rather than extreme primes. We (Moskowitz & Skurnik, 1999) concluded that these findings tease apart the different processes that produce contrast. The fact that extreme but not moderate exemplars yielded contrast suggests that a standard-of-comparison process was being used: The more extreme the standard relative to the judgment target, the more distinct it was, and the more likely it was that contrast would be produced. The finding that moderate but not extreme traits yielded contrast suggests that a correction process was used: The more extreme the prime, the less the prime–target feature overlap was, and the less likely it was that one would suspect an influence of the prime for which one needed to correct.

Cognitive Load and Contrast Effects

Stapel and colleagues (1996) state that contrast is "mediated by the *automatic* and *unconscious* use of contextually induced norms or anchors" (p. 439; emphasis in original). This is a perceptual phenomenon in which the perceptual system passively uses the context in which a stimulus is observed to assign meaning to it unconsciously. However, it has been asserted earlier that contrast may also be produced through the more effortful process of correction, in which judgment is adjusted in the light of a perceived bias. If the correction process produces contrast effects, this process should be dependent on having the *motivation* and *ability* to engage in correction. One way to test whether exemplars and traits trigger separate processing mechanisms responsible for contrast effects is to limit one's cognitive resources. If contrast effects persist, it suggests that the process is fairly automatic; if they do not, it suggests that the process is effortful. We (Moskowitz & Skurnik, 1999) did precisely this by priming concepts through exposing participants to either trait primes ("malicious," "malevolent," "unfair," "troublesome") or exemplar primes ("Bart Simpson," "Kurt Cobain," "Mike Tyson," "Dracula") and having them then read about a person acting in an ambiguously hostile manner. However, participants were placed under cognitive load prior to making their judgments. It was expected that the load would eliminate the ability to engage in the correction process. We found that trait primes did not lead to contrast effects under these conditions. This finding reveals that participants under cognitive load did not have the cognitive resources (ability) to engage in correction processes. However, exemplar primes did lead to contrast effects, despite the cognitive load. Exemplar primes could only lead to contrast effects under conditions of cognitive load if such a process is an efficient and effortless aspect of perceiving and categorizing behavior. These findings reveal that exemplars and traits are priming concepts, but that the manners in which these concepts are used to guide judgment are drastically different.

METACOGNITION

The research reviewed in this chapter is aptly summarized in Higgins's (1998) *aboutness principle*, which asserts that one seldom sees an outcome as if it "just occurs," but rather as being *about* something. The feeling that a concept has heightened accessibility, even if it is an implicit feeling, triggers attempts to figure out what the cause for that state is—what it is about. In this sense, priming effects are simply a case of misattributing, to a target, a perceptual readiness that should have been attributed to the *actual source* of the concept's increased accessibility. Essentially, research participants have information (in this case, traits or exemplars) accessible because the concepts have been exposed to them as part of an experiment. Yet these people misattribute the accessibility of the information to some other person (Donald) and assume that the source of the accessibility must be the other person's behavior (e.g., Li & Moskowitz, 2004a). The aboutness principle, and priming effects more generally, arise because people are thinking about why their cognition has given them a feeling/sensation that a particular concept has *fluency*—it feels available or perceptually ready (e.g., Jacoby, Kelley, Brown, & Jasechko, 1989).

We all can readily recognize that we think about our own cognition and thoughts, as well as assign meaning to the cognitive sensations we experience due to this self-reflection. We may feel dejected and say to ourselves, "I wonder why I feel so blue?" We may be trying to remember where the car keys are, and we think about what we were thinking when we put the keys away, to try to help us remember where we may have put them. There are dozens of examples we could generate of thinking about our thinking. In the example just provided, we have a cognitive sensation we consciously recognize (feeling "blue"), and this triggers cognition aimed at understanding the sensation. The act of thinking about thinking, or cognition about cognition, has been called *metacognition* (e.g., Flavell, 1979). Sometimes we have theories about our own cognition, such as "The reason I feel blue is that the weather is bad" (using a theory that grey skies make us blue). A theory about our mental states is one form of metacognition.

However, many of our cognitive processes occur implicitly. Does this mean we have no theories about them (because we are not aware they have occurred)? It is argued here that this is not the case; we also use theories to make sense of events we do not consciously detect. What is being proposed is that we perceivers use implicit theories about what it means to have implicit cognitive processes—theories about the meaning of our own implicit cognition. Priming effects, in this way, are a type of metacognition. They are our deployments of a theory that some other person's behavior is the cause for our own sensation of a particular concept as fluent. The rationale behind this argument is as follows: (1) Implicit cognitive processes happen all the time; (2) the output of these processes may be experienced as "sensations"; (3) we use sensations to make judgments; and (4) the judgments are based on the meaning assigned to these sensations via theories we hold about the meaning of the sensation. But the sensations are not really conscious to us; the processes producing the sensations are not aware to us; and the theories we use to make sense of the sensations are also used without our recognizing that we are applying theories (or knowing that we have theories about the sensation). Let us review a few examples to illustrate that the process of unconsciously theorizing about (undetected) mental sensations is one we use all the time.

The Availability Heuristic

The fact that introspection and thinking about one's thought processes may take place outside of conscious awareness is perhaps best evidenced by a phenomenon we have already discussed—the availability heuristic (e.g., Schwarz, Bless, et al., 1991; Tversky & Kahneman, 1973). As reviewed in Chapter 3, Schwarz, Bless, and colleagues (1991) demonstrated that the ease with which one can retrieve relevant examples about one's own behavior, rather than the absolute number of examples generated, is what determines how strongly one believes the behavior (and trait) in question characterizes the self. Participants asked to generate six instances of assertive behavior rated themselves as more assertive than participants who generated double that number of examples (12) of their own assertive behavior. This would sound odd if it was not also revealed that generating six instances of a behavior is considerably easier than the difficult task of trying to come up with 12 examples of one's behavior in a domain such as assertiveness.

Such data suggest that when people estimate the frequency or recency of events, they do so in part by considering the ease with which examples of the events come to mind. This information is used separately from any aspect of the content of the examples. In other words, people use the sensations associated with thinking (such as the ease of retrieval of examples from memory) as a guide for making judgments, apparently without awareness of using this information. The sensation of ease that accompanies retrieval of events is taken as a sign of the frequency or recency of the events themselves. In essence, the availability heuristic is a phenomenon whereby the experience of thinking qualifies the content of thinking.

Feelings of Familiarity

What does it mean to say that something feels familiar? What is this cognitive sensation? Jacoby and Whitehouse (1989) argue that the feeling that information is familiar derives from an attribution associated with the sensation of increased *fluency*. By calling the feeling of familiarity an attribution about the meaning of fluency, they are asserting that when information easily comes to mind, we humans experience this sensation and need to account for it. When asking (preconsciously) "Why has this sensation been detected?", one attribution that we make to account for this sensation is that the information is familiar. It comes to mind easily because it is something we have encountered before. Thus we use an implicit theory about the meaning of fluency, and this implicit theory delivers to us a feeling of familiarity.

How can such a metacognitive explanation of familiarity—that it represents an attribution for experiencing the sensation of fluency—be tested? Jacoby and Whitehouse (1989, Study 2) developed an extremely clever paradigm. Research participants were asked to study a list of words for a memory test that would occur later. When the test eventually occurred, it contained a list of words, some of which were new and some of which were from the studied list. The memory test simply asked participants to distinguish old words (those from the study list) from the new words not previously seen. However, there was one catch: During the test, each test word was preceded by a "context word." Thus, before participants saw the word for which they had to make the "new versus old" decision, another word appeared. In some cases, the context word was the very same word as the one appearing after it (the test word). In effect, just before deciding whether a word was either old or new, participants sometimes were presented with that exact word as a context word. This was done in order to create a potential reason for why a word might seem familiar. A word might seem familiar because it was on the original list and participants just could not recollect actually having seen it (leaving them with just the feeling of familiarity). However, the word might seem familiar not because it was on the original list, but because the participants had just seen it as a context word. If they had just seen the word as a context word, they would have a good theory about why they felt it looked familiar: It was familiar because the experimenter had just flashed it at them. If they had not just seen it as a context word, then how could they make sense of the fact that the word felt familiar? They could attribute it to the fact that they must have seen it earlier.

The experiment had one more twist that was essential for illustrating that attributions were being made for the feeling of familiarity. Half of the time, the context word was flashed so that it could clearly be consciously recognized. However, half of the time the word was flashed subliminally. This created the critical scenario. There were times where a new word was being presented as the test word, and this word was either just flashed subliminally or just flashed so that it was clearly seen. In each case, participants should be left with a sense of perceptual fluency relating to this new word. In the case where the word was clearly/consciously presented, the reason for this fluency would be obvious: Participants had just seen it. In the subliminal case, the reason for the fluency would not be clear, and this sensation would need to be defined. Thus a good test of whether or not people were making attributions about the feeling of familiarity was now available. The researches could look to see whether participants were more likely to call a "new" word "old" when the very same word had just been subliminally flashed (relative to when they called a "new" word "old" when it was preceded by the subliminal presentation of some other, nonmatching word). Attributing the fluency for a matching word to the fact that the word was previously seen would perfectly explain the fluency. Participants simply would mistakenly attribute the fact that they had seen the word before to the fact that it was on the study list, rather than to the fact that it had just been subliminally flashed (as they were not aware of this fact). This type of error should not occur for cases where the context word was presented so that it could be consciously detected. Jacoby and Whitehouse (1989) found precisely this pattern of data. Participants in the subliminal-context-word condition were more likely to mistakenly judge a new test item "old" if it had been preceded by a matching context word than if the context word had not matched the test word.

In this case, an experiential aspect of thinking—fluency of processing—was mistakenly attributed to prior presentation on the original study list. In essence, these people were thinking (making an attribution regarding the items' familiarity) about their thought processes (the experience of perceptual fluency), making this an implicit form of metacognition (as people were not aware of either of these steps). As a further example, in one experiment, participants received a list to study for a later memory task (Whittlesea & Williams, 2000). The list consisted of words, nonwords that were dissimilar to real words, and nonwords with word-like phonetic and orthographic features. During the recognition test, when participants had to pick out old items from a list that contained both old and new items, they were more likely to falsely claim that nonwords that seemed like real words were familiar (i.e., were in the study list). The moral from this research is that unexplained fluency induces a process aimed at explaining the fluency—that is, at linking it to a plausible event from which it originated (see also Whittlesea & Williams, 2001).

The False-Fame Effect

Feelings of familiarity are common in person perception. Often a person just seems familiar. The fluency that gives rise to the feeling of familiarity can come from people's having seen a person in the past and later failing to recall that they saw the person. Despite lacking any explicit memory, they have a feeling that the person is familiar (implicit memory). Jacoby, Woloshyn, and Kelley (1989) posited that when people experience this sense of familiarity, they attempt to attribute it to something. They ask themselves, "This person feels familiar to me. Why?" That is, if they do not explicitly recall having ever seen a particular name before, or met a person with that name before, the reason it feels familiar must be that they know the name for another reason. One explanation would be that the person is of some fame. Jacoby and colleagues found that research participants made this type of error. People who had actually seen a name earlier in the experiment, but had no memory of this, assumed a name that felt familiar to them was the name of a famous person. The researchers called this the *false-fame effect*, and it is a misattribution of the feeling of familiarity.

Banaji and Greenwald (1995) posited that if this effect represents an incorrect inference about the meaning of familiarity, then other factors that determine people's inferences about why someone might be familiar would have an impact on the false-fame effect. They argued that stereotypes about women would make it less likely for people to assume that a woman is famous. If people have the stereotype that women are unlikely to be important enough to attain fame, then feelings of familiarity associated with a female name would be less likely to be attributed to the fame of the person relative to when it is a man whose name feels familiar. The results showed both the basic false-fame effect and the gender effect in false fame. That is, the meaning of familiarity/fluency was different when participants had stereotypic expectancies that affected how that fluency was attributed.

The Illusion of Truth

We have just reviewed a phenomenon whereby people label perceptually fluent information as familiar and then try to make an attribution about why it feels familiar. We now turn toward examining the tendency people have to say that things that feel familiar are true. This occurs even if those things actually are false, and even can occur when people were explicitly told at one point in time that this information was false. Later they remember it to have been true if it feels familiar (e.g., Begg, Anas, & Farinacci, 1992; Begg, Armour, and & Kerr, 1985). Begg and colleagues called this inclination to see familiar things as "true" the *illusion of truth*. Begg and colleagues (1992) point out people rely on two independent types of information when deciding whether a statement is true. First, they may recall the statement clearly and accurately report whether the information is true or false. Second, they may use a feeling of familiarity; statements that feel familiar will seem true. The illusion of truth arises when explicit recall for information is poor, but the inability to remember the details does not affect the familiarity of the information. Hence, all people are left with is the feeling that the information is familiar (without remembering why or how, etc.). Skurnik, Moskowitz, and Johnson (2004) proposed that at this point perceivers use metacognition. The sensation of familiarity is responded to by the use of a theory about the meaning of familiarity. That is, the illusion of truth occurs because people have a theory about the meaning of the sensation of familiarity, which specifies that the sensation of familiarity is an indicator that the thing being said is true.

Why should people have a theory that familiarity indicates truth? Grice (1975) suggested that this is the case in discussing the conventions of communication (see "the maxim of quality" reviewed in Chapter 3). These conventions inform people that if something is said to them or something feels familiar to them (and therefore was said to them in the past), it is likely to be true, since communicators typically are trying to convey accurate and truthful information to one another. Gilbert, Krull, and Malone (1990, p. 605; emphasis in original) stated this quite well:

> Societies place a premium on candor, and it seems likely that the majority of information that people encounter, assess, and remember is, in fact, true. Thus, it may be that people generalize from ordinary experience and consciously *assume* that all ideas are true unless otherwise noted. In other words, the initial belief in the truthfulness of information may be a flexible, heuristic assumption.

There are many illustrations of the illusion of truth. Hasher, Goldstein, and Toppino (1977) asked research participants to study a list of unfamiliar trivia statements, some true and some not (e.g., "Zachary Taylor was the first U.S. President to die in office"). Two weeks later they returned to rate the probable truth of some new statements, as well as of some statements that were on the original list. The researchers found that the statements that participants had already seen (2 weeks earlier) were more likely to be rated true than new statements. This would hardly be an illusion if it turned out that all those statements they guessed were true were in fact true. However, people have the tendency to label familiar information that was explicitly labeled as false as being true! For example, Begg and colleagues (1992) had participants study trivia statements that were labeled true or false. Later, they were asked to rate a list of statements as true or false. The items on this second list were a mix of new items (not seen before) and items from the old list, some of which were previously indicated to be true, and some of which were previously indicated to be false. They found that participants were more likely to rate statements originally labeled false as true than they were to rate new and unfamiliar statements as true. The illusion of truth even applies to information that does not relate to prior knowledge. For example, Gilbert and colleagues (1990) found similar results when research participants were asked to learn "new" words from a (fictional) foreign language.

Mood as Information

How do people ascertain their affective reactions to people and events? According to Schwarz and Clore (1988), people may rely on their current mood in answering questions of the sort "How do I feel about _____?" For instance, people are usually in a better mood on sunny days, and in gloomy moods on overcast days. Remarkably, they found that people report higher life satisfaction on sunny than on cloudy days. This is more than people thinking, "I'm in a good mood; life is good." The effect we are talking about here is something quite distinct from people consciously reflecting on their moods in making a judgment. It is an unconscious use of an accessible mood state to evaluate something, including something as important as overall life satisfaction (see below). Often people are unable or unwilling to calculate a comprehensive answer to a complicated judgment question. This does not mean that they do not have a response to such a question. Instead, they may turn to their current mood state for an answer, assuming that they can use their mood as information reflecting their reaction to the object of judgment. Schwarz and Clore suggest that people use a "How do I feel about it?" heuristic by relying on their current mood state as a source of information. In a sense, the mood state is taken as the result of an assessment process that never actually took place. The mind notices its own affective tone and uses this information to guide other problem-solving activities. Therefore, people are using their feelings as information.

For example, Schwarz and Clore (1983) asked people how happy and satisfied they were with their lives on either especially sunny or rainy days. The result was that people reported greater life satisfaction on sunny days! They thought they were happier people in life when it just happened to be sunny out at that moment. The data also revealed that "sunny-day people" were in a better mood than "rainy-day people," suggesting that their mood was driving the difference in their responses. An even more striking aspect of this study was that the pattern of reported life satisfaction was reversed when people were first asked an incidental question about the weather that day, with sunny-day people then reporting lower life satisfaction than rainy-day people. Schwarz and Clore suggested that for complex and ill-defined judgments, such as assessing how satisfied people are with their lives, people use a theory telling them that their feelings or mood can be used as reliable information about their cognition. However, if people believe that the mood state has a different source (other than that resulting from their cognitive processing)—such as the weather—then the mood loses its informational value.

In summary, this section reveals that the theories we use to understand and categorize behavior are based not only upon the content that is accessible, but also on the subjective quality of mental experience. The claim is that *the experience of cognition (as opposed to the content of cognition)* serves as an input to judgment processes by being assigned a meaning from our implicit theory about the sensation. Metacognition (in this case, implicitly theorizing about the meaning of an implicit cognitive sensation) determines how we think and react to a person. Accessibility effects are a specific example of this type of metacognition.

CODA

Simple acts of identifying things—such as "What type of behavior did she just display—playful or aggressive?" or "What type of object is in that guy's hand—a gun or a wallet?") can be determined by what one is ready to see. However, accessible information does not always have an impact. The behavior being judged must be somewhat ambiguous and open to interpretation. The accessible constructs must be relevant to the judgment context. When accessible constructs do exert an influence, the type of influence exerted depends on a variety of factors. These include the features of the prime (whether it is an exemplar or a trait, whether it is extreme or moderate); the awareness one has of the prime's state of heightened accessibility or of its potential influence; and on the type of processing strategy in which the accessible construct gets used (it may be used as a standard of comparison, or it may be used as an interpretive frame that triggers the "set–reset" process). Thus contextual factors, such as the manner in which a construct is primed, affect the processes through which judgments are produced. The nature of assimilation and contrast effects is dependent on not merely what is activated, but how it is activated—even on relatively small variations in the information conveyed by a prime.

From this review, what can we conclude about the subliminal message in the anti-Gore political campaign commercial run by the Bush camp in 2000? "RATS" can be seen either as an exemplar of a hated animal or as a trait that means "sleazy." If the subliminal presentation of the word "RATS" triggered the concept of the animal, then we might expect absolutely no influence whatsoever. Animals are not relevant standards of comparison for judging people. However, if the subliminal message triggered the trait, then an influence might be seen. Since people were not aware of the prime's increased accessibility, we would expect the target (Gore) to be potentially assimilated into the primed trait. A relevant and ambiguous target would be seen as more sleazy due to the subliminal prime than if the prime had not existed. An irrelevant or unambiguous target would not be influenced by the prime. Thus, if a person did not have a firm opinion of Al Gore (Gore was ambiguous), and if Gore's behavior was ambiguously sleazy/opportunistic (it was relevant to the prime), then priming people with the word "RATS," and then presenting people with an image of Al Gore and asking them to form an opinion of him, should have caused those people without firm opinions (the undecided voters such campaign commercials are designed to influence) to form a negative opinion of Gore. Based on our existing knowledge, we would have to conclude that this campaign trick may have worked, but for a limited number of perceivers.

Although attempting to influence people without them knowing it may seem bad enough, sometimes the use of accessible constructs has worse—even tragic—consequences. For example, police officers may have notions of danger and threat accessible while walking the beat. This may make even the best-intentioned officers perceptually ready to see a threat in an ambiguous situation. One can only imagine what an officer who does not have the best intentions, and who harbors stereotypes toward particular groups, is perceptually ready to see. Consider the tragic tale of Amadou Diallo, a Black man shot dead in New York City when White police officers incorrectly identified an object Diallo was reaching for as a gun. It was, instead, a wallet. The officers, perhaps perceptually ready to see danger, interpreted Diallo's action as one that should prompt them to open fire on what turned out to be an unarmed man. The use of stereotypes that are perceptually ready is a dominant theme of the next chapter. However, it should be noted that most of the time, accessible constructs are used appropriately to help us make sense of the world. Their evolution in everyday psychology is most likely linked to their functionalism; they work, so we use them. If they repeatedly led to tragedy, we would not be so dependent on this process.

NOTES

1. Bargh, Bond, Lombardi, and Tota (1986) point out that temporary and chronic sources of accessibility can be present at the same time. The two separate influences can be antagonistic to each other (such as when one's chronically accessible construct is kindness, and one's tem-

porarily accessible construct is manipulativeness), or they can facilitate each other. Bargh and colleagues posit that when two constructs facilitate each other, the effects are additive, such that a chronically accessible construct can have its level of excitation (or the strength of its accessibility) heightened by an encounter with a stimulus that makes the same concept temporarily accessible. Thus the degree of accessibility, or the charge associated with a concept, is not determined solely by what has recently been encountered, but by what is chronically accessible, and the interaction of recent and frequent (chronic) sources of accessibility.

2. It is known from research in cognitive psychology that varying what features of a prime word are attended to can attenuate or eliminate semantic priming effects. Priming effects do not emerge when the priming task involves paying attention to specific letters within the prime words (Friedrich, Henik, & Tzelgov, 1991) or counting the number of syllables in the prime words (Parkin, 1979).

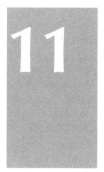

Stereotypes
and Expectancies

Most of us think of stereotyping and prejudice as the problem of select groups of "racists," "homophobes," "sexists," and so forth. In our everyday, naive understanding of the concept, stereotypes are negative and harmful, and the people who rely on them are seen as hateful and ignorant. We all recognize the probability that at some time we ourselves fall prey to using stereotypes, but most of us hold idealistic (almost egalitarian) views of ourselves that allow for these minor lapses to our otherwise fair-minded and tolerant treatment of others. The problem that we as individuals feel that stereotyping poses for society is felt to lie in others, and in the negative beliefs and attitudes those others harbor. Our own minor lapses hardly pose a threat to the social order. The fascists, authoritarians, and racists of the world are responsible for the unfair treatment experienced by so many.

However, how minor are our lapses into stereotyping as typical "egalitarian" persons? To what extent do those of us who would not identify ourselves as racists employ stereotypic views, beliefs, and attitudes in evaluating others? And to the extent that stereotyping may be far more common than we expect, must we define stereotypes as inherently negative, and the use of stereotypes as born of ignorance and hatefulness? Many of our common-sense and naive assumptions about the prevalence of stereotyping in ourselves and in our fair-minded friends are simply incorrect. E. E. Jones (1990) asserted that *stereotypes* are just expectancies that we hold about a category. Expectancies can range from specific information we know about (or think we know about) an individual, based on prior experience or hearsay about that individual, to more general types of information associated with the group or category to which that individual belongs. Stereotypes can be construed as category-based expectancies that we have learned from our own personal experiences and/or various socializing agents within the culture (parents, teachers, religion, friends, the Internet, TV, etc.). According to Jones, we have expectancies about every person with whom we interact; therefore, no observation, inference, or interaction is free from the influence of the expectancies that we bring to the person perception process. This makes stereotyping a far more common component of everyday thought than many of us would like to admit. In fact, our use of expectancies and stereotypes may be so routine that it comes to operate outside of awareness.

In this chapter, the everyday, mundane nature of stereotyping as part of the cognitive process is reviewed. The chapter examines how, as accessible constructs, stereotypes and expectancies influence social cognition from the earliest, preconscious stages of characterization and categorization to the more deliberate and effortful stages of impression formation where we are attempting to form accurate impressions and make important decisions about others (such as when we, as jurors, employers, teachers, friends, and lovers, are judging and evaluating others). Although obviously there are types of people who are motivated to hate others (especially to hate select groups of others who belong to minority groups), an analysis of these hateful persons will be left for another day and a different book (e.g., Adorno, Frenkel-Brunswik, Levinson, & Sanford, 1950; Allport, 1954; J. M. Jones, 1997; Sidanius & Pratto, 1999). The concern here is with an everyday type of stereotyping that we all practice and that goes unrecognized. This is not always negative, and it can be functional. But it is nonetheless stereotyping.

THE INVISIBLE NATURE OF STEREOTYPES AND EXPECTANCIES

We all have beliefs about the individuals and groups of individuals with whom we interact. Even a stranger is identified as belonging to a particular gender or racial group, and beliefs associated with that group will rush to mind (e.g., a man may be more likely to shake hands with another man, or to establish a particular type of personal distance, based on his beliefs about gender). These beliefs are derived from prior experience. The experiences on which we draw to provide these beliefs include things others have told us about the individual/group in question, inferences drawn based on what those others have said, and actual (at times limited) personal interactions at some point in the past with people from the group in question. The information gathered from these experiences provides for us *expectancies*—a set of probable actions and attitudes we can anticipate in others. Olson, Roese, and Zanna (1996, p. 211) defined expectancies as "beliefs about a future state of affairs"—beliefs drawn from past experience about the probability that some set of future events will come to pass. This bridge from the past to the future is what makes expectancies so central to everyday interaction.

Expectancies about groups of people can be defined as our beliefs about the probability that particular traits, features, characteristics, opinions, and behaviors will be observed in those people at some point during our (or someone else's) future interaction with them. In essence, *stereotypes* are expectancies about a social group, and about the extent to which the group's probable behaviors, features, and traits can be generalized from the group to individual members of the group. The term *stereotype* was first used in the social sciences by the journalist Walter Lippmann in his 1922 book *Public Opinion*, where he likened stereotypes to pictures in the head—images of how the world should be, which then serve to structure and guide how we actually come to see the world. Lippmann assumed that "reality" is highly complex, and that stereotypes serve a function of simplifying thought and perception to deliver meaning.

This is the perfect stereotype. Its hallmark is that it precedes the use of reason; is a form of perception, imposes a certain character on the data of our senses before the data reach the intelligence. (1922, p. 65)

In the great blooming, buzzing confusion of the outer world we pick out that what our culture has already defined for us, and we tend to perceive that which we have picked out in the form stereotyped for us by our culture. (1922, p. 55)

In this sense, Lippmann's use of the term *stereotype* is essentially equivalent to what we have earlier defined as a *schema*, except that it is a schema about a group of people. As Allport (1954) defined it, a stereotype is a set of beliefs about the personal attributes of a group that can structure the way we think about this group. It is a list or picture in our heads of the behaviors, characteristics, and traits that our culture has taught us a particular social group is likely to possess; it allows us to categorize and make predictions about the members of that category when forming impressions. If there seems to be a recurring emphasis on the functional role categories and schemas play in delivering meaning, and on the pragmatics of having such meaning for preparing behavior, keep in mind that Peirce, James, Lippmann, Bruner, Allport, and E. E. Jones share not only this functional/pragmatic approach to the use of categories, but an intellectual history as well. All these men were affiliated with Harvard University within 70 years of each other (and keeping in that tradition, Jones's former student, Dan Gilbert, moved to Harvard in the late 1990s).

Because expectancies and stereotypes are probabilities that we will see characteristics and behaviors when observing and interacting with others, these characteristics as represented in a stereotype may range from being 100% true to 100% false. A stereotype perhaps starts from a "kernel of truth" (Allport, 1954), so that a category begins being formulated on the basis of some experience; from this basis, the category widens and grows. The manner in which it builds, however, can be more or less rational, so it is filled with more or less accurate information. Ultimately, their accuracy does not matter to the definition; all that matters is that they represent (often socially shared) knowledge about that group, which we implement in action and judgment without much (if any) conscious reflection. Even expectancies that we hold with 100% certainty and that we automatically implement may turn out to be false in reality. In the realm of interacting with objects, an example of this is seen when we go to sit down on a chair. We expect that the object will support our weight; yet we do not engage in a conscious analysis of the structure of the chair, or in conscious generation of these expectancies. The expectancy is triggered unconsciously by the mere perception of the object. Any person who has ever had a chair collapse under him/her can attest to the fact that even probabilities we think are 100% certain need not be. As we have seen with the definition of schemas offered in Chapter 4, the characteristics and presumed behaviors that constitute an expectancy need not be perfectly accurate; still, the expectancy is functional all the same and is used to guide behavior, even if we do not realize it. Inaccurate, frequently used stereotypes (especially when use is unconscious) are what most people find troubling.

Stereotyping as a Functional Cognitive Process

The discussion thus far poses an interesting and important set of questions: What if stereotypes operate like any other pieces of information stored in our memory? What if stereotypes are simply collections of beliefs about, and behaviors expected to be performed by, members of social groups that we have learned from the culture and stored in memory? Simply knowing a stereotype, *regardless of whether we believe it to be true*, would then be sufficient for the stereotype to be triggered when we encounter a member of a stereotyped group. Just as our schema for eating in a fast-food restaurant would be triggered by entering a McDonalds', and just as our concept of "hostility" would be triggered by exposure to a fierce animal (or simply the word "hostile"), stereotypes that we have learned—even ones we have rejected as not very useful for describing individual people—could be triggered by a meeting with a member of a stereotyped group (Devine, 1989). If this knowledge stored in memory operates like any other knowledge stored in memory, the triggering of the concept should lead to spreading activation, so that a host of beliefs and expectancies associated with the stereotype should be triggered. A consequence of this should be that this wealth of information is now perceptually ready for making sense of and understanding the behavior of a person with whom we are interacting even though we consciously reject the stereotype.

In essence, when we encounter people, their group membership or memberships are often clearly marked by physical features that we cannot help detecting as part of basic and preconscious perceptual processes. Some physical features, such as gender and race, may be particularly likely to capture attention and be used to categorize people. Taylor, Fiske, Etcoff, and Ruderman (1978, p. 779) have offered an explanation as to why some characteristics are more likely to be used in categorizing another person:

> The main function of categorization is to reduce the complex object world to a more simple and manageable structure. . . . [People] may select salient social or physical dimensions to use as discriminating variables for grouping and managing person information. If this is true, certain variables such as race or sex would be likely candidates for such categories, since they are physically salient as well as useful social discriminators.

The stages of categorization and inference that proceed outside of awareness, and present to our conscious mind a world that is recognizable, coherent, and meaningful, come to rely on tried-and-true, salient, socially meaningful categories for classifying people. These categories are triggered, as discussed earlier, by features of the person being perceived (skin color, gender, attire, etc.). Therefore, even if we are not explicitly attempting to categorize a person, each person we meet is quickly and quietly placed into some primitive and broad "boxes": That is a woman, he is a man with Black skin, she is wearing a sari, his turban informs us he is a Sikh, and so forth. Once we have placed the person in a box, an inescapable part of this categorization process is the heightened accessibility of all the information in that box, including that which we have learned but rejected.

With categorization comes all the functions of a category, as reviewed in Chapter 3. First, it saves us from needing to figure out what a stimulus is that has a particular pattern of features (and from calculating what we can expect from it) each time we encounter it. Second, every person we categorize receives meaning from the class of things to which it has been assigned. That is, the category tells us what features we can expect that have not yet been exhibited, and allows us to know things about the person we have not yet seen in our own experience with this particular instance of the category. Attaining this meaning leads naturally to a third function of categorization: It allows us to make predictions about what to expect when interacting with the person. Once armed with expectancies and predictions concerning the people and things that cross our path, the next function of categorization is (let's hope) obvious: The act of categori-zation allows us to plan our behavior—to engage in what we feel are appropriate behav-iors that will bring about an expected consequence. As Allport (1954, pp. 20–21) stated, a stereotype "forms large classes and clusters for guiding our daily adjustments." As we shall see in Chapter 13, often we use expectancies to act in what we deem to be an appropriate way, rather than allowing the behavior of the person we are interacting with to determine our behavior. We may act rude to someone we expect to be hostile, with the expectancy (rather than any hostile behavior on the other person's part) being the cause of our action.

If we conceive of stereotypes in this manner, then stereotyping is no longer limited to the domain of hateful and ignorant persons. Rather, for each of us, stereotypes are constantly triggered and potentially bias our interactions with others. Our use of stereo-types, like our use of schemas, is a functional response to our simply being unable to process each individual as a complex and unique stimulus. We need help making sense of the world of other people, and we use these mental representations to fill in the gaps in a way that is ideally functional and accurate (or at least "good enough"). Granted, this bias is less severe than the hate that is often observed in highly prejudiced persons. But it is a prevalent and endemic bias nonetheless, and one that can allow social prob-lems to arise when our overgeneralizations are inaccurately and unknowingly applied to individuals.

Implicit Stereotyping

The functional nature of stereotypes reveals to us that, as Crosby, Bromley, and Saxe (1980) put it, we are far more likely to use them than we are apt to admit. This is not solely because we seek to hide the fact that we frequently use stereotypes from others (out of shame). In addition, we frequently use stereotypes and hide this fact from our-selves! Because of the unintended nature of stereotype activation and use, stereotyping often proceeds without our awareness, biasing us in ways we would never suspect and may vehemently deny. This is a denial born of ignorance, not shame. The use of stereo-types outside of awareness and without conscious intent is known as *implicit stereotyping*, and opens us up to the possibility of a more subtle form of bias than we typically con-strue when contemplating stereotyping.

Measuring/Assessing Implicit Stereotypes

One obvious problem in trying to measure/assess people's stereotypes is that people are concerned about what others think of them. Thus they offer opinions and beliefs in public that do not reflect their private beliefs. This is a problem of *reactivity*, where the obviousness of what is being measured makes people respond in a way inconsistent with their natural reactions and private beliefs. Knowing that they are being observed, such as when expressing opinions in public, can lead people to be overly concerned with how they present themselves to the individuals doing the observing. This allows them to cater to others in their views, promotes being accepted and liked by others, and protects self-esteem from the threat of being rejected or from holding unpopular views. In this way, stereotyping is a form of conformity. (However, some research suggests that people are more likely to express their private beliefs when asked about them publicly as opposed to privately—what McGuire [1964] called *bolstering*—especially if expressing ste-reotypes. See Lambert, Cronen, Chasteen, & Lickel, 1996.)

Self-presentation concerns can affect the expression of stereotypic beliefs in two opposing ways. In the first way, as discussed by Katz and Braly (1933), people may privately not agree with the stereotype, but may publicly express a belief in the stereotype so that they are seen as agreeing with their group. People often perceive that their group is more extreme than they themselves actually are. We have seen this in Chapter 1 when discussing the research of Robinson, Keltner, Ward, and Ross (1995). This perceived extremity of opinion from the group may serve as a pressure that causes people to express consenting views—they state publicly a view that is more stereotypic than what they privately believe. In the second way public and private beliefs may differ; people may believe in the stereotype privately, but may be unwilling to express this publicly. They may worry that expressing the stereotype may reveal some fact about their own biases that they are unwilling to admit to others. In this instance, the individuals are once again conforming to some expectation about the public view, but the altered belief is in the direction opposite to that described above—less stereotyping is being evidenced in public, rather than more.

However, the notion of common, everyday stereotyping of which people are unaware creates a separate problem for assessing people's stereotypes and for examining how those stereotypes bias them. How can researchers measure something people are concealing not simply from others, but from themselves? There are two broad reasons why people conceal private beliefs even from themselves (creating a divergence between what they say publicly and how they truly feel). The first is that they can't handle the truth—they do not want to face their own biases, so they repress and deny them. This may be especially true for people with a desire to be low in prejudice (what Dovidio & Gaertner, 1986, called *aversive racism*). This desire to avoid stereotypes may lead people to need to prove to themselves that they are not prejudiced. One way for them to do this is to exaggerate both their own sense of themselves as unprejudiced and their beliefs about the cultural stereotype (so that their own views seem positive in comparison). The second reason is that they don't know the truth—they have unconscious biases that lead them to distort what they express without even realizing it is a distortion.

A way to resolve the problem of measuring stereotyping—one that circumvents the fact that people may not be able to consciously access their true beliefs—is to use measures that do not explicitly address stereotyping. An *implicit measure* is one that taps a psychological event in a manner that conceals the true nature of what is being measured from the persons being tested (or taps reactions that people are unable to consciously control even if they were aware of what the measurement was tapping). Chapters 9 and 10 have already presented two examples of implicit measures in discussing priming effects. One involved asking people to form judgments about a person named Donald, without their realizing that their reactions to Donald allowed researchers to detect bias (e.g., Higgins, Rholes, & Jones, 1977). Even though explicitly asked for impressions of Donald, people did not explicitly recognize a link between their judgments and the factors that could be biasing those judgments. A second example involved processes of spreading activation, and the assumption that if some information has been triggered in memory, other information associated with it will be triggered as well, making people faster to respond to this information (e.g., Neely, 1977). Although people were explicitly asked to think about one concept, they did not explicitly recognize that this would facilitate responses to other words linked to that concept. Even if they did recognize this, spreading activation occurred so rapidly that people could not consciously control it; explicit awareness did not interfere with the implicit measure of association. Both these forms of implicit measures are popular, nonreactive ways to study stereotyping.

Measuring/Assessing the Implicit Activation of Affect

Stereotypes have been described here as knowledge structures—beliefs and expectancies about a group. However, distinct from the knowledge we possess about a category/ group are our *feelings* about the category/group. This is an important distinction, because the two (knowledge and affect) need not correspond with one another. We may have highly nonstereotypic beliefs about the qualities of a group (even rejecting the stereotype), while still harboring negative feelings regarding the group. And while beliefs about the qualities that describe a group may change over time, the negativity associated with the group appears to be more stable: The traits that make up the stereotype change, but they continue to carry a negative flavor (Devine & Elliot, 1995). The affect (often negative) associated with a group is what is known as *prejudice*. Whereas *stereotyping* and *prejudice* are often treated as synonyms, the distinction is clear—affect versus knowledge. Allport (1954, pp. 6–7) defined prejudice as "thinking ill of others without sufficient warrant. . . . An avertive or hostile attitude toward a person who belongs to a group, simply because he belongs to that group." It is a prejudgment, usually antipathy, that is difficult to overturn even in the face of evidence suggesting that the generalization of negative affect to members of specific groups is unwarranted.

Like stereotypes, prejudice may be difficult to detect because of strong social norms against expressing overgeneralized negativity toward others simply because they belong to one group or another. And, as with stereotypes, implicit measures have emerged that allow researchers to "tap" latent prejudice, even in people who truly believe that they do not hold such prejudice and who are convinced that they are "bias-free." A typical implicit measure of prejudice uses reaction times to stereotype-relevant stimuli at speeds where conscious processing cannot intervene. However, these experiments are less concerned with measuring reaction times to *knowledge* associated with the stereotype-relevant stimuli; rather, they focus on reaction times associated with affective responding. That is, these latter times are measures of attitudes and tap the positive versus negative associations linked to a category/group. Recall that Chapters 2 and 10 have discussed the *automaticity of attitudes*. It has been asserted there that every stimulus we observe (in this case, a member of a stereotyped group) is associated with specific types of evaluative responses, and that the process of having the affect or attitude associated with that person triggered occurs immediately and without awareness. This is true for all objects and people we encounter. Thus implicit prejudice would be revealed by the automatic activation of negative attitudes and affect, simply because a member of a stereotyped group has been seen. We may lack awareness that these negative feelings exist and are being activated. But if they are latently associated with the group in question, they should be triggered despite the fact that consciousness is uninvolved in the process.

Let us take a few classic examples to illustrate. Fazio and colleagues (1995) extended the research on automatic evaluation to the domain of racial prejudice. The technique was borrowed directly from Fazio, Sanbonmatsu, Powell, and Kardes (1986): The name of an attitude object is presented (the prime), and this is followed by a positive or negative adjective. The participant is to respond whether the adjective is "good" or "bad," with the speed of this evaluative response being facilitated if the affect has previously been triggered by the prime. In this study, the prime was a photograph of a face of either a White or a Black man. The adjectives were positive (e.g., "attractive," "likable," "wonderful") and negative (e.g., "annoying," "disgusting," "offensive") words that were irrelevant to the stereotypes of these groups. This allowed a test of whether positive or negative affect was immediately triggered upon seeing the face. The findings revealed that White participants were faster at making the evaluations when positive adjectives were preceded by White primes and negative adjectives were preceded by Black primes.

Wittenbrink, Judd, and Park (1997) used a sequential priming procedure in which White participants were primed by the subliminal presentation of a category (the group labels "Black" vs. "White"), and participants were immediately afterward asked to respond to words (a lexical decision task) that were either positive or negative in valence. Some of these words were in fact relevant to the stereotypes of Blacks and Whites, while some of the words were irrelevant to the stereotypes. The results revealed that participants responded faster to words with a positive valence when they followed the prime "White," yet they responded faster to words with a negative valence when they followed the prime "Black." And the effect was strongest when the words were stereotypical. That is, words relevant to the stereotypes of Blacks that were negative in nature were responded to particularly fast following the category label, as were words relevant to the stereotypes of Whites that had a positive valence and that followed the category label. This met the definition of implicit prejudice in that an affective response seemed to be triggered by the mere presence of a group label, with the participants remaining unaware of either the label's presence or their affective reaction to it.

The Implicit Association Test

Yet another measure of the implicit association between affect/attitude and a particular group is the *implicit association test* (IAT; Greenwald, McGhee, & Schwartz, 1998). How does the IAT work? It presumes that associations in the mind can be detected by mapping two tasks (judging a face and judging the valance of a word) onto a single pair of responses. If both tasks require one and the same response, then an association between the two tasks should make the response easier. To be more specific, mapping two tasks onto one response means asking people to make two different decisions by doing exactly the same thing. For example, if participants have to indicate whether a face is White or Black by pressing the "s" key on a keyboard when a White face appears and the "l" key on a keyboard when a Black face appears, researchers now have a specific response to seeing a Black face—pressing the "l." Now, if a second task is also required—pressing a key on a keyboard when a positive word is seen, and a different key when a negative word is seen—researchers can map these responses onto the earlier responses if the same two keys on the keyboard are used. Thus participants can be instructed to press "l" each time a negative word appears and "s" each time a positive word appears. In this instance, the Black face requires making a response that is the same response required of negative words (pressing "l"). In studies using the IAT, these are usually referred to as *compatible* responses, because the affect believed to be associated with a particular group requires that one respond by using the same action as is used for detecting that particular group. When detecting a certain group requires a response that is mapped onto an unexpected affective response (such as when indicating one has seen a Black person requires pushing the same button as responding to positive words), then the responses are referred to as *incompatible*.

The IAT proceeds through stages. First, people are trained to make each response separately. For instance, in Stage 1 they learn to press a certain key each time they see a person from a certain group. Then in Stage 2 they learn to press a certain key each time they see a positive word versus a negative word. Then people are asked to combine the two tasks so that they have to do both of them in an alternating fashion. On one trial they are making distinctions between types of groups, while on the next trial they are making distinctions between positive and negative words. The juxtaposition of the two tasks and the mapping of the responses allow researchers to detect whether an implicit association exists.[1] For example, if Black faces are implicitly associated with bad feelings in White participants, it should be easier for them to press the key indicating that a Black face has been seen if the same key is being used to indicate that a bad word has been seen. The implicit association should be revealed by a facilitation in response times when compatible responses are being mapped together.

Greenwald and colleagues (1998) provided several concrete illustrations of this effect. In one experiment, one group of Japanese American students and one group of Korean American students performed an IAT in which two tasks were mapped together. The first task involved pressing one button when a Japanese surname was presented, and another when a Korean surname was presented. The second task involved pressing one button when a word was considered to be pleasant, and another button when a word was considered to be unpleasant. The logic was that if Korean participants had implicit negative feelings toward Japanese people (and vice versa), then the Korean participants would be faster to respond to negative words when doing so required pressing the same button as responding to Japanese surnames (as opposed to when it corresponded to a Korean surname). Similarly, they would be faster to respond to positive adjectives when these adjectives were mapped onto the same response as detecting Korean surnames. Japanese participants would show the same implicit bias, but in favor of their group and against Koreans (i.e., faster responses when negative adjectives were responded to with the same action as Korean surnames). This was precisely what was found. It was easier (participants were faster) to perform a task when the responses were mapped together and the affect triggered during one response was consistent with the affective evaluation being made by the other response. Koreans were slower to detect Japanese surnames when doing so required the same response as detecting positive words; Japanese people were slower to detect Korean surnames when doing so required the same response as detecting positive words. In another experiment by Greenwald and colleagues, this same pattern of findings was revealed in White subjects who were asked to detect whether a name was that of a Black person or not. If the button participants pressed to indicate that a Black name had been seen was the same button they pressed to detect a positive word, White participants were slower than if the button they pressed was the same button to detect a negative word. This indicated an association between negative affect and Black names in these White people—an association they did not intend to reveal and did not know they had expressed.

What Is an Implicit Association between Affect and a Group?

A debate has emerged surrounding exactly what the IAT measures. When attitudes toward a group are assessed explicitly (by asking people), then it is clear what is being measured—people's evaluation of the group. However, does an association between negative affect and members of a group mean that people endorse such a negative evaluation? Does it mean implicit prejudice toward that group? Or could it be that it simply means people have learned that in their culture these two things are typically associated, though they may not personally endorse such feelings? The IAT may simply measure the associations that are present in a cultural environment. Karpinski and Hilton (2001, p. 776) state that "according to the environmental association model of the IAT, a high score on a White/Black IAT, for example, should not be seen as indicating that the individual has more favorable evaluations of Whites compared with Blacks. Instead, the score may simply indicate that the individual has been exposed to a larger number of positive–White and negative–Black associations."

Alternately, rather than assessing true attitudes, the IAT may simply reflect lack of familiarity with one of the groups in question (Brendl, Markman, & Messner, 2001). Japanese have less exposure to Koreans than to other Japanese people. Whites have less exposure to Blacks than to Whites. Can the effect be explained by mere familiarity (a lack of experience with one group, due to its lower frequency of being encountered)? Perhaps White people are not prejudiced against Blacks; they just dislike Black surnames they are not very familiar with (Dasgupta, Greenwald, & Banaji, 2003). However, some research has indicated that familiarity does not seem to be the root of the IAT effect. For example, Rudman, Greenwald, Mellott, and Schwartz (1999) controlled for the degree to which people were familiar with the primes. One experiment examined automatic pro-Christian attitudes among Christian college students and found, as expected, a bias toward Christian surnames on the IAT (relative to Jewish surnames). The ability to rule out familiarity as an explanation for the IAT comes from the fact that the names selected to represent each of the groups were selected because they were equally familiar to research participants. But this issue is not yet settled. Brendl and colleagues (1999) proposed that IAT data patterns need not be interpreted as reflecting implicit prejudice, but as indicating difficulty of the task. That is, the incompatible trials of the IAT may be perceived by participants as harder than the compatible trials. Participants may try to avoid error on these harder trials by adopting a stricter criterion before responding (raising their response threshold). Thus the slowdown observed may not be attributable to prejudice, but to efforts to be more careful on what people perceive as a harder task.

At this writing, a new argument against the validity of the IAT is brewing—one that questions its psychometrics (Blanton & Jaccard, 2004; Blanton, Jaccard, & Gonzales, 2004). The argument is essentially that the IAT is a measure of relative attitudes. It measures a person's evaluative ratings of two different attitude objects in relation to one another—such as a Japanese person's ratings of Korean names relative to Japanese names, or a White person's ratings of Black faces/names relative to White ones. This is not a controversial statement; it merely summarizes how the IAT works (i.e., it produces a single score meant to capture the difference in evaluation between the two attitude objects). Indeed, the creators of the IAT recognize this fact, and argue that measures of relative evaluations, such as the IAT, are not limited by this state of affairs. Instead, as Greenwald and Farnham (2000, p. 1023) have stated, "the IAT can nevertheless be effectively used because many socially significant categories form complementary pairs, such as positive–negative (valence), self–other, male–female, Jewish–Christian, young–old, weak–strong, warm–cold, liberal–conservative, aggressive–peaceful, etc." Blanton and colleagues (2004) argue that while this may seem reasonable, it requires that researchers using the IAT embrace a restrictive and unrealistic conceptual model. It requires them to accept the idea that the influence of the evaluation of one attitude object (e.g., negative evaluations of Blacks) is equivalent to the influence of its opposite in the difference score that is being calculated (e.g., positive evaluations of Whites). That is, by creating difference scores, researchers assume equal weighting of the two things contributing to the difference score. The authors describe two easy-to-imagine scenarios in which this assumption underlying the IAT would not be true: (1) Racism in Whites is contributed to more by their negative evaluation of Blacks than it is by their positive evaluations of Whites; and (2) racism in Whites is driven by negative evaluations of Blacks, and the extent to which this is true increases as they feel more positively about Whites. In this way, the use of a difference score in calculating the IAT effect would not be capturing the true nature of a person's attitude. As Blanton and Jaccard (2004) have put it, the measure would lack a rational zero point; therefore, its predictive validity (its usefulness as a predictor of prejudice) would be called into question. The next few years will undoubtedly see an explosion of research examining the validity of the IAT. This is an increasingly important issue, as the number of research articles using the IAT has grown in a very few years to over 100 published papers (with increasing numbers being applied in nature).

Aversive Racism as an Implicit Type of Bias

Given changing social norms, it is far more uncommon to hear people in modern-day Western society (relative to the decades immediately prior to and immediately after World War II) express overtly negative beliefs about groups that are stereotyped by their cultures. Part of this is due to the fact that people are simply, as discussed above, conforming to these norms and not publicly expressing the racist views they hold in private. However, part of this is due to the fact that people do truly have new, more modern beliefs that oppose being prejudiced—beliefs they try (with varying degrees of success) to uphold both in public and in private. *Aversive racism* is a more modern type of intergroup bias, one in which people who truly uphold beliefs that oppose the old stereotypes are also latently holding negative feelings toward the group. These feelings persist despite the change in beliefs and the conscious rejection of the stereotypes.

Focusing on an American example, Gaertner and Dovidio (1986) have proposed that many White Americans are conflicted and ambivalent about race. They value being fair and unbiased, as these are cherished components of the American creed. However, they also harbor resentful feelings about character flaws they see in stereotyped groups, and hold feelings of unease regarding being around such groups. These feelings lead to avoidance so as not to feel anxiety or discomfort. Guarding against an embarrassing transgression, such as saying something offensive or "politically incorrect," only heightens the anxiety. Yet the very same people, often unaware of their negative feelings, are consciously quite dedicated to the idea of egalitarianism. Their bias is subjugated and is not visible to themselves or others. Only through implicit measures would it be revealed. They have the biases not of the overt and hostile racists of old, but of persons who desire to be egalitarian, fair, and nonbiased. They are perhaps even consciously working quite hard to accomplish this, but these efforts are undermined by an unconscious bias that seeps out in the implicit measures. This ambivalence is not overtly expressed. It comes out "through the cracks" (1) when behavior and attitudes in domains not clearly related to race are examined; and (2) in situations where there are no clear norms about how to behave.

Issues Mask Bias

McConahay and Hough (1976) assert that stereotyping can be observed by asking White persons about beliefs regarding abstract types of issues they do not realize are linked to race (such as welfare reform, political beliefs about Black candidates, affirmative action, school busing programs, etc.). They may oppose a mayoral candidate who is Black, using his positions on issues as a justification for their opposition to him. They may convince themselves that the candidate has unacceptable positions on issues, despite the fact that a White candidate with the same positions on the same issues would be deemed acceptable. When people use socially acceptable reasons (such as political issues and beliefs) to protect themselves from recognizing their own biases, then they can be described as being aversive racists. For example, McConahay and Hough's White research participants truly believed that it was school busing they opposed, not the percentage of Black kids in their school district being increased. When opposition to a legitimate issue—busing—is used to mask opposition to a group of people, we have the more modern form of racism.

A more recent example is illustrated by a discussion concerning Black athletes I heard in April 2003 on WFAN radio (a sports talk station in New York City). A caller accused the hosts of the show (Mike Francessa and Chris Russo) of being racists because, this caller claimed, the hosts consistently used Black athletes as examples when attempting to illustrate how athletes these days lack a "work ethic," "solid preparation," and "discipline" (i.e., they are prone to behavioral problems). The reaction of the hosts was one of indignation at the suggestion; they screamed in rage in their own defense at the helpless caller. What was their defense? It was that their favorite athletes all were African American, and that there was absolutely no way a person could admire African American athletes as much as they did and be called racists. This defense was, given the scientific evidence, a bad one. The issue is not whether these hosts knew and liked African American individuals. This alone would not prove that they were not aversive racists. And the use of this as evidence made their indignation misleading to people listening. It suggested that so long as the hosts liked individual members of a group, they could not have dislike for the group as a whole. It failed to address the possibility that they could have unrecognized and very subtle biases. One possible way such bias could emerge was by being masked by what seemingly were legitimate attitudes. There certainly are Black athletes who lack a work ethic, and there certainly are admirable Black athletes. This was not what the radio hosts needed to worry about. To determine whether their indignation was justified, they would need to assess whether they had an implicit bias, and they could not determine this by examining their explicit attitudes. The question of interest was this: Did they use legitimate attitudes as an *opportunity* to trash Black athletes?

Now the question of whether these radio hosts were truly exhibiting subtle racism is one I cannot answer. Perhaps they were correct to have such indignation because they were being wrongly accused. The reason the issue is raised here is that their defense was one used by aversive racists—"Some of my best friends are Black [or Jewish, Arabic, etc.]." It is indeed very possible to maintain the sort of positive attitudes toward members of a minority group these men claimed to have and still harbor subtle feelings of bias toward the group more generally. The issue is not whether the Black athletes used as examples displayed negative behaviors (we can always pick out examples, such as the Kobe Bryant rape accusation, or the Allen Iverson tirade against practicing). It is the *systematic* use of the same types of illustrations, using the same group repeatedly to describe a negative behavior. To determine aversive racism, we would need to ask not whether the hosts liked or disliked specific Black people. We would need to ask whether they disproportionately described Blacks when chid-

ing lazy, poorly behaving athletes, using the legitimate issue to let negative affect
toward the group seep out.

Norms Are Unclear

Many situations have clear rules informing people how to act and how to be politically
correct. However, in some situations the rules are not clear; here bias appears, and
implicit stereotypes leak out. Gaertner (1973) demonstrated this by looking at the willingness of Whites to offer help to a person in need, and manipulating whether the person in need was White or Black. Furthermore, they manipulated whether the White
person faced with the decision to "help" was a conservative or a liberal. Liberals and
conservatives were called at home by a motorist whose car had broken down and who
was supposedly trying to reach an automotive shop, but had dialed the research participants at home by mistake (the "motorist" was not really trapped on the side of the road,
but worked for the experimenter). The motorist was identified as Black or White by his
dialect. The motorist identified himself as being out of coins (and, since they did not
exist at the time, without a cellular phone), and asked each participant to help out by
calling the garage (with the phone number actually being the number at the laboratory,
allowing the researchers to keep track of who decided to help).

The logic of the experiment was that liberals would be particularly likely to strive to
avoid racism, and thus their overt behavior should be more helpful than that of conservatives. However, an aversive form of stereotyping should reveal itself when the rules
about how to behave were not clear, particularly in liberals. Explicit stereotyping was
measured by the degree to which participants actually agreed to help a motorist who
explained his dilemma. Choosing to help a Black person to a lesser degree than a White
person, under the very same conditions, would be a sign of overt prejudice. How was
aversive stereotyping measured? Sometimes when a wrong number is received in ordinary life, people hang up quickly without talking to the person (who obviously did not
mean to call them). In this research, hanging up early (before the person could explain
his dilemma) would be a situation not governed by any clear rules. Therefore, implicit
stereotyping could be detected by a greater tendency to hang up early on Black callers
than on White callers. The results showed that when the rules about how to act were
clear (the motorist had time to explain his dilemma), liberals helped more than conservatives when the motorist was Black (but the two were equally helpful to a White motorist). However, when the rules were unclear and no normative pressures existed, liberals
were more likely to hang up the phone on a Black person early, before he had a chance
to explain his dilemma, than on a White person. Liberals also hung up early on a Black
caller more often than conservatives did. Thus people who were consciously motivated
to be nonbiased, and who acted on those beliefs in many circumstances, had implicit
stereotypes jumping to the fore when their guard was let down.

The Activation of Stereotypes

The placement of an individual into a category creates meaning by triggering associated
beliefs and affect linked to this category. In Chapter 3, this has been called an *inference*—
a process of triggering knowledge and affect stored in memory that is associated with
the category in question. When that knowledge includes a well-organized set of beliefs
and expected behavior the culture has taught us, then the categorization process can

lead to the triggering of the social stereotype. A consequence of this is that regardless of whether we have egalitarian values, anti-stereotypic personal beliefs, and a dedication to fairness, a stereotype can still be triggered without our knowing it, simply because we "know" the stereotype. And if it is triggered without our knowing it, we can be biased by its accessibility even if we reject the stereotype. In Chapter 10, this has been called a *priming effect*—the undetected influence of accessible information. If we are not aware of the accessibility or its impact on us, an accessible stereotype can affect our judgments despite our consciously rejecting stereotypes. However, the impact of the activated stereotype on judgment would depend upon exactly what gets activated. We have seen in Chapter 10 that priming "hostility" activates associated concepts that then get used in social judgment. However, stereotypes are not single traits, but hosts of traits and characteristics. Can the entire structure be triggered, making each of these traits perceptually ready?

Dovidio, Evans, and Tyler (1986) performed a clever experiment illustrating spreading activation of stereotypes that leads to the implicit accessibility of stereotypes. Participants were asked to respond to pairs of words on a monitor by pressing a button marked "yes" if the second word in a given pair could possibly be conceived of as a trait possessed by a member of a particular group, with the group being the first word presented in the pair. Thus they might see the pairing of "White–ambitious" or "Black–athletic." Given that any trait can conceivably be seen as being possessed by some member of a given group, this task was not explicitly about stereotypes. It would not be stereotypical to say that a specific White person could be ambitious or that a specific Black person could be musical. However, the speed of responding "yes" to a word pair was a measure of how readily participants were willing to associate the trait with the group—whether they made an implicit association linking the stereotypical trait to the group. Thus, if people were faster to respond when the pairings were stereotypical, it would reveal an implicit activation of the stereotype that would otherwise not have been expressed. This was precisely what Dovidio et al. found.

Exactly what gets triggered is a matter of debate. Some theorists follow a *spreading activation model*, which holds that all information associated with a stereotyped feature is triggered in the lexicon and becomes perceptually ready upon attending to that feature (e.g., Devine, 1989). Other theorists propose a *parallel-constraint-satisfaction model* (e.g., Kunda & Thagard, 1996; reviewed in Chapter 9), which asserts that not all information that is stored in the lexicon associated with a particular category (such as a stereotype) is triggered by encountering a person exhibiting behavior that fits that category (or a member of a stereotyped group). Instead, expectancies and context bolster the activation of some information while simultaneously (in parallel) inhibiting or constraining the activation of other information. For example, if a Black fireman is detected by a White observer, the information that gets triggered will be constrained by the context. If he is seen at a fire, perhaps the concepts associated with the category "fireman" (traits such as "helpful," "brave," "friendly") will inhibit competing traits that are associated with the category "Blacks" (traits such as "hostile," "threatening," "lazy"). If he is seen at a protest march, perhaps the categorical traits associated with the race stereotype will inhibit the traits associated with his occupational stereotype. Each model answers this important question: Does information associated with a stereotype get triggered as part of the process of categorizing a person as a member of a particular group? Each model answers it in the affirmative. Yet they differ regarding what information must get activated, with one model predicting that some of the information we might think would be activated actually gets inhibited and is less likely to come to mind. However, momentarily ignoring the important subtleties associated with whether all information is activated versus some information is activated while other information is inhibited, let us turn to an issue raised by both models.

The description of the cognitive processes in each of these models raises this question: Is stereotyping inevitable? But this is not really a meaningful question, because *stereotyping is not really one mental process*. It starts with the *identification* of features possessed by an individual, and proceeds to fitting those features to some preexisting category. Once *categorization* has occurred, there is a spreading of activation within the category to all/some of the related components that are linked to (associated with) the stereotype (if one exists). This results in the *activation* of the stereotype. If the stereotype is activated, there is perceptual readiness. Finally, if we are to conclude that stereotyping has occurred, there must additionally be stereotype *use*. The stereotype is incorporated into the perceiver's responding, altering the type of judgments, impressions, emotions, and behaviors that are associated with the person being perceived. Thus the question is really multitiered: Is the triggering of a stereotype inevitable, given that a perceiver has categorized a person as belonging to a particular group? And is the use of a stereotype in the perceiver's judgment and action inevitable, given that a stereotype has been triggered? Are these processes automatic?

For activation of a stereotype to be inevitable/automatic, it must be more than unintended and proceeding outside of the perceiver's awareness. It must also be triggered by the mere detection of group membership (meaning that the stereotype must be activated upon encountering an individual from the group in question), and the triggering of related information must be unstoppable, even if the perceiver tries to control it (these features of automaticity have been reviewed in Chapter 2). Questions of stereotype inevitability will be addressed more fully in the next chapter. For now, let us simply review one experiment to illustrate the point. Devine (1989) conducted what is considered to be a seminal experiment examining the question of whether stereotypes are automatically activated. After reviewing this evidence that stereotype activation is automatic, let us dedicate the rest of this chapter to reviewing the evidence that stereotypes, once activated, are used in judgment and memory in a fairly routine, effortless, habit-like, and efficient manner.

Evidence for Automatic Stereotype Activation

Stereotypes not only arise from personal experience with exemplars, but are culturally shared beliefs transmitted to all of us in a culture through socialization forces (e.g., parents, media, peers, teachers). This process begins as soon as we are able to understand speech, even before we understand abstract concepts like race and gender (Aboud, 1988), and continues throughout life. Because of an unyielding association between certain groups and certain traits/behaviors, Devine (1989) proposed that stereotypes come to operate like habits, being triggered by appropriate cues in the environment. The mere presence of a group member will automatically activate the concepts with which the group has been habitually associated. Stereotypes are posited to be more than subtle biases that *may be* triggered and have an impact on our judgments. They are beliefs that *must be* triggered whenever we categorize a person as belonging to a group—the triggering is inevitable:

The present model assumes that . . . because the stereotype has been frequently activated in the past, it is a well-learned set of associations that is *automatically* activated in the presence of a member (or symbolic equivalent) of the target group. The model holds that this unintentional activation is equally strong and equally inescapable for high- and low-prejudice persons. (Devine, 1989, p. 6; emphasis in original)

Much as one cannot look at the sky and have concepts relating to the color "blue" fail to be triggered, a non-Arab presumably cannot look at an Arab and have concepts relating to "oil" fail to be triggered. By this account, any concept linked to the stereotype of Arabs, including negative and erroneous conceptions, would be triggered by necessity. As an automatic process, stereotype activation would occur without the non-Arab observer intending it, without the observer being constrained by cognitive load and limits to processing resources, without his/her being aware of spreading activation, and regardless of whether he/she is an egalitarian person. Either a high- or a low-prejudice observer would have the stereotype triggered by virtue of the fact that each type of person knows the stereotype. Personal beliefs that lead to either acceptance or rejection of the stereotype would play no part in the triggering of the stereotype. All that would matter is that the observer has learned the association between the group label and the stereotype that exists in the culture.

To test this assertion, Devine (1989, Experiment 2) used high- and low-prejudice people as research participants. The prediction was that while low-prejudice people might be able to prevent themselves from using a stereotype if they were aware of its existence, they would not be able to stop the stereotype from being activated. And if the stereotype was automatically activated (without awareness and without the ability to control it), then there might be many times when people would be unable to prevent themselves from using a stereotype (because they did not know it was relevant to their current thinking). This would be evidenced by their forming judgments consistent with the stereotype. If participants did not know that the impressions they were forming were even relevant to stereotyping (an implicit measure of stereotyping), then any impact on those judgments in which people interpreted behavior as more consistent with the stereotype would have to be due to the fact that the stereotype had been activated. Devine argued that under these conditions, stereotypes would bias the judgments of low-prejudice people just as powerfully as they biased the judgments of high-prejudice people—thus revealing that the stereotype had been activated just as powerfully for low-prejudice people, despite their personal beliefs.

To test this idea, at least two conditions would need to be in place. First, there would have to be a stimulus whose mere presence would potentially trigger the stereotype (supposedly equally for low- and high-prejudice people). Second, there would have to be a measure of stereotype accessibility in which stereotype activation could be assessed without participants being aware that stereotypes were being assessed (an implicit measure). To satisfy these two conditions, Devine (1989) followed Bargh and Pietromonaco's (1982) subliminal priming procedure, reviewed in Chapter 10. The first condition was met by presenting participants with stereotype-relevant stimuli. To ensure that participants did not know the experiment concerned stereotypes, these stereotype-related stimuli were presented such that participants never consciously saw them; stereotypes were activated by a *subliminal* presentation of stereotype-related words. One hundred words were subliminally presented. White participants either "saw" a list that contained 80 words relevant to the stereotype of African Americans and 20 neutral words, or a list with 80 neutral words and 20 stereotypic ones. Importantly, one specific word that is part of the stereotype–the word "hostile," or any synonym of it–was never shown in these lists. This was done to illustrate that the stereotype would be triggered through a process of spreading activation. Even though the word "hostile" was never presented, it is associated in a semantic network with the words that *were* presented (by virtue of the fact that they are all part of one structure–a stereotype of African Americans). The presented words were expected to lead to the increased accessibility of the entire stereotype, including elements of the stereotype that were not initially present.

To satisfy the second condition, people were asked to perform a second task ostensibly unrelated to the previous task (where words were being subliminally flashed). Thus, in an unrelated context, people were asked to make judgments of a person acting in a manner that was ambiguous along a behavioral dimension associated with the stereotype. Specifically, they were asked to read about a man named Donald (race unknown), who acted in a way that was ambiguously hostile. They then formed an impression of Donald, including making some ratings of how hostile they found him to be, and some ratings that involved traits not relevant to the stereotype. If the stereotype was accessible and contained notions of hostility, then being "ready" to see hostility should have an impact on how people interpreted the behavior. They should see Donald as more hostile when they had been primed with word lists that were 80% (vs. 20%) stereotypic. This priming manipulation should not have an impact on judgments made of Donald on traits not relevant to the stereotype. In summary, the only way people could rate Donald as more hostile was if that concept had somehow been triggered, which in this case could only have occurred through the activation of the stereotype.

The results supported these predictions. Only judgments of Donald's hostility were affected by the primes. Hostility, an item related to the stereotype, was seen as descriptive of Donald, but traits unrelated to the stereotype were not seen as descriptive of Donald. And this tendency to judge Donald in line with the stereotype occurred only when the stereotypic items had been presented 80% of the time (as opposed to 20% of the time). This impact on judgment could only have been caused by the heightened accessibility of the concept "hostility" in the mind of the perceivers. This heightened accessibility occurred even though the word "hostile" was never presented, and even though none of the words that were presented were consciously seen (people were not aware that they had been exposed to any words). Finally, and most importantly, this finding did not interact with the prejudice level of the perceivers. *Low- and high-prejudice people were equally likely to have their stereotypes triggered.* This was indicated by the fact that people in each group were equally likely to have their impressions of Donald biased in the direction of the stereotype when they had been (subliminally) exposed to items related to the stereotype. The mere presence (not even the conscious presence) of items related to the stereotype was enough to activate the stereotype. Devine (1989) claimed this to be uncontrollable because it occurred even for people explicitly trying to control being prejudiced (the low-prejudice people).

The findings of Devine (1989) do not suggest that people are doomed to *use* stereotypes once activated; they simply suggest that stereotypes are inevitably *activated*. However, the finding that stereotypes are automatically activated paints a somewhat sobering picture–because, although stereotype activation does not necessitate that people use those stereotypes in their judgment, people often do (as we shall soon see). Stereotype use is fairly pervasive, especially because people do not realize their stereotypes are triggered or are affecting them (as is the case when stereotypes are primed, which, unfortunately, may happen each time a member of a stereotyped group is seen).

STEREOTYPE USE: STEREOTYPES AS HYPOTHESES THAT BIAS JUDGMENT

Once a stereotype has been triggered, must it be used to guide the way an individual thinks and acts? Because stereotyping is a type of top-down/schema-driven thinking, the properties that govern the use of stereotypes are redundant with the properties that govern such thinking (as described in Chapter 5, and then applied to accessible information in Chapters 9 and 10). To review, people rely on stereotypes because the outer world is too complex for the limited abilities of the processing system—this is the principle of limited capacity. As a means to navigate around this constraint, people develop the strategy of using as little mental effort as possible, thus preserving their limited resources for instances when they are truly needed—this is the principle of least effort (cf. Sherman, 2001). As with other forms of top-down processing, stereotyping leads people to incorporate new information into the existing stereotype. People assimilate information into the stereotype, casting a stereotypic light on the behavior of those they encounter. This stereotypic hue is cast over social cognition at the most basic levels, determining what grabs people's attention, how they perceptually analyze (interpret) and encode the features to which they choose to attend, and what types of information they use when forming impressions. With this dedication to the stereotype, the clinging to the existing structure, comes a *confirmatory bias*: Information is processed in manner that confirms the existing stereotype. As Allport (1954, p. 21) states, "so long as we can 'get away' with coarse overgeneralizations we tend to do so. (Why? Well, it takes less effort, and effort, except in the area of our most intense interests, is disagreeable.)"

The research reviewed below illustrates the ubiquitous and unintended influence of stereotypes. However, what this review also reveals is that the use of stereotypes, though often occurring without intent or without awareness that a stereotype is even having an impact, is something that people can control if they become aware of the stereotype's influence. Thus *stereotypes act like hypotheses, and people are not wont to use hypotheses without first attempting to test them and assess their validity*. However, this will not guarantee that people are bias-free. First, people may not be aware that hypotheses (in the form of stereotypes) are influencing them. Second, even if they become aware of this, the principles of least effort and limited capacity suggest that the amount of evidence they need to gather in order to support a hypothesis may be trivial—thus making the hypothesis likely to have an impact, regardless of what the reality of the data may be. As Allport (1954) stated, "there is a curious inertia in our thinking" (p. 20).

Mere Categorization and the Perception of Category Differences

The idea that stereotypes bias judgment assumes that the content of the stereotype serves as an expectancy, and that perceivers are perceptually ready to see this expectancy. Tajfel and Wilkes (1963) proposed that the mere assignment of a category label to a group with a set of associated features was capable of biasing how individual members of the category were judged. Categorization would lead perceivers to see features associated with the stereotype of the group, even when there was no evidence to support that this given instance of the category had those features. To perform a first, basic test of this proposition, Tajfel and Wilkes asked perceivers to make judgments not of people, but of a group of lines! Obviously, the implications of how stereotypes bias judgment are important, because they have an impact on how people judge other people. But the fact that people were not used in this experiment doesn't move our discussion off track and make the point less interesting; it makes it even more powerful. People, and their behavior, are very subjective targets for perceivers. The behavior they perform requires interpreting. But something as clear-cut as a line should not be judged differently simply because it has been labeled as being in one group versus another. If these researchers could illustrate differential and biased perceptions emerging from a stereotype about a group of lines, it only augments the point that perceptions of something more subjective, like people, will be biased as well.

In their experiment, Tajfel and Wilkes (1963) presented a series of eight lines to research participants, with the lines grouped into two sets of four lines. The participants were asked to judge the difference in length between two consecutive lines. For half of the people, the lines were grouped according to membership in a category that had meaning. The first four in the series were labeled as part of Group A, and the meaning attached to them was that lines from Group A were short. The last four lines in the series of eight lines were labeled as part of Group B, and the meaning attached to them was that lines from Group B were long (see Figure 11.1). Thus participants formed stereotypes that Group A lines were shorter than Group B lines. The other half of the participants saw the same eight lines, in exactly the same order, but membership in Group A versus Group B now did not coincide with line length. Each group had long and short lines. Thus these participants did not form stereotypes about what it meant for a line to be in Group A versus Group B. Remarkably, when the lines were labeled as being part of a group that had meaning, the difference between the longest line in Group A (Line 4) and the shortest line in Group B (Line 5) was seen as greater than when these very same lines were being judged without this frame of reference. People with a stereotype exaggerated the difference between lines from two different groups, perceiving these groups to be more different than they actually were. Why? Because when people had a simple stereotype about what it meant to be in a group, it biased their judgment of line length, even though the lines were sitting right under their noses and open to inspection. Mere categorization as a member of Group A led a line to be

Grouping of lines where group membership has meaning (features are associated with the group, and these features form a stereotype – A is short, B is long).

Grouping of lines where group membership has no meaning (features associated with the group do not lead to stereotype formation).

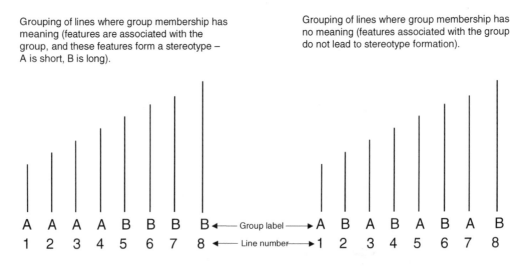

FIGURE 11.1. Mere categorization to a trivial, stereotyped group causes distortion.

seen as more different from its neighboring line in Group B only when a stereotype was associated with the groups.

The next step for Tajfel and his colleagues was to apply this logic to judging people. We all have a sense that we favor the groups we belong to, and perhaps treat more unfairly the groups we do not belong to. But is this because there is real conflict, dislike, and competition between groups? Just as categorizing lines led to seeing exaggerated differences between the lines in different groups, Tajfel and colleagues maintained that the mere act of categorizing people would have a similar effect. However, they went even further. They predicted behavioral differences: The mere act of labeling people into groups should lead to attempts to maximize the differences between the groups in how they were treated. This would occur, they predicted, even when the groups were trivially determined, making them defined in as a bland and meaningless a way as two groups of lines. Simply being in two different groups should cause an exaggeration of the differences between them. To test this, Tajfel and colleagues performed a series of studies using what they called *minimal groups*. A minimal group is based on no meaningful criteria at all, and is, from the group members' perspective, a trivial and pointless feature of their personalities they happen to share with others.

Tajfel, Billig, Bundy, and Flament, (1971, p. 174; emphasis in original) concluded that when minimal groups are created, the simple act of being in a group creates a bias where people behave in ways that differentiate their (trivial) group from others:

> When the subjects have a choice between acting in terms of maximum utilitarian advantage to all (MJP) combined with maximum utilitarian advantage to members of their own group (MIP) as against having their own group *win* on points at the sacrifice of both of these advantages, it is the winning that seems more important to them.

Tajfel and colleagues found that when given the choice to behave (allocating rewards in a game) in a way that would provide the most rewards for their own group, people rejected this opportunity. They also rejected the opportunity to be fair and allocate the points with equal benefit to all (perhaps a logical choice, since the groups were totally meaningless). What did they choose to do instead? They allocated rewards in such a way that the difference between their group and the other group was the greatest, even if it meant getting fewer rewards for their own group. For example, people would rather have a mere $7 allocated to their group and see another group get nothing (a difference of $7), at the expense of getting $20 for their own group, if it would mean that the other group would get $16 (a difference of only $4)! People acted in ways confirming that differences were perceived to exist between the groups, even though the groups were meaningless, trivial, and minimal. They would basically throw away large sums of money just to guarantee that members of some other trivial group would get a lot less than them rather than just a little bit less then them (or more than them).

Outgroup Homogeneity

The discussion of minimal groups gets our discussion slightly ahead of itself with its focus on behavior. We will return to discussing the effects of stereotypes on behavior at the end of this section. For now, let us stay focused on the major point illustrated by Tajfel and Wilkes (1963)—that stereotypes associated with group membership lead to a perceptual–judgmental effect of seeing exaggerated differences between groups. The minimal-group research has shifted the discussion from trivial stereotypes about lines to trivial stereotypes about people. Let us now take the next step and start moving toward examining whether more meaningful stereotypes about people lead to the same types of effects as those observed by Tajfel and Wilkes.

First, Taylor and colleagues (1978) examined the hypothesis that, as a result of categorizing people into meaningful social groups, "within-group differences become minimized and between-group differences become exaggerated (e.g., Blacks are seen as similar to each other and different from Whites)" (p. 779). Taylor and colleagues asked research participants to listen to a discussion between six people, three of whom were White and three of whom were Black. Participants heard each person make a statement and later had to try to recall which person had said what. Their logic was that because race is a salient characteristic, people would categorize the discussants according to race. And once the discussants were divided into groups, individuals within a given group would be confused with one another, while the chances of confusing two people from different groups would be substantially smaller. To examine this prediction, the researchers calculated the number of errors people made in remembering who said what, and classified those errors into two types: errors where a person from one group was confused with another person from that same group, and errors where a person from one group was confused with a person from another group. They found that people made a much higher rate of intracategory relative to intercategory errors. Differences between members of two groups were sharpened. This replicates the Tajfel and Wilkes (1963) research, using social groups instead of lines.

Let us now take this question one step further. Do members of meaningful social groups perceive greater differences between their group and other groups? We have already seen one example of this in the research of Robinson, Keltner, Ward, and Ross (1995) where liberals felt that conservatives held more extreme views than liberals (and vice versa). In an earlier demonstration, Linville and Jones (1980) reported that people made more extreme ratings of members of an outgroup, for both positive and negative evaluations, relative to members of their own group. Their research participants were asked to play the role of an admission board member and evaluate applications to a law school. The applications varied on two dimensions: The application was either strong or weak, and the application was submitted by either a White or a Black applicant. They found that when White participants made judgments of two identical applications, they made more extreme evaluations for Black versus White applicants. A weak application was seen as weaker when submitted by a Black versus a White person; a strong application was seen as stronger.

Linville and Jones (1980) posited that one reason for such perceived differences when judging two identical people from two different groups is the degree of complexity with which perceivers think about the groups. Linville and Jones argued that when more features are incorporated into perceivers' thinking, and a more complex/differentiated set of issues is brought to the processes of evaluation and judgment, less extreme judgments are made. In fact, Linville and Jones illustrate that when perceivers focus their attention on six features associated with a stimulus, they make less extreme evaluations of the stimulus than when they focus on only two features associated with the stimulus. The logical extension of this line of reasoning is that one reason people make more extreme evaluations of members of other groups, relative to members of their own group, is that they have more simplistic and less differentiated mental representations about other groups. For example, lawyers see fine distinctions in the type of law practiced—distinctions they fail to make when thinking about the types of psychology practiced by psychologists (who somehow are all just seen as clinicians). The French see

Americans as being "all alike," yet see themselves as subtle, complex, and highly differentiated. Allport (1954, p. 134) summarized this in stating that an outsider will see a Lutheran simply as a Lutheran, "but to an insider it makes a difference whether he is a member of one Synod or another." People from many disparate cultures have been known to comment about members of outgroups that "they all look alike to me." When perceiving members of other groups, people do not process the individuality of each face as well as they do when fixing a gaze on ingroup members.

This perception of a highly differentiated and complex ingroup contrasted with a simple and undifferentiated outgroup has come to be called *outgroup homogeneity*. Linville, Salovey, and Fischer (1986) have argued that stereotyped categories become more differentiated when people become more familiar with a group. People are more familiar with members of their own group, and therefore have more highly differentiated categories with which to make distinctions between people. The basic idea is that categories or schemas about other groups can range from being highly complex to overly simplified. When they are complex, people can think of many different features or subtypes that can exist within the group. When they are simple, people tend to produce extreme evaluations and see members of the group as homogeneous. This is the outgroup homogeneity effect.

Linville and Jones (1980, Experiment 3) provided a demonstration of the outgroup homogeneity effect and its link to category complexity. They tested the idea that White research participants would have more complex sets of beliefs about White people than about Black people. They gave participants a set of 40 cards, each of which had a trait word printed on it. Participants were asked to sort the cards so that traits that went together, or should be grouped with one another, were in the same pile. They were asked to form as many groups as they thought was necessary, and to continue until they had formed all the groups that they thought were important. Half of the participants were told to think of the groups they were forming as representing the characteristics of White people, while the other half were asked to think of them as the characteristics of Black people. As predicted, people formed more piles with the cards when they were thinking about White people (all participants, as noted above, were White). They were able to come up with more dimensions for describing members of their own group than for describing members of the outgroup.

There are limitations to this effect, and one can easily imagine instances in which it is important to see one's own group as fairly uniform and of one mind, while other groups are perceived as fractious and ill defined (Linville, 1998). This is particularly true when ingroup membership is made salient and social identity needs are high. When it is important to see oneself as belonging to a group, it is often useful to see this group as providing a uniform set of well-defined positive qualities that can reflect on the self. Ingroup homogeneity is also likely to emerge when evaluations are being made on dimensions or traits that are highly relevant to the ingroup. Thus, when nurses make ratings of nurses and doctors, they see the doctors as more homogeneous when they are rating qualities that have very little to do with nurses but that have a lot to do with doctoring. However, when making judgments about attributes relevant to nursing, nurses now rate their group as more homogeneous than they rate doctors (Brown & Wootton-Millward, 1993). These limitations to the effect raise important questions: Why are there differences in how differentiated people's views of the ingroup and outgroup are? What conditions and goals determine when the difference is evidenced by greater homogeneity seen in outgroups versus greater homogeneity seen in ingroups? What cognitive processes drive people's thinking about groups and can cause such differences in differentiated thinking? These questions are important, but are simply too detailed to review in a chapter such as this. Linville (1998) provides an excellent overview of the research in this domain that can address these questions.

Stereotypes Bias Spontaneous Trait Inferences

Most behaviors are open to interpretation. As seen in Chapter 10, the same behavior can be interpreted as reckless or as bold, as confident or as conceited. The type of trait people spontaneously infer when they observe behavior should be determined by stereotypes associated with the group membership of the person performing the behavior. Thus people should be more likely to spontaneously infer the trait "lazy" when hearing about a person who hung around the corner all day if the person hanging around is a member of a group for which laziness is a stereotypic trait. Even implicit inferences—those people do not intend to form and are not aware they have formed—can be biased by stereotypes and the expectancies associated with stereotypes (Otten & Moskowitz, 2000).

This point—that expectancies influence implicit inferences about what categories and traits best describe the behavior—is essential to Trope's (1986a; Trope & Pesach-Gaunt, 1999) model of attribution, reviewed in Chapter 7. Trope argues that behavior can have multiple meanings, and that an expectancy (stereotype) can disambiguate behavior by determining which one of the many potential ways a behavior could be categorized will be the one used to describe the behavior. Even implicit processes of categorization, behavior identification, and inference are biased by expectancies and stereotypes. For example (and see Chapter 7 for a detailed review), when the situation leads perceivers to expect that a person will be frightened, or they have a stereotype leading them to expect that a person will be frightened, this expectancy makes them more likely to categorize the behavior they see as an instance of a person being frightened, even more so than if the expectancy had not existed (e.g., Trope & Alfieri, 1997). Thus people are more likely to make an inference that confirms an expectancy they already hold (e.g., Newman & Uleman, 1990).

It is not only behavior that has multiple possible interpretations. Even traits can have multiple meanings, so that the same trait can mean two different things when performed by two different people. "Aggressive" can mean "hostile and violent," or it can mean "argumentative and pushy." Kunda, Sinclair, and Griffin (1997) argue that stereotypes serve to constrain the meaning of traits, limiting the possible meanings. While "aggressive" can potentially mean two different things, when the word is seen as linked to a group for whom aggressiveness has a very specific meaning, the stereotype will dictate the meaning attached to the trait. In fact, Kunda and colleagues propose that the opposing meaning(s) will be inhibited by the stereotype. Thus an aggressive lawyer will be seen as argumentative and pushy, but unlikely to punch and curse (and vice versa for an aggressive construction worker). "The different connotations that the trait aggressive takes on when applied to these two groups may be due to other knowledge contained in the relevant group stereotypes" (Kunda et al., 1997, p. 722). That is, the other components of the stereotype of a group like lawyers (such as being educated, competitive, and highly verbal) are associated with aggression as well, but only with a particular form of aggression. Thus it is only this meaning of aggression that gets triggered when one sees the trait in the context of group behavior, rather than all of the possible meanings. The stereotype disambiguates the meaning of the trait.

To illustrate that spontaneous trait inferences (STIs) would be biased by stereotypic expectancies associated with group membership, Otten and Moskowitz (2000) took a tack of making this point in the most dramatic fashion possible—when the groups were totally meaningless and void of specific attributes. It was shown that labeling a person as being a member of a trivial ingroup, using the minimal-group procedure described earlier, altered the types of STIs people formed. Participants were more likely to spontaneously infer positive traits about an ingroup than an outgroup member. The way in which the behavior was interpreted and the traits inferred were dictated by the group membership of the person performing the behavior.

The impact of stereotypes on STIs has also been illustrated by Wigboldus, Dijksterhuis, and Van Knippenberg (2003), moving out of the domain of minimal groups and into the domain of groups with real traits and attributes associated with group membership. They provide evidence that categorizing people according to stereotypes not only facilitates making STIs that are compatible with the group stereotype, but inhibits the likelihood of making inferences when the behavior being observed implies a trait that is inconsistent with the stereotype. The procedure used the probe reaction time procedure of Uleman and colleagues (1996). Wigboldus and colleagues manipulated stereotype consistency between the group membership of the actor in the sentence (professor or garbage collector) and the behavior performed by that actor (". . . won the science quiz"). The sentences were followed by probe words, and participants had to indicate if each word was in the sentence preceding it. The researchers found that responses to the trait words (e.g., "smart") implied in the behavior descriptions were faster when the actor in the sentence belonged to a group whose stereotypic traits were inconsistent with the behavior. This suggests that participants did not make the inference implied by the behavior (since trait inference in this paradigm is indicated by responses being slowed on the probe recognition task). In a follow-up experiment, Wigboldus and colleagues used a subliminal priming method to activate the actor's group membership. The stereotype of the primed group was either inconsistent with, consistent with, or neutral in regard to the traits implied by the behavior. Participants were slower to indicate that the trait probe was not part of the sentence when the subliminally flashed group labels were consistent with the behavior in the sentence rather than inconsistent.

Shifting Standards of Comparison

Most of us would agree that the words we use to describe people and things are relative in nature and depend on the context in which the word is used. A large melon will be smaller than a small chair. The standard used for defining large and small shifts as the category shifts. If this seems reasonable, why should we not assume the same when discussing adjectives that describe people? Different categories of people should potentially create different referents, so that the same trait might mean something different when we are describing one category of people than another. A personal trait might take on new dimensions when we are discussing a Black person versus a White person or a woman versus a man. For example, when we describe someone as "an athletic White man," this might convey different information, because of a shifted standard of comparison, than when we say "an athletic Black man." An "analytical woman" might be very different from an "analytical man." Stereotypes may be thought of as standards or referents against which subsequent information is imbued with meaning; they may even alter the way in which the same trait is experienced (Manis, Nelson, & Shedler, 1988). If we refer back to Figure 10.4, categories may be thought of as setting the comparison standard against which the meaning of a trait is evaluated.

Biernat, Manis, and Nelson (1991) illustrate that one consequence of this state of affairs is that our verbal descriptions of people may not accurately reflect our true beliefs. Men and women who are described in exactly the same terms (e.g., "analytical") may be perceived very differently. What is meant by "analytical" when judging a woman is something different from when that description is applied to a man, because the standard or referent shifts. Rather than using the same standard, such as the average person, when judging how analytical (or assertive or independent) a man versus a woman is, we may use the average woman when judging women and the average man when judging men. If the trait being judged is relevant to the stereotypes of these groups, than the average person would look very different if the person is a woman versus a man, and thus a very different standard for evaluating the person will be used. Thus our description may suggest that we are unbiased (we see a woman as very analytical and a man as very analytical), but the description does not really reflect what we mean or how we experience those traits in one group versus the other. We may still think of a given woman as much less analytical than a given man, even though we have seemingly judged them identically. What a prejudiced person might mean is "She's very analytical, for a girl."

To illustrate this use of stereotypes even when judgments seemingly suggest that stereotypes are not being used, Biernat and colleagues (1991) had research participants make judgments of women and men. Participants saw a picture of a man or a woman and needed to make a judgment—how tall was this person? This judgment could be made on either an objective scale or a subjective scale. For example, an objective scale would be estimating height in feet and inches. A subjective scale would be judging whether the person was short or tall relative to the average person. The prediction was that when using a subjective scale, a perceiver might describe a woman as tall and a man as tall, to equal degrees. The same word would be used to describe each ("tall"), and it might perhaps appear that this person perceived no difference between the groups on this dimension. However, the objective scale would indicate whether people really did perceive a difference. The women might be rated as smaller than the men when estimates were made in feet and inches, despite the fact that they were called "tall" just as often as the men in subjective ratings. Such a finding would suggest that the participants were using different standards when making the subjective judgment. Shifting standards would be the only logical explanation as to why people subjectively described the two groups equally, given that on objective measures they rated the two groups differently.

The data were in support of this "shifting-standards" hypothesis. When making judgments in feet and inches, the participants saw men as significantly taller than women. However, when they were instructed to make judgments by evaluating each person's height relative to a typical person, the difference noted on the objective measure was reduced by 80%. It seemed as if they were now employing different standards when making the judgment for women than for men. The "typical" person was the "typical woman" when participants were judging women and the "typical man" when they were judging men. Since stereotypes suggest that the typical woman is shorter than the typical man, the standard being used for judging women should be shorter than that used for judging men. The objectively short woman would seem taller when the relatively shorter subjective standard was used. This would mean that the use of similar terms to describe people from two different groups did not necessarily mean that participants really saw them equally.

Biernat and Manis (1994) illustrated this shifting-standards effect in judgments made about members of a wide variety of social groups. Stereotypes that men are more competent than women, that women have better verbal skills than men, that Whites have better verbal skills than Blacks, and that Blacks are more athletic than Whites were all shown to exist when an objective measure was used to assess the various attributes. However, when subjective measures were used, they led people to use different evaluative standards when comparing individual members of a group against the attribute in question. This led to an apparent lack of stereotyping. Whites were judged as just as "athletic" as Blacks on a subjective rating of athleticism. The suggestion is that what it meant to be "athletic" shifted when a Black person was used as a standard of evaluation (because the perceivers had a stereotype about Blacks and athletic performance). It would require greater levels of athleticism for a Black person to achieve the same rating that a White person received; thus each group was judged relative to the standards created within that group, not by the same standard. In this way, people may seem not to be using stereotypes when in fact they really are, and at quite a basic level—in establishing the referents or contexts in which their evaluations of others are occurring (see also Biernat & Kobrynowicz, 1997).

Biased Attributions by Perceivers

Are our powers of attributional reasoning used to confirm our existing stereotypes about a group? Chapter 8 has discussed research by Taylor and Jaggi (1974) in which Hindu research participants (office clerks in southern India) were asked to evaluate Muslims performing either positive or negative behavior in four different contexts—such as giving shelter to someone in a rainstorm (vs. failing to do so), or helping someone who was injured (vs. not helping). For each behavior, the participants had to rate what caused the Muslim to act in this way. Participants could choose from among a list of internal and external causes. The findings revealed a pattern of biased attributions—ones that confirmed existing stereotypes. Internal attributions were more likely to be used to explain the behavior of a Muslim when it was negative as opposed to positive. Thus negative behavior was seen as caused by the traits and characteristics of the person, whereas positive behaviors were attributed to external pressures that forced the Muslim to act positively.

A similar pattern of distorted attributions to confirm stereotypic expectancies was found by Duncan (1976). Duncan was looking at how White Americans judged the cause of the very same action performed by either a Black or a White person. Whereas Taylor and Jaggi (1974) examined behavior that was either clearly positive or negative and found a biased pattern of responding, Duncan focused on behavior that was ambiguous. Rather than finding that people could use attributions to put a negative cause behind a positive act, Duncan found that the very way in which an act was interpreted in the first place (as either positive or negative) depended upon what participants' stereotypes led them to expect to see. Duncan asserted that stereotypes could be made accessible by encountering a member of a stereotyped group, and that the stereotype, once accessible, would serve as an expectancy, providing hypotheses about what the person would be likely to do and say. When perceivers then observed that person behaving in an ambiguous fashion, the accessible stereotype would guide the way in which the behavior was interpreted. So long as the behavior could be construed as being relevant to the stereotype, it would be interpreted in a manner confirming the stereotype.

Duncan's (1976) hypothesis was that since the cultural stereotype held by White Americans dictates that Blacks are more prone to violent acts than Whites (notions of violence and hostility consistently emerge in White people's lists of the stereotypic traits of Black Americans—e.g., Devine & Elliot, 1995), it would be reasonable to assume that the concept of violence would be more accessible when Whites were viewing a Black person than when viewing a White person. Thus, with the expectancy from the stereotype that Black people are violent, White people might be more likely to categorize a behavior by a Black person as violent than the same behavior performed by a White person: "The threshold for labeling an act as violent is lower when [Whites are] viewing a Black actor than when viewing a White actor" (Duncan, 1976, p. 591). To illustrate this bias in attribution, Duncan told research participants that three people had been scheduled for each experimental session. Two were said to be asked to engage in a discussion, while the third person observed the interaction from a television monitor in another room. In actuality, the (White) participant doing the observing was the only person truly there during the session. The other two individuals, who the participant believed were in the next room, were on videotape. Participants were told that the experimenter was developing a new rating scale for interpreting interpersonal behavior, and the participants therefore were asked to make ratings at six points during the experiment using this scale. In actuality, the ratings being made were assessing the participants' interpretation of the causes for the behavior they were observing. In addition, the interaction was recorded in such a way so that the moment that the final rating was being called for from each participant, one of the two people being observed shoved the other. The experimenter deliberately chose this behavior because of its ambiguity; the shove could be seen as an act of hostility or as an act of playfulness among friends (think of the character Elaine on *Seinfeld*).

The question of interest was this: How would this ambiguous shove be interpreted? What made the question interesting were the manipulations in the experiment. Some participants observed an interaction between two White people; others observed an interaction between two Black people; a third group of participants observed a Black person and a White person interacting where the White person shoved the Black person; a fourth group observed a Black person and a White person interacting where the Black person shoved the White person. Thus White people were observing the same ambiguous behavior, and what varied were the races of the people involved in the interaction. Participants were asked to rate the extent to which the behavior was caused by either the situation, the issue being discussed, the person doing the shoving, or the person getting shoved. The results were striking. When a Black person shoved a White person, the participants labeled this act as violent 75% of the time. However, when a White person shoved a Black person, it was seen as violent only 17% of the time. If it was not violent, what then? The act was labeled as playful 42% of the time (as opposed to being labeled as playful only 6% of the time when a Black person shoved a White person). Duncan (1976) found a similar pattern when examining whether situational or dispositional attributions were formed. When a Black person was doing the pushing, personal attributions were high and situational attributions were low; when the pusher was White, there were low personal attributions and high situational attributions. This study provides evidence that the perception and categorization of acts vary, depending on the expectancies that are brought into the perceptual situation by perceivers via their stereotypes. Duncan calls this evidence for "differential social perception": White people are likely to label the very same act as more violent when it is performed by a Black person than when the act is perpetrated by a White person.

Now that we have illustrated that people label the same behavior differently, depending on the group membership of the person who performs it, a host of relevant social behaviors can come under the purview of confirmatory judgment. Three of these are examined here. First, police officers could be biased in how they label the behavior of a suspect, altering what they believe they see to be a crime; an extreme example of this (mentioned briefly at the end of Chapter 10) was the tragic case of Amadou Diallo, a Black man shot on a dark New York City street after White police officers misidentified the object in his hand as a gun, rather than a wallet. Second, jurors could potentially be biased in how they evaluate the case against a particular defendant, with drastically different verdicts reached based on the interpretation assigned to the evidence (driven by jurors' stereotype-based hypotheses). Third, managers might evaluate employees differently based on stereotypes of group membership, without being aware that their negative evaluations would have been less negative had the employee simply been from a different group.

In the case of Amadou Diallo, an ambiguous act in the dark (a man reaching for something in his pocket) was interpreted as a dangerous and threatening act by police officers, who chose to react to the perceived threat with gunshots (41 shots). Although this reaction seems excessive to most people (it is hard to justify shooting one man 41 times), perhaps the initial act of perception seems warranted. Imagine yourself as a police officer, a walking target, searching the streets for a dangerous suspect. You come across a man who could be that suspect, and you order him not to move. He does not listen, but instead reaches into his pocket. You now are under extreme time pressure, with less than 2 seconds to decide what to do. And in this instance you perceive a threat, a gun. It is easy to imagine an argument in defense of the officers that would take on this tone. This scenario only becomes relevant to our discussion of stereotyping if we can make the case that the ethnicity of the person encountered by the police changed what they thought they perceived and how they responded in reaction to that perception. Would they have been slower to fire on a White man? Would they have given a White man a second warning? Would they have been less likely to have believed the man was reaching for a gun, and less likely to have believed the object he pulled out actually was a gun, if the man had been White? Does differential perception of Black and White people alter our perception of the objects they are holding, contribute to whether we interpret them as threatening, and lead to drastically different behavior, which in the Diallo example included a greater likelihood of shooting a Black man? It was exactly these questions that Katie Couric, host of NBC's *Today* show, put to two social psychologists (Chick Judd and Tony Greenwald) on a December morning in 2002.

The answer can be found in the research of Correll, Park, Judd, and Wittenbrink (2002), who asked White research participants to play a video game in which they had to shoot at people who appeared on a screen if and only if those people posed a threat. They posed a threat if they held a gun. However, to shoot a person who did not pose a threat (who did not hold a gun) would be quite damaging. For example, correctly shooting someone holding a gun would win the person 10 points. However, shooting someone who was holding a nonthreatening object (a cell phone, a wallet, a can) would result in a loss of 20 points. Harsher yet, failure to shoot at someone who was holding a gun resulted in a loss of 40 points. Thus a premium was placed on not failing to shoot a bad guy, because failing to shoot an armed man was believed to create a motivation analogous to what a police officer faces every day—the danger of being killed. However, this desire to avoid a harsh consequence could result in a greater likelihood of false alarms where an innocent was accidentally shot. As we might expect, along with varying whether a given "target" was carrying a gun or some other, nonthreatening object, the researchers also varied the race of the target. Thus sometimes a White man appeared holding a gun, and other times he was holding a cell phone. Sometimes a Black man appeared holding a gun, and other times he was holding a wallet. The game was played in this manner for 80 trials (i.e., 80 targets appeared that participants had to either shoot or not shoot, based on their perception of the object in his hand). Over a series of experiments, a consistent pattern emerged. People were more likely to shoot an unarmed target if he was Black than if he was White. People were also more likely to correctly shoot an armed target if he was Black than if he was White. Speed of responding also supported the prediction. People were faster to fire at an armed Black man than an armed White man, and they were faster to decide not to fire at an unarmed White man than at an unarmed Black man. In summary, the decision to shoot may be determined by the perception of threat, and the perception of threat may be determined by a target person's group membership and processes of differential perception.

In another domain of extreme importance where confirmatory perception exerts itself outside the laboratory, the courtroom provides a fertile ground for stereotyping to influence attributions. The whole function of the trial in the American judicial system is to come up with an attribution—namely, to figure out who is to blame for some event. A particular individual is accused of being responsible, but this individual is to be presumed innocent until proven guilty. The prosecuting attorney is attempting to convince the jurors that they should attribute the cause of the crime to something related to the person being charged. Biases in judging the causes for events could well play an important role in determining how jurors reach verdicts. A defendant for whom jurors have a negative stereotype may be judged more harshly or deemed more likely to have committed a crime (the movie *12 Angry Men* provides an excellent illustration of this type of bias). More subtly, the way in which jurors interpret the evidence may be different for one defendant than for another. They may be more likely to make internal attributions for the negative actions, or even ambiguous actions, of a defendant whose behavior could potentially be linked (assimilated) to cultural stereotypes, as we have seen in the Duncan (1976) research. Typically, if the cause is seen as dispositional, the punishment is more severe. In addition, the amount of mental effort jurors are willing to exert in evaluating the evidence may be different for defendants from some social groups. When jurors have strong stereotypes, they may no longer be as likely to do their job as jurors and weigh the evidence as carefully as possible, falling prey instead to the bias to rely on judgments based on less effort (because the stereotypes that result in less effort allow them to feel confident enough in their evaluations without needing to exert more effort).

Bodenhausen and Wyer (1985) examined exactly these types of issues relating to a member of a stereotyped group who is accused of a crime. The question of concern was whether stereotypes are used as heuristics for making decisions about (1) interpretation of the evidence (which is likely to involve a great deal of ambiguity and be open to interpretation and subjectivity), (2) punishment for the criminal act, (3) the likelihood of recidivism, and (4) the willingness to grant parole. There are at least two broad ways in which the perception of why a defendant committed a crime can be guided by stereotypes. First, as a heuristic, a stereotype is immediately triggered by a heuristic cue (the group membership of the individual on trial), and is used from the very start as a least effortful way of making sense of the individual's action. Second, a stereotype may be turned to only after people thoroughly examined the information in a detailed and effortful way and are still left wanting an explanation—one the stereotype can then provide (they attempt to follow the instructions of the judicial system and weigh evidence carefully, turning to the stereotype only as a default when examining the evidence is insufficient).

How can we tell whether jurors are using stereotypes, and if they are, through what cognitive processes stereotypes are invoked—as heuristics or as the last resort? The first part of this question can be answered by modeling an experiment on Duncan (1976)—by giving different participants the same behavior to observe and manipulating the race of the person performing the behavior. For example, Bodenhausen and Wyer (1985) asked White participants to make decisions about guilt, punishment, and likelihood of recidivism for a criminal, whose case was described to them through a court transcript. The person was signaled to be either White or Hispanic (via the name and birthplace of the criminal—e.g., Juan from Puerto Rico). The crime committed by this person was also manipulated so that it was either consistent with or inconsistent with cultural stereotypes. Thus the crime was either an Enron-style white-collar crime, or a crime of a physical nature (beating up another person in a fight). Some participants read a scenario where a Puerto Rican committed a white-collar crime; some read a scenario where the Puerto Rican was involved in a barroom brawl; some read about a White man committing a white-collar crime; and, finally, some read about a White man whose crime was fighting in a barroom brawl. If stereotypes were being used as heuristics, then actions consistent with a stereotype should be judged in a stereotypic way, whereas actions not relevant to the stereotype should be judged in a manner unaffected by the stereotype. This logic hinged on principles reviewed in Chapters 9 and 10—that people are most likely to use accessible information, such as a stereotype, when the behavior they are observing is both open to interpretation (ambiguous) and relevant to the accessible information. A crime consistent with a stereotype would meet both of these criteria. A crime inconsistent with a stereotype would not meet these criteria (since it would not be relevant to the stereotype). According to this logic, the stereotype of Puerto Ricans would not be really relevant to a behavior concerning an accounting scandal. But it would be relevant to behavior concerning a fight. Thus, if participants used stereotypes as heuristics in their judgments of defendants, they should be more likely to make judgments of guilt and arrive at harsher penalties if a defendant was a member of a stereotyped group and the alleged crime could be construed as relevant to that stereotype.

The results supported this conclusion. People did not simply eschew stereotypes because they were asked to make judgments that were of real importance to another individual. Instead, when a member of a stereotyped group committed an infraction that was consistent with the stereotype of that group, the action was more likely to be seen as a stable quality of that person—the individual was seen as more personally responsible for those acts. The stereotype allowed the perceivers to see the crime as a more natural feature or characteristic of the criminal than when no relevant stereotype existed. The consequences of this were quite stern. When a crime was relevant to the stereotype that existed in mainstream U.S. culture regarding the defendant's group, perceivers recommended more severe punishment, judged the action as more likely to recur, and asserted that the person deserved harsher punishment to deter future infractions. Thus, when a White man and an Hispanic man both got arrested for being in a fight, the Hispanic man was judged as more likely to have been responsible and was therefore likely to get harsher punishment. The very same crime was perceived and judged in different ways as a function of defendants' ethnicity.

To assess the cognitive process that produced these results, Bodenhausen and Wyer (1985) used a memory measurement. The review of systematic and heuristic processing in Chapter 5 has revealed that when people process systematically, they pay greater attention to information, especially to arguments or facts that are relevant to the task at hand. This leads them to have better memory for such information (see Chapter 4). When people process heuristically, attention to details and facts is less important; instead, there is a superficial matching of information to the triggered heuristic that guides what they see, and therefore what they can later remember. Therefore, if stereotypes were being used as a last resort, only after having exhaustively analyzed the details of the information provided (the evidence), then the research participants should have good recall for the arguments and data about the case that were presented as the evidence. If they were heuristically processing, they should not be making fine-grained analyses of this information. Their recall should not be particularly better for information pertinent to the case.

To put this to the test, Bodenhausen and Wyer (1985) included various types of information in the transcripts summarizing the case. First, there was demographic information, irrelevant to why the crime occurred. Second, there was information describing events that happened after the transgression occurred, while the person was in prison. This information had nothing to do with why the transgression happened, but might be relevant to deciding about whether the person was rehabilitated and whether the transgression might occur again. Finally, there was information describing events in the person's life around the time the crime occurred that might be used to provide insight as to why it occurred. This information included some stereotype-consistent and some stereotype-inconsistent facts about the person. If participants were using stereotypes as heuristics, they should have no preferential recall for any of these types of information, because they were not scrutinizing the information in enough detail to realize that some of it was more relevant for making a good decision. However, if participants were systematically processing, they would have noted that some of this information was relevant to making an evaluation in an accurate manner, and they would have better recall for these types of information, having taken the time to scrutinize it carefully.

Sadly, the data revealed that people were not taking the time to scrutinize the information carefully when a stereotype was perceived as being consistent with a crime (their memory for the information was generally poorer than when there is not a relevant stereotype to fit the crime). Instead, they processed heuristically, paying no more attention to relevant information that could address why the crime occurred than they did to irrelevant information. They were superficially scanning the materials for some evidence that supported their stereotypes and using that evidence to guide their judgment, without even thinking in too much detail about that information. In fact, even when information inconsistent with a stereotype was provided, people were able to ignore it; their judgments were still biased, and their memory for the facts showed no trace of such information having been used (or at least any more so than perfectly irrelevant information).

Let us examine one last case of biased attributions, once again turning to an existing social problem to make the case: men's use of stereotypes in how they judge women (e.g., Fiske, 1993a). This particular form of biased attribution, and the psychological research that illustrates it, have even informed Supreme Court rulings on sexual harassment (e.g., *Price Waterhouse v. Hopkins*), with researchers called in to testify to the court about how such processes operate and can influence an employer's evaluations of employees without the employer realizing it or consciously intending it (Fiske, Bersoff, Borgida, Deaux, & Heilman, 1991). The first thing to establish is that, like ethnic stereotypes, gender stereotypes bias people's attributions.

Banaji, Hardin, and Rothman (1993) performed an experiment in which research participants were asked to read about a person who was acting in a manner that was mostly not relevant to gender stereotypes, but whose actions included a small subset of behaviors that were weakly related to the stereotype of women (e.g., the trait of dependence). Thus the behavior was ambiguous and open to interpretation. After reading about the behavior, the participants were asked to make judgments about the person and rate the degree to which the person could be described as "dependent." For half of the participants, the person performing this behavior was named Donald, signaling that he was male. For the other half of the participants, the person was named Donna, and was thus clearly female. Banaji and colleagues also manipulated the extent to which gender stereotypes were accessible at the time people were evaluating the behavior. Using the standard paradigm of asking participants to perform two "unrelated" tasks prior to reading about Donald/Donna, the participants were first asked to perform a task that they thought was unrelated to the judgment task, but that actually was being used to prime the stereotype of women. Specifically, half of the participants were primed to think about the trait of dependence, while half of the participants were primed with concepts neutral in regard to the stereotype.

The judgments reported by participants provided a clear illustration that stereotypes were guiding judgment. A man was never judged as highly dependent, based on the behavior described in the story; in fact, the more notions of dependence were accessible, the less likely a man was to be judged as dependent. However, a woman who performed ambiguous behavior that was at best weakly related to the domain of dependence was interpreted in a stereotype-confirming manner when the stereotype had been previously triggered. Thus, when notions of dependence had been primed in the first task, ratings of Donna indicated that participants saw her as highly dependent, thus fitting the stereotype of women. Interestingly, when participants had not been primed with notions of dependence, ratings of Donna did not suggest that she was particularly dependent. It appeared as if the name alone was not enough to initiate the use of the stereotype. Stereotype use required that the stereotype be made accessible prior to the encounter with the person, thus ensuring that it was activated and being used to interpret the actions of Donna.

Swim, Borgida, Maruyama, and Myers (1989) published a meta-analysis of research on how gender stereotypes bias evaluations of women. Somewhat surprisingly, "the size of the difference in ratings between female and male target persons was extremely small" (p. 419). Swim and colleagues, however, did not conclude that this means gender stereotypes do not exist or are not frequently used. For one thing, it is impossible to know whether gender stereotypes were even being triggered in the majority of the studies evaluated. While participants in those experiments certainly knew that they were evaluating either a woman or a man, this information may not have been enough to trigger stereotypes. As we have seen above, in the research of Banaji and colleagues (1993), stereotypes did have an impact on judgments of women, but only if they first were made accessible. Second, the use of gender stereotypes may depend on whether the performance dimension being evaluated is relevant to the stereotype. Recall that

Bodenhausen and Wyer (1985) found that an ethnic stereotype was not used if the behavior provided about the person was not relevant to the stereotype. Gender stereotypes should operate with the same limitations. People should not uniformly rate women as inferior to men, but should rate them as inferior only in domains where the stereotype specifies that women should be seen as weaker. In addition, as we have reviewed in Chapter 5, when information that is highly diagnostic and that opposes a stereotype is encountered, people stop relying on stereotypes and begin to process in a more individuating fashion. Thus we would need to keep in mind whether the information being received fits this description. Third, in keeping with the argument raised earlier about shifting standards, it is impossible to know whether people are seeing men and women equally or using a different standard when reporting their subjective evaluations. The conclusion that gender stereotypes are not being used must be tempered by the fact that they may very well be used in more objective ratings.

Thus, while there is much existing evidence to support the fact that people's gender stereotypes bias their evaluations, this is not a clear and simple conclusion that we can draw. It will depend on a host of factors that similarly govern the use of any stereotype. The behavior being interpreted must be somewhat ambiguous; the perceiver must not be highly motivated to be accurate or fair; the behavior being evaluated must be able to be construed as relevant to the stereotype; and gender must be at least salient enough for the individual to be categorized according to gender, and for the stereotype linked to that category to be potentially activated. Unfortunately for many women, these precise conditions are often met in the workplace. Women may be present in smaller numbers and thus likely to be categorized according to gender. If they are not present in smaller numbers, the job may be fairly sex-typed, making gender roles likely to be triggered. Work environments are typically a constant source of cognitive load, with people racing to get many tasks done; thus they often have no incentive to engage in systematic processing, but instead have a need for structure that promotes heuristic processing. These conditions may make gender stereotyping even more likely in the work environment than in the laboratory. This leads us to the real-world examples provided by Fiske (1993a).

One way gender stereotypes can be used that leads to potential discrimination is this: They may lead men to describe women in very restrictive terms that are consistent with the roles specified by their stereotype of women. This can create a hostile work environment by leading men to exhibit an inability to react to women in ways that deviate too much from the description specified by the stereotype. This leads men to think of women not primarily as coworkers, but as potential sexual partners; not as competent computer programmers, but as bad at math and computing; and so on. Fiske (1993a) describes the case of Lois Robinson, a welder at a Jacksonville shipyard who was constantly made the target of lewd comments and exposed to obscene material pasted and written on the walls, depicting women in demeaning ways. Stereotypes in this way serve to *describe* women in ways that create a hostile environment and anchor any interpretation of their behavior close to the cultural stereotype.

A second way stereotypes bias judgment is not in the way they describe women, but in the way they *prescribe* women. Fiske (1993a; see also Fisk et al., 1991) describes the case of an accomplished accountant, Ann Hopkins, who was denied promotion to partner at her firm because her achievements were attributed to an overaggressiveness and "bitchiness" rather than to competence and high levels of skill. The evaluators were men. The Hopkins case reveals to us that a woman is not always interpreted as being consistent with the stereotype; she was not seen as weak and emotional, but as hard, cold, and tough. The male evaluators were not using the stereotype to describe her, but to fence her in. Prescriptive stereotypes limit the type of behavior that is seen as acceptable and detail how a woman *should* act, as prescribed by the stereotype of women. The men in Hopkins's firm were using the stereotype in a prescriptive (not descriptive) way, adjusting their opinion of Hopkins to preserve the stereotype, with her behavior being interpreted differently from the same behavior performed by a man.

Perceptual Confirmation and Biased Hypothesis Testing

Chapter 3 has reviewed an experiment by Darley and Gross (1983) that illustrated how stereotypes about a person can be made accessible and then guide judgment, despite the person not being aware of this influence. Research participants watched a videotape of a little girl named Hannah; half of them saw her play in an affluent neighborhood, while the other half watched her play in a poor neighborhood. The play area depicted in the videotape essentially activated the stereotypes of "rich" and "poor" people. Participants were next described as seeing another videotape of the girl performing at school and taking a test said to assess her academic ability. Importantly, this videotape was made in such a way so that Hannah's performance on the test provided no conclusive evidence regarding her academic abilities. She was seen answering both difficult and simple questions correctly, as well as failing to answer such questions correctly. This meets our definition of an ambiguous behavior. What Chapter 3 has not indicated was that this described only half of the experiment. Another set of participants had the categories "rich" and "poor" primed, but then proceeded to make judgments about the girl's academic ability without the benefit of having observed her ambiguous performance on the test. Essentially, they were asked to make judgments without any information on which to base that judgment.

The findings revealed that the effects of stereotypes on judgment, which we have been reviewing in this chapter, do not occur inevitably and automatically. Instead, people only exhibit evidence of bias when they have what they believe to be a valid basis for making a judgment—some evidence on which to base their judgment. When participants in this study were asked to make a judgment of the child's ability based solely on knowing she was rich or poor (without having seen any information about her academic ability on the second videotape), their ratings of her academic ability were not biased. If they were told she was in the fourth grade, they rated her ability as being at a fourth-grade level, regardless of whether they had been primed with the stereotypes of "rich" or "poor." Participants were not licensed to assert any type of impression, because there did not exist any relevant behavioral information on which to base any assertions about the girl's performance. However, as soon as information relevant to academic ability was provided, the stereotypes came rushing to judgment. As we would expect if people were relying on accessible categories to make judgments, the people primed with "rich" judged her to be above average in academic ability, while the people primed with "poor" rated her below average in academic ability.

Based on their findings, Darley and Gross (1983) proposed a two-step process through which stereotypes exert their impact. Initially, perceivers develop a hypothesis about what might cause the behavior they are observing, and this hypothesis is usually based on a stereotype. However, factors such as their goals or the pressures of the situation may cause them to want to be somewhat diagnostic, or to have a valid opinion (they must feel licensed to use this stereotype). Thus people typically refrain from using their hypotheses/stereotypes until tested. Thus, if they are asked for a judgment prior to having engaged in such a test, they should not have an evaluation they are willing to offer in one direction or the other. Next, perceivers put the hypothesis to the test, endorsing the stereotype and allowing it to bias judgment only after gathering supporting, hypothesis-confirming information. This suggests a somewhat happy conclusion: People only judge other people according to a stereotype if they feel that there is some evidence on which to base a judgment or if they deem the target "judgeable." The somewhat unhappy qualification of this statement is that the amount of evidence it takes for perceivers to decide that a target is "judgeable" is quite small, because they have a hypothesis-confirming bias. Even ambiguous behavior that does not provide clear evidence for the stereotype is taken to be evidence supporting the stereotype. People do not seek evidence that would disconfirm the stereotype. They pursue the easier strategy of seeking to keep rather than revise their existing beliefs—a confirmation effect. In the Darley and Gross experiment, Hannah was judged in a stereotypic way when all that was provided was vague feedback about her ability.

Yzerbyt, Schadron, Leyens, and Rocher (1994) have summarized this effect by describing people as not seeking to be informed, but seeking the *illusion of being informed*. Yzerbyt and colleagues offer a slightly different interpretation of Darley and Gross's conclusion. Rather than perceivers requiring a test of their hypotheses, and only forming a biased impression after such a test has occurred, they simply require a feeling that the target is worthy of being judged; the perceivers feel entitled to judge the person. To test this, these researchers led participants to believe they had been informed about what another person was like, when in fact no such information was provided. The participants had the illusion of having information, and thus were provided with the sense that they were entitled to judge the person, even without hypothesis testing. Thus category information alone would not be enough to trigger a biased judgment, because it would not provide the sense of "social judgeability" that people require to assert their stereotypes into judgments. However, if participants believed they received individuating information about the person, they should feel entitled to make a judgment and to use stereotypes. How did Yzerbyt and colleagues make people think they had such information? They told some people the information was being subliminally presented (outside of conscious awareness) throughout the experiment. The results showed that people with the illusion of being informed about the person were more likely to use stereotypes in forming impressions. If they perceived having some evidence to support their views, they felt licensed to use their stereotypes.

Subtyping

As seen in the Darley and Gross (1983) study, people engage in a biased form of hypothesis testing that allows them to confirm their stereotypes. To allow themselves to feel as if they have "justifiable evidence" for their stereotypes, even if the evidence is inconclusive, people ask these questions: "Can the behavior I have observed be seen as evidence in support of a hypothesis I already have about the person? Does it support my stereotype?" Darley and Gross found that people are all too willing to answer "yes" to this question and infer that the observed behavior supports the stereotype (hypothesis) that they are supposedly "testing." They see supporting evidence everywhere, even when the behavior of others is ambiguous at best.

Kunda and Oleson (1995) have proposed that when the evidence is not so ambiguous, and it instead provides information that suggests the stereotype is not useful for describing this person, people ask a different question that *still allows them to maintain their stereotypes*: "Do I have evidence for concluding that this person is unrepresentative of his/her group?" Therefore, even when a person's behavior clearly violates the stereotype, people again seek evidence in support of a hypothesis, except this time the hypothesis is that this person is atypical of the group. If this hypothesis is supported, there is no need to revise the stereotype. This individual is instead classified as an exception to the rule, or as a unique case of the stereotyped group—a *subtype*. As Kunda and Oleson put it, "when people encounter group members who violate a group stereotype . . . they 'fence off' these members by assuming that they constitute a distinct subtype of the group" (p. 565).

Kunda and Oleson (1995) review two general points about subtyping. First, more subtyping (less stereotype change) occurs when the disconfirming information that exists is concentrated in a small number of people. When the evidence is spread out across many people, it is more difficult to readily assign this large group of people to some subtype. Second, subtyping is promoted when the "deviant" person—the one who is acting in a manner inconsistent with the stereotype—is atypical of the group in general. That is, the more dimensions on which this person is inconsistent with the group stereotype, the more likely he/she is to be subtyped, and the less the perceiver needs to revise the group stereotype. The more stereotype-disconfirming attributes there are that make a person atypical of the group, the more reasons (or potential justification) the perceiver has for subtyping the person and separating him/her (fencing him/her off) from the group more generally.

In their research, Kunda and Oleson (1995) predicted that when a person acted in a way inconsistent with a stereotype (here, the stereotype of lawyers as extraverts), the stereotype would not always be revised. Instead, the person might be seen as different from the rest of the group, to whom the stereotype would still be applied. Perceivers might point to any possible rationale to justify labeling the person as different from the group. Even irrelevant information about the person would get creatively used to justify not altering the global stereotype. Some people in the experiment (the control group) simply rated how extraverted lawyers were. But how would people rate lawyers on this dimension when they encountered a lawyer who was an introvert? Would they change their stereotype of lawyers so that lawyers were now rated as less extraverted? They might, but the interesting prediction here was that irrelevant information about the lawyer, provided along with the information that he was an introvert, would stop people from altering the stereotype and instead promote subtyping this lawyer (because people would use it to support a theory about why this lawyer was more introverted than other lawyers).

Some participants were provided with irrelevant information (irrelevant in that it had nothing to do with how introverted he was). For example, the introverted lawyer was said to work for a small firm. Other participants were given no additional information (they were told only that he was an introvert and a lawyer). Finally, people indicated their beliefs about lawyers by rating the group (i.e., they indicated on a scale of 0–10 how extraverted lawyers were). Despite the fact that people were told the person was an introvert, their ratings of how extraverted lawyers were differed as a function of whether additional information was provided. When additional (but irrelevant) information was provided, people saw lawyers as more extraverted than when no additional information was provided, and just as extraverted as people in the control group. Thus, when no additional information existed, people generalized from this lawyer to all lawyers, altering their global stereotype. However, creating a subtype by making use of whatever information was available (e.g., he was in a small firm) protected the stereotype from being altered. How does subtyping work to preserve and protect stereotypes?

By allowing any information inconsistent with the stereotype of the group more gener-ally to be seen as unique to the subtype of the group. Spike Lee's film *Do the Right Thing* illustrates this process well. A young Italian American character explains to a Black coworker how it is possible for an Italian American like himself to hate Blacks, but have all his idols be black men (Michael Jordan, Prince, etc.). His explanation amounts to lit-tle more then subtyping. Blacks are, he explains, "niggers," whereas these few excep-tions are something different. They are, he explains, "more than Black." They are a sep-arate category, and their positive acts, therefore, do not alter his perception of the group more generally.

Biased Attributions by Members of Stereotyped Groups

How does the fact that people routinely use stereotypes in judging others affect the attributions of those others who are so often the recipients of those stereotyped judg-ments? Such "targets" of bias develop expectancies that people will be biased against them, promoting an attributional style that helps them to confirm that they are in fact the targets of stereotypes. Dion and Earn (1975) had Jewish research participants per-form a ticket exchange task with three non-Jewish students. Some of the Jewish partici-pants were asked to provide background information that made the other (non-Jewish) players aware of the fact that they were Jewish. Other Jewish participants provided triv-ial background information. After completing the task, all the players were told that they had failed severely compared to the other players. They then made ratings of both themselves and their opponents. These ratings revealed that the Jewish participants attributed their failure to anti-Semitism and reported feeling more aggression, sadness, anxiety, and egoism—but only when the other people in the game were aware that the participants were Jewish. An attributional style emerged in which failure was seen as caused by the bias of others, not the participants' own shortcomings.

Kleck and Strenta (1980) illustrated the same point, using persons who appeared to have a negatively valued physical condition. Participants were told that the experiment-ers were interested in how people would be affected by interacting with individuals who have a variety of physical conditions. They were randomly assigned to one of three con-ditions: people with a facial scar, people with epilepsy, and people with an allergy. Par-ticipants assigned to the epilepsy and allergy conditions were asked to lie on a fake bio-graphical essay, and to indicate to another person that they had either "a mild allergy" or "a mild form of epilepsy." Each person in the facial scar condition had a cosmetic scar applied to his/her face. Thus each participant thought he/she would be interacting with a person who believed them to have one of three physical conditions. In reality, the interaction partner never received the fake biographical information. In addition, the partner never saw the scars on the faces of people in the scar condition, because an experimenter secretly wiped the scar off each person's face before the interaction occurred. The findings revealed that the participants in the scar and epilepsy groups perceived that their "medical conditions" caused the interaction partner to act nega-tively toward them. In reality, the behavior could not have been determined by such ste-reotypes, because the partner did not really know what type of condition each partici-pant supposedly suffered from.

In a similar vein, Crocker, Voelkl, Testa, and Major (1991) had African American students receive positive or negative feedback from a White evaluator. Half of the par-ticipants believed that the evaluator knew their race (because the evaluator was said to be watching them through a one-way mirror), and the other half believed that the evalu-ator did not know their race (because the blinds on the one-way mirror were pulled shut). The participants were then shown either a very favorable or a very unfavorable response from the evaluator. The participants then rated how various factors may have influenced the evaluator's responses toward them, including how much they felt they had been the recipient of a stereotypical reaction from this other person. The findings revealed that when African American participants thought that they could be seen by the evaluator, they believed the unfavorable feedback was especially likely to have been caused not by the evaluator disliking them personally because of the traits and behaviors described on the forms, but because of stereotyping. The only condition in which the African American participants did not attribute prejudice to their evaluator was when positive feedback was received and the evaluator was unaware of their race. Thus when they thought the other person knew their race, even in the condition in which they received positive feedback, they were likely to discount the feedback. Major and Crocker (1993) proposed that members of stereotyped groups are placed in a unique conflict when attempting to understand why they are treated as they are by other people in their social world. The members of these groups are faced with *attributional ambiguity*, because they are unsure whether the feedback they receive from others reflects a bias against their own social category/group memberships. They resolve this ambiguity by assuming that others are biased against them.

However, Taylor, Wright, and Porter (1994) report a finding that is almost the opposite of this attributional ambiguity finding. They suggest that members of stereotyped groups may actually minimize the prejudice that they feel personally affects them, even though they are well aware of the problem at the societal level. Instead of seeing stereotyping against them everywhere they look, they instead refuse to see stereotyping against them, and are unlikely to use discrimination as an explanation for negative feedback that they receive! This has been dubbed the *personal–group discrimination discrepancy*. Their research shows that the only time members of stereotyped groups attribute negative feedback to prejudice is when it clearly is attributable to prejudice, and the bias cannot be denied. If there is ambiguity, then (unlike what Major and Crocker suggest) Ruggiero and Taylor (1995) find that members of stereotyped groups minimize perceptions of prejudice and take responsibility for the failure, rather than blaming it on the bias of others.

How can we reconcile these diametrically opposed findings? Operario and Fiske (2001) hypothesized that the types of attributions formed by members of stereotyped groups regarding the bias inherent in other people may depend on how strongly the members identify with their group. According to Operario and Fiske (2001, p. 551), individuals who are highly identified with their group in the sense that they "derive personal and emotional meaning from their social category" should be more likely to attribute negative feedback to prejudice in an ambiguous interpersonal situation than group members who rate themselves low on group identification.

THE CONFIRMATORY BIAS IN MEMORY

Imagine you are asked to read about one person describing another person's house to a third party. This person mentions all types of details, from structural issues, to exquisite artwork, to alarm systems. Now imagine you are told that the two people discussing this house are burglars. It is quite likely that the information you attend to, encode, and later remember will be quite different than if you are led to expect that the two people are interior designers (e.g., Anderson & Pichert, 1978). What you remember is biased by how information is being encoded—what subset of the information your stereotypes and schemas direct you to. However, what you remember is not only determined by what you put into memory (and whether it is distorted in favor of stereotype-consistent information), but what you pull out of memory. Even if you encode this information in a perfectly nonstereotypic way, you may still retrieve selectively only the stereotype-consistent bits of information when looking back on the event/person.

Illusory Correlation

Illusory correlation (discussed in Chapter 3) is a term introduced by Chapman (1967) to describe the fact that people sometimes see two things as being related when in fact there is no relationship between them at all. Two events are deemed as more likely to co-occur than another two events that co-occur just as frequently. A basis for an illusory correlation exists whenever previous experience suggests a relationship between two things. Hamilton and Rose (1980) have proposed that stereotypes cause illusory correlations, because a stereotype is such a perceived relationship between two things—group membership and some traits/behaviors. They predict that if one of the items in the correlation is activated, such as group membership, then people will pay more attention to the other, such as the traits and behaviors expected to accompany it. Thus, because perceivers expect a correlation, they come to see a correlation that isn't really there, believing that they see more evidence in support of the stereotype than they actually do. Even if stereotype-consistent behaviors occur just as often as, and no more often than, irrelevant behaviors, people will think the consistent behaviors actually occurred more than they did. Similarly, if stereotype-inconsistent behaviors are just as likely as irrelevant ones, people will come to see them as less prevalent. They will perceive a correlation (albeit a negative one) when it does not really exist. This then gets reflected in later recall for the evidence. Their memory will be that a large amount of stereotype-consistent and a small amount of stereotype-inconsistent behavior were observed.

Depth of Processing

As reviewed in Chapter 4, deeper, more elaborate processing of information at the encoding stage leads to better retrieval of that information later, when memory for the information is being tested (Craik & Lockhart, 1972). And the relationship between some new piece of information and a schema has been shown in Chapter 4 to determine how elaborately it is processed. Information consistent with a stereotype/schema is not processed as deeply as information inconsistent with the stereotype. This has been shown to lead to the unusual finding that people recall information about a person that does not play a heavy role in what they think about the person. They use the information consistent with the stereotype fairly effortlessly in their judgment, while expending mental effort to make sense of the incongruent information. This greater depth of processing leads to better memory for information inconsistent with the stereotype, despite the confirmatory bias observed in their judgment (e.g., Hastie & Kumar, 1979).

However, there are also times (notably, when people's expectancies are weak or are first developing) in which both recall and judgment show a confirmatory bias, with stereotype-consistent information being recalled better than stereotype-inconsistent information (for a review, see Chapters 4 and 12). Rothbart, Evans, and Fulero (1979) have provided evidence of this confirmatory bias in memory, and attributed it to the

manner in which information is processed at encoding. They asked research participants to memorize a set of 50 behaviors. Of these 50, 17 were *friendly* behaviors, 17
were *intelligent* behaviors, 3 were *unfriendly*, 3 were *nonintelligent*, and 10 were irrelevant
to these domains. Two key variables were then manipulated. First, half of the people
were told these behaviors described a group that was generally friendly, while half of
the people were told the behaviors described a group that was generally intelligent. Second, half of the people were given this stereotype about the group before receiving the
information, and half were given the expectancy after having read all 50 behaviors.
Rothbart and colleagues predicted that if a confirmatory bias existed in memory, they
should see better recall for the information consistent with the stereotype. In addition,
if this was due to the depth of processing that occurred at encoding, then the bias
should only emerge when people were given the expectancy before reading the behavior, so that the stereotype was accessible at the moment they were encoding the information.

This was precisely what was found. Participants who were given the stereotype
prior to receiving the behavioral information were later shown to remember information in a biased way. If told the group was intelligent, they recalled more intelligent than
friendly behaviors. If told the group was friendly, they recalled more friendly behaviors.
In addition, when asked to estimate how many of the 50 behaviors were relevant to the
stereotype (remember, there were 17 friendly and 17 intelligent behaviors actually presented), there was a tendency to estimate in a way biased by the stereotype. If participants were told the group was intelligent, then more of the behaviors were assumed to
be about intelligence than friendliness (and vice versa). However, this pattern of confirmatory recall did not emerge when the stereotype was presented after the list of behaviors was read. This suggested that confirmatory memory bias, in this experiment, happened because of information processing occurring while the behavioral information
was being encoded.

Reconstructed Memory

The research reviewed above on illusory correlation and depth of processing showed
that stereotypes bias memory because they alter the way information is initially
encoded. Thus what is stored in the mind and available to be remembered is different
when a stereotype is present versus not present. As such, the processes of retrieving
information from memory are not truly biased, but memory is biased because it is
reflecting biases that took place when the information was initially being interpreted.
Another way in which stereotypes may affect recall is to lead perceivers to selectively
recall information that fits their stereotypes. They may not even know that a person is a
member of a stereotyped group when they first encounter that person, but then they
may get this information later on. Do people, upon learning a stereotype, use their
retrieval processes in a biased way to reconstruct events from the past to fit what they
currently think? If what they currently think is a stereotype, it will change what they
actually remember about the past. To demonstrate this selective reconstruction of past
events, Snyder and Uranowitz (1978) presented participants with a fictional description
of a woman called Betty K. The case history of Betty followed her from birth through
school and into adulthood. It provided information about her early home life, her relationship with her parents, her social life in high school and college, and so forth. However, her history was carefully constructed so that while it in no way suggested Betty was
a lesbian, some of the statements could be seen as perfectly consistent with the stereo-

type of lesbians (e.g., "Though she never had a steady boyfriend in high school, she did go out on dates"). The participants were told that their task was to form an impression of Betty.

Participants were later asked to remember the facts about Betty by taking a multiple-choice test. However, there was one twist. Just before taking the memory test, half of the people were told that Betty later became a lesbian; the other half were told that she was later married to a man. The test contained items meant to detect whether the stereotype was biasing memory. For example: "In high school, Betty (a) occasionally dated men, (b) never went out with men, (c) went steady, (d) no information provided." The answer that would show biased recall would be "b," since this is part of the stereotype of lesbians and was not stated in the case history. If people who thought Betty was a lesbian responded "b" more often than people who thought she was heterosexual, then this would be evidence that their recall of the facts was being twisted. As predicted, the researchers found that when given the label "lesbian" for Betty, people made more errors on test items that were potentially relevant to lesbianism. They inaccurately recalled receiving information in the original story that was consistent with Betty's being a lesbian but was not actually presented.

What do the Snyder and Uranowitz (1978) findings reveal about how memory works? One possibility is that the participants twisted their memory of information so that it came to be seen as consistent with a stereotype. Thus, even though a stereotype was not available in memory as the information about Betty was being encoded, its later activation reorganized the memory structure so that information consistent with the stereotype of lesbians was more likely to be retrieved. A second possibility is that people were simply guessing on the multiple-choice test and using their stereotypes to help them guess. In essence, memory was not affected at all, just the responses people made. A third possibility is that the stereotype made the perceivers desire to see the target person as consistent with the stereotype, thus leading them to reanalyze the behavior of the person in a stereotype-confirming manner. A fourth possibility is that the participants used stereotypes to generate a set of stereotype-consistent possible behaviors, based on the stored representation of the stereotype and not on the actual information about the person. In this case, people would have made more errors on the multiple-choice test not because they selectively altered their prior beliefs about Betty or because the stereotype made congruent information more available in memory, but because they generated new behaviors based on their stereotype, which they then added to what they thought was information provided about the person (Belleza & Bower, 1981). It is likely that all of these processes can occur under different circumstances.

CODA

The cognitive process in stereotyping, as suggested by Allport (1954), assumes that stereotyping is much like any other inference or judgment we humans make. We label a person as belonging to a group (categorization), and then we have a set of beliefs and characteristics (inferences) triggered that we see as belonging to that group. This is our stereotype for that group. Just as we often use implicit personality theories to assume that a person we have labeled as a liar may also be untrustworthy, we often use our stereotypes to assume that a person who is a member of Group X is likely to have the characteristics we associate with people from Group X.

According to Allport (1954), the cognitive process in stereotyping has several features. First, stereotypes are triggered so that the most dominant association to a cue is what is activated by the presence of that cue. Second, contradictory evidence is likely to be rejected. Third, evidence conflicting with a stereotype may be distorted so it is seen as confirming the stereotype. Fourth, stereotypes resist change; rather than altering stereotypes in the face of disconfirming evidence, we see exceptions and create subtypes. Stereotypes have an impact on how we identify a new object or person, especially when his/her behavior is ambiguous and open to interpretation. We apply stereotypes more readily than other, competing explanations for behavior. Finally, we can recall evidence consistent with our stereotypes more readily than we can recall other types of behaviors we have observed that are either irrelevant to or inconsistent with the stereotypes. In summary, stereotyping is not merely the product of disturbed individuals or unconscious forces that haunt the psyche. The basic building blocks for prejudice—reactions to others in stereotypic and categorical ways—are by-products of very normal perceptual processes.

In conclusion, stereotype use may not be technically inevitable, because (1) processes of hypothesis testing alert us that the stereotype is not licensed to be used in a given instance, or (2) our goals make us desire to exert greater processing effort (as reviewed in Chapter 5). But the reality—given our motives to rely on effortless processing, and given the functionality of the stereotypes—is that we usually find ways to confirm our hypotheses and to use stereotypes, even when we become aware of them. This fact, compounded with the notion that we are often not even aware stereotypes are influencing us in the first place, is what makes stereotyping such a pressing social issue.

Note

1. Given that it measures associations between positive affect and some category, the IAT presents a potentially useful way to test self-esteem accurately. Without the bias of the conscious need to feel positively about the self, the IAT could be used to assess the implicit association of positive or negative affect with the self-concept (Greenwald & Farnham, 2000).

12 Control of Stereotypes and Expectancies

Stereotyping has been said to result from two distinct processes, each of which can occur rather effortlessly and mindlessly (without conscious awareness or intent). The first process is the triggering (activation) of the stereotype, given the presence of people who are members of a stereotyped group (or the symbolic equivalence of their presence, such as mention of their group membership, a description of a person from the group, imagining interacting with someone from the group, etc.). The second process is the decision whether to use that stereotype (e.g., in one's impression and memory of a given person). Just as with the activation of stereotypes, the use of stereotypes in guiding one's judgment and memory can occur implicitly, reflecting a search for stereotype-confirming information. Even something as effortful-sounding as "hypothesis testing" (where the hypothesis is one's stereotype) can occur in a fairly effortless and somewhat biased fashion.

Just because the use of stereotypes can be effortless and mindless, must it be inevitable? Granted, people are often not aware of stereotypes' impact on their judgment, and may even cling to a belief that they exert no impact (naive realism). But does this mean that people cannot be made aware of such a bias and then decide to try to prevent the use of stereotypes in their judgment? A large body of research illustrates that even if the first process (stereotype activation) is inevitable, there need be no reason to assume that the same is true of the second process (stereotype use). Stereotype use may often proceed outside of awareness, but people are nonetheless capable of controlling stereotypes if they intend to. Even before research was able to support this idea, most people have accepted it as fact, believing that they have the will and the way to be fair-minded. The foundation of the American creed is that if they intend to, people can prevent themselves from stereotyping. The U.S. Constitution and civil rights laws demand it of them (as well as the Judeo-Christian ethic that forms the basis of the American creed); the laws of the land in America dictate that all people are created as, and should be treated as, equals.

Chapter 5 has reviewed two general sets of factors that prevent people from engaging in heuristic/stereotypic/top-down processing. The first is that the evidence or data may cause people to doubt the validity of their beliefs and opinions formed on the basis of heuristics, schemas, and stereotypes. That is, the evidence/data cause their confidence in a stereotypic judgment to be shifted below some hypothetical sufficiency threshold. The second is that people may adopt goals that raise the level of confidence they desire, so that stereotypes, and the judgments formed on the basis of stereotypes, are no longer deemed acceptable or sufficient. Instead, increased desire for accuracy and judgmental confidence will lead to putting increased effort toward personalizing the target individual and engaging in deliberative and systematic processing. In this chapter, these two themes are explored again and applied to stereotyping. After exploring how stereotypes are controlled once they are activated, the discussion will shift toward a second, more proactive form of stereotype control—examining whether the activation of stereotypes can be controlled.

HOW STEREOTYPE-INCONSISTENT INFORMATION UNDERMINES STEREOTYPING

What triggers systematic processing, as opposed to an overgeneralized application of stereotypes? As reviewed in Chapter 5, one factor is that a person may be led to experience doubt, or a lack of confidence, in judgments that were formed based on theory-driven types of thinking (such as stereotypes). Judgmental confidence is often undermined by the behavior of the person the perceiver is interacting with, especially if that behavior is counterstereotypic or inconsistent with the expectancies the perceiver has brought to the interaction. Such behavior is memorable and shapes judgment.

A Paradox

Chapter 11 has reviewed evidence that memory is biased in a stereotype-confirming manner. This introduces a seeming paradox, because that conclusion is at odds with the conclusion just drawn (above) and explored in some detail in Chapter 4—that people have better memory for stereotype-inconsistent information. The mental energy (depth of processing) required to make sense out of the inconsistent information (coherence building) is said to make it especially likely to be attended to and remembered (e.g., Bargh & Thein, 1985; Sherman, Lee, Bessenoff, & Frost, 1998). How can one set of research findings indicate that memory is biased toward stereotype-confirming information, while another set of findings suggests that memory is biased toward stereotype-incongruent information? What situations trigger systematic processing of inconsistent information so that such information is better recalled (vs. leaving people to use stereotypes in guiding what is remembered and showing a bias for stereotype-confirming information in memory)? Once this has been answered, the logical next question is whether systematic processing influences not only recall, but impression formation, thus delivering stereotype control.

Memory Bias Revisited: Stereotype Strength

Stangor and Ruble (1989) argue that a factor determining whether one elaborately evaluates stereotype-inconsistent information, and thus reveals a bias toward better recall for such information, is how well developed the stereotype is. Even if a stereotype is weak, not well formed, or still developing, it may have enough of a mental structure for one to try to keep the stereotype together and have it guide one's impressions (as opposed to rejecting the young stereotype altogether). However, for such a young stereotype, high enough "fences" have not yet been built to allow one simply to disregard inconsistent information. Thus, for a developing stereotype, there might be one set of findings: Stereotypes guide judgment, but stereotype-inconsistent information predominates in memory because of the effort one has to exert to incorporate it into the stereotype in a manner that allows the structure of the stereotype to remain unscathed. Stronger, well-developed stereotypes, however, may enable one to reject stereotype-inconsistent information altogether, or at least to rationalize it away with relatively little effort needed. For example, one may be better able to discount such information, or make attributions to the situation rather than to the disposition of the person (e.g., Crocker, Hannah, & Weber, 1983). In contrast to the findings with weak stereotypes, strong stereotypes would guide both judgment and memory in a stereotype-confirming way. As Stangor and Ruble (1989, p. 20) put it, "strong expectations will lead perceivers to 'filter' or ignore inconsistent information, in an attempt to maintain the established expectancy intact . . . they rely on 'top down' rather than 'bottom up' processes to guide impression formation."

Stangor and Ruble (1989) tested the idea that stereotype strength determines the stereotype's impact on memory. They created two fictitious groups—one described with behaviors that were predominantly extraverted, and one described with behaviors that were predominantly introverted. They then had research participants read 60 behaviors about these groups, asked them to form impressions, and also tested recall for the behaviors. However, for some of the participants there was an opportunity to first form an expectancy about the groups. They first read a separate set of behaviors strongly suggesting that one group was composed of extraverts, the other of introverts. After having formed the expectancy, they then read and evaluated the set of 60 behaviors. Thus one group of participants was developing an expectancy as they were reading the 60 behaviors; the other group had already formed an expectancy before exposure to these behaviors. According to the logic outlined above, the people with the more developed expectancy should be more likely to show a stereotype-confirming bias in memory. This was what was found. When people had formed an expectancy prior to reading the "target information," they recalled proportionately more extraverted than introverted behaviors about the group that was extraverted (and more introverted behaviors about the introverted group)—a stereotype-confirming bias. However, when there was no expectancy developed beforehand, there was no stereotype-confirming bias in memory. The proportion of extraverted behaviors recalled did not differ from the proportion of introverted behaviors.

As a caveat before this section ends, it should be stated that there is not overwhelming evidence for this point that stronger stereotypes always lead to memory being biased in favor of consistent information. There have not been many experiments on this issue; also, some of the experiments in support of this idea rely on age (the length of time one has known the stereotype) as a reflection of strength, and age need not be the same thing as strength. Indeed, some of the research could be seen as promoting the opposite conclusion regarding the relationship between stereotype strength and bias. Srull (1981) showed that perceivers who observe individual targets (specific people as opposed to a group of people) have greater memory for items inconsistent with their expectancies. Srull argued that perceivers have stronger expectancies for consistent behavior to be performed by individuals than by collectives or groups.[1] Thus Srull's findings show superior recall for inconsistent information when expectancies are strong, if we accept that expectancies held toward individuals are stronger than expectancies held toward groups. In contrast, the Stangor and Ruble (1989) work shows superior recall for inconsistent information when expectancies are weak. In summary, there seems to be an association between stereotype strength and memory for consistent versus inconsistent information; however, researchers have not yet perfectly worked out all the moderating factors that determine the nature of this association.

Memory Bias Revisited: Behavior That Is Diagnostic of Nonstereotypic Concepts

The results of Stangor and Ruble (1989) might lead us to conclude that elaborate, systematic, personalized processing of information is only possible when a stereotype is still developing or is weakly held. Does this mean that for minorities and other stereotyped groups that face strong and long-standing biases, there is little hope that stereotype-inconsistent and expectancy-disconfirming information will be noticed, be processed, or have influence? The literature suggests that this is not the case, as does intuition. In the United States, part of the rationale for desegregating schools, school busing programs, and the landmark 1954 *Brown v. Board of Education* case was that contact among members of disparate groups would expose them to counterstereotypic behavior—and with exposure to such behavior, stereotypes would change and prejudice would be reduced, along with discriminatory behavior. Because of these policies, we may all intuitively accept that coming into contact with people who behave in ways that violate our stereotypes will allow those stereotypes to change.

However, such contact and such exposure to counterstereotypic behavior do not guarantee that stereotypes will not continue to bias how we judge others and what we recall. As Allport (1954) noted, the case is not so simple as merely bringing people together. Contact between people at a superficial level may do little to reduce prejudice and stereotypes, and can even at times lead to increased prejudice (even if behavior inconsistent with the stereotype is routinely performed and seen). Thus children who are bused to schools for the purpose of providing contact, but who then self-segregate themselves at lunch in the cafeteria, in the gym, and in the social groups they form, are not coming into meaningful contact. The *contact hypothesis* (Allport, 1954; Pettigrew, 1997) asserts that several ingredients need to be in place to promote positive effects due to contact: The people in contact must have interactions with each other; they must have equal status in these contact situations; they should pursue common goals; and the situation they are in should promote a norm of equality between groups (i.e., there should be social support that sanctions all groups as equals). Finally, *the behavior observed in the course of the contact must provide the data—the counterstereotypic behavioral evidence—that will allow the stereotype to be dispelled.*

However, as we have seen, people with stereotypes strongly in place seem to have a harder time recalling stereotype-inconsistent information (relative to consistent information). They are also more likely to perceive behavior that is slightly ambiguous in a way that is consistent with their stereotypes. Thus, in addition to contact bringing people together, the behavior that is enacted by the stereotyped group must be clear and consistent enough to challenge the existing stereotypes and break the stereotype-confirming biases in judgment and recall (e.g., Hamilton & Rose, 1980; Locksley, Hepburn, & Ortiz, 1982). For example, work on illusory correlation has shown that even when people are exposed to information that does not suggest a relationship between a particular type of behavior (such as assertiveness) and a particular group of people (such as salespeople), such a relationship is perceived anyway. Illusory correlations do not merely occur because people see an imaginary positive correlation between stereotype-related behaviors and members of stereotyped groups, but because people also see a *negative correlation between counterstereotypic behaviors and stereotyped groups*. They may underutilize disconfirming information even when it exists, recalling mostly instances that support what they think they know. For instance, people who have the stereotype that Jewish people are cheap will fail to incorporate into their impressions or to recall the many instances presented to them when Jews were not acting in a stingy fashion. This is an illusory, negative correlation being perceived between Jews and noncheapness.

Perhaps the way to prevent people from forming illusory correlations like these is to expose them to stereotype-inconsistent information, such as through intergroup contact. But will they detect and process the inconsistent information? Hamilton and Rose (1980) conducted an experiment to examine this using the stereotype of "salesmen" (the term "salespeople" was not yet in widespread use) as "loud and extraverted." They presented to research participants a description of a salesman that included counter-stereotypic behavior: The salesman acted quietly. The participants also received a description of a person for whom, according to the stereotype, quiet behavior was not unexpected and inconsistent—an accountant. This person was also described with information that included behaviors signaling he was quiet. However, even though both the salesman and the accountant were described with behaviors that included actions indicating quietness, the behaviors describing the salesman as acting quietly were seen more often than the behaviors describing the accountant as quiet. The counter-stereotypic behavior should have been particularly salient in this context; not only did the salesman act in a stereotype-inconsistent way, but he acted that way more often than someone for whom such behavior would be expected. Under this condition, the participants *did not show a stereotype-confirming bias in memory*. The proportionate recall advantage for stereotype-consistent information was not found, and an illusory, negative correlation did not emerge.

Hamilton and Rose (1980) interpreted this to mean that the participants were not merely attending to and analyzing stereotypic information, but counterstereotypic information as well. However, incorporating the inconsistent behaviors into processing would require the exhibited behavior to be not only counterstereotypic, but highly salient ("relative to a quiet person, he acted quietly"). Stroessner and Plaks (2001) provide a review of the illusory-correlation research that reveals this to be a robust finding. Contexts in which counterstereotypic information is salient lead to the undermining of illusory correlation. This can occur when the information is frequently observed (as in Hamilton & Rose, 1980), or when it is distinctive enough to capture attention and trigger elaborate processing (McConnell, Sherman, & Hamilton, 1994). The type of information that is best recalled may depend on whether the behavior being enacted is diagnostic of counterstereotypic action, and on whether it is salient and distinct. Distinctiveness of behavior causes its thorough processing, making it more memorable.

Entitativity

The salience and distinctiveness of the behavior are not the only features of the data that can determine whether stereotype-inconsistent information is recalled. The nature of the group to which the individual performing those behaviors belongs is also influential. One such feature of the group is its *entitativity*—that is, the extent to which a group is perceived as a coherent social entity. Groups are collections of individuals. But they take on qualities that are more than the sum of the individual parts. Groups have meaning and are perceived as, to varying degrees, real entities (e.g., Allison & Messick, 1988; Hamilton, 1991). According to Yzerbyt, Rogier, and Fiske (1998, p. 1091), "the basic idea is that, whereas some groups seem to display a high degree of groupness, others show little coherence . . . people perceived as being close and similar to each other, organized, and sharing a common fate, are likely to be appraised as forming a real group." In essence, entitativity is the "groupiness" of the group—how closely tied together it seems to be.

How does a group's sense of coherence and "groupiness" influence how people interpret stereotype-inconsistent information? Yzerbyt and colleagues (1998) propose that people expect more similarity among the members of a real group than an aggregate of individuals. The "groupier" the group, the more similar people think the group members should be (and the more likely people are to expect them to act in a stereotype-confirming way). The more similar the group members should be to each other, the more surprising and attention-grabbing it will be when one of them acts in a way that violates the stereotype. Because people process information more deeply when they need to make sense of it and reconcile it with existing beliefs, they should need to think more deeply about inconsistent behavior from a group high in entitativity. The inconsistent behavior somehow seems more inconsistent and incoherent when coming from such a group.

However, just because entitativity increases people's recall of stereotype-inconsistent information, it does not mean they are likely to use that inconsistent information in their judgments. The discrepancy between what people recall and what they say about others has already been reviewed in Chapter 4. Entitativity may only deepen this disjunction. Although people are more likely to recall inconsistent behaviors of groups that seem more entity-like, they may also attribute stereotypic traits to such groups. One reason for this is that people cling to the belief that real groups share real attributes and characteristics, so they may be more likely to try to find such shared traits, even when there are salient inconsistencies. Yzerbyt and colleagues (1998) found that people did in fact make greater amounts of dispositional attributions to entitative groups: Research participants were less sensitive to situational information and more prone to committing the fundamental attribution error when a group was high in entitativity.

Memory Bias Revisited: Attributions

Crocker and colleagues (1983) have already made a similar argument that relates the types of attributions people form after having been exposed to stereotype-inconsistent information to the type of processing they engage in. These authors point out that despite the presence of inconsistent information, people form remarkably stable impressions of others. Stereotypes seem resistant to change in the face of discrepant information that people cannot help attending to and processing deeply. Why would this be the case? Crocker and colleagues suggest that people recall the incongruent information because they have spent mental effort using attributions to discredit it. The motive to have a consistent schema and maintain coherence is said to be so strong that it leads people to use attributional reasoning to preserve the schema (or stereotype). Stereotype-congruent behaviors may get attributed to a target person's stable personality, whereas incongruent behaviors are attributed to the situation and do not require people to alter their impressions of persons from that group. While people may be able to recall stereotype-inconsistent information, they do not use it in their impressions, because they have formed attributions that deem the information not dispositionally relevant. This explanation is consistent with the attribution literature, where it has been found that situational attributions are more effortful than the automatic-like dispositional ones (see the discussion of the correspondence bias in Chapter 7). Thus the reason stereotype-inconsistent information is less likely to be used in forming impressions, but is more likely to be recalled, is that the effort spent to preserve an attribution to the stereotypic disposition of the member of the stereotyped group (effort to explain away inconsistencies) makes the inconsistent behavior more memorable.

This review of the factors that lead to increased recall for information inconsistent with a schema/stereotype returns us to a paradox introduced in Chapter 4: A disjunction exists between people's memory for stereotype-inconsistent information and their reliance on stereotype-consistent information in their judgments. This creates a potential problem for their ability to exert control over stereotype use. If one way in which people's stereotype use is contained is by observing others behaving in ways that are inconsistent with the stereotype and having their sense of confidence in relying on the stereotype undermined, it requires that they actually allow the inconsistent information observed in others to be a source of doubt for trusting their stereotypes. It is possible that people exert a great deal of effort to shield themselves from experiencing such doubt, and that this effort is what results in the heightened memory for stereotype-inconsistent information. Thus people may never feel that their confidence in the use of stereotypes is threatened, even when they have seen evidence that a person being perceived acts in ways that violate a stereotype (and even when they have dedicated mental energy to focusing on the inconsistent information, thus making it memorable). For stereotype-inconsistent behavior performed by others to have an effect on people's ability to control stereotyping, that behavior not only must trigger systematic and effortful processing, but must undermine their confidence in relying on stereotypes when judging others. When do people use stereotype-inconsistent information in *forming* an impression, so that a target individual is responded to according to the behaviors and characteristics he/she displays, rather than those the perceivers expect to see?

Confirmatory Judgment Revisited: Inconsistent Behavior Can Lead to Nonstereotypic Judgment

Several factors have now been reviewed that determine whether people will detect, attend to, and elaborate on stereotype-inconsistent information: (1) making situational attributions for inconsistent behavior, (2) observing inconsistent behavior from highly entitative groups, (3) having weak stereotypes regarding the group in question, and (4) the observed behavior being relatively distinct and unique. However, in each of those instances the effortful processing engaged in is being used to elaborate on inconsistent information, thus making it more memorable, while simultaneously *preventing the inconsistent information from having an impact on judgment.* The discussion turns now to examining the question of when there is not a disjunction between what people remember and what types of impressions they form. When do people remember others in a way that is consistent with the impressions they have formed of those others? One obvious instance in which memory coincides with judgment is when people form stereotypic judgments of others and have stereotypic memory of these others. Thus Chapter 11 has described many instances of people having a stereotypic bias in their recall, such that stereotype-consistent information was both what they remembered and what they used in judgment. However, to control stereotyping, exactly the opposite set of affairs would need to be observed in perceivers. Control over stereotype use would be evidenced when the mental effort that had been exerted in thinking about inconsistent behaviors from members of stereotyped groups worked its way into influencing the impressions people form. If people not only had better recall for stereotype-inconsistent behavior, but allowed that behavior to be used in shaping the judgments they formed, there would be a conjunction between recall and judgment, thus creating control over the use of the stereotype.

Before we consider how stereotype-inconsistent behavior triggers the use of mental effort in forming stereotype-free impressions, one last point must be made clear. Using effort to think about inconsistent information, and allowing that effort to have an impact on judgment, do not guarantee that judgments will be stereotype-free. At times the effort used to think elaborately about stereotype-inconsistent information does have an impact on judgment, but in a way that will preserve, rather than control, stereotype use. The effort exerted may be used to construct a stereotype-consistent impression in which the extra effort is used to make the inconsistent behaviors seem as if they fit with the stereotype. For example, Asch (1946) showed that people attempt to make a coherent impression, and that a unified/coherent impression is produced by people even when traits are observed that do not fit well together (when some of the traits are inconsistent with the set as a whole). Asch and Zukier (1984) followed this up by showing that research participants who were asked to form impressions of another person who had displayed traits that were clearly antagonistic to each other were still able to resolve this inconsistency in the person's behavior and form a unified impression. "Each person possesses a multiplicity of qualities, dimension, and aspects; consequently, a unitary impression implies that one fits these diverse features to one another in a coherent fashion—it does not suffice to treat them as a mere heap. One has to comprehend (or sense) how they belong together" (Asch & Zukier, 1984, p. 1230).

How did Asch and Zukier's (1984) participants resolve the case of clashing dispositions (when there was an inconsistency among traits)? One strategy was to "segregate" inconsistent traits so that an inconsistent trait was assigned to a "separate sphere" of the person. Rather than modifying the entire structure, participants included the traits that did not seem to fit, but held them separate from other traits. This was perhaps similar to subtyping, reviewed in Chapter 11. An exception was being made that would allow perceivers to grant that the inconsistent behavior was descriptive of the person, without altering the entire set of traits believed to describe the group more generally.

Another strategy people used to resolve having been exposed to inconsistent behaviors was to make a distinction between the inner and the outer person—that is, to invoke what Asch and Zukier (1984) called the *depth dimension*. Thus a person might exhibit a trait on the outside, but the perceivers might conclude that it did not reflect the true, inner person. This strategy would allow the perceivers to account for an inconsistent behavior, but would not require them to change or alter the stereotype. They could attribute the behavior to a superficial feature of the person. A third strategy Asch and Zukier detected in their participants was the use of "means–end" thinking, in which the inconsistent behavior was seen as a means by which some other goal was achieved. Thus the behavior could be explained as perhaps not really counterstereotypic at all, because it helped the observed person to attain something that (according to the stereotype) people belonging to that group would want. Finally, perceivers might engage in *interpolation*, whereby they added some new information that could link the inconsistent information to the rest of the structure. For example, the stereotype of Jewish people contains notions of intelligence and ambition. What would happen if perceivers learned that a particular Jew displayed a set of traits that included intelligence and a lack of ambition? Rather than simply incorporating the lack of ambition into the judgment (and changing the stereotype), perceivers might interpolate, adding information to explain the apparent inconsistency. For example, they could argue that this Jewish person had been ambitious in the past, but had met with failure so often that now the person was unambitious. In this way the added information would resolve the inconsistency and would not require altering the stereotype of Jews. The person, despite being unambitious now, was imagined to have been very ambitious at some previous time, with a good explanation generated for the change.

This brief review of ways to resolve the inconsistency perceived in others reveals that substantial mental effort is exerted toward detecting and thinking about inconsistencies, and using that effort in the judgments people form. But it is used to make the existing stereotype stay relevant, rather than to control its use. This finally brings us to the goal of this section—to illustrate that one way to control stereotype use is to detect the stereotype-inconsistent behavior in others. Inconsistent behavior will trigger elaborate processing aimed at including that inconsistent behavior in the impression in a way that does not rationalize it away or marginalize it. The judgment formed is nonstereotypic, not an expanded stereotypic one. For example, Gill (2004) found behavior that contradicts a stereotype undercuts the use of that stereotype, depending on whether a descriptive or prescriptive stereotype is being contradicted. Behavior inconsistent with a prescriptive stereotype still resulted in biased judgment. However, the same behavior shook perceivers free from descriptive stereotyping. Male participants asked to make hiring decisions showed a gender bias despite the fact that women applicants enacted masculine roles, but this bias evaporated when measures of descriptive stereotyping were used.

Minority Influence: Being Consistently Inconsistent

If stereotyped minority groups never triggered more elaborate types of thinking in perceivers than those afforded by cultural stereotypes, then social change would never be observed. Instead, minorities are sometimes successful at shaking perceivers from the constraining tunnel vision of their stereotypes, opening the perceivers' minds to a more effortful style of processing information about the minorities, and inducing them to form impressions not anchored by the stereotypes. Moscovici (1976, 1985a) suggested that this occurs when a minority consistently adheres to its minority view, refusing to yield to the social pressure of the majority. To support this position, Moscovici (1976) initially drew on historical examples of minorities that maintained a deviant outlook (i.e., relative to the majority, their positions were unexpected), yet subsequently changed majority opinions despite lacking power (e.g., the Baptists and Quakers of 18th-century England, feminists, ecologists, the American civil rights movement). Why does this strategy work? Because such conviction is said to be attention-grabbing and hard to "explain away." A person/group persevering with a minority view in the face of a dominant group is seen as confident and unyielding, and with time this confidence is perceived by others and may cause those in the majority to begin doubting the confidence and conviction with which their own views are held. Indeed, even basic processes such as color perception may be challenged when a minority offers an opinion that deviates from the majority. Moscovici, Lage, and Naffrechoux (1969) found that when a clearly blue patch of light was consistently called "green" by one person in a group, the other people in the group started to doubt their own color perception. People virtually never called the color patch "green" when simply asked for its color when alone. But when a consistent minority called it "green," suddenly other people started to call it "green" as well! (Although this occurred on only 8.4% of the trials in the experiment, it was still a big increase from 0%.)

Moscovici's logic is that perceivers initially reject minority viewpoints rather categorically and without much systematic appraisal. The implication is that for minority group members to exert influence and have others see them in nonstereotypic ways, those people perceiving them must be shaken from their reliance on categorical and heuristic thinking (e.g., Baker & Petty, 1994; Bohner, Erb, Reinhard, & Frank, 1996; Crano & Chen, 1998; de Dreu & de Vries, 1996; Erb, Bohner, Schämlzle, & Rank, 1998; Kruglanski & Mackie, 1990; Moskowitz, 1996; Moskowitz & Chaiken, 2001; Pérez, Falomir, & Mugny, 1995; Trost, Maass, & Kenrick, 1992; Wood, Pool, Leck, & Purvis, 1996). Clinging to a minority view over time and in the face of pressure to yield is one way to do this. It should undermine perceivers' confidence in their attitudes and cognitions, making them more susceptible to thinking elaborately about the minority group and reexamining the issues. Moscovici (1985a) referred to this as a *validation process that leads to influence.* Another way to shake people from a reliance on categorical thinking, as suggested by dual-process models, is for members of a stereotyped minority to act in a manner inconsistent with the prevailing stereotype.

For example, when minority behavior is highly diagnostic, it leaves little room for majority interpretations to be foisted upon it (Moskowitz, 1996). Here, *highly diagnostic* means that the behavior clearly implies an interpretation incongruent with an existing stereotype/heuristic prescribing the behavior of the minority. When encountering such behavior, majority group perceivers should need to devote processing effort to make sense of this unexpected state of affairs. Confidence in their heuristic-based beliefs and evaluations should be undermined by the clear and counterstereotypic behavior they have witnessed. This confidence gap, and its associated elaborate processing, should make the perceivers susceptible to rejecting their preconceived expectancies/stereotypes and coming to have fuller appreciation for the minority as a group, the complexities of their views, and the inapplicability of the stereotype. In one study (Moskowitz & Chaiken, 2001), such a confidence gap in the mind of perceivers was created by using just this formula—specifically, by exposing perceivers to a member of a minority group who, during a short monologue, expressed attitudes incongruent with the perceivers' expectancies. Other perceivers, however, experienced no such confidence gap. They listened to a minority group member expressing attitudes congruent with prior expectancies. For these latter participants, heuristic-based judgments should be sufficient. Perceivers were asked to evaluate the minority, to rate agreement with the issue the minority person had discussed, and to list the thoughts they had while listening to the person speak. An expectancy-violating minority group member was predicted to trigger systematic processing, whereas a minority person who acted in a manner consistent with expectancies would not shake the perceivers from the comfort of their heuristic processing.

The results supported these predictions. A minority person who violated expectancies was viewed by perceivers more positively than one who confirmed expectancies. This triggered systematic processing and resulted in a greater chance of the perceivers' being influenced by the minority. Systematic processing (actively evaluating arguments and issues raised in the monologue) was revealed in two ways. First, the types of thoughts participants had while listening to the monologue from the "incongruent" minority group member were more focused on the details of the argument—the issues raised in the monologue. Second, systematic processing was measured by assessing whether perceivers had detected the *quality* of the arguments offered in the monologue. Some participants heard a monologue that was extremely well formed, while others heard one with weak arguments. People who heard the "congruent" minority group member did not differ in their ratings as a function of the quality of the arguments. It appears as if they were not attending to the content in enough detail to detect its quality. However, people who heard the "incongruent" minority person were persuaded by this person only if the positions were well articulated. The ability to detect differences in argument quality is a tried-and-true method of illustrating that people are doing more than superficially attending to others, but instead are scrutinizing them in a systematic and effortful way (Eagly & Chaiken, 1993).

In summary, before a minority can exert influence, first it must not be categorically rejected. Unlike majorities, which are typically seen as legitimate by virtue of the consensus that surrounds their positions (Eagly & Chaiken, 1993), the typical reaction to minorities is to view them as illegitimate. Thus the strategy at the heart of minority influence is triggering a switch in the mind of the majority perceiver from heuristic to systematic processing. Unless the perceivers' negative expectancies and heuristics are challenged, minority positions will be disregarded and uninfluential. Behavior that is inconsistent with a stereotype can have this effect. But it is not the only method. Both Baker and Petty (1994) and Wood and colleagues (1996) illustrated that systematic processing of stereotyped minorities can be triggered by the feelings of surprise, threat, or curiosity aroused by finding out that a minority group member agrees with majority group perceivers. This too is a type of inconsistency, since these perceivers perhaps assume that minorities will not think and act like them (and when they do so, it is inconsistent with what had been expected).

Ignoring Base Rates

Locksley and colleagues (Locksley, Borgida, Brekke, & Hepburn, 1980; Locksley et al., 1982) also found evidence that people attend to, and readily make use of, information not linked to the stereotype of the group, but to the specific qualities of the person being perceived. This occurs if the behavior is highly diagnostic, with *highly diagnostic* again meaning that the behavior has a clear, unambiguous meaning that identifies it as counterstereotypic. Locksley and colleagues have argued that stereotypes are typically only used as a last resort, when there is no other information available about a member of a stereotyped group (and possibly used when the only individuating information available is not highly diagnostic). It is their claim that practically any time people are provided with behavioral information signaling that a target person is behaving in a nonstereotypic way (i.e., stereotype-inconsistent information), they abandon their stereotypes in favor of basing their interpretations on the inconsistent information.

Although experiments such as Darley and Gross's (1983) examination of confirmatory hypothesis testing seem to suggest that people use stereotypes if given the slightest bit of stereotype-confirming evidence, Locksley and colleagues suggest that when good, stereotype-disconfirming evidence is provided, this bias disappears. Although this may seem contradictory to the pervasive influence of stereotypes described up until now, it must be kept in mind that the types of stereotypic biases reviewed in Chapter 11 have been explained from the start to be most likely in ambiguous situations. People have been described as active constructors of reality, with perception being an interaction between what is actually there (the data) and what perceivers bring to the situation (expectancies, stereotypes, and perceptual readiness). Chapters 1, 5, 10, and 11 have explicitly stated that when the situation provides clear and unarguable data, then biases have less impact on what people perceive. Locksley and colleagues simply add that when a person from a stereotyped group clearly and unambiguously acts in a nonstereotypic way, then perceivers will not try to force a stereotyped interpretation on them. What is less clear from their research is just how stereotype-discrepant the behavior has to be. Their research has tended to hit participants over the head with counterstereotypic behaviors, making it difficult to know what would happen in more complex situations when some behaviors are counterstereotypic and some are irrelevant (or even when some behaviors support the stereotype, as was the case in Darley and Gross's research on confirmatory hypothesis testing).

For example, Locksley and colleagues (1980) showed participants a transcript of a conversation between two people. One person described him-/herself as having acted assertively (or passively) in three separate situations. No other individuating information was provided. The people having the conversation also had their first names mentioned, in order to signal their gender to participants. The results show that participants were not likely to base judgments of how aggressive the self-describing person was on stereotypes of how aggressive versus passive women and men are. Instead of using the sex stereotype, they based judgments on the individuating information.

Why are people controlling stereotypes when stereotype-inconsistent information is being presented? Locksley and colleagues (1980) suggest that people do not stereotype when individuating information is present because they are making a mistake! There is a well-established finding that when people know prior probabilities, and should use those prior probabilities when making predictions, they often throw those probabilities out the window and base their predictions on recently encountered examples and information. In Chapter 3, this was called the *base rate fallacy*, because base rates are neglected: "Research on the subjective use of prior probabilities indicates that they are often neglected when consistent, individuating target case information is available" (Locksley et al., 1982, p. 24). For example, if you know that 80% of the people at a party are librarians, and you are asked to guess whether Linda, a woman you met at the party, is a librarian, you should guess yes. However, if she exhibits a behavior that is not typical of the stereotype (such as telling loud, crude jokes), you are likely to ignore the probabilities. You ignore the base rate of encountering a librarian in favor of relying on one piece of behavioral "evidence." Similarly, when predicting how likely it is one will encounter a Black person in Munich, you should use the percentages. If only 1% of Munich residents are Black, you should not predict that there is a 10% chance you'll bump into a Black person. However, if you have just recently encountered a Black man while strolling through the English Garden, you will be swayed by the recent evidence rather than by the known probabilities or base rates. Locksley and colleagues argue that stereotypes operate the same way, in that a stereotype is no more than a set of prior probabilities in your mind about certain traits being associated with certain types of people. If a nonstereotypic behavior is encountered, you will be prone to forget the probabilities and mistakenly use the recently encountered information.

However, a different explanation can be offered for why people in Locksley and colleagues' (1980) research have failed to use stereotypes—an explanation that matches the rationale we have been building in this section. In the research of Locksley and colleagues, the potential for an impact from the stereotype is quite obvious. Moreover, the individuating information is salient and impossible to ignore. It may be that people recognize the potential for bias and try to correct for it by using the individuating information. That is, salient and diagnostic information hits people over the head and forces them to realize that the stereotype is not valid. A woman who has acted assertively on three separate occasions just cannot be described as passive, no matter what the stereotype says. People recognize this and adjust their impressions accordingly, to fit the data.

The studies reviewed thus far suggest that if the victims or targets of stereotypes can behave in clear ways that are diagnostic of violating a stereotype, then they may personally be prevented from being stereotyped by others. An important question then becomes this: If many individuating behaviors are present, and if the social information available is complex, do people use or ignore the individuating information? In other words, how uniformly counterstereotypic must behavior be to challenge the use of the stereotype? Locksley and colleagues (1982) provided initial evidence relevant to answering this question. Their participants were given information about 12 men and 12 women, and then had to rate how assertive each one was. In the information they were given about each person, they were told about four past situations the person had been in relevant to assertiveness. Participants were then asked to guess how assertively each of the targets acted in a fifth situation. Instead of simply overwhelming people with four instances of assertive behavior, the experimenters manipulated this factor. Some people read about targets who had four assertive prior incidents; some read of three assertive prior responses and one passive one. Some read information that was passive in half of the situations and assertive in the other half. Finally, some read of three passive and one assertive prior responses. The results showed that people did not rely on stereotypes, even when there was a mix of stereotype-consistent and -inconsistent information. Rather than clinging to the stereotype-consistent information, they did not form stereotypic judgments. Thus the data suggest that people stop stereotyping as soon as *any* individuating information is provided.

Although this research did not "hit people over the head" with an excessive amount of counterstereotypic information, it could be that the experiment was quite obviously about stereotyping, thus making people sure to individuate. Or, as Deaux and Lewis (1984) point out, it could be that giving people information about how assertive someone was, and then asking them to judge how assertive that person was, would almost by necessity force them to use the information just provided rather than the stereotype. Perhaps in settings that are not so clearly about stereotyping, and where the behavior being judged is not the very same behavior just provided by the individuating information, people will need a more overwhelming amount of contradictory evidence before no longer relying on stereotypes.

A DISSOCIATION MODEL OF STEREOTYPE ACTIVATION AND STEREOTYPE USE

The correction models reviewed in Chapters 5, 7, and 10 reveal that when people suspect an unwanted influence is being exerted on their judgments, they attempt to remove the biasing impact of this influence through conscious effort. What motivates this effort? Sometimes the data are so clear and unambiguous that they force a reevaluation and validation of beliefs. For example, in minority influence, either (1) the minority group members must act unyieldingly consistently, or (2) their behavior must disconfirm expectancies held by the perceivers. To Allport (1954, p. 384), this state of affairs places a "preponderance of responsibility" on members of a stereotyped group; it is incumbent on them to act nonstereotypic for people to be nonprejudiced. But must motivation to engage in systematic processing be initiated by a minority's behavioral strategy? Sometimes the selected goals of the perceivers are what motivate them to be fair and unbiased in how they evaluate others. People can, of their own accord, be motivated to remove the impact of stereotypes from their judgment by engaging in systematic processing when they choose to. As discussed in Chapter 5, systematic processing can be motivated by raising the *sufficiency threshold*. In the case of controlling the effects of expectancies and stereotypes, this would mean adopting goals that promote accuracy and fairness when judging others (independently of the behavior of those others).

Many people have incorporated egalitarian ideals and goals relating to fairness into their value system. Despite embracing these ideals, there are numerous reasons such goals/values are not in place when judging others. The correction model described in Chapter 10 requires putting these goals in place: People become aware that their responses are in violation of these important values, and this motivates them to rectify the situation and correct their thinking. Devine (1989) has described a *dissociation model* similar to the correction model, where people become aware of a possible influence of activated stereotypes on their impressions/evaluations and seek to dissociate/remove/correct this influence:

> Nonprejudiced responses are, according to the dissociation model, a function of intentional, controlled processes and require a conscious decision to behave in a nonprejudiced fashion. . . . For those who have integrated egalitarian ideals into their value system, a conflict would exist between those ideals and expressions of racial prejudice. The conflict experienced is likely to be involved in the initiation of controlled stereotype-inhibiting processes. (p. 15)

Thus, even when people intend to be nonbiased and not allow stereotypes to influence their impressions, they often are not aware of such biases because of the automatic components that trigger the stereotype and make it perceptually ready. However, if they become aware of the fact that their impressions may be biased, people can consciously intend to remove that influence.

According to the dissociation model, awareness of bias is triggered by perceivers' detecting a discrepancy between their nonprejudiced belief/value system and the possibility that a stereotype is leading them to think and act in a biased way. As with any negative feedback system of control (see Figure 2.5), a discrepancy between a desired state (being egalitarian) and the current state (being biased by a stereotype) creates a psychological tension and compensatory efforts aimed at reducing that tension. In this case, the tension is experienced as feelings of compunction and guilt, and the compensatory response is a correction process aimed at removing the stereotype's influence from judgment. As with any correction model, people must not only be aware of a bias, but be motivated to eliminate it, have a theory about how such a bias is influencing them, and have cognitive resources to engage in the processes that will overturn this unwanted influence (see Figure 12.1). This leads to an obvious question: What motivates people to control a stereotype, especially if they are not aware of the stereotype's influence?

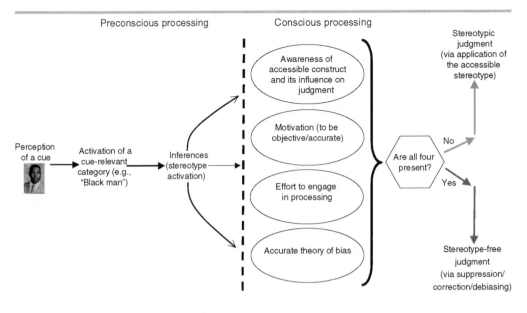

FIGURE 12.1. A dissociation model of stereotyping and correction processes in stereotyping.

Stereotype-Relevant Discrepancies Produce Compunction

Devine (1989) found that stereotypes were equally likely to be activated for low- and high-prejudice people. What then distinguishes these two types of people? Devine, Monteith, Zuwerink, and Elliot (1991) suggest that for low-prejudice persons, the activation and use of stereotypes is distasteful and undesired. They see their egalitarian values, standards, and beliefs as discrepant with stereotyping. The dissociation model predicts that because of this discrepancy with their value system, they first experience compunction/guilt (as specified by self-discrepancy theory; Higgins, 1987). Next they are motivated to eliminate those feelings of compunction by reaffirming their sense of self in this domain (as specified by self-completion theory; Wicklund & Gollwitzer, 1982). High-prejudice people, however, do not unilaterally reject prejudice. Although they may detect a discrepancy between the way societal standards assert they should act and their own biased/stereotypic responses, this discrepancy is not experienced as a tension. They have no remorse or guilt, because they have violated no internal standard. As both the self-discrepancy and self-completion theories predict, if people receive negative feedback in a domain that is not relevant to them, they experience no psychological tension, no sense of incompletion, and no motivation not to use stereotypes (no compensatory responses).

Self-discrepancy theory (Higgins, 1987) states that detecting a discrepancy within the self leads to specific types of emotional reactions. Higgins proposes that you experience different "selves"—the self you ideally "ought" to be, the self you believe you "should" be, the person you actually are, and so on. These various selves can align to varying degrees, so that the person you are is either consistent with or discrepant from the person you (1) want to be, and (2) ought to/should be. A discrepancy between who you actually are and who you feel you should be will lead to feelings of guilt (see Figure 12.2). Devine and colleagues (1991) proposed that low-prejudice persons' motivation to inhibit stereotypes arises from feelings of guilt caused by the recognition that they have failed to live up to an important value, or have recently failed at being persons who reject stereotypes. As Devine and colleagues put it, "nonprejudiced beliefs and prejudiced thoughts and feelings may coexist within the same individual" (p. 817), and when they do, the ability to respond in a nonprejudiced way requires that one first become aware of one's prejudiced thoughts and then be motivated to remove them from one's current thinking in favor of "the conscious, intentional activation of nonprejudiced beliefs" (p. 817). Realizing this discrepancy between how they should be and how they actually are should lead to guilt, but only for low-prejudice people. High-prejudice people will presumably not hold a sense of how they "should" act that is in any way discrepant with the use of stereotypes. Therefore, any discrepancy they detect will be between with how they act and with how others might think they should act, and this discrepancy will not be related to feelings of guilt.

Devine and colleagues' (1991) participants were asked to indicate (according to their personal standards) how they should act in a variety of interactions with members of an outgroup. They then were asked to indicate how they actually, if being perfectly honest, would act (or have acted in the past) when interacting with members of the outgroup. These answers were then subtracted from each other to produce a discrepancy score—the degree to which how a participant actually acted differed from how he/she should act. Affect was then assessed by having people rate their feelings on a series of scales asking them about a wide range of emotions (anxious, guilty, depressed, etc.). People were also divided into high- and low-prejudice "types" in order to examine whether the emotional reactions associated with a discrepancy would differ for the two groups. The findings revealed that for low-prejudice people, the greater the discrepancy score, the more guilt experienced. However, high-prejudice people did not experience guilt even when they reported a discrepancy between how they should and would

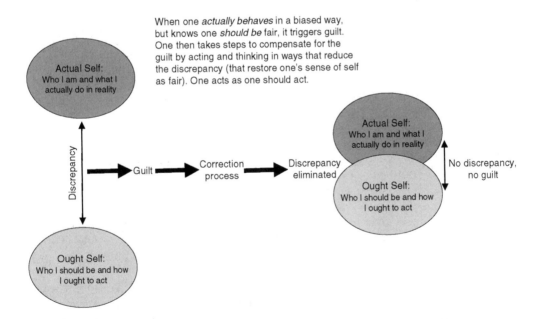

FIGURE 12.2. Possible selves and the impact of discrepancies between the actual and ought selves.

act. Their personal standards allowed them to be prejudiced. The data also revealed that high- and low-prejudice people had fairly equal ratings of what they believed societal expectancies/standards were. Devine and colleagues concluded that all people seem to believe society lets them get away with some amount of prejudice, but for low-prejudice people their personal standards do not. These standards are what cause them to feel guilt. They have not violated the societal standard, but they have violated their own standards. High-prejudice people have upset neither the societal standard nor their personal standards, so they feel no compunction and are unmotivated to change their ways.

Compunction Motivates Conscious Control

The notion of compensatory acts arising from detecting a discrepancy between actual and ideal actions is critical to Monteith and Voils's (2001) *self-regulation model of prejudice*. In this account, noting that one has acted in a manner discrepant with one's egalitarian ideal triggers an affective response, which then initiates control attempts aimed at reducing the discrepancy and alleviating the negative affect/guilt. Monteith (1993, Experiment 1) triggered a discrepancy in participants by telling them they had acted in a biased way toward gay men. Participants were first asked to evaluate what they believed was an application to law school from a man who was labeled as either gay or straight. People who read the application of a gay student were told by the experimenter that their evaluations of this candidate revealed an anti-gay bias (i.e., they had evaluated him in a negative manner simply because he was gay). Measures were then taken to see whether negative affect and compensatory responses followed. First, ratings of guilt were higher for participants who were experiencing a discrepancy (replicating Devine et al., 1991). In addition, a thought-listing task was used to measure the extent to which participants continued to ruminate on their discrepancy. Participants who were feeling guilty reported a greater number of thoughts about their discrepant feelings/behavior. Finally, when given an essay to read about why discrepancies occur and what can be done to reduce them in the future, these participants took longer to read the essay and had better memory for the evidence discussed in the essay during a later memory test. These responses were compensatory, in that they allowed these individuals to specify the conditions that produced the discrepancy and establish coping strategies to be utilized in the future.

In a separate illustration of how guilt motivates conscious attempts to correct for, or compensate for, the undesired use of stereotypes, Monteith (1993, Experiment 2) asked participants to evaluate some jokes. Two of the jokes were irrelevant to the stereotypes of gay men, but two other jokes invoked these stereotypes. Participants who were low in prejudice did not have a problem with the "irreverent" jokes, unless these participants had recently been made to face a discrepancy between their egalitarian strivings and their actual behavior. Participants who had been made by the experimental procedures to experience a prejudice-related discrepancy were more unfavorable in their evaluation of the jokes (in an ostensibly unrelated study concerning humor) than people who did not experience a discrepancy.

Monteith and Voils (2001; see also Monteith, Ashburn-Nardo, Voils, & Czopp, 2002) have posited that the mechanism producing this type of stereotype control is one in which an association is created between the cues that trigger the negative affect (e.g., for a straight White person, the presence of a Black or gay person), the experience of the negative affect (guilt, shame), and the action that caused the negative affect (acting in a nonegalitarian fashion toward members of the group). Through these associations, the cues come to serve as a warning that a discrepant response may follow, and this triggers a *behavioral inhibition system* (BIS) that will allow for control over the unwanted response: "When [cues for control] are present in subsequent situations, the BIS should be activated again, causing heightened arousal and a slowing of ongoing behavior (i.e., behavioral inhibition). Consequently, the response-generation process should be slowed and executed more carefully" (Monteith & Voils, 2001, p. 382). With time and practice, the cues may serve to stop stereotyping from ever occurring. The presence of a stereotype-relevant cue, rather than triggering an attempt to correct for a bias that has already occurred, may inhibit stereotypes and prevent the stereotype's activation.

Outcome Dependency and Accountability Promote Dissociation via Accuracy Goals

If we were to rely on people becoming aware of their biases and feeling guilty about those biases in order to prevent stereotyping, we would run into the dangers that (1) people would not be aware of these biases because they are activated unconsciously and influence them without their knowing it; and (2) people would not feel guilty enough at the realization that such biases exist, or at least guilty enough to be motivated to act on reversing, altering, or correcting whatever biased impressions have already been formed. What goals other than guilt reduction lead to decreased stereotyping?

Chapter 5 has reviewed, in some detail, research on *accountability* (e.g., Tetlock, 1983) and *outcome dependency* (e.g., Neuberg & Fiske, 1987). As noted there, these motives make people form impressions of others in a way that does not rely on schemas and theory-driven/top-down processing. Instead, such goals make people desire greater confidence in their judgments than stereotypes usually permit. When people adopt goals that make them desire accuracy from the outset, rather than waiting to be made guilty about their lack of accuracy, stereotype control can occur via the same processes of dissociation and correction discussed above (for a review, see Fiske & Neuberg, 1990). Although cues in the environment may continue to trigger stereotypes in a fairly effortless and mindless way, people with accuracy goals are motivated to attempt to make certain that no bias is evidenced in their judgment as a result of accessible stereotypes.

For example, Neuberg and Fiske (1987; reviewed in Chapter 5) found that when people were motivated to be accurate (due to outcome dependency), they were less likely to form impressions of a schizophrenic person that reflected the stereotype of such persons, and were more likely to spend time evaluating information describing the individual qualities of a specific schizophrenic person. Neuberg (1989) extended this to the important domain of job interviews, examining the impact of stereotypes on the behavior of both the person doing the interviewing and the person being interviewed. However, the important point for our current discussion is that these biases due to stereotypes found during job interviews were found to be controlled when the person doing the interviewing had a goal that was incompatible with using stereotypes. Naturally, one would think that interviewers, especially on job interviews, would have the goal of being fair and nonstereotypic. But apparently such stereotypes are triggered and operate during job interviews nonetheless, and it requires an explicit goal to control this phenomenon in order to rein it in.

How were stereotypes in a job interview assessed? First, Neuberg (1989) reasoned that people would ask confirmatory questions that might elicit answers that could only affirm the stereotype. It was assumed that people who held stereotypes would seek to confirm those stereotypes through the way in which they gathered information and tested hypotheses. A job interview is merely one forum for gathering information and testing hypotheses about a person, so if a stereotype exists about a group to which that person belongs, the confirmatory processes of hypothesis testing reviewed in Chapter 11 should predominate. In addition, Neuberg predicted that these biases on the part of the person doing the interviewing would work their way into the behavior and responses of the person being interviewed. If the interviewee was continually asked about stereotype-relevant issues, he/she would be more likely to respond in a way that might confirm the stereotype. The interviewer's behavior would restrict the interviewee's ability to respond and would lead him/her to produce expectancy-confirming responses in the course of the interview (see the review of the self-fulfilling prophecy in Chapter 13). However, these stereotype-confirming processes should be *attenuated when interviewers had accuracy goals*. An interviewer with the explicit goal of being fair and accurate should attempt to gather more comprehensive and less biased information, and this would lead the person being interviewed to produce more complex and expectancy-inconsistent behaviors. These behavior, in turn, would then give the interviewer cause for either changing the stereotype, or at least seeing it as being irrelevant to this individual.

Could interviewers be given goals that would allow them to remove biases in their interviewing style that they weren't even aware existed? Neuberg (1989) asked each research participant to interview two job applicants. The interviewer first received negative, job-relevant information about one of the applicants, thus establishing a negative expectancy about him. No information was provided about the other candidate. The negative expectancy informed the interviewer that the job candidate was (among other traits) not very self-motivated, good at solving problems, or skilled in interpersonal interaction. The job was described as requiring a person with strengths in these dimensions, thus making the expectancy damaging to the candidate's chance of getting the job, unless those expectancies were dispelled during the interview process. Half the interviewers were given explicit goals to be accurate in their interview; the other half were given no explicit goals. The interviews then occurred, and the interviewers rated the job applicants. In addition, the interactions were audiotaped, so there was also a measure of the behavior of the interviewers (the questions they asked, the number of speech errors they made while conducting the interview) and the responses of the interviewees.

The results revealed that people without a goal to be accurate formed more negative impressions of the person for whom they had a negative expectancy than someone for whom they had no expectancy. People with accuracy goals, however, did not show this bias. Their initial negative expectancies were dispelled over the course of the interview process (given that the expectancies were false, an accurate interview process would have allowed the negative expectancy to be overturned and corrected). What sorts of behaviors were indicative of attempts to be nonbiased and accurate? People with accuracy goals were found to listen more to the person they had a negative expectancy toward than to the person they had no expectancy toward. They also provided more encouragement with the questions they asked (e.g., they were more likely to interject affirming things like "mmm-hmm"). Finally, people with accuracy goals asked more open-ended, novel, and positively framed questions. A positively framed question allowed the individual to discuss positive events; an open-ended question could not be answered with a simple "yes" or "no"; and a novel question introduced a topic unrelated to the expectancy. Consequently, being asked more open-ended types of questions and more novel questions led interviewees to act in ways that were more favorably received. The interviewee was also evaluated by neutral observers. When the applicant was responding to someone who had a negative expectancy but an accuracy goal, the person was rated as favorably as a person being interviewed by someone with no expectations.

Thought Suppression: The Ironic Increased Incidence and Hyperaccessibility of Stereotypes

You might think that asking people not to use stereotypes would be a viable strategy to get them to try to be accurate and to remove stereotyping from their judgments and evaluations. If you wanted people not to use stereotypes in their evaluations, simply asking them not to should produce the desired result. And your common-sense intuition would be partially correct. Asking people to avoid or suppress a particular thought, such as to avoid thinking about stereotypes when evaluating another person, meets with initial success. However, there are counterintuitive and ironic side effects associated with asking people to suppress their stereotypes. Specifically, *thought suppression* (trying to suppress, or not to think, a specific thought) leads to an even greater incidence of that thought in consciousness than if the thought has not been suppressed, as mentioned in Chapter 10. If I asked you to attempt to avoid thinking about a "white bear" at all costs, you might meet with initial success, but soon would find images of white bears entering your head where they never would have without my initial instruction.

Thus *attempts at mental control do not always meet with success, and may have the ironic or paradoxical effect of producing an even greater incidence of unwanted thoughts.* According to Wegner's (1994) theory of *ironic processes of mental control*, any attempt to suppress a thought (or engage in mental control) activates two concurrent processes: an intentional operating process and an "ironic" monitoring process. The monitoring process is tuned to detect failures of mental control; it looks for references to the unwanted thoughts. In order not to think a specific thought, one must constantly monitor the mind to make sure that the unwanted thought is not entering consciousness. This creates the unusual demand to hold in mind, at some (preconscious) level, the very thought that is not to enter the mind. The operating process, on the other hand, seeks items inconsistent with the unwanted thought that can serve as distractors, making the mind full so that undesired thoughts cannot enter. In order not to think a specific thought, one is best served by distracting oneself with thoughts of something else.

Wegner (1994) suggests that the operating process requires cognitive resources, because one is engaged in an active search for ideas, people, and objects to think about that can replace the unwanted thought in one's mind. This active search requires mental energy, whereas the monitor's task is simpler and is relatively free from capacity restrictions. The monitoring process is engaged in preconscious scanning of the mind, which does not engage much of one's limited processing resources. Because of its relative effortlessness, the monitoring process should continue to function efficiently even when there are other drains on attentional resources. The operating process, however, would be disabled by such processing drains. It is in this differential use of processing resources where Wegner claims suppression can fail. The unwanted thought, rather than being purged, ends up ironically being more prevalent. Ironic effects emerge because during attempts at mental control, the introduction of concurrent tasks or other drains on resource availability can disable the operating process, leaving the monitoring process running unchecked. The unwanted thoughts on which the monitoring process is focused then become relatively more accessible; the operating process, having been shut down, is no longer able to prevent the monitoring process's successful searches from reaching consciousness.

Wegner, Erber, and Bowman (cited in Ansfield & Wegner, 1996) presented evidence to support the automatic nature of the monitoring process and the ironic return of suppressed thoughts. Participants were given a sentence stem to complete. Some were asked to do so by avoiding being sexist. For the sentence stem "Women who go out with many men are . . . ", an example of a sexist answer was "sluts" and a nonstereotypic response was "popular." The availability of cognitive resources (and thus the ability of the operating process to do its job) was manipulated by having half the participants complete the sentence quickly, while the other half were not placed under time pressure. Participants who were asked to be nonsexist and under time pressure responded with more sexist responses than people who were never asked to suppress sexist thoughts. Wegner (1994) concluded that "the very attempt to control prejudice may initiate ironic automatic processes that promote prejudice. The discovery of automatic activation of stereotypes under conditions of load may be less an expression of the individual's basic prejudice than it is an indication of the individual's attempt to avoid prejudice" (p. 47).

Two alternative explanations for this *rebound effect*, where unwanted thoughts bounce back more powerfully after attempts to suppress them, are reviewed by Macrae, Bodenhausen, Milne, and Jetten (1994). First, Macrae, Bodenhausen, and colleageus (1994, p. 812) state that "during suppression, perceivers are assumed to form associations in long-term memory between the unwanted item and each of the selected distracters. When these distracters are encountered on a subsequent occasion, they simply serve to cue or trigger the unwanted thought." Thus, just as the presence of features such as skin color or gender can trigger a stereotype because of a history of being associated with it, when one attempts to replace an unwanted thought with some distracting thought, the two become associated. If this happens, the later presence of the previously irrelevant thought now comes to trigger the stereotype because of the newly formed association.

Second, these authors suggest that the monitoring process's scan for and detection of the unwanted thought constitute a form of repetitive priming, generating greater accessibility of the suppressed thought. During thought suppression, a representation of the to-be-suppressed thought must be held up as an object in awareness in order to deny such thought's entrance into consciousness. Once the operating process is disengaged, residual activation persists, and the suppressed construct remains accessible (Macrae, Bodenhausen, et al., 1994). As in any opponent-process system that involves simultaneous excitation and inhibition, the removal of the restraining force leads to the temporary hyperaccessibility of the inhibited construct or thought. Thus, attempting to suppress a stereotype should lead to initial success, but as soon as the intention to suppress the stereotype is removed, the stereotype should be accessible. In fact, it should be even more accessible than if one had never tried to suppress the stereotype in the first place. This accessibility advantage for unwanted thoughts following attempts to suppress them led Wegner and Erber (1992, p. 909) to declare that the suppressed thoughts are *hyperaccessible*: "To the degree that intentional concentration marshals as much accessibility as can engineered by conscious means, the finding that suppression under cognitive load yields greater levels of accessibility constitutes evidence for a higher degree of access—hyperaccess."

To examine the ironic effects of stereotypes, Macrae, Bodenhausen, and colleagues (1994) asked participants to write a story about a day in the life of a person depicted in a photograph. Half of the participants were asked not to use stereotypes about the group this person belonged to when writing the story. The other half were given no explicit instructions. They then received a photograph of a skinhead, a group for whom participants had clear social stereotypes. All participants next had to write a second "day in the life" story, but this time there were no instructions to suppress the stereotype. The results were quite interesting. Though people successfully suppressed the stereotype when asked to on their first essay, the use of the stereotype came roaring back on the second essay, when the goal to suppress the stereotype was no longer in place. In fact, the second essays written by the people who had previously been suppressing were more stereotypic than the essays written by people who were never asked to suppress the stereotype. It was as if the stereotype was not only ready to be used, but was even more likely to be used than it was for people already using it!

An implicit measure of stereotype accessibility (response times on a lexical decision task) verified this assumption. One way to assess whether a stereotype is accessible is to look at how quickly people respond to words relevant to the stereotype. If the stereotype has been triggered in the persons' minds, they are fast to recognize words relevant to that stereotype. Macrae, Bodenhausen, and colleagues (1994) found that people who had suppressed their stereotypes of a skinhead in an earlier task (when writing about a day in the life of a skinhead) later showed evidence of increased accessibility of the stereotype. For example, despite showing a reduction in the use of stereotypes in their essays (the essays were less stereotypic than those of people not suppressing the stereotype), participants asked to suppress responded more quickly to stereotype-relevant words on a lexical decision task (indicating whether a string of letters was a word or not). The facilitated ability to recognize stereotype-relevant words suggested that the stereotype was more accessible to suppressors than the people who had, moments earlier, just gone ahead and used the stereotype in the essays they had written.

Debiasing social thought involves attempts by individuals to exert control over the content and nature of their cognitive processes. Mental control allows the individuals to direct cognition in the service of currently held goals, such as the goal to be accurate, the goal to suppress the use of a stereotype, and the goal to correct for the use of some stereotype that is wracking them with guilt. Attempts at controlling stereotypes, however, can fail, if the conditions for mental decontamination/correction are not met: (1) when people lack awareness that the stereotypes is exerting any bias; (2) when they lack the cognitive capacity to engage in the processes that allow for stereotype control; or (3) when they have an incorrect theory about how they are being biased (see Figure 12.1). The thought suppression work reveals yet another way in which effortful attempts to control stereotyping can fail—by ironically causing the undesired thought to rebound, and paradoxically making it hyperaccessible rather than less accessible.

Perspective Taking versus Thought Suppression

Rather than ending our review of stereotype control on this less than optimistic note, let us emphasize that despite the fact that control over the use of stereotypes can fail, it also can, and often does, succeed. People can be made aware of their hypocrisies and shortcomings in the domain of fairness and egalitarianism, and such awareness does motivate them to act and think in a way consistent with their beliefs. People can adopt goals that make them desire to be accurate, and such goals allow them to overturn the biases that would otherwise have emerged from accessible stereotypes. *Perspective taking* is a further goal that could potentially curb the use of stereotypes—a goal that does not require one thinking of the self as a hypocrite (or feeling guilty over one's shortcomings as a fair person), and does not require one suppressing a thought (and hence being susceptible to the stereotype rebounding into judgment with greater force). Perspective taking could produce the positive consequences of stereotype suppression (i.e., limiting the expression of stereotypical content) without the ironic side effect of the stereotype becoming hyperaccessible.

One experiment (Galinsky & Moskowitz, 2000) adapted the procedure of Macrae, Bodenhausen, and colleagues (1994). All participants were shown a photograph of an elderly man and were asked to write an essay about a day in the man's life. Before constructing their narrative essay, one-third of the participants were given no additional instructions; one-third were assigned to the suppression condition; and one-third were asked to adopt the perspective of the individual in the photograph and imagine a day in the life of this individual as if the participants were that person. After writing the essay, participants were told that they would be performing an unrelated experiment involving a lexical decision task. They were informed that strings of letters would flash briefly on a computer screen and it was their job to determine, as quickly as possible, whether the letters constituted a word in the English language. Some of the words were relevant to the stereotype of elderly persons ("lonely," "dependent," "traditional," "forgetful"); others were control words irrelevant to the stereotype.

The findings revealed that both stereotype suppressors and perspective takers wrote less stereotypical essays about the elderly man than people in the control condition did. Thus both goals led to less use of the stereotype when participants were evaluating, judging, and making predictions about a specific member of the group in question. However, Macrae, Bodenhausen, and colleagues (1994) found that although people wrote less stereotypical essays, the stereotype was hyperaccessible and was perceptually ready to pounce back into judgment. To examine this, Galinsky and Moskowitz (2000) measured participants' mean response time to stereotype-consistent words relative to stereotype-irrelevant words on the lexical decision task. As expected, stereotype suppressors responded significantly faster to stereotype-consistent words than to irrelevant words, and they responded faster to stereotypic words than people in the control condition did. The stereotype was more accessible when participants were asked to suppress than when they were given no instruction at all. How did people who were taking the perspective of the individual fare? Was the stereotype accessible for them? Perspective taking did not lead to the hyperaccessibility of the stereotype. Reaction times to stereotype-consistent words were slower for perspective takers than for suppressors, and did not differ reliably from those for people in the control condition. In addition, perspective takers revealed no facilitation for responding to stereotype-consistent words relative to stereotype-irrelevant words.

Thus, without guilt, and without the irony of making stereotypes more accessible, perspective taking was able to reduce the expression of and the accessibility of stereotypes. This latter point brings us to a separate question regarding the control of stereotyping. We have been assuming that the increased accessibility of a stereotype must follow the exposure to a member of a stereotyped group. We have also seen that some contextual forces can make this tendency even more likely. Because of this immediate, passive activation of the stereotype, the manner in which to control stereotyping has been described in a fairly reactive way. Once the activation occurs, a person reacts to it. However, here we see a contextual force that makes the activation of the stereotype seem less likely: Stereotypes were less accessible in the Galinsky and Moskowitz (2000) study when people took the perspective of another person.

Chapter 11 has suggested that a rosier picture of human nature would be provided by the conclusion that people are capable not only of correcting for stereotyping after activation of a stereotypic construct, but of controlling the activation of the stereotype in the first place. Blair (2001) likens the control of stereotyping to medical models that seek control of disease. Although it is important to have *reactive forms of control* that allow for reduction in symptoms once they have been triggered, it is equally important to have *proactive forms of control* that prevent the triggering of the symptoms in the first place. Can people exert such proactive control over stereotyping?

PROACTIVE STEREOTYPE CONTROL: CONTROL OF STEREOTYPE ACTIVATION

The desire to paint a rosier picture of human nature is a legitimate reason to initiate a research program (provided that the science can substantiate the desired conclusion!). In recent years, researchers have attempted to paint such a picture—not only because they want to believe that humans are not doomed to have stereotypes inevitably triggered, but also because they think that the evidence for such inevitability is not beyond doubt. Methodological concerns have been raised regarding Devine's (1989) conclusion, bolstering the desire to see whether an opposing conclusion might be found.

What are some of these methodological concerns? First, the failure to find a difference between the activation of stereotypes in low- and high-prejudice people in one experiment does not mean that no differences in activation really exist. In addition, the particular way Devine (1989) labeled such people (using a measure of so-called *modern racism*) may have been poor at identifying people who really could control stereotype activation. Perhaps some other measure of individual differences would reveal differences in stereotype activation if such a measure could tap the extent to which people were truly committed to low-prejudice/egalitarian ideals. Second, recall the Devine procedure from Chapter 11. The lists of words that were used to activate the stereotype contained words that, while not synonyms of hostility, were hostile in tone—words such as "nigger." It could be that the low- and high-prejudice people were not having stereotypes activated, but having feelings of hostility triggered by these types of words. Third, perhaps stereotypes are not activated by the mere presence of members of stereotyped groups. Devine's participants did not see or meet real people; they read words, and perhaps it is difficult for White people to think of anything but the stereotype when they read the word "Black man" or "nigger." But they may think of a variety of things when they see or meet a Black man, and it may not be the stereotype. We have already discussed this point in Chapter 10. The thoughts triggered upon meeting someone may be different from the thoughts triggered upon reading about that person's category label, thus forcing the category label to be brought to mind (when it otherwise might not). A Black fireman need not trigger the concept "Black" when a White person meets him, but can it help triggering this concept when the White person reads the words?

Increased Stereotype Activation as a Sign of Control

One way to illustrate that stereotype activation can be controlled is to take a less intuitive approach. People usually think of control as the inhibition and suppression of an unwanted thought or behavior. But people are also exerting control when they pursue a desired state. Thus control of stereotype activation would be illustrated by evidence that the process can be increased in people who have goals that make them desire to have stereotypes triggered. What would make a person who is not particularly high in prejudice want to have stereotypes triggered? One answer to this question is self-esteem threat.

As reviewed in Chapter 8, any threat to one's identity is posited to trigger the goal of repairing the threatened self-image, of attaining self-affirmation (e.g., Steele, 1988). This lowered state of self-esteem can be repaired by stereotyping others (e.g., according to Tajfel & Turner's [1979] *social identity theory*). Essentially, the argument is that the response of derogating others when one is experiencing a lowered state of self-esteem is learned through experience and repetition, and eventually it comes to operate automatically. The threat to identity triggers the goal of repairing the threat, and this is repaired by stereotyping others (Fein & Spencer, 1997; see also Spencer, Fein, Wolfe, Fong, & Dunn, 1998). In this way, stereotype activation is a form of *automatic self-affirmation*. Being undermined in some self-relevant domain, or experiencing lowered self-esteem, leads to implicit stereotype activation because stereotype activation will help one to repair the threat to the self.

Spencer and colleagues (1998) illustrated this by giving participants false feedback about their performance on a "new intelligence test." Half were informed that they did well on the test, and half that they did poorly. They were then taken to participate in an ostensibly new experiment where they were asked to do a word completion task. The task asked them to look at words with several letters missing, and to fill in the blanks to form a word. There was one trick. Some of the words were part of the stereotype of Asians (e.g., "shy," "short," "polite"). The experimenters were really interested in seeing whether stereotypes were activated by people's responses to these words. Thus, looking at the stimulus "P_L_ _E" and completing it to form the word "polite" would indicate stereotype activation. However, completing it with the word "police" would not. Why would stereotypes be activated? Because the person who was presenting these incomplete words to the participant was an Asian American. In fact, for half the participants there was an Asian person presenting the words, and for half there was a White person. Thus, if stereotypes of Asians were being automatically triggered, people should form stereotypic completions on the task; this would occur when there was an Asian person but not a White person presenting the words.

The results showed that people who received negative feedback versus positive feedback performed no differently on the task when a White person was presenting the words. No stereotype should have been activated, and no activation was evidenced. However, if the stereotype was automatically activated, people should have been showing evidence of stereotype activation when they encountered the Asian person. However, this was only found to be the case among participants who had just been told they did poorly on the intelligence test. People who did well on the test did not show evidence of stereotype activation. Thus stereotype activation is not the normal state, and it is not automatically triggered whenever one encounters a member of a stereotyped group. Instead, Spencer and colleagues (1998) argue that a threat to self-esteem must exist, and that stereotype activation is a form of compensatory cognition—a response to threat aimed at self-affirmation.

Cognitive Load

Gilbert and Hixon (1991) proposed that since an automatic process is one that is not disrupted by cognitive load or limits to one's processing resources, then if stereotype activation is constrained when attentional capacity is restricted, it cannot be inevitable and automatic. A distracting cognitive load could shift salience away from race and other features that might normally trigger a stereotype. To illustrate this, Gilbert and Hixon used the word completion task described above. The procedure was identical to that of Spencer and colleagues (1998), except that instead of participants being given negative feedback before performing the task, they were placed under a state of cognitive load while performing the task. The load task was to try to memorize an eight-digit number during the course of the experiment. The prediction was that participants under load would not show stereotype activation, despite the fact that the words were being presented by an Asian woman. However, participants who were not under load would show evidence of stereotype activation, reflected by the number of word completions finished in a stereotypic manner. The results supported this prediction. Participants under cognitive load and exposed to an Asian person formed the same number of stereotypic completions as people who encountered a White person, and these were reliably fewer than the number of stereotypic completions formed by people not under load who had encountered an Asian person. The conclusions was that stereotypes are not automatically activated every time perceivers come into contact with a member of a stereotyped group; activation is at least dependent on the perceivers not being "cognitively busy" (for a discussion of load effects on stereotyping, see also Li, 2004).

Feature Detection

Livingston and Brewer (2002) point out that stereotypes are abstract group representations that contain sets of traits and behaviors, but that these are distinct from other types of representations of social groups. One of these other types may be racial attitudes (liking for the group), which may be quite distinct from stereotypes about the characteristics and traits of the group (e.g., Fazio & Dunton, 1997; Wittenbrink, Judd, & Park, 1997). Another may be the physical features associated with typical exemplars of the group, such as a large nose or dark skin. Livingston and Brewer argue that what gets activated when perceivers encounter a member of a stereotyped group may not be the abstract representation. In fact, the activation of stereotypes may vary, depending on whether the perceivers focus on the category the person comes from (the abstract group representation) or the concrete perceptual features of the person, such as skin color and facial features. Livingston and Brewer make this point eloquently:

> Faces are ontologically ambiguous; they can serve as symbolic representations of abstract social categories (concepts) or as configurations of concrete physical features per se (percepts), independent of any higher order semantic meaning. Hence, one question that arises is whether automatic responses to faces necessarily reflect category-based evaluations of the abstract social groups that the faces represent (e.g., African Americans) or whether they reflect cue-based, affective responsiveness to concrete, physical features. (p. 5)

It may well be that perceivers do not always respond according to a person's group membership, but according to specific facial features. It could be that the *evaluative reaction to specific physical/facial features*, rather than a stereotype of the group, is what gets triggered. It is wholly possible that this is why participants in Gilbert and Hixon's (1991) research failed to have stereotypes activated when under cognitive load. Perhaps cognitive load focuses attention on specific cues and features in the environment, rather than on general category labels and abstract stereotypes associated with those labels. Although people can report those categories when later asked, this may simply be because they have encoded the features that allow them to make such a designation, not because they have encoded the person according to those abstract categories.

High- versus Low-Prejudice Belief Systems

Perhaps one way to control stereotype activation is by developing a history of responding in a fashion that rejects the stereotype and endorses a counterstereotypic belief system. This point leads naturally to a discussion of a distinction that must be drawn between *cultural stereotypes* and *personal beliefs*. If a cultural stereotype is inaccurate, and one worries that the use of beliefs based on this stereotype can bias one's judgment, memory, and behavior, one can create a set of personal beliefs about the group that departs from what the culturally shared stereotype dictates. One may either reject the cultural stereotype in one's personal beliefs or endorse the stereotype (Devine & Elliot, 1995). However, regardless of whether or not the cultural stereotype is rejected in one's personal belief system, one's knowledge of that cultural stereotype does not dissipate. Even people who find the cultural stereotype offensive (such as low-prejudice people and members of the groups that are negatively affected by those stereotypes) still have the knowledge of that stereotype stored in memory and can easily have that stereotype triggered, as well as report what that rejected stereotype looks like (e.g., Devine, 1989). To illustrate this, Devine and Elliot (1995) identified two groups of White research participants who reported drastically different personal beliefs about the group "African Americans." They labeled these high- and low-prejudice people. They then asked both groups to describe the cultural stereotype of African Americans. They found that despite holding opposing personal beliefs about this group, both high-prejudice and low-prejudice people reported exactly the same cultural stereotypes. If people do not believe in something, this does not mean that they have no mental representation of it that can be retrieved from memory, or that they cannot describe it according to a shared stereotype.

However, the question of current concern is whether people who have developed a belief system that rejects the stereotype can have these beliefs automatically triggered instead of the stereotype. This can be examined by attempting to identify certain types of people who reject stereotyping, and have been able to break the implicit mental association between cues relevant to the stereotyped group and the cultural stereotype. Devine (1989) attempted to do this by labeling people as low- and high-prejudice, but, as reviewed earlier, perhaps the method for labeling people was not a successful one. Would a different method of identifying people reveal that the stereotype is not triggered when a member of the stereotyped group is encountered?

Lepore and Brown (1997) performed a near-exact replication of Devine (1989), with a few methodological modifications, to make the point that negative stereotypes need not be automatically triggered. They posited that chronic belief systems that either promoted or denounced group stereotypes would determine whether stereotype activation would occur. Thus, although people with low-prejudice belief systems would know the social stereotype, this construct would be unlikely to be activated for such people. To test this, White participants were presented with category labels for the group "Black people" via a subliminal priming procedure. Then subsequent judgments of a target person, who behaved in an ambiguous manner along a stereotype-relevant behavioral dimension, were examined. Lepore and Brown found that while high-prejudice people interpreted a target person more negatively after subliminal exposure to the stereotype of Blacks, low-prejudice people did not. The activation of this negative stereotype was said to be not inevitably activated, but prevented by a nonprejudiced belief system.

Expectancies and Associations

Blair and Banaji (1996) examined whether expectancies could disrupt stereotype activation. In their research, participants saw a prime word (a trait) followed by a name. The name was either clearly male or clearly female, and the task was to classify the name as male or female. The logic was that if stereotypes are automatically activated, and this activation cannot be disrupted, then pairings of female names with stereotypically female traits (the primes) should always be responded to faster than female names paired with words not relevant to the stereotype. In an attempt to illustrate that activation of the stereotype could be controlled, Blair and Banaji manipulated participants' expectancies regarding the pairings of words and names, hoping that these expectancies could disrupt stereotype activation. Some participants were told to expect counterstereotypic pairings (e.g., "ambitious–Betty," "sensitive–Brian"), while others were told to expect stereotypic pairings (e.g., "ambitious–Brian," "sensitive–Betty"). If a stereotype is activated, it should facilitate responses to the classification task. The results showed that such facilitation occurred when people expected to see stereotypic pairings. But when people were led to develop the expectancy that they would see counterstereotypic pairings, they no longer showed this facilitation effect. That is, when an actual pairing was presented that had a trait consistent with the female stereotype paired with a female name, people were not faster to classify the name. The counterstereotypic expectancy seemed to have disrupted the activation of the stereotype.

Kawakami, Dovidio, Moll, Hermsen, and Russin (2000) took a slightly different tack in examining whether stereotype activation could be controlled. They reasoned that if stereotype activation is a case of association, with concepts linked to a category being triggered, perhaps people could be trained to have associations to a category other than the stereotype. Allport (1954, p. 21) suggested this possibility when he asserted that whatever association to a category that is *most dominant* is what gets triggered: "A person with dark brown skin will activate whatever concept of Negro is dominant in our mind. If the dominant category is one composed of negative attitudes and beliefs we will automatically avoid him." What is most dominant could be the stereotype. But stating it this way leaves open the possibility that it might not be. Something other than the stereotype might be triggered because it, not the stereotype, is the dominant response. The development of an association between a stereotype-relevant stimulus and a nonstereotypic construct, and the possibility for this association to be more dominant than the one to the stereotype, were examined by Kawakami and colleagues (2000).

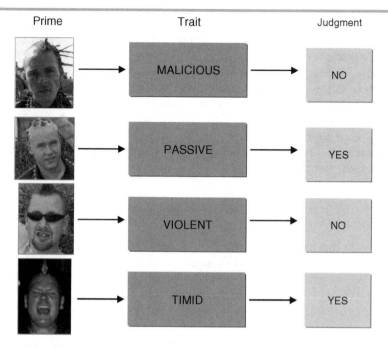

Prime	Trait	Judgment
	MALICIOUS	NO
	PASSIVE	YES
	VIOLENT	NO
	TIMID	YES

FIGURE 12.3. Counterstereotype association training (repeated for 45 minutes).

Kawakami and colleagues (2000) provided people with *counterstereotype association training* (see Figure 12.3). Participants completed a lengthy training session in which nonstereotypic associations to an outgroup were learned through repeated pairings. The training task forced people to practice responding "No" each time they encountered a stereotypic trait being paired with a member of a stereotyped group. For example, the participants had to press a button marked "No" on the keyboard each time they saw a picture of a skinhead paired with a trait stereotypic of skinheads (e.g., "malicious," "crude"). In addition, they were to press a key marked "Yes" on the keyboard each time they saw a picture of a skinhead on the monitor paired with a trait not stereotypic of skinheads (e.g., "passive," "timid"). They practiced developing these new associations for 45 minutes (six blocks of trials with 80 trials per block), training themselves to reject the stereotype. They found that despite a lifetime of having learned to associate the stereotype with the group, the training created new associations that led to disruption of stereotype activation.

Chronic Motives and Goals: Preconscious Control

Yet another way people can prevent stereotypes from being activated is through volition (Moskowitz, Gollwitzer, Wasel, & Schaal, 1999). The goals to be an egalitarian person and to be nonbiased in one's dealings with members of stereotyped groups were posited to be able to result in control over stereotype activation (as such activation is antithetical to these goals). This research focused on people who had such dedication to these goals that these goals were said to be chronically held (see Chapter 9). For people dedicated over the course of their lives to being egalitarian toward members of a particular group, an association was posited to have developed between members of that group and the goals. If this pairing of goals and stimuli was repeatedly pursued, it could lead to the development of an automatic link between the goals and the stimuli (Bargh, 1990) in much the same way the cultural stereotype might be linked to the stimuli. Moskowitz and colleagues posited that if the associative link between the goals and the stimuli was more dominant for these individuals than the association between the stimuli and the stereotype, then the goals rather than the stereotype would be automatically triggered in the presence of the stimuli. In fact, the stereotype, in line with the parallel-constraint-satisfaction model reviewed earlier, might even be inhibited by the goals rather than activated by the stimuli (members of the stereotyped group).

To test this hypothesis, male participants were identified who possessed chronic goals to be egalitarian to women. Their responses were to be contrasted with those of men without such chronic goals. (Note that such people were not prejudiced people; they simply had not dedicated their lives to attaining an egalitarian ideal. The nonchronic participants were presumed to be average, fair-minded men.) The task was a simple one—to pronounce a word aloud as soon as it appeared on the computer monitor. As you may have guessed, these words did not appear in isolation. They appeared as part of a string of events, with the most important fact being that a picture of a member of a stereotyped group preceded the appearance of the word. Thus participants would see a picture of a person (either a woman or a man) paired with a picture of an object, followed by a trait (either a stereotype of a woman or a trait not part of the stereotype), and were simply to pronounce the word as fast as possible so reaction times could be recorded. Participants were told that this task was part of an experiment on recognition memory; they had no idea the study was about stereotyping. They thought the study concerned memory for the pictures that appeared, with words being presented simply to try to interfere with their memory. Thus the complete procedure involved two images appearing on the monitor simultaneously—one of a person's face and one of an object—followed by a word. After pronunciation of the word, one more image appeared, and participants were asked to decide whether this image matched the image seen earlier in that trial (see Figure 12.4). To conceal further that the task was about stereotyping, there were well over 100 of such trials, with only 20 of them containing pairings of stereotypic words with the faces.

If the stereotype had been activated automatically by the photograph (a woman's face), responses to the stereotype-relevant trait (words related to the stereotype of women) would be facilitated, but no such speed-up in reaction times would be found for words that were irrelevant to the stereotype. Similarly, responses to words related to the stereotype would be facilitated only if they were preceded by a woman's face and not by a man's face. In support of the hypothesis that stereotypes are automatically activated, individuals who were not chronic egalitarians exhibited a speed-up in response times to stereotype-relevant words (vs. stereotype-irrelevant words) following photographs of women (but not following photographs of men). However, in support of the idea that stereotype activation is not automatic, but can come to be controlled if one desires to do so, individuals with chronic goals to be egalitarian toward women did not exhibit this facilitation and were shown not to have stereotypes of women activated. In fact, the evidence suggested that such people were actually inhibiting the activation of stereotypes. Rather than an increased likelihood of stereotypes being activated, there was a decreased likelihood. Furthermore, Moskowitz, Salomon, and Taylor (2000; see Chap-

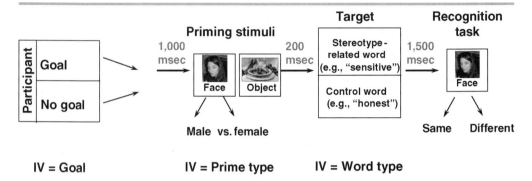

FIGURE 12.4. A pronunciation task to investigate chronic goals and stereotype activation. IV, independent variable; DV, dependent variable.

ter 9) found similar control over stereotype activation in a study examining the stereotype of African Americans. It was additionally found that along with the stereotypes failing to be activated, a photograph of an African American activated an alternate construct—egalitarian goals. Thus a link between the goal and the stimulus appeared to have been formed and was capable of being automatically activated. In essence, for chronic egalitarians, an encounter with a member of a stereotyped group leads to the inhibition of stereotypes and the triggering of egalitarian goals instead.

Preconscious Compensation

Finally, to underscore the point that not only certain types of individuals (those low in prejudice, those who are chronic egalitarians, etc.) can control stereotype activation, recent research (Moskowitz, Li, & Kirk, 2004) illustrated that individuals without chronic goals can be given temporary goals to be egalitarian and exhibit similar control over stereotype activation. Some participants were asked to reflect on a time when they had failed to act in an egalitarian manner, thus undermining their sense of self in this domain. This feeling of incompletion, or need for affirmation, should produce compensatory responses aimed at restoring the sense of self in the damaged domain. Participants who, in contrast, had contemplated a recent success at being egalitarian should not feel this esteem threat or sense of hypocrisy. It was found that participants who had been undermined engaged in compensatory responses to attempt to restore their sense of self in this domain, and these responses were at the preconscious level! People with the goals to be egalitarian triggered in this way were able to prevent the activation of stereotypes. Using a procedure similar to that in the Moskowitz and colleagues (1999) study illustrated in Figure 12.4, White research participants were shown pictures of either African American or White men as part of a memory test. Following the pictures were briefly flashed strings of letters that were to be identified as either words in the English language or nonsense syllables. The words, on the trials of interest, were either related to or irrelevant to the stereotype of Blacks. The usual finding—that people responded faster to words relevant to the stereotype following a Black face—was found only for participants who had not been asked to contemplate a previous instance of being unfair. People who had fairness goals triggered by contemplating such a prior experience failed to show activation of the stereotype. Stereotype activation was preconsciously controlled.

In order to assess whether this was truly due to a preconscious goal, White participants in a follow-up experiment were asked to respond to words related to the goals of being egalitarian (e.g., "tolerant," "fair," "just," "egalitarian") and to words irrelevant to such goals. The people whose fairness goals had been undermined in the session responded faster to the words relating to egalitarianism following a Black face (but showed no such facilitation following a White face), relative to people who had not been undermined in this domain. And such detection occurred preconsciously: People were detecting these goal-related words at facilitated speeds, even though the stimuli were being presented (and responded to) too quickly for conscious control to have been directing attention (and too quickly for people even to recognize them as words).

Finally, to verify that indeed *goals* to be egalitarian were disrupting stereotypes and facilitating responses to words relating to egalitarianism, Moskowitz and colleagues (2004) looked to see not only whether people were faster at recognizing words relating to the concept "egalitarian," but whether they started scanning their environment for stimuli that would allow them to address their goals. Some research participants were made to reflect on a prior time in their lives when they had acted in a manner opposed to the values of fairness and egalitarianism. This was believed to trigger goals of being fair, and attempts to compensate (correct) for their prior behavior. If this truly was an instance of trying to compensate for goal states that participants desired to attain, people should initiate processes (both behavioral and cognitive) aimed at restoring the damaged domain and attaining the goals (e.g., Gollwitzer, 1993). One way this could be evidenced would be through detecting goal-relevant stimuli in the environment faster than people who were not attempting to compensate and who did not have fairness goals. To assess this, participants were provided with a visual search task: Four images of men were flashed on four quadrants of a screen, and the participants had to detect which man was not wearing a bow tie. This man was always White. However, the three other men (all wearing bow ties) were sometimes all White, and sometimes were two White men and one Black man. The logic was that when a Black man was embedded among the stimuli, the White participants, who had the goal to be egalitarian and fair toward Black men, would be scanning the environment, preconsciously, for stimuli relevant to their goals. A Black man would present just such an opportunity. Thus these participants should be distracted by this image, and their response time in detecting the man not wearing the bow tie would be slowed by this momentary attention to the goal-relevant stimulus. This was precisely what was found. When goals to be fair had been temporarily introduced, it made people more likely to detect stimuli in the environment relevant to those goals than people who did not have such goals triggered.

Thus the triggering of a stereotype may be easy, effortless, unintended, and likely to occur for most people. But it is not inevitable. However, the ability to stop the process—through either developing chronic goals, or undergoing extensive training—is not meant to imply that stereotyping is any less of a social problem. From a vast literature, we see that people use stereotypes often, and often without knowing that such biases are at play. The ability to control stereotypes is theoretically important and could have strong practical implications. But at the current time, the far greater tendency seems to be for people to have stereotypes triggered fairly effortlessly when they encounter members of stereotyped groups.

CODA

We have seen two distinct ways to control stereotyping. The first has been described as a reactive form, where the effects of stereotypes, once activated, are rooted out of people's cognitive and behavioral responses to members of stereotyped groups. People exert cognitive effort to think more deliberately, systematically, and elaborately about the individual qualities of a person, rather than employing a gross application of a cultural stereotype. People are attempting to correct for bias or to dissociate bias from judgment, adjusting their beliefs about an individual to reflect (what they believe is) a more accurate form of evaluation.

Chaiken and Trope's (1999) edited volume on dual-process models has revealed a theme in the literature in psychology—that correcting, modifying, and adjusting for the effects of automatic processes requires conscious intent. And to successfully implement such intent is dependent on one possessing (1) awareness that a biasing influence exists; (2) a theory about that influence and in what direction the influence pushes judgment, evaluation, and decision making; (3) the motivation to remove this unwanted influence; and (4) the cognitive resources (capability) to carry out the capacity-straining processes of correction and judgment modification. Implicit in this approach is the assumption that control is effortful—that intentional acts are born of consciousness, requiring awareness and cognitive resources to be pursued. It assumes that preventing unwanted responses and controlling bad habits require overturning the outputs of automatic processes. Motives and goals may be deployed to enhance, facilitate, inhibit, suppress, mold, adjust, or correct the inputs to consciousness that are provided automatically by the cognitive apparatus. But strategic processes are seen as occurring sequentially later, and as requiring greater cognitive effort, than automatic processes.

However, the exact conditions that undermine the occurrence of effortful processing are precisely those that exist in life outside the laboratory (Bruner, 1957). Time pressure (e.g., Kruglanski & Freund, 1983), working on multiple tasks simultaneously and thus overburdening cognitive capacity (e.g., Bargh & Thein, 1985; Gilbert & Hixon, 1991; Macrae, Bodenhausen, et al., 1994), and serving goals other than objectivity and accuracy (e.g., Chaiken, Liberman, & Eagly, 1989; Jones & Thibaut, 1958; Sedikides, 1990) are omnipresent conditions of social life. If exerting control is constantly met by these potential pitfalls to control, what allows people to pursue their goals without constant failure? Will attempts to control stereotyping fail? One answer to this question is that the ends people desperately desire become pursued so routinely that the effort dedicated to the pursuit becomes smaller and smaller as skill at the pursuit develops. The routinization of important activities leads these activities to become almost invisible, despite the initial effort required. Consciousness and effort are not required to intentionally control the activation of a stereotype. Thus, rather than the "hard" process of overturning, modifying, correcting, and adjusting the outputs of automatic processes, a second route to controlling stereotyping is available. People can engage in processes capable of interfering with and inhibiting the activation of the stereotype in the first place.

Note

1. Srull's data match the findings of Rothbart, Evans, and Fulero (1979), reviewed in Chapter 11, where a group was the target of perception and expectancy-consistent information was better recalled.

From the Intra-
to the Interpersonal

BRIDGING THE GAP
FROM COGNITION TO BEHAVIOR

It is a general principle in Psychology that consciousness deserts all processes when it can no longer be of use ... if we analyze the nervous mechanism of voluntary action, we shall see that by virtue of this principle of parsimony in consciousness the motor discharge *ought* to be devoid of sentience. If we call the immediate psychic antecedent of a movement the latter's *mental cue*, all that is needed for invariability of sequence on the movement's part is a *fixed connection* between each several mental cue, and one particular movement. For a movement to be produced with perfect precision, it suffices that it obey instantly its own mental cue and nothing else, and that this mental cue be incapable of awakening any other movement. Now the *simplest* possible arrangement for producing voluntary movements would be that the memory-images of the movement's distinctive peripheral effects, whether resident or remote, themselves should constitute the mental cues, and that no other psychic facts should intervene.

—JAMES (1890/1950, pp. 496–497; emphasis in original)

In many places in this book, it has been asserted that social cognition has a major impact on our behavior. That is, the cognitive processes guiding who and what we attend to, what we encode, how we structure that information in memory, whether (and when) it gets retrieved from memory and becomes accessible, and whether (and how) accessible information is used in our judgments and evaluations determine how we behave. Social cognition prepares us for social interaction and instructs us as to what is appropriate behavior. This assumption ties social cognition to issues of instrumentalism and functionalism (e.g., Allport, 1954; Bruner, 1957; James, 1890/ 1950; Jones, 1990), extending it beyond epistemology. It is not only concerned with how we attain meaning and the nature of the knowledge attained about others, but with how that knowledge is *used*. However, for the most part, the topics in this book have stayed within our heads as perceivers, examining how we see the social world. Let us now explore some of the ways these social cognition processes work their way out of our heads and into action.

To begin, consider the following example. Imagine you are locked up in the basement of the Stanford University psychology building, as part of an experiment in which you have agreed to play the role of a prisoner. Patrolling the halls is another student whom you recognize (he is someone who studies near you in the library), playing the role of a prison guard in the experiment. Your scripts and schemas tell you precisely the roles for each of these categories of people, and you enact the script. But something unusual happens in the basement to you and the library guy. You both start becoming your roles. Your expectancies about role-appropriate behavior end up becoming the reality of the situation. All too soon, the script is real and your behaviors are guided by the mental representation. The famous "Zimbardo prison experiment" shows the all-too-real effects of mental representations, such as scripts and roles, on human behavior. Zimbardo (1971, p. 3) stated:

> At the end of only six days we had to close down our mock prison because what we saw was frightening. It was no longer apparent to us or most of the subjects where they ended and their roles began. The majority had indeed become "prisoners" or "guards," no longer able to clearly differentiate between role-playing and self. . . . We were horrified because we saw some boys ("guards") treat other boys as if they were despicable animals, taking pleasure in cruelty, while other boys ("prisoners") became servile, dehumanized robots.

The Zimbardo prison experiment suggests that categorizing people in the environment according to roles will produce the behaviors consistent with those roles (schemas). It is reminiscent of the work on scripts and mindlessness discussed in Chapters 2 and 4, where specific behavioral responses are said to be stored as part of mental representations. Triggering these mental representations thus predisposes people to act in ways consistent with the expectancies suggested by the schemas. The present chapter elaborates on three ways that behavior emerges from social cognition processes, and that might account for the actions of the "prisoners" and "guards." The first is the role that expectancies play in how individuals construe what is appropriate behavior when they encounter other people relevant to those expectancies. The second is the way social cognition processes influence motivation, which then influences behavior. The third is an unmediated impact of category activation, such that the behaviors stored as part of mental representations become triggered as part of categorization and lead directly to production of the behaviors that have been triggered.

As is the case with much of social cognition, the cognition–behavior link is not always as consciously controlled as we would like to think. Ideally, by now you have accepted that a good portion of your judgment and evaluation and meaning is determined by preconscious processing, much of which you do not intentionally control or are not even aware of. In each of the three ways in which behavior emerges from social cognition processes that will be reviewed here, you will be asked to take an even larger step toward embracing the degree to which automaticity influences your everyday life by considering the possibility that your behavior is implicitly determined. This is what James was proposing in the quote that starts this chapter. Action can be initiated upon the mere detection of appropriate cues associated with that action, without any conscious decision to act needing to intervene. But let us first start with a less controversial notion. Chapters 11 and 12 have dealt with how expectancies guide thinking. It is not too great a leap of faith to imagine that in addition to guiding cognition, they guide action.

CONSTRUAL AND BEHAVIOR

The most obvious determinant of how one acts is how one construes the social environment. The "realities" of the situation are important only in that they may have an impact on how one construes those realities. This book has started by discussing the active construction of reality; it ends by pointing out that the actively constructed perception of others will dictate how one acts toward those others. Certainly the features and behaviors of others may influence how they are construed, but construal, as seen throughout the book, is not so purely determined. It is instead affected by one's goals, mind-sets, expectancies, stereotypes, and accessible knowledge. In turn, an interaction between two (or more) people is defined by how these people respond and react to each other; the construal of a given person is now shaped not only by his/her own expectancies, goals, and so forth, but by the behavior of the person with whom he/she is interacting.

Darley and Fazio (1980), as well as Jones (1990), describe social interaction as a sequence of events—a complex "dance" or set of exchanges between people. In this *interaction sequence*, the construal of others is said to be affected by the goals and the expectancies of the perceiver, which give meaning to the behavior of the person being perceived. However, the perceiver often remains unaware even of the fact that expectancies regarding the other person exist—let alone of the fact that such expectancies are influencing behavior toward that other person, or the other's behavior in return. Of course, if one does not think *one's own* acts are being influenced by expectancies, how could it be that one's expectancies influence how the *other person* is acting and thinking? This would seem impossible. But it is not impossible; it is all too probable, because people operate with false assumptions. They are wrong to think they do not have expectancies, and (if they are aware that they have them) wrong to think these expectancies do not bias how they think and act. And finally, people are wrong to assume that these biases have no impact on the people with whom they interact. In fact, people's actions, guided by their expectancies, constrain the nature of interactions by revealing information about themselves to others, and thus setting parameters for how these interactions will unfold. As Olson, Roese, and Zanna (1996, p. 211) put it, "the concept of 'expectancy' forms the basis for virtually all behavior. . . . Every deliberate action we take rests on assumptions (expectancies) about how the world will operate/react in response to our action."

The Interaction Sequence

The effect of construal on the interaction sequence is felt at several points. The sequence begins with the goals that each individual brings to a particular encounter. Thus before any stimulus is encountered, before the perceiver detects the presence of another person, and before he/she detects the particular features of that person, there is the individual perceiver with his/her set of chronic (long-standing) goals at that given point in time. In addition, there are the goals that are triggered in the perceiver by his/her current placement in that particular social environment. Expectancies are involved at this extremely early stage, as the perceiver has expectancies about the likelihood of attaining those goals, what types of people and stimuli will be relevant to helping him/her attain those goals, and what sort of efficacy the perceiver has in regard to those goals. These expectancies relating to attaining goals will have an impact on how the perceiver interprets the situations and stimuli around him/her; what situations the perceiver chooses to enter; whom the perceiver chooses to interact with; and what types of features, behaviors, and characteristics of that person the perceiver chooses to pay attention to. Each of these choices involves selecting from multiple alternatives, and goals establish expectancies that dictate which choices are made. As one example, many people have the goal to be fair persons who treat others in a nonbiased manner. Upon entering a situation, they may evaluate it to determine whether it affords an opportunity to pursue that goal (e.g., whether this situation is consistent with expectancies about what types of situations will allow them to pursue this goal successfully).

In the second step of the interaction sequence, the perceiver has selected a person to interact with (the interactant) and has detected certain features and behaviors of that person, which then allow the perceiver to form an initial impression of the interactant. From this initial impressions flow a set of expectancies about the interactant—perhaps expectancies based on a stereotype about the person's group membership(s). These initial expectancies may be somewhat tentative, with the perceiver unsure as to whether they are a valid basis for evaluating the other person (and they may subsequently become either confirmed and strengthened or undermined and attenuated); yet they still provide a basis for an initial reaction (Jones, 1986). Alternatively, the expectancies may be quite confidently held and provide for the perceiver what is felt to be a firm basis for subsequent action. Thus, as an example, a (Gentile) perceiver detects that the interactant is Jewish, and this triggers the associated expectancies and beliefs (stereotypes) that are associated with this group in the perceiver's mind, as specified by the cultural stereotype of Jews. Stereotypes are not required for expectancies to be triggered, as any concept can have expectancies associated with it. Thus, the perceiver may simply form the initial (spontaneous) impression that the interactant has certain traits, and with the concepts of these traits come associated sets of beliefs and behaviors—expectancies. In the current example, the perceiver relies on the expectancies linked to the stereotype of "Jew."

The third step of the sequence takes us back to Bruner's (1957) notion of *predictive veridicality* (discussed in Chapter 3). Here, an inference is a means to anticipate behavior and formulate appropriate behavior in response to the expected action of others. Based on the impression formed and the expectancies/stereotype triggered at the prior step, the perceiver acts toward the interactant in ways that are designed to achieve his/her goals and that are consistent with the expectancies the perceiver has generated about the interactant. *Thus actions toward another person are not necessarily a response to the actions of that person, but are generated as a response to the perceiver's own anticipation of that person's actions–his/her expectancies of what the interactant will be like.* The interaction is now tainted, with the perceiver exhibiting a behavior dictated not by real data observed in another person, but by what the perceiver expects to see and hopes to achieve through the interaction. To continue with the present example, if the perceiver enters a situation with the goal of being a fair person, and the situation is having lunch with a new acquaintance, the sequence could unfold as such: The perceiver detects that his/her new acquaintance is Jewish, and this triggers a stereotype that includes the notion that Jewish people are cheap. The perceiver may or may not endorse this stereotype, but it comes to mind nevertheless, and with it come expectancies about how well the person will tip, whether or not he/she will expect the perceiver to pay for the lunch, and so on. Even if the stereotype is only weakly held, it may provide a conservative basis for the perceiver's initial behavior ("Just to be safe, I'll act as if this person is cheap"). In order to meet his/her goal of being a fair person and to be consistent with this expectancy, the perceiver decides that the best way to treat the server (assuring he/she gets a good tip and is thus treated fairly) and the best way to treat the new acquaintance (to assure that he/she does not feel put out by needing to pay and is thus being treated fairly) is to offer to pay for the lunch. In this case, the perceiver's expectancies about how the interactant will behave, in combination with the perceiver's goal, have dictated the response. The actual behavior of the other person is not the most powerful force. The interactant has done nothing but eat lunch and look Jewish. But in so doing, he/she has triggered all sorts of expectancies in the mind of the perceiver that dictate, along with that perceiver's goals, how the perceiver acts in this social interaction.

In the next step of the sequence, the interactant interprets the meaning of the perceiver's action and responds with what he/she feels is an appropriate response. Thus the interactant's behavior is not purely driven by his/her own traits, wants, opinions, and so forth, but is in some good measure simply a reaction to the action the perceiver has generated (which, as just seen, has resulted from the perceiver's expectancies and stereotypes). In the current example, the Jewish interactant may not pay for lunch—not because he/she is cheap, but because the perceiver has offered to pay, and the interactant considers it rude or offensive to deny the perceiver this request. Finally, in the last step of the sequence, the perceiver interprets the meaning of the action just offered by the interactant, reacts in kind, and bolsters (or alters) the expectancy based on the action just observed. Figure 13.1 illustrates the steps in this process.

To finish the example, with the Jewish person now having not paid for lunch, the perceiver interprets his/her act of acquiescing to the offer to pay for lunch as confirmation of the expectancy that this person is cheap (and Jews are cheap). The perceiver has bolstered that expectancy, and will perhaps use this interpretation of the action to dictate how he/she acts next. Darley and Fazio (1980) refer to this as *behavioral confirmation*: The expectancy held about another person has led the other person to act in a way that confirms the expectancy. This may be more familiar to you as the *self-fulfilling prophecy*.

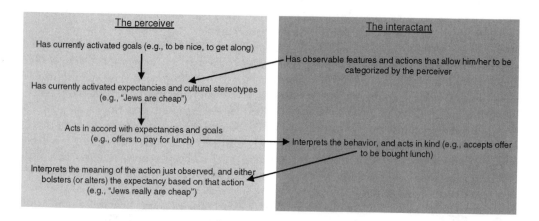

FIGURE 13.1. A social interaction sequence (driven by the expectancy "Jews are cheap").

The Self-Fulfilling Prophecy

According to Merton (1948, p. 423; emphasis in original),

> the self-fulfilling prophecy is, in the beginning, a *false* definition of the situation evoking a
> new behavior which makes the originally false conception come *true*. The specious validity
> of the self-fulfilling prophecy perpetuates a reign of error. For the prophet will cite the
> actual course of events as proof that he was right from the very beginning.

In other words, a perceiver's expectancies can actually cause someone else to act in line
with those expectancies. Perhaps the most famous example of the self-fulfilling prophecy is the "Pygmalion in the classroom" studies of Rosenthal and Jacobson (1968).

Rosenthal and Jacobson (1968) gave expectancies to school teachers about the
intellectual abilities of their students. This is not unusual, as most teachers know
whether they are teaching an advanced, average, or remedial class, and also have data
about specific students' abilities within each type of class. However, in this case the
expectancies were lies! The teachers were told that students had various intellectual abilities as derived from the students' scores on an IQ test. What the teachers did not know
was these scores were not at all accurate; instead, students were randomly assigned to
an ability level. Thus the experiment could now investigate whether expectancies came
to cause the very behavior that was expected, even though the expectancy was false.
Would a teacher's expectancies about the intellectual abilities of a student lead that student actually to develop those abilities? Would a student who spent a year with a teacher
who believed the student had intellectual potential actually come to have a higher IQ?

Teachers were told that some students in the class were identified by a test as
"bloomers," or kids who would soon show strong increases in intellectual performance.
All students had their actual IQ recorded by the experimenters at the start of the school
year. They hypothesized that the processes in the interaction sequence, described
above, would cause children labeled as bloomers to bloom. Teachers would have expectancies triggered about those students' superior ability. These expectancies might cause
a teacher to call on a student more often, or to challenge the student more. In addition,
the teacher might be more likely to interpret an ambiguous answer as evidence for the
student's ability and to respond in kind, with affirmation and positive reward. The student, in turn, might start working harder to meet these increased pressures, or to continue to attain the positive feedback. Eventually this cycle would contribute to the actual
intellectual development of the student, relative to other students of equal skill. The
results were consistent with this idea. Students labeled as bloomers had significantly
larger increases in their IQs than students who were not labeled as bloomers.

Another dramatic example of how a perceiver's expectancies can actually cause
another person to exhibit the very behaviors associated with the expectancies was provided by Snyder, Tanke, and Berscheid (1977). They asked college men to have a
"getting-acquainted" conversation with a woman over the telephone. These conversations were recorded, and the portion spoke only by the woman was later played back to
a different set of research participants to see how those participants rated her general
warmth, sociability, and friendliness. The researchers predicted that the expectancies of
the men in the conversation would have an impact on how warmly and sociably they
spoke to the woman, which would in turn determine how warmly and sociably the
woman spoke back to each man. Thus each man's expectancy would be responsible for

the behavior of the woman. But there was one trick: The men did not realize that they were acting particularly warm or sociable, or that an expectancy of any type was affecting their behavior. Because they did not realize this, they would think that the warm and sociable behavior on the part of the woman was mostly due to her being a warm and sociable person.

How could an expectancy be created that would lead men to act in a way that was warm and sociable, without realizing they were acting in any particular way? It was quite simple. Snyder and colleagues (1977) showed some of the men a picture of the woman that revealed her to be extremely attractive. The remaining men were given a picture that led them to expect they were talking to a physically unattractive woman. The results supported the self-fulfilling prophecy: The woman who was labeled as attractive to the men in the telephone phase of the experiment was judged as being more sociable and warm by the research participants in the second phase of the experiment, who had no information about her appearance and who heard only what the woman had said on audiotape. The expectancies of one group of men led to consistent behavior being performed by a woman, and this behavior was detected by a separate group of men who had no expectancies. The expectancies of the first group of men elicited the confirming behavior.

One final demonstration of how perceivers' beliefs, expectancies, and stereotypes of others can end up producing the actual behaviors that they expect to see was provided by Word, Zanna, and Cooper (1974). They started with the assumption that expectancies are linked with specific types of nonverbal responses, through which one unknowingly communicates with those to whom the expectancies apply. The more positive one's expectancies, the more positive a host of nonverbal behaviors there will be. These include closer interpersonal distance (being closer to a person while conversing), more eye contact, a shoulder orientation that is more direct, and leaning into the person. The opposite behaviors are found when stigma and negative stereotypes are associated with a person: One tends to terminate discussions sooner, have greater interaction distances, make less eye contact, and so forth. Word and colleagues examined whether these expectancy-derived behaviors would be detected by members of stereotyped groups, and whether this would cause them to respond to those behaviors with reciprocal behavior (thus fulfilling the prophecy by confirming the stereotype).

Their experiment required that a so-called "team" of four research participants work on a task together. Three of them were not really participants, but confederates working for the experimenters. The task assigned to the group was to pick a fifth member for their team. Each participant (a White man) was chosen to interview the person, using a list of 15 questions provided for him. The applicant, who was either a Black man or a White man, was also a confederate who was trained to give the same responses to the questions regardless of what the participant did (keep in mind that all participants were asking the same set of 15 questions). The issues of interest were what sort of nonverbal cues the interviewer gave off during the interview, and whether stereotypes associated with Black men would have an impact on how the person chose to behave while conducting the interview. The behavior of the participant was measured through things such as physical distance (as measured by how far the person sat from the interviewee after bringing a chair over), forward lean, eye contact (proportion of time looking into person's eyes), and shoulder orientation. In addition, interview length and speech error rate were measured. The results, as we might predict, revealed that participants acted in different ways during the course of an interview. Although there was no explicit racism, there were subtle, nonverbal behaviors that differed in how interviewers interacted with a Black versus a White person. White interviewers sat farther from a Black man than a White man; they leaned less closely toward him; they looked less often into his eyes; they made more errors in speech; and they conducted shorter interviews.

What effect would being the recipient of such nonverbal cues have on a person's reciprocal performance to the interaction partner? In the context of a job interview, the reciprocal behavior could be perceived as an inferior performance and might lead to the person not getting the job. To examine this issue in the context of this research, Word and colleagues (1974) conducted a second experiment in which White research participants were being interviewed by a White confederate who was trained how to conduct the interview by the experimenters. The interesting twist to this experiment was that half the time, the interviewers used the nonverbal behaviors and style of interacting that had been discovered to be associated with how White men acted toward Black men. The other half of the time, the interviewers used the nonverbal behaviors and style of interacting that had been discovered to be associated with how White men acted toward White men. The interviews were then videotaped, and they were rated by judges who did not know the hypotheses of the experiment. Only the interviewee was seen on each tape. The judges rated the person's composure and performance. The results showed that when people were treated with differential nonverbal cues, they reacted in kind. White people treated by interviewers the way Blacks were typically treated (with less eye contact, shorter interview times, more speech errors, and apparent distance) were evaluated as doing less well in the interview. They mimicked the behavior they received from others—committing more speech errors, seeming more distant, and so forth. In essence, they performed worse during an interview because of the behavior of the interviewer. The interviewer produced behaviors in others that came to fulfill the negative expectancies, although both parties were naive to this influence.

Stereotype Threat

Word and colleagues (1974) showed how stereotypes lead to deficits in the performance of members of a stigmatized group—deficits that have nothing to do with the actual ability of the group members. These deficits are implicit responses to the behaviors of others, and these behaviors are biased by the stereotypes the others hold. Steele (1997) points to a different type of behavioral deficits in the members of a stereotyped group. Although these deficits are also linked to the stereotypes of their group that are held by others, in this case an expectancy embodied in others' behavior does not cause reciprocal behavior on the part of the group members. Instead, the members of the stereotyped group simply perceive the existence of bias in the situation (including in other people), and this perception causes behavioral deficits. That is, *a belief that others have negative expectancies of (and negative behaviors aimed at) the group causes the group members to perform below their actual ability because they feel threatened by this stereotype.* People from stigmatized groups worry that others will reduce them to being nothing more than the stereotype, and will judge them exclusively in terms of it. They have anxiety that their own behavior might actually allow others to confirm existing stereotypes of the group. Although it is true that all people suffer from performance anxiety and fear of being evaluated negatively, this is an additional, and quite distinct, form of anxiety—the pressure of holding the fate of the group on their backs and of expecting to face a world that is biased against them. It is more than performance anxiety; it is stereotype threat. Steele has defined *stereotype threat* as an anxiety or threat that arises when one is in a situation or doing something for which a negative stereotype about one's group applies. This predicament threatens one with being negatively stereotyped, with being judged or treated stereotypically, or with the prospect of conforming to the stereotype. Called stereotype threat, it is a situational threat—a threat in the air—that, in general form, can affect the members of any group about whom a negative stereotype exists (e.g., skateboarders, older adults, White men, gang members). Where bad stereotypes about these groups apply, members of these groups can fear being reduced to that stereotype. (p. 614)

Steele (1997) outlines two debilitating effects of stereotype threat. The first is a decrease in performance on tasks relevant to the threat. If the stereotype involves notions of poor intellectual ability, then expectancies that others hold biased views of the group on this dimension will cause group members to perform poorly on tests of intellectual ability. If the stereotype is that the group lacks athletic ability, then the expectancy that others will see them as poor athletes will lead group members to perform worse than they would have had they not contemplated the expectancies of others. The performance deficit is domain-specific, linked to acts that are relevant to the stereotype. The second debilitating effect is called *disidentification*: "a reconceptualization of the self and of one's values so as to remove the domain as a self-identity, as a basis of self-evaluation. Disidentification offers the retreat of not caring about the domain in relation to the self" (Steele, 1997, p. 614). The real deficit here is that the threat associated with an expectancy that others are stereotyping can undermine motivation. This leads group members to withdraw from caring about the behavior. When the behavior is as important as intellectual ability, this threat is quite damaging. Steele argues that it will have the strongest impact on the people who care most about the domain. Thus, ironically, the very best students may start to care less and less about school as they disidentify with this domain, shrinking from the anxiety associated with the negative expectancies. For fear of fulfilling the stereotype that the group is "stupid," even the smartest among them may start to withdraw from intellectual pursuits because of this threat.

As an example, Spencer, Steele, and Quinn (1999) recruited for an experiment female and male students who were good at math, and who strongly identified with it. They took a very difficult math test (items were taken from the advanced math Graduate Record Examination [GRE]). Women, though equally qualified and able, performed worse than men. However, when they took an advanced literature test, women performed the same as equally qualified men. Presumably, these effects emerged because the women felt stereotype-threatened in the domain of math, where, according to the cultural stereotype, women are challenged. No such threat exists in the literature domain, so no deficits in performance arose in that domain. In an interesting follow-up to this point, Spencer and colleagues attempted to manipulate threat. The logic was that if women could take a difficult math test under conditions in which they were *not* led to contemplate the negative expectancies associated with their group in this domain, then they would perform up to their ability and do as well as men. However, if those expectancies existed, the stereotype threat induced would undermine performance. To manipulate threat, the researchers told some participants that the math test they were taking generally shows gender differences, thus creating a condition of stereotype threat for the women. Other participants were told that the math test has in the past shown no gender differences, implying that the stereotype would not be relevant in this situation (and hence no threat). As expected, when threat was removed from the situation, women performed as well as men. The expectancy caused performance deficits that could be defeated by the removal of the expectancy/stereotype.

Steele and Aronson (1995) performed a similar set of experiments with African Americans. Black and White research participants took a test resembling the GRE or the Scholastic Aptitude Test (SAT), under conditions that either promoted stereotype threat or minimized it. To promote it, participants were told that the test was diagnostic of intellectual ability (a domain that is relevant to the stereotype of Blacks). To minimize threat in the situation, participants were told that the test was not diagnostic of intellectual ability. Black and White students of equal intellectual ability performed differently if the test was supposedly a measure of intellectual ability, with Blacks doing worse. However, if they took the same test thinking that it was not about intellectual ability, the two groups scored the same! Blacks were scoring lower on the test not because they were less able, but because the anxiety associated with the performance was heightened—the burden associated with the expectancy was greater for them. Do group members need to be told explicitly that a test is about intellectual ability for these negative deficits to appear? What does it take to trigger the threat? Apparently, not much. Steele and Aronson performed one experiment where all they did was ask some participants to record their race on a demographic questionnaire just before taking the test, while others did not indicate race. Black students showed a deficit in performance only when race was indicated. Thus making race salient was enough to trigger stereotype threat and its related deficits. Simply asking about race lowered the scores of African American students who otherwise would have scored higher, and not reliably differently from White students of similar ability.

Finally, does one need to be a member of a stigmatized group to experience stereotype threat? Stone, Lynch, Sjomeling, and Darley (1999) cleverly illustrated how the very same task can be threatening to an ethnic minority group when framed one way, but threatening to members of the majority group when framed a different way. Stereotypes regarding athletes have an impact on both White and Black men. For Whites, there is the "Larry Bird" stereotype—having lots of on-court smarts/intelligence, but not being especially gifted athletically (in terms of speed, grace, agility, etc.). For Blacks, the opposite stereotype exists—the naturally gifted athlete who lacks intelligence. Stone and colleaguess' Black and White research participants were given an athletic task to perform (putting). Some were told the task measured natural athletic ability; others were told that it measured "sports intelligence"; and still others were not given any information relevant to stereotypes about Whites or Blacks ("the task you are performing is for a study on sports psychology"). In the "sports psychology" control condition, both Blacks and Whites did the same on the golf task. However, stereotype threat emerged in the other conditions. Black participants performed worse when the task was framed as being about sports intelligence as opposed to natural ability, while White participants suffered only when told that the task measured natural athletic ability (as opposed to "sports intelligence"). How the task was construed altered the behavior of the participants drastically, and in different ways for Blacks and Whites.

Expectancies and Construal of the Environment

Anxiety associated with possibly fulfilling a negative cultural stereotype is one way to explain the decreased performance observed in members of stigmatized groups in domains relevant to the stigma. Although this may often be the cause of performance deficits, there is another plausible account as to why behavior may be undermined when stereotypes are brought to mind. Perhaps fear of fulfilling the stereotype is not the cause; perhaps the stereotype itself alters the manner in which the situation is construed. Like the behavior of people, situations are often ambiguous. In order to act appropriately in response to a situation, one must first identify and categorize it to know what is appropriate. For example, when one is in a doctor's office waiting to pay a bill after having been examined, and the person collecting the money behind the glass window is yammering away on the telephone with what appears to be a personal call, how is one to construe this situation? Does it call for patience or assertiveness? Does it call for politeness or rudeness? How one acts is determined by how the situation is construed. As another example, when one is taking a test like the SAT, how is one to construe this situation? Is it an opportunity to display one's abilities and intellectual acumen, or is it an opportunity to possibly destroy one's hopes for college admission and to put one's inadequacies into an official document? In a final example, perhaps one is on the way to the store and comes across a person passed out on the sidewalk. Does one stop to help or walk on by? The answer probably depends on how the situation is construed. Is the person in trouble and in need of help? Is he/she drunk or a victim of assault?[1]

Accessible Stereotypes

The notion that situations need to be construed, and that construal determines behavior, can be used to explain why members of a stereotyped group underperform on tasks relevant to their particular group stereotype. Let us return to our stereotype threat example. It could be that thinking about the group stereotype alters the way in which one frames the task at hand. For example, perhaps a test like the SAT is now seen as a chance to do poorly rather than a chance to do well, and this anxiety makes one choke. Why would the stereotype of African Americans make one frame the test as an opportunity to do poorly? The stereotype contains the notion of poor academic achievement. Having this concept primed might then lead one to use that concept to frame the task when it otherwise might not be. Thus the difficulty is not fear of fulfilling the stereotype, just the tendency to construe the situation (a test) in an anxiety-provoking way.

One way to illustrate this would be to show that effects that resemble stereotype threat (such as reduced performance on a test like the SAT) occur for White research participants when they are primed with the stereotype of African Americans. White participants could not have the anxiety of fulfilling the stereotype, because the stereotype of Blacks is not relevant to them. But they do have knowledge of the stereotype that could be triggered and then could have an impact on behavior through altering how the test is construed. As an example, Wheeler, Jarvis, and Petty (2001) had non-African American research participants work on a task that had questions taken from the math section of the GRE. Half of the participants first had stereotypes of African Americans primed by writing an essay, for an ostensibly separate experiment, about a day in the life of Tyrone Walker (a name meant to signal to participants that the person was Black). The other half wrote about a day in the life of Erik Walker (a name not suggesting that the person was Black). Remarkably, non-Black participants who wrote about Tyrone scored lower on the math test than participants who wrote about Erik. Here is an example where behavior on a test was modified by a stereotype of another group that happened to be accessible, altering how the situation is construed.

Accessible Theories

Bushman, Baumeister, Philips, and Collen (2001) have proposed that the accessibility of a theory about the meaning of a behavior will determine how people construe the appropriateness of the behavior at a given point in time, and determine whether they perform a behavior (or not). For example, if people have a theory that venting their anger will make them feel better, they should act aggressively and express their anger (this is the logic of catharsis). On the other hand, if they believe that venting anger will not make them feel better, they should not tend to aggress against others. The accessible theory of what it means to be aggressive will determine whether the act is displayed or not. Bushman and colleagues' research participants were asked to read a bogus newspaper article informing them about scientific research that either supported or refuted the notion of catharsis (i.e., venting anger improves mood). This was used to manipulate the accessible theory about the behavior "aggressiveness." Then each participant was asked to write an essay that would be read and reviewed by another research participant. The person providing the feedback was actually a confederate working for the experimenters who provided negative and insulting feedback. Finally, in a competitive task, the participant was given the opportunity to punish the insulting person who was providing the feedback. The participant's behavior on the competitive task was the measure of interest (the participant was able to inflict an unpleasant blast of noise on the other person, and the duration and intensity of the blast were the measures of aggression). The findings revealed that those who read the pro-catharsis article gave more punishment and more severe punishment (acted more aggressively). Believing that aggressive action was cathartic and could restore their mood led people to use aggressive behavior against others more than when the same behavior by those others was being construed by perceivers who believed that aggressive behavior would not be useful for mood restoration.

Accessible Traits

Carver, Ganellen, Froming, and Chambers (1983) examined not only how the meaning of aggressiveness can alter behavior, but whether the mere accessibility of the trait "aggressive" would determine how aggressively people acted. Whereas behavior is typically assumed to require conscious deliberation, in the form of either a self-selected choice to pursue a goal or an explicit instruction to adopt a goal to behave a particular way, the authors were able to illustrate that people could act aggressively simply by being primed with the trait "aggressive." Carver and colleagues used a sentence construction task (e.g., Srull & Wyer, 1979) with words related to aggression so that the concept would be primed. Participants then performed a task where they had to shock another person every time that person incorrectly answered a question. The duration of the shock was longer for participants primed with aggression. Although not as dramatic as the Milgram (1963) experiment (see Chapter 1), where participants persisted in shocking others at ever-increasing levels and despite the victims' screams, this research demonstrates the impact of passive primes on (shocking) behavior.

Neuberg (1989) revealed a similar effect of accessible traits on behavior by examining how people act in the *Prisoner's Dilemma game*. The game gets its name from the options available to two criminal suspects being interviewed in separate rooms at the police station. Each prisoner has two options: to confess or not to confess. Each choice carries with it some ramifications, but the ramifications are also dependent on what the "partner" does. If one person confesses and turns in the other, and the other refuses to blow the whistle, the police may reward the person who confessed and punish harshly the other prisoner, on whom they can now pin the crime. However, if both suspects blow the whistle, they are now both in danger of a penalty, but not as severe as when only one of them is alone to take the fall for the crime. Thus, if one person does not confess and the other does, the first one is now in deep trouble. Finally, if neither person blows the whistle on the other, then the chance of being convicted is extremely low. This is a dilemma, because the appropriate action depends on how each prisoner construes what the partner will do. If a prisoner believes the partner will squeal, then it is in his/her best interest to squeal as well—this way, the penalty for the prisoner will be more lenient. If, however, the prisoner believes the partner will not talk, then it is in his/her best interest not to talk also. But if this is wrong and the partner does talk, the prisoner is now in serious trouble. In the absence of knowing what the partner will do (since the two persons are in separate rooms), the prisoner needs to decide how to act under conditions of uncertainty. An analogous situation can be created in the lab. Money is awarded to people who play a game where there are two possible moves: to cooperate with the partner or to compete with the partner. An analogous payoff structure can be created to the prisoner's dilemma by giving one person a huge reward for choosing the competitive option if (and only if) the partner has chosen the cooperative option (and for that person, there is no gain). If, however, both people choose to cooperate, then there is loss for both people; if both people choose to compete, the losses to each are more severe yet (see Figure 13.2). Thus choosing to compete is a risk that may have big rewards or big losses. In the absence of knowing the partner's choice, how should one act?

Neuberg (1989) found that one variable determining how research participants would act in the Prisoner's Dilemma situation was whether they had previously been primed with notions of competitiveness. The logic was that primed concepts would have an impact on how participants construed the situation (as one calling for cooperativeness or competitiveness), and that this would guide what they deemed to be appropriate behavior. To make things even more intriguing, the primes in this case were presented subliminally. Thus items that participants could not even consciously detect

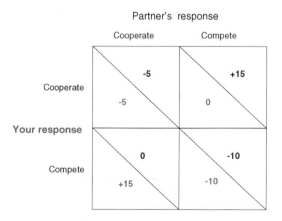

FIGURE 13.2. The possible rewards in the Prisoner's Dilemma game.

might determine how they acted. Research participants were subliminally exposed to words as part of a task they believed was about perceptual decision making. For half of the participants the words were relevant to competitiveness, and for the other half they were neutral words. Next, participants were asked to perform a supposedly unrelated task—the Prisoner's Dilemma game. The important measure was the degree to which participants selected a competitive strategy. The measure was made on each participant's second move of the game—after he/she had a chance to make one decision (cooperate or compete) and see how the partner responded to that move (cooperate or compete in return). The partner's first move was cooperative for half of the research participants and competitive for the other half. The second move was chosen as the dependent measure, because it was felt that until a participant had seen the partner respond, the situation was not one open for construal; the participant would need some information to interpret before being able to spin that interpretation one way or the other. The results were actually a little more complicated than a simple finding that primes influenced behavior. Priming participants with the trait "competitive" had no effect if the persons had a natural inclination to cooperate. Thus it was hard to turn cooperative persons into competitive persons by priming them (natural inclination was assessed by looking at what people did with their first move of the game). However, if participants were not cooperative sorts by default, then the prime had a powerful effect. People primed with "competitive" were more likely to compete on the second trial than people exposed to neutral concepts as primes. This was true regardless of the partner's move. Other research has similarly suggested that how one construes the behavior of an interaction partner is an important determinant of whether one cooperates with that person (e.g., Smeesters, Warlop, Van Avermaet, Corneille, & Yzerbyt, 2003; Van Lange & Semin-Goossens, 1998).

Accessible Exemplars

It stands to reason that if priming people with a trait leads them to assimilating their own behavior to match the primed trait, then, given what we have learned in Chapter 10, priming people with an exemplar should be expected to trigger contrast rather than assimilation. Thus people should act in the manner opposite that implied by a prime if the prime is an exemplar. Dijksterhuis and colleagues (1998) found exactly this. In one study, Dutch research participants were primed with an exemplar of an elderly person, the Dutch Queen Mother. It was found that participants, when primed with this exemplar, walked faster following the prime—a contrast effect. In another experiment, Dijksterhuis and Van Knippenberg (1998) replicated this finding, using intellectual performance. People were primed with one of two exemplars relevant to intelligence: a famously brilliant person (Albert Einstein) and a famous person not known for intellectual prowess (Claudia Schiffer). Performance on a task tapping intelligence was better when participants were primed with Schiffer, but deteriorated when they were primed with Einstein—a case of behavioral contrast.

Accessible Goals

Chapter 10 has concluded that subliminal primes in a political commercial may affect judgment if the target of judgment is ambiguous. However, subliminal advertising is meant to alter not only judgment of a product, but behavior toward the product. In the 1960s, a famous experiment was unleashed on the consuming public. A researcher infiltrated a movie theater to investigate the effects of subliminal advertisements on what sort of products people purchased at the refreshment stand. It was reported that the words "Drink Coke" being subliminally flashed in a movie theater led sales of Coca-Cola to go up by 18%. Why would people leave their seats to buy Coke following this subliminal message? The answer is "They would not." It turns out that the famous data reporting this finding were fabricated.

Strahan, Spencer, and Zanna (2002) suggest that this does not mean that behavior is never influenced by a subliminal prime. However, for subliminal priming to alter how you behave, you must first have the goal to behave. The prime could then influence your behavior if the concepts primed are consistent with the actions needed to attain the goal. For instance, you would not get up and drink Coke if you were not thirsty, but if you were already thirsty and contemplating a trip to the refreshment counter, a prime might influence your selection. But even if you were thirsty, you might not choose to drink Coke unless the cognitions relevant to Coke that were made accessible were particularly linked to the goal—such as its being a particularly thirst-quenching beverage. If the advertisement said something like "Drink Coke. It's the real thing," this would not prime concepts relevant to the goal of quenching you thirst, so the advertisement would be useless. But "Drink Coke. It quenches your thirst" might work. Thus action can be affected by a prime that is relevant to that action if the goal to act is also triggered. Of course, you may now also be wondering, "If people already have the goal to act a particular way, why would priming influence whether or not they act?" Strahan and colleagues (2002, p. 557) state that "in our view it would not be adaptive for people to pursue every goal every time it is activated." People have many goals active at any point in time, and which ones they actually pursue depend on their level of commitment to each goal, which ones are more feasible to attain in this situation, and so on. Priming can prioritize one of the goals and have an impact on whether the current environment is construed as likely to yield successful attainment of the primed goal.

To illustrate that priming a goal can have an impact on behavior if and only if people are already motivated to act, Strahan and colleagues (2002) examined whether priming people with "thirsty" would increase beverage consumption, but only among people who were already thirsty. Research participants believed they were participating in a marketing experiment assessing various foods and beverages. They were asked not to eat or drink for 3 hours before the experiment. At the lab, the participants first performed a taste test and ate some cookies. Next, half were asked to cleanse their palates by drinking water; the other half did not have this opportunity. Participants were now in two groups—a thirsty group (those who did not drink for 3 hours, ate cookies, and did not get a chance to drink) and a not-thirsty group (those who had a drink in the experiment). Next, participants were asked to perform a lexical decision task, and in this task they were being subliminally primed. Half of the participants were primed with words relevant to thirst, and the other half were primed with neutral words. Finally, the four groups of people (thirsty and primed with thirst words; not thirsty and primed with thirst words; thirsty and primed with nonthirst words; and not thirsty and primed with nonthirst words) were asked to perform a second taste test comparing two beverages (both were really Kool-Aid). The measure of interest in the experiment was how much Kool-Aid the participants had to drink, which was measured by seeing how much was left over when they left the room. The hypothesis was that the subliminal prime would have an impact on behavior (drinking Kool-Aid) only if the persons already had the goal in place (they were thirsty). This was what was found. When participants were not thirsty, priming did not matter. However, when people were thirsty, they drank more when primed with thirst-related concepts as opposed to neutral concepts.

This research shows that priming concepts related to action only guides behavior if goals relevant to the act are also primed. In this case, the goal of quenching thirst was primed before subliminal primes were presented by asking people not to drink for 3 hours before the experiment. However, it is also the case that a goal can be primed as implicitly as trait concepts (as seen in Chapter 10), and once subtly primed can have an impact on behavior. As Bargh (1997) put it,

> Once activated, functionally transparent or automated skills can interact with the environment in a sophisticated way, taking in information relevant to the goal's purposes, and directing appropriate responses based on that information, without the need for conscious involvement in those responses. The auto-motive model of goal-directed action (Bargh, 1990) added just one assumption to this idea: The entry point or trigger that starts the goal into operation can itself be subsumed and removed from conscious choice. (p. 29)

Fitzsimons and Bargh (2003) demonstrated how priming a goal, as opposed to a person's consciously selecting a goal, can alter how the person construes the environment (thus altering behavior to be in accord with that construal). They proposed that mental representations of interpersonal relationships (e.g., mother, best friend) include the specific interpersonal goals relevant to those relationships (e.g., achievement, helping, understanding). The goal relevant to a relationship can be implicitly activated by a person simply thinking about the relationship partner. Because the goal is part of the representation, triggering the representation will trigger the goal. Despite the person not consciously deciding to pursue a goal, its activation through its association to the activated representation of the significant other can now have an impact on responding.

In Chapter 9, two experiments by Fitzsimons and Bargh (2003) have been reviewed—each illustrating that the priming of different relationship partners altered the way in which people behaved, so that behavior was consistent with the goals associated with the specific relationship partner who had been primed (people primed with their mothers achieved more; people primed with their friends helped more). How can we be certain that the priming influenced the activation of a goal (rather than having an impact on behavior for some other reason)? Fitzsimons and Bargh made this point by assuming that if priming a participant's mother activates a relationship-relevant goal (i.e., achievement), then the participant should view a set of behavior ambiguously relevant to achievement as more achievement-oriented than a person primed with a different relationship partner (e.g., a friend) should. Any impact on behavior should be caused by the triggering of the goal associated with that specific partner, which should determine how the current situation is construed (which in turn should determine what actions are appropriate). To demonstrate this, participants were asked to visualize either their best friends or their mothers, and to write about the appearance of these partners in a couple of lines. Next, participants read a vignette about a college student whose behavior was ambiguously related to being successful at school, and rated the extent that they believed the target person was motivated to be successful at school. Participants primed with their mothers saw the target person as more motivated to succeed than those primed with their best friends. Thus goals seem to alter the way other people are construed, and this difference in construal guides how people act, even if they are not aware a goal has been primed.

For anyone ever concerned with weight watching, goal priming has implications for how one chooses to eat. Eating behavior is certainly one important domain of behavior that people dedicate a lot of time to regulating. Fishbach, Friedman, and Kruglanski (2003) investigated the behavioral effects of implicit goal priming in the domain of dieting. Participants were primed with either dieting goals or control goals. Diet primes were introduced by asking participants to work in a room with magazines and photographs about weight watching, while control participants were in a room with magazines and pictures irrelevant to this goal. As a dependent variable, participants were asked to choose between a chocolate bar and an apple as a departing gift upon completing the experiment. Diet-goal-primed participants were more likely than controls to choose the apple rather than chocolate. Therefore, priming can "lead us not into temptation."

Finally, Aarts, Gollwitzer, and Hassin (2004) have argued that the priming of a goal can be "caught" from other people. Goals are contagious, such that seeing someone else performing a goal-relevant behavior can prime that goal in a perceiver (even though it is not explicitly stated). They label this process of automatically adopting the goals that others seem to be pursuing as *goal contagion*. Once a goal is activated through goal contagion, it can influence behavior without the perceiver's awareness of this influence (or awareness that a goal-relevant behavior has even been observed in the other person, let alone triggered in the self and governing the self's action). However, perceiving a goal-directed behavior in another person is not proposed always to lead to the perceiver adopting that goal. The perceiver must value the goal before the goal will be caught from others. In a test of this impact of goals on behavior, research participants read about the behavior of a person who went to work on a farm. For half of the participants the person was described as going to do volunteer work, whereas for the other half the person was described as working for money to pay for a vacation planned with some friends. Next, a message appeared on the computer screen telling participants that another task would follow and that following that task, if time permitted, they could perform yet another task to earn cash. The question of interest was whether the participants who had read about someone with the goal of making money would now adopt this goal and then have it influence their behavior. In this case, the behavior would be to try to fly through the second task to ensure that there was time for the money-making task.

Aarts and colleagues (2004) further predicted that the extent to which participants valued the goal would moderate the effect. While all students like money, some are more in need of it than others. Therefore, they predicted that the speed with which people found their way to the final task (the cash-earning task) would be moderated not only by the goals implied in the behavior of the person they read about, but by the financial status of the research participants. People short on cash should be more susceptible to catching the goal (they should have a reduced "immune system," so to speak). Results supported the hypotheses. Participants who read about someone with the implied goal of making money were faster in working their way through the experiment when they had a high need for money, but not when they had a low need for money. Goals were primed by observing others, and they then had an impact on behavior because of this interpersonal exchange when participants valued the goal pursuit. We may conclude that we need not have a fear of starting to act like others who behave in non-normative and maladaptive ways. We do not adopt the goals of a freak, a creep, or a weirdo. We are not inclined to experience goal contagion following socially undesirable behavior (unless we already value that behavior).

Attributions of the Perceiver

Perhaps the clearest way to illustrate that how one construes an event determines how one behaves is to manipulate construal more directly. The previously described studies manipulated what information was accessible and predicted that this accessibility would alter construal. Seligman, Finegan, Hazlewood, and Wilkinson (1985) performed an experiment in which the attributions made by perceivers were directly manipulated and their impact on behavior was observed. Research participants were the customers of a take-out pizza place who were waiting for delivery of a pizza. The participants were not aware they were in an experiment; they simply wanted pizza and called the pizza place to order one. Each person was informed that the pizza would be at his/her door in 45 minutes. Ten minutes later, participants were phoned back and told that the pizza would either be late or early, and the reason for its being late or early was also manipulated. Half of the people were told that traffic conditions were the reason. Half were told that the reason was the delivery driver's ability (or lack of it) to keep up with the deliveries in a timely fashion. In essence, people were given two different construals for the same event. A pizza being late (or early) was either due to uncontrollable forces of traffic or due to the abilities of the delivery guy. How did these construals affect behavior? The dependent measure in the study was tipping. The prediction was that people would tip more when the pizza arrived early rather than late, but this was dependent on making an internal attribution, since tips are a reflection of satisfaction with a person providing a service. If the delivery time was construed to be linked to uncontrollable forces, the tip should not be dependent on when the pizza arrived. In support of the prediction, when a person attribution was made, the tip was larger when the pizza was early than when it was late. When a situational attribution was made, there was no difference in how people acted based on when the pizza arrived—the tip was the same for a late pizza as it was for an early one. We may conclude that how we act toward others is determined by the intentions and causes we think underlie their actions.

Accessible Self-Standards

Throughout this book, several ways in which behavior can be used to compensate for some perceived shortcoming have been revealed. In Chapter 2, this has been described in terms of a negative feedback loop, in which a shortcoming in a goal pursuit provides the drive for behaving in ways that will rectify the shortcoming. In Chapter 12, the self-regulation model of prejudice (Monteith & Voils, 2001) has been applied to similar ideas governing behavior. Failing to act in a nonprejudiced way is a failure to attain a desired goal for many people. This triggers feelings of guilt that then serve as the drive for acting in ways to rectify the perceived shortcoming. People step up their efforts to be egalitarian and fair.

Embarrassment, guilt, and shame, as motivators of compensatory responses, could be conceived of as reactions people have when they detect themselves being hypocrites. When people detect a discrepancy between how their values/beliefs dictate they should act and how their perception of reality reveals they actually do act, this amounts to little more than detecting their own hypocrisy. Their actions do not back up their words. *Hypocrisy* is essentially the discrepancy between people's behavior and a standard that has been established (usually by themselves) relating to that behavior. Just as perceiving a discrepancy between some current state and a goal can lead to compensatory behavior, hypocrisy should also be a powerful motivator of compensatory behavior. This was evidenced in the research of Stone, Aronson, Crain, Winslow, and Fried (1994). Stone and colleagues were working within the framework of cognitive dissonance theory, where it is well established that when behavior is incongruent with attitudes (creating a state of cognitive dissonance), either the behavior or the attitudes must be altered to bring an end to the aversive state. Although much research has been conducted looking at how people change their attitudes to rationalize their dissonant behavior, less work has been done examining how people alter their behavior as a means to rectifying the dissonance between a desired state and the actual state of affairs. As Monteith and Voils (2001) illustrated in the domain of prejudice, behavioral responses can be initiated to compensate for such discrepancies and to reduce the tension associated with people's own undesirable behavior. Stone and colleagues illustrated this exact point by making people aware of the hypocrisy between their own stated beliefs and their own past behavior.

Research participants were asked to make a videotape where they were advocating to others the importance of a specific prosocial behavior: They were asked to speak about the importance of using condoms during sex to prevent the spread of AIDS (in other research, people have been asked to make arguments promoting the conservation of water, the use of sunscreen to prevent skin cancer, and the importance of recycling). By itself, making such a plea would not create dissonance and would not be hypocritical, because it was probably not inconsistent with participants' beliefs/values. No standard was violated. However, the researchers predicted that hypocrisy would be experienced and dissonance would be aroused when participants were made aware that their own past behavior was not always consistent with what they had just stated—that they did not "practice what they preach." This was done by having people contemplate times in their own lives when they acted in ways inconsistent with the behavior they had just advocated on the tape. Stone and colleagues (1994) found that after hypocrisy was created in people, they subsequently acted in a manner that would reduce the dissonance associated with this hypocrisy. The experimenters provided participants with the opportunity to purchase condoms at the end of the experiment, and participants made aware of their hypocrisy on this issue were more likely to engage in behavior that addressed reducing the hypocrisy (purchasing condoms).

But were people simply attempting to make themselves feel good in this research, or were they attempting to address the specific problem at hand and reduce the discrepancy in the domain in question? This question relating to feelings of hypocrisy has important implications for stereotyping. The former option suggests that people who feel guilty or hypocritical about their stereotyping of others may perform any positive action that will let them feel good about themselves, even if it has nothing to do with the domain (stereotyping) that has caused their sense of hypocrisy. The latter option suggests that people must make responses in the exact domain that has caused their cognitive strife, and this prediction suggests that they must act in a nonstereotypic way to reduce hypocrisy in the domain of stereotyping. To investigate this question, Stone, Wiegand, Cooper, and Aronson (1997) offered more than one behavioral strategy for "feeling good" to participants—one irrelevant to their hypocrisy and one relevant to it. Following the procedure of Stone and colleagues (1994), participants were made aware of the hypocrisy that existed between their own practice of safer sexual behavior relevant to AIDS and their advocacy for the use of condoms in the videotape they made for the experiment. Some participants were then offered an opportunity to "feel good": They were asked whether they would donate the payment they received for being participants in the experiment to a shelter for homeless persons. Other participants were offered the opportunity to donate to the shelter, but they were also provided with the opportunity to use their payment to buy condoms. The results showed that when participants were made aware of their hypocrisy and then were only asked to donate money, 83% donated to the shelter. However, when the opportunity to buy condoms was present along with the opportunity to donate to a homeless shelter, 78% chose to purchase condoms, and only 13% chose to donate to the shelter.

We can conceive of participants in these studies as detecting that their behavior did not meet some standard that had been made accessible. For example, when the standard was the personal goal of being an egalitarian person, acts of prejudice triggered compensatory behavior. When the standard was being the type of person who practices what he/she preaches, hypocrisy would trigger behavior aimed at alleviating the hypocrisy. However, if some different standard had been used against which to assess the behavior, perhaps a different form of behavior would have been observed. If the behavior did not violate the standard being used, then no shortcoming would have been perceived, and no compensatory behavior would have been needed. For example, Stone and colleagues' (1994) research participants were not displaying any desire to purchase condoms when not asked to contemplate their own past behavior. The absence of a discrepancy with a standard led to drastically different behavior than when participants' current options as to how to behave were construed in the context of their past behavior as a relevant standard.

Stone (2001) proposed that the various "selves" posited by self-discrepancy theory (see Chapter 12) can each be used as a standard for evaluating one's own behavior. If the "ought" self is primed, this should establish a different standard than if the "actual" self is primed. These differences in one's accessible standards should lead to differences in how one construes one's own behavior (and how one subsequently behaves in response to that construal). For example, if one advocated the use of condoms for an experimenter in the way participants did for Stone and colleagues (1994), and was then reminded of one's past failures at consistently using condoms, this would trigger feelings of hypocrisy and lead one to behave in ways to rectify the feeling. However, if one was using a normative standard for evaluating one's past behavior (e.g., making salient the idea that, like many others, one had not been consistent in this regard), the construal of the past behavior might be quite different than if a more personal standard had been accessible. Behavior would change as the accessible standard changed, because the way in which one construed one's own past actions would be quite different in the two contexts (e.g., Stone, 2003).

Construing the Past by Relying on Peak Experiences and End Experiences

The impact of past behavior on current and future behavior is not limited to the way in which the construal of prior action can lead to feeling hypocritical. Varey and Kahneman (1992) argue that the construal of the past also can determine future behavior by contributing to decision making. In deciding whether to perform a particular behavior, we typically first assess the *utility*, the *hedonic consequences*, of engaging in that behavior. In other words, we ask, "Will I like it? Is it pleasurable or aversive?" To make this decision, we look to past experience. However, there are two mental processes, each fallible, that can make our assessment of how much we enjoyed our prior behavior inaccurate: memory and evaluation. First we have to recall the event accurately; then we have to make accurate evaluations of the recalled information.

Varey and Kahneman (1992) focused on two ways in which misremembering the past alters the evaluation of the action, and changes our construal of its hedonic consequences. As perceivers of our own past, we focus too heavily on *peak experiences* and *end experiences*. That is, we overweight our evaluation of a memory with the hedonic experience associated with the very end of the episode and at the very height of the emotional impact of the episode. Thus, if we are recalling a pleasurable experience, such as a trip to the amusement park, we may recall the exhilaration of the trip at its peak (such as how we felt when we were cascading down the roller coaster) and at its end (such as how we felt when we were riding our favorite roller coaster one last time before leaving the park). We neglect to adequately recall the hours of waiting in lines, the overpriced food, and the disgusting bathrooms. This leads us to remember the nice event as more pleasurable than perhaps it really was. More curiously, we use the same overreliance on peak and end experiences to distort our memory for painful past behaviors. Many painful experiences taper off so that the pain diminishes gradually. If we rely too heavily on the end experience, we may recall the hedonic consequences of a painful event in a biased way, so that they are seen as not too bad.

Redelmeier and Kahneman (1996) provided evidence illustrating how people will misremember a painful medical procedure by relying too heavily on recall for the peak and end experiences. Patients undergoing a colonoscopy were asked to evaluate the pain they were experiencing minute by minute during the procedure. They also were asked to evaluate the experience after the fact (both immediately after the procedure and 1 month later). The recollected evaluation of the procedure was determined best not by the length of the actual procedure (e.g., how long they had to undergo the painful experience), but by the combined experiences of the pain felt at the peak moment and at the end of the procedure.

This bias in construing the hedonic consequences of past behavior will lead us to actions in the future that are determined by this construal of the past. For example, we paradoxically should be more likely to choose to have a colonoscopy if, the last time we had one, the procedure took 45 minutes as opposed to 30 minutes. If the extra 15 minutes were unpleasant, but were characterized by diminishing unpleasantness, then our recollection of the experience will be that the 45 minutes of discomfort and pain were not as bad as the 30 minutes of discomfort and pain, even if at their peak the pain was exactly the same. Why? Because it ended better. Thus we would be more likely later to choose a colonoscopy 45 minutes long over one 30 minutes long, even though the former experience is objectively worse—just as painful during the first 30 minutes, with 15 extra minutes of diminishing pain tacked on. Overrelying on the prior experience at the end (how we felt when the procedure finished) causes a change in the construal of the event; in this case, it does so in an irrational manner, so that we choose to engage in painful behavior that lasts longer.

Kahneman, Fredrickson, Schreiber, and Redelmeier (1993) illustrated this phenomenon in the lab. Research participants were asked to have two unpleasant experiences that were identical at the peak, but that differed in the end. First, each participant had to immerse a hand in freezing cold water (the moderately painful temperature of 14 degrees Celsius) for 1 minute. The second experience was identical to the first, with two exceptions: the duration of the experience, and the temperature of the water for the end of the experience. The participants each held a hand in freezing cold water at the same temperature for the same amount of time (one minute), but then had to keep the hand in the water for an additional 30 seconds while the temperature was raised slightly to the still uncomfortable level of 15 degrees Celsius. This long trial had all the discomfort of the short trial, plus an extra 30 seconds of discomfort. However, the extra discomfort was slightly more bearable than that in the preceding minute. Finally, participants were told that there would be a third trial and they could choose how to act. Would they want to repeat the short or the long trial? Remarkably, people chose to act in the more painful way, with 69% choosing the longer trial. Kahneman and colleagues proposed that memory for the longer event was biased by the end experience. Even though it was just as painful at its peak, and even though the peak amount of pain was equivalent in length, and even though the extra time was uncomfortable (not even close to pleasant, just less uncomfortable), participants still chose the longer-lasting episode. The construal of the event was biased by the way it ended, and the construal then shaped behavior. Clearly, when using prior acts as information about how much we enjoyed an experience, and using that information to help us make decisions about how we should act in the here and now, we make bad decisions because of the fallibility inherent in the mental operations.

Social Change Strategies

Chapters 5 and 8 have introduced *social identity theory*, a theory suggesting that one uses social comparison processes to evaluate one's own group against relevant other groups (e.g., Tajfel & Turner, 1986). This theory maintains that a simple striving for a positive identity to be linked with one's social group can give rise to ethnocentrism and other forms of prejudice. The model posits several stages in the rise of prejudice and conflict: (1) The need for positive social identity can be satisfied by having the group one belongs to positively evaluated (since part of self-identity comes from group memberships); (2) the group to which one belongs has both positive and negative connotations, and one's goal for the outcome of social comparison processes is to reveal one's own social group to be positive and distinct; and (3) when these comparisons are negative, one seeks to do something about it. One can either denigrate the comparison group(s) or take action to alter the contributions to identity made by one's own group.

What determines how one behaves when social comparison processes provide one with a negative social identity? Tajfel and Turner (1986) propose that an important factor is the manner in which one construes the environment as a group member. Beliefs about *social mobility* versus *social change* influence the strategies one uses to change negative social identity and to relate to others (as individuals vs. members of a group). When the borders of society are construed to be free and open, then social mobility is seen as viable. Perceived social mobility may lead to the belief that one might have the ability to change a group's lot in life through individual effort. One perhaps believes that "if enough individuals act as I do, the lot of the entire group would be lifted up." This belief system leads one to seek individualistic strategies of change for negative social identity and to treat others more as individuals than as group members. Although "going mobile" can alleviate the negative contributions to identity, one may not construe social mobility as possible, such as when the borders between groups are perceived to be impermeable. Responses to this state of affairs are collectivistic strategies one can adopt as a reaction to negative social identity, such as mobilizing one's group to instigate change. Construing one's environment as impermeable, with lines of group membership clearly drawn, dictates a group-based rather than an individual-based approach to changing status. One should respond to others in ways that define those others in terms of group memberships (rather than reacting to them as individuals; see also Taylor & Moghaddam, 1987; Wright, Taylor, & Moghaddam, 1990).

The belief system of "social mobility" is based on the assumption that the society in which the individuals live is a flexible and permeable one, so that if they are not satisfied, for whatever reason, with the conditions imposed upon their lives by memberships in social groups or social categories to which they belong, it is possible for them (be it through talent, hard work, good luck, or whatever other means) to move individually into another group that suits them better . . . At the other extreme, the belief system of "social change" implies that the nature and structure of the relations between social groups in the society is characterized by marked stratification, making it impossible or very difficult for individuals, as individuals, to divest themselves of an unsatisfactory, underprivileged, or stigmatized group membership. (Tajfel & Turner, 1986, p. 9)

Tajfel and Turner (1986) describe several behavioral strategies that one can enact to attempt to change a negative social identity when social mobility is not construed as possible. One possibility is to shift the dimension on which social comparisons between groups are made. If the group comes off negatively when we compare against another group along Behavior X, then let us now collectively decide that Behavior X is irrelevant and start valuing Behavior Y instead—a behavior where the ingroup is better than the comparison group. A second collectivistic strategy is to assign a more positive value to attributes the group already possesses, rather than accepting the negative value assigned by others. This is known as *redefining* the attributes associated with the group, such as when the slogan "Black is beautiful" emerged following the civil rights movement in the United States. A third behavioral strategy for altering negative identity has been discussed in Chapter 12 during the review of minority influence. Members of minority groups can initiate change in how others think about their group (perhaps altering the negative perceptions that are contributing to negative social identity) by a direct challenge to the views of the dominant group. Moscovici (1985a) believed that successful influence occurs through conflict, not compromise; it is dependent on minority group members' consistently, persistently, and tenaciously adhering to their "unique" minority view and refusing to yield to the majority: "Stringent intransigence often typifies the attitude of individuals who have had a great impact on our ideas and behavior"(p. 29).

Finally, one last "social change" strategy to address a negative social identity is to change the group used as the standard of comparison. Rather than using a dominant group that will reflect negatively on one's own group, one chooses a different standard for comparison in which one's group is now the superior one (downward social comparison). This can create a positive self-image, but may result in repressing the shortcomings of one's own group. Perhaps a more serious cost is that such a strategy may lead one to treat the group serving as the standard of comparison unfairly. That is, this strategy can lead people to raise their esteem by seeing themselves more positively than others, leading them to derogate other minority groups. For example, Francophones in Canada constitute a numerical minority in every province except Quebec, and are considered a political outgroup because the seat of power is largely occupied by Anglophones. It is not uncommon to hear French Canadians denigrating immigrant groups. However, this process has cost them politically: As the immigrants get to vote, they will not vote for Francophone candidates, ultimately preventing Francophones from achieving their goals.

To test whether construing the environment as closed (i.e., viewing groups as having impermeable boundaries) would lead to collective action, whereas perception of group boundaries as open would lead to a more individualistic strategy, Wright and colleagues (1990) assigned research participants to groups. They were asked to perform a decision-making task as part of one group, but the group had a disadvantaged status relative to another group in the experiment. Participants were told that promotion to the better, more sophisticated decision-making group could occur if their performance warranted it. The members of the "better" group subsequently unilaterally rejected some of the participants from joining their ranks. Thus the experimenters had manipulated the perceived level of openness of the boundaries between the groups. The participants who were told that the "better" group was impermeable chose a different behavioral response from that selected by people who believed it was open. As the theory predicts, construing of the borders between groups as closed led to collective action: Research participants wrote letters of protest and urged the other members of their group to ignore the decisions made by the so-called "superior" group.

THE AUTO-MOBILE MODEL

Speeding with Ned

During my first year as a member of the faculty at Princeton University, the psychology department hosted a conference to honor its beloved former member, E. E. (Ned) Jones. Aside from his important work on such issues as correspondent inference, actor-observer bias, stigma, outgroup homogeneity, self-handicapping, and ingratiation (all reviewed in this book), he was a storied mentor of many of the other researchers whose work has been reviewed in this book. One of them, Dan Gilbert, used the opening of his talk at the conference to relay a story. The young Gilbert, we were told in the talk, had found himself in the passenger seat speeding at 90 miles per hour along the New Jersey Turnpike with his advisor, Jones, when a common occurrence was observed: A police car had someone pulled over on the side of the road. Gilbert observed how all the drivers on the road acted in the same, predictable way upon seeing the police car—they slowed down. Except for Jones, who acted in an unpredictable way; he sped up. To Jones, getting caught speeding or getting away with speeding was a game—a matter of guessing where the police were—and to play the game well meant adjusting his speed accordingly at the right moments. Slowing down at the sight of the engaged police officer, Jones explained, was just irrational behavior. Police cars, young Gilbert was told, need to be spread out over miles and miles of turnpike. Slowing down just before you reach one is rational, but you don't know where they will be, and they are not evenly spaced out. That is what makes the game challenging. However, there is one instance where it is not so challenging. When you see a cop busy on the side of the road, it is rational to assume that another won't be encountered in the immediate future. This is the time to adjust speed upward, not downward, Jones explained to Gilbert, since the moment after passing an engaged officer is the one moment during the trip when you are least likely to see a cop. Gilbert (personal communication, 1995) relayed Jones's words: "Speeding by the cop is the best move you can make. . . . But most people don't, because they're too reflexive. They react in ways they recognize as totally illogical even when they're perfectly capable of drawing a logical conclusion. . . . It never ceases to amaze me."

The story tells us of one man's passion for understanding the detours people take from rationality in their attempts to speed toward attaining meaning, construing their environment, and deciding how to act. But what might have amazed Ned Jones even more, had he lived just another few years to see it, was research telling us that perhaps other drivers are not being so irrational. Rather than using the wrong rules in construing their environment, the other people may be acting without using rules at all. It is possible that they are slowing down not because they are incorrectly construing their environment or acting without rational thought, but instead because they are *behaving without the influence of any thought*. Such behavior is not mindlessness (see Chapter 2), where people are using minimal thought or following simple rules. The suggestion is that such behavior is automatic, unmediated by thought of any kind other than the triggering of a mental concept that has stored within it a representation of the behavior. A remarkable line of recent research indicates that often people act simply because mental representations that include the action have been triggered (e.g., Bargh, Chen, & Burrows, 1996). To return to Gilbert's story, it could be that drivers' knowledge of the concept "state trooper" includes the fact that they should be cautious around them. However, this fact is not consciously brought to bear in construing the situation; instead, the unmediated impact of such knowledge on behavior means that seeing the police car triggers the concept "state trooper." Once triggered, it initiates behavior linked to that concept, such as being cautious and driving slowly. Rather than thinking irrationally and slowing down at precisely the wrong moment because of bad decision making under pressure, people act without thinking at all. They start slowing down without knowing why or deciding to do it. These drivers are being *auto-mobile*—acting automatically. Whereas an *auto-motive* (Bargh, 1990) has been said to be an automatically triggered goal that can guide behavior by altering intentions and volition, being auto-mobile eliminates the need to implicate volition in action. Behavior follows its own mental notion.

Ideomotor Behavior

This explanation for what determines our behavior is somewhat hard for most of us to accept. The idea that we act without even knowing we are acting, or being involved consciously at any stage of the decision to act, is even more amazing than the idea that we act in nonrational ways. It removes our individual wills from the equation altogether. We behave because the mere presence of a cue in our environment that is relevant to some construct is followed immediately and unhesitatingly by the behavior, without the intervention of construal processes or consciousness (Dijksterhuis & Bargh, 2001). The logic behind this assumption is derived from James (1890/1950), as evidenced by the quote that has begun this chapter. In his chapter on the will, James (p. 522) posed the question of whether the representation of a behavior can be directly triggered by a cue in the environment: "Must there be an additional mental antecedent, in the shape of a fiat, decision, consent, volitional mandate, or other synonymous phenomenon of consciousness, before the movement can follow?" James answered his own question by turning to the notion of *ideomotor action*, or the "sequence of movement upon the mere thought of it. Wherever movement follows *unhesitatingly and immediately* the notion of it in the mind, we have ideo-motor [*sic*] action" (p. 522; emphasis in original).

One excellent way to illustrate that the will is not involved in the production of behavior is to show that people act in the exact opposite of the way that they intend! If people are consciously willing not to do something, only to find themselves engaging in the undesired act, there is a good chance that they are behaving automatically. Elegant and easy-to-grasp examples are offered by James (1890/1950). First is the example of a woman who, in the early morning, finds herself getting dressed despite her conscious thoughts having last placed her in bed dreading the cold awaiting outside the covers. Her will has her desiring to be in bed, yet thoughts of work and the chores of the day ahead impel her to be getting dressed before she has even realized she is no longer in her desired place snugly under the blanket. A second example is the "stuffed" man who, after finishing a big dinner, further stuffs nuts and chocolates into his mouth on perceiving them on the table. James also gives the example of the host retiring to his bedroom to dress for his dinner party, only to find himself moments later in his pajamas and in bed, instead of in his tie and walking down the stairs to await his guests. The cues in each of these situations are triggering the behaviors associated with those situations, not the behaviors the individual is willing. Recent research has illustrated what James proposed—that it is not only judgment that is determined by accessible information, but *behavior*.

In a classic illustration, Bargh and colleagues (1996) examined whether the accessibility of a construct would lead individuals to behave in a manner consistent with behavioral representations that were part of that construct. In one of their experiments, participants were subtly exposed to words linked to the stereotype of old people ("Florida," "old," "wrinkle," "ancient," "wise"). None of these words implied the concept of "slowness," which is also part of the stereotype. The idea was that this task would prime the stereotype of elderly people, and activation would spread so that all components of the stereotype would now have a heightened state of accessibility, including the concept of "slowness." With the behavioral component "slowness" now primed, people would come to act in a way consistent with the mental representation: They should start to move more slowly!

Unlike in research on assimilation and contrast effects reviewed in Chapter 10, the perceivers' judgment of some ambiguous person was not of interest in this experiment. Rather than asking the research participants to read about and form an impression of a man named Donald, the researchers simply told them that the experiment was over. The measure of interest was how quickly or slowly the participants walked from the experimental room, down the hallway, toward the elevator. Unbeknownst to participants, an experimenter timed their trek down the hallway. People primed with the elderly stereotype now acted like elderly people in at least one regard: They walked more slowly than people who had not been primed with this stereotype. The subtle priming of the stereotype altered how people behaved without their realizing that their behavior had been influenced in any way. It would be difficult to explain this result in terms of their construing the situation differently, such as a hallway that called for them to walk more slowly. Rather, the mental act seems to have become the physical act. In subsequent experiments, Bargh and colleagues illustrated this phenomenon of behavior following the mere thought of the behavior by priming participants with subliminal images of African Americans. The prime was predicted to have an impact on action by triggering the stereotype associated with the prime. The researchers found that once the stereotype was unknowingly triggered, one aspect of the stereotype (aggression) found its way into the actions of the participants: They acted more aggressively, despite the fact the stereotype was not relevant to them (since the participants were White). Therefore, people seem to be acting what they are thinking, even without realizing they are thinking it.

It might now seem feasible to introduce yet another way effects that look like what we have called *stereotype threat* might come about. It could be that if the stereotype of African Americans is triggered, the component of the stereotype having to do with poor academic ability would lead one simply to act in this way, unmediated by construal of the test-taking situation. Wheeler, Jarvis, and Petty (2001) propose that many of the findings in the stereotype threat literature could be explained via this ideomotor mechanism, as opposed to the idea that people fear fulfilling a negative stereotype and are debilitated by this specific form of anxiety. This does not mean that stereotype threat does not occur. It means that in addition to stereotype threat, there are other reasons to be careful that people are not primed with stereotypes relevant to intelligence when taking tests. In a clever illustration of this ability for test-taking performance to be guided by accessible constructs, Dijksterhuis and van Knippenberg (1998) primed research participants in the Netherlands with stereotypes of groups known to be associated with either intelligent or moronic behavior. People were asked to think either about professors or about soccer hooligans, and then to take a test. The people for whom college professors (the intelligent group) were accessible subsequently performed better on the test, while people asked to think about soccer hooligans performed worse. Something seemingly unmovable, such as intellectual ability measured by performance on a test, was shaped by the primes people were exposed to before taking the test. Apparently, people act smarter when primed with stereotypes of smart people.

Against the Will: Unwanted Action

Ansfield and Wegner (1996) argue that there is a feeling usually associated with actions that we have decided to pursue: "Some sort of sensation, an internal 'oomph,' goes with the effort of doing . . . the feeling is not there when we simply think about an action" (p. 482). However, not all actions lead us to experience this feeling of doing. Following James (1890/1950), many behaviors are performed even when they are explicitly being avoided and suppressed. If we are explicitly trying to disavow a behavior, yet it occurs nonetheless, there must be an automatic component to the behavior that is not dependent on the conscious or phenomenal will. Such behaviors that occur against the will should lack this feeling of doing. Ansfield and Wegner review a series of historically well-known phenomena (which many of us are familiar with from our own experience) that seemingly occur without the influence of the conscious will. The list includes pendulum swings with magical powers (such as predicting a baby's gender when held over the mother's belly), divining rods, Ouija boards, automatic writing, and seance tables that move. However, Ansfield and Wegner are quick to rob these phenomena of their mysticism. They cite, as an example, Mischel Chevreul's claim that the movement of the "wise pendulum" is dependent on the psychological state of the person holding it. For the pendulum to work its magic, it has to be suspended by the arm of a person in a manner allowing the muscular movement of the person to guide the swing. Thus what is magical is not the power of the pendulum, but the power of the person holding it to guide the pendulum movement without any awareness that his/her muscles are moving or having any impact on the pendulum. "Just thinking about a circular or left-to-right swing pattern, for example, seems to be sufficient for many people to have that pattern occur . . . when a person is thinking about the hour of the day and swings a ring by a thread inside a glass, it often strikes the hour even while the person has no conscious sense of doing this" (Ansfield & Wegner, 1996, p. 483).

This is an excellent example of ideomotor action: Mere thought of movement causes the movement in the absence (and denial) of a conscious will to act. This is how Carpenter (1884, pp. 284–287), clearly an inspiration to James (1890/1950), described the "mystical" pendulum swing:

If "a fragment of anything, of any shape," be suspended from the end of the fore-finger or thumb, and the Attention be intently fixed upon it, regular oscillations will be frequently seen. . . . This will occur, notwithstanding the strong Volitional determination of the experimenter to maintain a complete immobility in the suspended finger. . . . [The movement] is entirely derived by his expectation of the given result. For if he be ignorant of the change which is made in the conditions of the experiment, and should expect or guess something different from that which really exists, the movement will be in accordance with his Idea, not with the reality. . . . [This is an] example of the general principle, that, in certain individuals, and in a certain state of mental concentration, the expectation of a result is sufficient to determine—without any voluntary effort, and even in opposition to the Will (for this may be honestly exerted in the attempt to keep the hand perfectly unmoved)—the Muscular movements by which it is produced.

Wegner, Ansfield, and Pilloff (1998) revisit the theory of ironic processes of mental control (reviewed in Chapter 12) as a way to account for the occurrence of automatic behavior. The theory proposes that operating and monitoring processes make up a control system. Whereas the operating process is effortful and conscious, the monitoring process is unconscious and less demanding of effort. The operating process aims toward achieving desired end states, whereas the monitoring process searches for failure in order to signal that control is needed. When one has the goal to avoid a thought or action, the monitoring process can have the ironic effect of creating the unwanted act or thought. Chapter 12 has reviewed how this process can give rise to the increased accessibility in the mind of the very thoughts one is trying to avoid, especially when one is under cognitive load.

Wegner and colleagues (1998) turned toward examining ironic effects on action. Some research participants were told not to move a pendulum in a specific direction (horizontally); others were asked to hold it steady. The task was performed either under cognitive load or without load. It was predicted that load would produce an ironic effect, such that there would be an increase in unwanted pendulum movement. A video camera was placed underneath a glass plate on which a grid was centered in order to measure the pendulum movements. In the condition where participants were instructed to prevent pendulum movement, they were told, "Your task is to not let the pendulum move, keeping it as steady as possible. The pendulum should be held as steady as possible over the center spot, and you should not let it move in the direction of the parallel horizontal line on the page in front of you." In the condition where participants were instructed to hold the pendulum steady, the instructions made no mention of the forbidden direction. The results showed that when participants were under cognitive load and given explicit instructions not to move the pendulum along the x axis, the exact opposite behavior emerged. More movement was observed on the x axis than on the y axis. These results suggest that trying not to perform a simple action can create ironic effects.

THE DYNAMIC PERSONALITY

Much of our discussion of social cognition has centered around perceivers' attempts to infer dispositions in the people they observe. Armed with these inferences, perceivers can make predictions about these others' behavior, thus informing their own decisions about how to behave. There is an important assumption built into this logic, one not yet discussed. The assumption is that people actually do act in a manner consistent with their dispositions. That is, a *direct relationship between traits and behavior* is assumed, with behavior being *stable across time and consistent across situations*. Knowing the personality of another person is believed to indicate something about how the individual will act: The kind person will act kindly; the honest person will not steal or lie; and the aggressive/violent person will be threatening and a danger to others. Consider the following quote from the former Mayor of New York, Rudolph Giuliani, who was answering a question about Presidential candidate John Kerry's positions regarding fighting terrorism during a March 7, 2004, interview on the NBC-TV show *Meet the Press*:

> I honestly don't know what Senator Kerry's approach is to the war on terrorism. He voted against the Persian Gulf war in the early '90s; he voted for the Iraq war; he voted against sufficient funding for the Iraq war after that; he seems to be in honest confusion about what his position is. The best case I can have on it, listening to the debates in the Democratic primaries, is that Senator Kerry doesn't have a real position on the war on terrorism; it changes. . . . What would be missing is that steady, very consistent approach, which President Bush has had.

The assumption that basic consistencies or invariances constitute the core of personality and guide behavior from situation to situation is made not only by laypersons trying to perceive their social world, but by many psychologists studying the nature of personality. Mischel and Peake (1982; Mischel, 1973), however, challenged this notion, claiming that there is a striking lack of consistency in behavior across situations. For instance, Mike Tyson may be a violent personality type with an aggressive disposition, but he is not a constant threat to people. He acts kindly, he cries, he is at times gentle. Some situations evoke aggressiveness and violence, but others (many others) do not. Consistency in John Kerry should not be assessed by whether his votes on specific issues change, but by the degree to which those changes are logical, given the situations and goals when each vote was taken. It would be foolish to vote the same if circumstances change. Morf and Rhodewalt (2001) describe personality as being *dynamic*, in that it involves a reciprocal transaction between a person (and person-centered variables such as emotion, motivation, and cognition) and the constraints/affordances presented by the situation. Because of this dynamic, the same person's behavior will vary across situations.

Behavioral Signatures

According to Mischel and Shoda (1995), the essence of personality—and hence the relationship between personality and behavior—can be captured by the idea that situations provide affordances for action, and that only in the interaction between the current situation and the traits of the person can a pattern of consistent behavior be observed. Dispositions, rather than driving the same behavior across all situations, specify appropriate ways to act IF certain conditions are met or IF certain environmental conditions are in place. IF-THEN relations are seen as the basic units of personality. IFs refer to situations or conditions, and THENs to the responses exhibited in them. The unique pattern of IF-THEN relationships that exist for a person (IF Condition X is in place, THEN we expect to see Behavior Y associated with Trait Z) is likened to a signature. It is a distinct way of identifying a person, with behavior contextualized so that personality expresses itself differently, for each person, in different situations. Consistency in behavior should be expected, because personality does exist. But it does not exist as an invariant property of the person that superimposes itself on the environment. It is a subtle interaction of the forces within the person and the affordances of the situation.

The unique pattern of trait-relevant behavior as evidenced in specific contexts has been labeled by Mischel and Shoda (1995) as a *behavioral signature*. The logic of behavioral signatures dictates that there is not a direct relationship between traits and behavior, but an indirect one that can even allow for the same personality trait to cause the same person to act in totally different ways in different situations (as well as explaining how two different people can act differently in the same situation). Behavior can even reverse itself from one situation to another. This is not evidence that people are inconsistent. They are being internally consistent with their traits; those traits just express themselves differently when different situations arise (the THEN changes when the IF changes). The "acquired meaning" of a given situation, or the individual's construal of the situation, will determine how the person acts (Mischel & Shoda, 1995).

Paradoxically, we can expect people to act sometimes in ways that seem inappropriate or opposed to their so-called personality traits IF the situation they are in triggers goals and intentions that make that behavior appropriate given their construal of the event. Rather than labeling people as inconsistent or as not acting according to their traits based on some observable behavior, what we need to do to evaluate consistency in behavior (the ability to be true to traits) is look to see whether the behavior is consistent with a goal that may have been triggered, given the construal of the environment. Let us get less abstract. A person may be categorized as a sociable and extraverted type, yet may be observed acting like a wallflower at a party. Do we conclude that this behavior is inconsistent with his/her personality? Not before we examine the goals of the person triggered by his/her construal of the event. What we see as "a party" may be construed by the person as a "social obligation for my boss, who has bullied me into attending this gathering." The next day we may see the same person in what seems to be a psychologically similar situation, acting as if he/she wants to fight for the right to party. Is this reversal inconsistent? Not if we understand that the event is now being construed by the person as "a chance to meet interesting new people" and thus has triggered a different set of goals.

Personality Types as Signatures

Morf and Rhodewalt (1993) provide a beautiful illustration of how a person can act in a seemingly irrational way, but when we look at the IF-THEN relationship specified by that person's construal of the situation, the paradoxical behavior makes sense. It is consistent with what that person's personality would imply. Knowledge of the behavioral signature makes the behavior meaningful and perfectly predictable, despite seeming unpredictable when examined without the benefit of the behavioral signature. Morf and Rhodewalt examined people with narcissistic personalities. These are persons with a grandiose sense of self-importance, who are preoccupied with fantasies of unlimited achievement, talent, and success. Such persons have a strong sense of entitlement, require admiration from others, and are arrogant and haughty, despite also being capable of envying those who seemingly have something they do not. Morf and Rhodewalt propose that such a personality type has linked to it goals to be superior to others, and these chronic goals should lead such persons to search for situations that afford them the opportunity to pursue the goals. They look for chances to exert their superiority and avoid situations that present threat to that superiority, such as those that can present failure in an important domain. Thus how narcissistic persons act is dependent on how the situation interacts with these goals and intentions associated with the personality type. Two logical IF-THEN behavioral signatures can now be used to describe these persons: (1) IF there is an opportunity to promote the self, THEN start self-promoting at all costs, even at the expense of others; (2) IF there is a threat to the self, THEN start behaviors aimed at compensating for the failure and at restoring the exaggerated sense of positive regard, thus lessening (or undoing) the threat.

In one experiment, Morf and Rhodewalt (1993) had research participants receive (false) feedback about how well they performed on a task relative to another person. This constituted a threat, because the other person was described as being superior on the task. How would participants respond to such a threat? We would predict that they would act in ways to restore the positive sense of self. But what types of specific behaviors might we expect to see in narcissistic relative to non-narcissistic participants? If narcissistic individuals intend to be superior, how does this intention work its way into action? One way in which people restore a positive sense of self after having been threatened by a negative social comparison is to denigrate the person who is seemingly superior. Another strategy is to attempt to rationalize away the failure by minimizing the importance of the failure: Its domain is seen as less relevant, thus minimizing its impact. Morf and Rhodewalt expected that narcissistic participants would be especially prone to engage in these types of behaviors. Participants (half narcissistic and half non-narcissistic), after being told that another person was superior to them, were then asked to evaluate the other person on a personality measure. Half of the people were told that these evaluations were being made in private and would only be seen by the experimenter. Half were told that the evaluations were going to made in public and that the partner would be seeing these evaluations.

Most people would not engage in the behavior of saying negative things about another person if they knew that the other person was going to see that information (especially if the only thing the other person did wrong was to perform well on some task). It would create too great a source for interpersonal conflict. Narcissistic participants, however, were predicted to act in a way that would appear paradoxical if one did not understand their behavioral signature. They should provide negative evaluations of the other, regardless of whether the other person would see it or not. Their strong sense of entitlement and their need to be superior would create too great an intention to reduce their feelings of threat, leading them to get nasty and personal directly to the other person. The findings revealed that the narcissistic participants derogated the other person much more than the non-narcissistic ones did, and that this was much greater in the *public* condition (think of the journalist Bill O'Reilly). Even non-narcissistic participants derogated another person who outperformed them when ratings were made in private. But in public, they modified their ratings to conform to conventions of politeness and not to look overtly envious. Narcissistic persons did not bother moderating their reactions in public. Their goals in this situation (their IFS) specified behavior (their THENS) that warranted an attack on the other person's character.

Another example of seemingly paradoxical behavior that can be explained if one understands the behavioral signature is provided by the work of Downey and colleagues (e.g., Downey & Feldman, 1996; Downey, Freitas, Michaelis, & Khouri, 1998). This research examined the behavior of people with a personality type labeled as *rejection sensitivity*. If persons are sensitive to being rejected by others, then it would seemingly make sense for such persons not to engage in behaviors that might bring about rejection from others. However, this is not the case. Why? The intended behavior of such people is to avoid rejection. This makes them chronically engaged in a search of the environment for indications that they might be rejected; they are thus perceptually ready to perceive rejection from others, especially from relationship partners, with whom the fear of being rejected may be strong. The IF specified by interactions with significant others then becomes skewed toward detecting rejection and ultimately seeing rejection in the behavior of others, even when another person would not construe the interaction in such a way. The behavior then is dictated by the perceived rejection, and these persons engage in a host of behaviors aimed at reducing the perceived rejection. These behaviors then may actually cause their significant others to start to actually reject the person. Perhaps the story of Marilyn Monroe is a good example. Despite being perhaps the most publicly desired woman of the 20th century, Monroe apparently had such fear of relationship partners' saying "Goodbye, Norma Jean" that it caused her to act in overly clingy and jealous ways. Her last husband, the writer Arthur Miller, apparently started writing in his diaries within weeks of marriage that he was unaware of what he had gotten himself into, as his every act was being perceived by his wife as a sign of rejection.

Downey and colleagues (1998) illustrated this phenomenon by having people sensitive to rejection discuss a conflict situation with their significant others. The rejection-sensitive people were observed to engage in a host of negative behaviors that could only serve to make others reject them: They denied responsibility for the conflict; they put down their partners; they voiced displeasure and disapproval; they acted in a disgusted manner; they withdrew affection; they displayed sadness and depression; and, perhaps worst of all, they whined incessantly. The very behaviors that would seem to create the state their personality type suggested should be avoided were the behaviors being enacted. Were these people inconsistent? Does personality not exist? No. Personality exists within the behavioral signatures of an individual that tie the goals, wants and expectancies of the individual to the situation, thus linking behavior to the construal of the situation and others, as filtered through processes of active construction. As Morf and Rhodewalt (2001) assert, much of the active construction in which people engage takes place in the social arena, and involves goals and intentions that influence their interactions with other people. This is what can give rise to seemingly paradoxical behavior, as the goals of an individual may override what norms suggest would typically be appropriate behavior when interacting with another person. Thus, a narcissistic individual, who desires to be admired by others, paradoxically will be more likely than other people to insult another person in public, thus causing exactly the opposite outcome (being disliked) because this behavior serves the goal of undoing a perceived threat. The person sensitive to rejection will act in ways that are sure to make others be rejecting.

CODA

Rather than focusing exclusively on factors inside the person or in the environment, psychology is an increasingly interactionist discipline. Psychologists now envision internal dispositions interacting with environmental inputs to affect ongoing thoughts and feelings in a continual and dynamic manner. These interactions unfold over time, as factors within the individual affect the choice and the interpretation of situations, and as individuals change their social situations. Conversely, factors in the situation not only trigger individual affective and cognitive inclinations in the short run, but over time, also change aspects of the person.

—KENRICK ET AL. (2002, p. 347)

With this quote, we arrive at a resting place for the book. As individuals, we engage in a host of cognitive processes in the service of various goals. Social cognition involves the processes triggered when we are engaged in the social world, and the various domains of behavior linked to the presence (either real or imagined) of others. The social world needs to be construed and constructed, rather than merely perceived. We are social animals engaged in social cognition. Separating the processes of person perception from object perception is this fact that within the various domains of social behavior and social cognition are domain-specific motives, goals, expectancies, stereotypes, and so forth, which influence how we construe the social world and create a sense of reality.[2] The relevant goals, expectancies, stereotypes, and so on that are triggered will be uniquely associated with the situations in which we are located. Reality is actively built by the triggering of cognitive, motivational, and affective inclinations that direct our perception, attention, encoding, recall, judgment, and behavior. These are not only determined by the chronic states of accessibility we perceivers carry around from situation to situation, but by the social situation and the goals inherently tied to the various domains of social life. The responses that emerge may be based on our employing prior theories, expectancies, stereotypes, schemas, scripts, exemplars, and heuristics (as these have evolved because of their functionality and adaptiveness for us), but they may be based on a more elaborate and extensive analysis. In sum, responses to the social world represent interactions of persons (us) with situations.

Finally, as we have seen in this chapter, another force that differentiates interpersonal perception and behavior from object perception (and behavior directed at objects) is the fact that with person perception the objects being perceived are in turn perceivers. They are construing and making sense of the people in their social world, including us. Person perception and interpersonal interaction are special epistemological problems, in that they involve the construal of active agents who are in the midst of their own construals—even construals of us as we perceive them. At best, we can only attempt to discern the internal qualities of the people we attempt to perceive, to make predictions (which are more or less veridical) about how they are likely to act, and to plan our own behavior appropriately. This level of uncertainty rarely greets us in the world of objects. I know what a brick rocketing toward my head will do, and I am likely to know why it is speeding in my direction. People we perceive are only partly and imperfectly discernible, and they feel the same way about us. Interpersonal perception is a dance of mutual construal and prediction. It is an imperfect process, and we rely on whatever cognitive tools we have evolved to help us get through the dance without stepping on too many feet. We often get tripped up, and we are often smooth as silk, but it is a process that relies heavily on leaps of faith in the form of automatic processes that tell us what to do—even if, as Wilson and Brekke (1994) so comprehensively illustrated, we cannot adequately report what we have done or why we have done it. Life in the social world is a barrage of mutual construals, directed by goal-driven, expectancy-riddled, schema-based cognitive processes, both effortful and automatic, that allow us to perceive what others are like, just as they are perceiving us, and guide us through the dance that is the interaction sequence.

NOTES

1. The construal of the situation is determined by many forces. In Chapter 1, it is said to be influenced by the explicit framing of the situation. A situation described in terms of risk will

be reacted to differently than the same situation described in terms of loss will be. These subtle changes in how the very same situation is described alters what concepts are made accessible and are used in construing the situation and, in turn, determining what course of action is appropriate for that given construal (e.g., Tversky & Kahneman, 1981). In Chapter 2, one's goals are said to alter the way in which a situation is interpreted, with different means and opportunities becoming salient dependent on one's accessible goals. In Chapters 9 and 10, the construal of the situation is said to be dependent on whatever accessible information happens to be ready to be used for interpreting what one sees, regardless of whether the reason the information is accessible is that it represents a chronic concern or that it was recently encountered. In Chapters 11 and 12, stereotypes have been shown to create expectancies that alter how one perceives an ambiguous social event (e.g., Darley & Gross, 1983; Devine, 1989; Duncan, 1976).

2. Researchers have recently attempted to parse the social world into specific types of domains that have specific goals linked to the domain-specific problems of adaptation and function. Bugental (2002) refers to domains as "the bodies of knowledge that act as guides to partitioning the world and that facilitate the solving of recurring problems faced by organisms within that world" (p. 187). Bugental carves up the social world into five domains with specific sets of social problems and goals linked to solving those problems. These domains are (1) the attachment domain (dealing with joining others for reasons of safety); (2) the hierarchical power domain (dealing with issues relating to social power); (3) the coalition group domain (dealing with issues relating to identity, belongingness, and relatedness); (4) the reciprocity domain (dealing with the obligations of being part of a collective, such as responsibilities to others); and (5) the mating domain (dealing with selecting, attaining, and maintaining relationships for sexual purposes and survival of the gene pool). Kenrick and colleagues (2002) describe six key domains of social life, each specifying social goals that will determine how the environment is construed and which behaviors one intends to pursue.

References

Aarts, H., Gollwitzer, P. M., & Hassin, R. R. (2004). Goal contagion: Perceiving is for pursuing. *Journal of Personality and Social Psychology, 87,* 23–37.

Abelson, R. (1981). Psychological status of the script concept. *American Psychologist, 36,* 715–729.

Aboud, F. E. (1988). *Children and prejudice.* Cambridge, MA: Blackwell.

Adorno, T. W., Frenkel-Brunswik, E., Levinson, D. J., & Sanford, R. N. (1950). *The authoritarian personality.* New York: Harper & Row.

Alba, J. W., & Hasher, L. (1983). Is memory schematic? *Psychological Bulletin, 93,* 203–231.

Albright, L., Kenny, D. A., & Malloy, T. E. (1988). Consensus in personality judgments at zero acquaintance. *Journal of Personality and Social Psychology, 55*(3), 387–395.

Alicke, M. D. (1985). Global self-evaluation as determined by the desirability and controllability of trait adjectives. *Journal of Personality and Social Psychology, 49*(6), 1621–1630.

Allison, S. T., & Messick, D. M. (1988). The feature-positive effect, attitude strength, and degree of perceived consensus. *Personality and Social Psychology Bulletin, 14*(2), 231–214.

Allport, G. W. (1937). *Personality: A psychological interpretation.* New York: Henry Holt.

Allport, G. W. (1954). *The nature of prejudice.* Cambridge, MA: Addison-Wesley.

Allport, F. H., & Lepkin, M. (1945). Wartime rumors of waste and special privilege: why some people believe them. *Journal of Abnormal and Social Psychology, 40,* 3–36.

Ambady, N., Hallahan, M., & Conner, B. (1999). Accuracy of judgments of sexual orientation from thin slices of behavior. *Journal of Personality and Social Psychology, 77,* 538–547.

Ambady, N., & Rosenthal, R. (1992). Thin slices of expressive behavior as predictors of interpersonal consequences: A meta-analysis. *Psychological Bulletin, 111*(2), 256–274.

Ambady, N., & Rosenthal, R. (1993). Half a minute: Predicting teacher evaluations from thin slices of nonverbal behavior and physical attractiveness. *Journal of Personality and Social Psychology, 64*(3), 431–441.

Andersen, S. M., & Cole, S. W. (1990) Do I know you?: The role of significant others in general social perception. *Journal of Personality and Social Psychology, 59,* 384–399.

Andersen, S. M., & Glassman, N. S. (1996). Responding to significant others when they are not there: Effects on interpersonal inference, motivation, and affect. In R. M. Sorrentino & E. T.

Higgins (Eds.), *Handbook of motivation and cognition: Vol. 3. The interpersonal context* (pp. 262–321). New York: Guilford Press.

Andersen, S. M., Glassman, N. S., & Gold, D. A. (1998). Mental representations of the self, significant others, and nonsignificant others: Structure and processing of private and public aspects. *Journal of Personality and Social Psychology, 75,* 845–861.

Andersen, S. M., & Klatzky, R. L. (1987). Traits and social stereotypes: Levels of categorization in person perception. *Journal of Personality and Social Psychology, 53,* 235–246.

Anderson, C. A., & Deuser, W. E. (1993). The primacy of control in causal thinking and attributional style: An attributional functionalism perspective. In G. Weary, F. Gleicher, & K. L. Marsh (Eds.), *Control motivation and social cognition* (pp. 94–121). New York: Springer-Verlag.

Anderson, C. A., Horowitz, L. M., & French, R. (1983). Attributional style of lonely and depressed people. *Journal of Personality and Social Psychology, 45,* 127–136.

Anderson, C. A., & Sedikides, C. (1991). Thinking about people: Contributions of a typological alternative to associationistic and dimensional models of person perception. *Journal of Personality and Social Psychology, 60,* 203–217.

Anderson, J. R. (1993). Problem solving and learning. *American Psychologist, 48,* 35–44.

Anderson, J. R., & Bower, G. H. (1973). *Human associative memory*. Washington, DC: Winston.

Anderson, M. C., Bjork, R. A., & Bjork, E. L. (1994). Remembering can cause forgetting: Retrieval dynamics in long-term memory. *Journal of Experimental Psychology: Learning, Memory, and Cognition, 20,* 1063–1087.

Anderson, N. H. (1965). Adding versus averaging as a stimulus combination rule in impression formation. *Journal of Experimental Psychology, 70,* 394–400.

Anderson, N. H., & Hubert, S. (1963). Effects of concomitant verbal recall on order effects in personality impression formation. *Journal of Verbal Learning and Verbal Behavior, 2,* 379–391.

Anderson, R. C., & Pichert, J. W. (1978). Recall of previously unrecallable information following a shift in perspective. *Journal of Learning and Verbal Behavior, 17,* 1–12.

Ansfield, M. E., & Wegner, D. M. (1996). The feeling of doing. In P. M. Gollwitzer & J. A. Bargh (Eds.), *The psychology of action: Linking cognition and motivation to behavior* (pp. 482–506). New York: Guilford Press.

Aronson, E. (1968). The theory of cognitive dissonance: A current perspective. In L. Berkowitz (Ed.), *Advances in experimental social psychology* (Vol. 4, pp. 1–34). New York: Academic Press.

Aronson, E. (1988). *The social animal* (5th ed.). New York: Freeman.

Asch, S. E. (1946). Forming impressions of personality. *Journal of Abnormal and Social Psychology, 41,* 258–290.

Asch, S. E. (1948). The doctrine of suggestion, prestige and imitation in social psychology. *Psychological Review, 55,* 250–276.

Asch, S. E. (1952). *Social psychology*. New York: Prentice-Hall.

Asch, S. E., & Zukier, H. (1984). Thinking about persons. *Journal of Personality and Social Psychology, 46,* 1230–1240.

Ashmore, R. D. (1981). Sex stereotypes and implicit personality theory. In D. L. Hamilton (Ed.), *Cognitive processes in stereotyping and intergroup behavior* (pp. 37–81). Hillsdale, NJ: Erlbaum.

Atkinson, J. W. (1964). *An introduction to motivation*. Princeton, NJ: Van Nostrand.

Baker, S. M., & Petty, R. E. (1994). Majority and minority influence: Source–position imbalance as a determinant of message scrutiny. *Journal of Personality and Social Psychology, 67,* 5–19.

Baldwin, J. (1991). Nobody knows my name: More notes of a native son. New York: Vintage. (Original work published 1961)

Baldwin, M. W. (1992). Relational schemas and the processing of information. *Psychological Bulletin, 112,* 461–484.

Baldwin, M. W., Carrell, S. E., & Lopez, D. F. (1990). Priming relationship schemas: My advisor and the Pope are watching me from the back of my mind. *Journal of Experimental Social Psychology, 26,* 435–454.

Banaji, M. R., & Greenwald, A. G. (1995). Implicit gender stereotyping in judgments of fame. *Journal of Personality and Social Psychology, 68*, 181–198.

Banaji, M. R., Hardin, C. D., & Rothman, A. J. (1993). Implicit stereotyping in person judgment. *Journal of Personality and Social Psychology, 65*, 272–281.

Bargh, J. A. (1982). Attention and automaticity in the processing of self-relevant information. *Journal of Personality and Social Psychology, 43*, 425–436.

Bargh, J. A. (1984). Automatic and conscious processing of social information. In R. S. Wyer, Jr. & T. K. Srull (Eds.), *Handbook of social cognition* (Vol. 3, pp. 1–44). Hillsdale, NJ: Erlbaum.

Bargh, J. A. (1989). Conditional automaticity: Varieties of automatic influence in social perception and cognition. In J. S. Uleman & J. A. Bargh (Eds.), *Unintended thought* (pp. 3–51). New York: Guilford Press.

Bargh, J. A. (1990). Auto-motives: Preconscious determinants of social interaction. In E. T. Higgins & R. M. Sorrentino (Eds.), *Handbook of motivation and cognition: Foundations of social behavior* (Vol. 2, pp. 93–130). New York: Guilford Press.

Bargh, J. A. (1992). Does subliminality matter to social psychology?: Awareness of the stimulus versus awareness of its influence. In R. F. Bornstein & T. S. Pittman (Eds.), *Perception without awareness* (pp. 236–255). New York: Guilford Press.

Bargh, J. A. (1994). The four horsemen of automaticity: Awareness, intention, efficiency, and control in social cognition. In R. S. Wyer, Jr. & T. K. Srull (Eds.), *Handbook of social cognition* (2nd ed.): *Vol. 1. Basic processes* (pp. 1–40). Hillsdale, NJ: Erlbaum.

Bargh, J. A. (1997). The automaticity of everyday life. In R. S. Wyer, Jr. (Ed.), *Advances in social cognition* (Vol. 10, pp. 1–62). Hillsdale, NJ: Erlbaum.

Bargh, J. A., & Barndollar, K. (1996). Automaticity in action: The unconscious as repository of chronic goals and motives. In P. M. Gollwitzer & J. A. Bargh (Eds.), *The psychology of action: Linking cognition and motivation to action* (pp. 457–481). New York: Guilford Press.

Bargh, J. A., Bond, R. N., Lombardi, W. J., & Tota, M. E. (1986). The additive nature of chronic and temporary sources of construct accessibility. *Journal of Personality and Social Psychology, 50*, 869–878.

Bargh, J. A., Chaiken, S., Govender, R., & Pratto, F. (1992). The generality of the automatic attitude activation effect. *Journal of Personality and Social Psychology, 62*, 893–912.

Bargh, J. A., & Chartrand, T. L. (2000). The mind in the middle: A practical guide to priming and automaticity research. In H. T. Reis & C. M. Judd (Eds.), *Handbook of research methods in social and personality psychology* (pp. 253–285). New York: Cambridge University Press.

Bargh, J. A., Chen, M., & Burrows, L. (1996). Automaticity of social behavior: Direct effects of trait construct and stereotype activation on action. *Journal of Personality and Social Psychology, 71*, 230–244.

Bargh, J. A., Gollwitzer, P. M., Lee-Chai, A., Barndollar, K., & Trötschel, R. (2001). The automated will: Nonconscious activation and pursuit of behavioral goals. *Journal of Personality and Social Psychology, 81*, 1014–1027

Bargh, J. A., Lombardi, W. J., & Higgins, E. T. (1988). Automaticity of chronically accessible constructs in person ? situation effects on person perception: It's just a matter of time. *Journal of Personality and Social Psychology, 55*, 599–605.

Bargh, J. A., & Pietromonaco, P. (1982). Automatic information processing and social perceptions: The influence of trait information presented outside of conscious awareness on impression formation. *Journal of Personality and Social Psychology, 43*, 437–444.

Bargh, J. A., & Pratto, F. (1986). Individual construct accessibility and perceptual selection. *Journal of Experimental Social Psychology, 22*, 293–311.

Bargh, J. A., & Thein, R. D. (1985). Individual construct accessibility, person memory, and the recall–judgment link: The case of information overload. *Journal of Personality and Social Psychology, 49*, 1129–1146.

Bargh, J. A., & Tota, M. E. (1988). Context-dependent processing in depression: Accessibility of negative constructs with regard to self but not others. *Journal of Personality and Social Psychology, 54*, 924–939.

Barsalou, L. W. (1983). Ad hoc categories. *Memory and Cognition, 11*, 211–227.

Barsalou, L. W., & Medin, D. L. (1986). Concepts: Static definitions or context-dependent representations? *Cahiers de Psychologie, 6*(2), 187–202.

Bartlett, F. (1932). *Remembering.* Cambridge, UK: Cambridge University Press.

Batson, C. D. (1991). *The altruism question: Toward a social-psychological answer.* Hillsdale, NJ: Erlbaum.

Batson, C. D. (1998). Altruism and prosocial behavior, In D. T. Gilbert, S. T. Fiske, & G. Lindzey (Eds.), *The handbook of social psychology* (4th ed., Vol. 2, pp. 282–316). Boston: McGraw-Hill.

Baumeister, R. F., & Leary, M. R. (1995). The need to belong: Desire for interpersonal attachments as a fundamental human motivation. *Psychological Bulletin, 117*, 497–529.

Baumeister, R. F., & Steinhilber, A. (1984). Paradoxical effects of supportive audiences on performance under pressure: The home field disadvantage in sports championships. *Journal of Personality and Social Psychology, 47*(1), 85–93.

Beck, A. T. (1967). *Depression.* New York: Harper & Row.

Beck, A. T. (1976). *Cognitive therapy and the emotional disorders.* New York: International Universities Press.

Begg, I. M., Armour, V., & Kerr, T. (1985). On believing what we remember. *Canadian Journal of Behavioural Science, 23*, 195–213.

Begg, I. M., Anas, A., & Farinacci, S. (1992). Dissociation of processes in belief: Source recollection, statement familiarity, and the illusion of truth. *Journal of Experimental Psychology: General, 121*, 446 458.

Belleza, F. S., & Bower, G. H. (1981). Person stereotypes and memory for people. *Journal of Personality and Social Psychology, 41*, 856–865.

Berglas, S., & Jones, E. E. (1978). Drug choice as a self-handicapping strategy in response to noncontingent success. *Journal of Personality and Social Psychology, 36*, 405–417.

Berkowitz, L. (1984). Some effects of thoughts on anti- and prosocial influences of media events: A cognitive-neoassociation analysis. *Psychological Bulletin, 95*(3), 410–427.

Berry, D. S. (1990). Taking people at face value: Evidence for the kernel of truth hypothesis. *Social Cognition, 8*, 343–361.

Berry, D. S. (1991). Accuracy in social perception. Contributions of facial and vocal information. *Journal of Personality and Social Psychology, 61*, 298–307.

Biernat, M., & Kobrynowicz, D. (1997). Gender and racebased standards of competence: Lower minimum standards but higher ability standards for devalued groups. *Journal of Personality and Social Psychology, 72*(3), 544–557.

Biernat, M., & Manis, M. (1994). Shifting standards and stereotype-based judgments. *Journal of Personality and Social Psychology, 66*, 5–20.

Biernat, M., Manis, M., & Kobrynowicz, D. (1997). Simultaneous assimilation and contrast effects in judgments of self and others. *Journal of Personality and Social Psychology, 73*, 254–269.

Biernat, M., Manis, M., & Nelson, T. E. (1991). Stereotypes and standards of judgment. *Journal of Personality and Social Psychology, 60*, 485–499.

Birnbaum, I. M. (1972). General and specific components of retroactive inhibition in the A-B, A-C paradigm. *Psychology in the Schools, 9*(4), 364–370.

Birnbaum, I. M. (1973). Retroactive inhibition in two paradigms of negative transfer. *Journal of Experimental Psychology, 100*(1), 116–121.

Blair, I. V. (2001). Implicit stereotypes and prejudice. In G. B. Moskowitz (Ed.), *Cognitive social psychology: The Princeton Symposium on the Legacy and Future of Social Cognition* (pp. 359–374). Mahwah, NJ: Erlbaum.

Blair, I. V., & Banaji, M. R. (1996). Automatic and controlled processes in stereotype priming. *Journal of Personality and Social Psychology, 70*, 1142–1163.

Blanton, H. (2001). Evaluating the self in the context of another: The three-selves model of social comparison, assimilation, and contrast. In G. B. Moskowitz (Ed.), *Cognitive social psychology: The Princeton Symposium on the Legacy and Future of Social Cognition* (pp. 75–88). Mahwah, NJ: Erlbaum.

Blanton, H., & Jaccard, J. (2004). *Zeroing in on the IAT: Analysis of the condition needed to justify IAT rational zeros.* Manuscript under review.

Blanton, H., Jaccard, J., & Gonzales, P.M. (2004). *Decoding the Implicit Association Test: Perspectives on criterion prediction.* Manuscript under review.

Block, J., & Block, J. (1951). An investigation of the relationship between intolerance of ambiguity and ethnocentrism. *Journal of Personality, 19,* 303–311.

Bodenhausen, G. V., & Wyer, R. S. (1985). Effects of stereotypes on decision making and information-processing strategies. *Journal of Personality and Social Psychology, 48,* 267–282.

Bohner, G., Erb, H. P., Reinhard, M. A., & Frank, E. (1996). Distinctiveness across topics in minority and majority influence: An attributional analysis and preliminary data. *British Journal of Social Psychology, 35*(1), 27–46.

Borgida, E., & Howard-Pitney, B. (1983). Personal involvement and the robustness of perceptual salience effects. *Journal of Personality and Social Psychology, 45,* 560–570.

Boring, E. G. (1953). *A history of introspection. Psychological Bulletin, 50,* 169–189.

Bousfield, W. A. (1953). The occurrence of clustering in the recall of randomly arranged associates. *Journal of General Psychology, 49,* 229–240.

Bradley, G. W. (1978). Self serving biases in the attribution process: A reexamination of the fact or fiction question. *Journal of Personality and Social Psychology, 36,* 56–71.

Bransford, J. D., & Johnson, M. K. (1972). Contextual prerequisites for understanding: Some investigations of comprehension and recall. *Journal of Verbal Learning and Verbal Behavior, 11*(6), 717–726.

Brendl, C. M., Markman, A. B., & Messner, C. (2001). How do indirect measures of evaluation work? Evaluating the inference of prejudice in the implicit association test. *Journal of Personality and Social Psychology, 81*(5), 760–773.

Brewer, M. B. (1988). A dual process model of impression formation. In T. K. Srull & R. S. Wyer (Eds.), *Advances in social cognition* (Vol. 1, pp. 1–36). Hillsdale, NJ: Erlbaum.

Brewer, M. B. (1991). The social self: On being the same and different at the same time. *Personality and Social Psychology Bulletin, 17,* 475–482.

Broadbent, D. E. (1958). *Perception and communication.* New York: Pergamon Press.

Broadbent, D. E. (1977). The hidden preattentive processes. *American Psychologist, 32*(2), 109–118.

Brown, R., & McNeill, D. (1966). The "tip of the tongue" phenomenon. *Journal of Verbal Learning and Verbal Behavior, 5,* 325–337.

Brown, R., & Wooton-Millward, L. (1993). Perceptions of group homogeneity during group formation and change. *Social Cognition, 11*(1), 126–149.

Bruner, J. S. (1957). On perceptual readiness. *Psychological Review, 64,* 123–152.

Bruner, J. S., Busiek, R. D., & Mintrum, A. L. (1952). Assimilation in the immediate reproduction of visually perceived figures. *Journal of Experimental Psychology, 43,* 151–155.

Bruner, J. S., & Goodman, C. D. (1947). Value and need as organizing factors in perception. *Journal of Abnormal Social Psychology, 42,* 33–44.

Bruner, J. S., Goodnow, J. G., & Austin, G. A. (1956). *A study of thinking.* New York: Wiley.

Bruner, J. S., & Postman, L. (1948). Symbolic value as an organizing factor in perception. *Journal of Social Psychology, 27,* 203–208.

Bruner, J. S., & Tagiuri, R. (1954). The perception of people. In G. Lindzey (Ed.), *Handbook of social psychology* (Vol. 2, pp. 634–654). Cambridge, MA: Addison-Wesley.

Bugental, D. (2002). Acquisition of the algorithms of social life: A domain-based approach. *Psychological Bulletin, 126*(2), 187–219.

Bumiller, E. (2002, September 16). White House letter: Did President 43 say to 41, "You be Dad, I'll be son"? *The New York Times,* p. 15.

Bushman, B. J., Baumeister, R., Philips, F., & Collen, M. (2001). Do people aggress to improve their mood?: Catharsis beliefs, affect regulation opportunity, and aggressive responding. *Journal of Personality and Social Psychology, 81*(1), 17–32.

Cacioppo, J. T., & Berntson, G. G. (1994). Relationship between attitudes and evaluative space: A critical review, with emphasis on the separability of positive and negative substrates. *Psychological Bulletin, 115*(3), 401–423.

Cacioppo, J. T., Berntson, G. G., & Crites, S. L., Jr. (1996). Social neuroscience: Principles of psychophysiological arousal and response. In E. T. Higgins & A. W. Kruglanski (Eds.), *Social psychology: Handbook of basic principles* (pp. 72–101). New York: Guilford Press.

Cacioppo, J. T., Gardner, W. L., & Berntson, G. G. (1997). Beyond bipolar conceptualizations and measures: The case of attitudes and evaluative space. *Personality and Social Psychology Review, 1*, 3–25.

Cacioppo, J. T., & Petty, R. E. (1982). The need for cognition. *Journal of Personality and Social Psychology, 42*, 116–131.

Cantor, N., & Fleeson, W. (1991). Life tasks and self-regulatory processes. In M. Maehr & P. Pintrich (Eds.), *Advances in motivation and achievement* (Vol. 7, pp. 327–369). Greenwich, CT: JAI Press.

Cantor, N., & Fleeson, W. (1994). Soical intelligence and intelligent goal pursuit: A cognitive slice of motivation. In W. Spaulding (Ed.), *Nebraska Symposium on Motivation* (Vol. 41, pp. 125–179). Lincoln: University of Nebraska Press.

Cantor, N., & Kihlstrom, J. F. (1987). *Personality and social intelligence.* Englewood Cliffs, NJ: Prentice-Hall.

Cantor, N., & Malley, J. (1991). Life tasks, personal needs, and close relationships. In G. J. O. Fletcher & F. D. Fincham (Eds.), *Cognition in close relationships* (pp. 101–125). Hillsdale, NJ: Erlbaum.

Cantor, N., & Mischel, W. (1977). Traits as prototypes: Effects on recognition memory. *Journal of Personality and Social Psychology, 35*, 38–48.

Cantor, N., & Mischel, W. (1979). Prototypes in person perception. In L. Berkowitz (Ed.), *Advances in experimental social psychology* (Vol. 12, pp. 3–52). New York: Academic Press.

Carey, S. (1985). *Conceptual change in childhood.* Cambridge, MA: MIT Press.

Carlston, D. E. (1980). The recall and use of traits and events in social inference processes. *Journal of Experimental Social Psychology, 16*, 303–328.

Carlston, D. E., & Skowronski, J. J. (1994). Savings in the relearning of trait information as evidence for spontaneous inference generation. *Journal of Personality and Social Psychology, 66*, 840–856.

Carlston, D. E., & Skowronski, J. J. (1995). Savings in relearning: II. On the formation of behavior-based trait associations and inferences. *Journal of Personality and Social Psychology, 69*(3), 429–436.

Carlston, D. E., & Smith, E. R. (1996). Principles of mental representation. In E. T. Higgins & A. W. Kruglanski (Eds.), *Social psychology: Handbook of basic principles* (pp. 184–210). New York: Guilford Press.

Carpenter, W. G. (1884). *Principles of mental physiology, with their applications to the training and discipline of the mind and study of its morbid conditions.* New York: Appleton.

Carver, C. S., Ganellen, R. J., Froming, W. J., & Chambers, W. (1983). Modeling: An analysis in terms of category accessibility. *Journal of Experimental Social Psychology, 19*(5), 403–421.

Carver, C. S., & Scheier, M. F. (1978). Self-focusing effects of dispositional self-consciousness, mirror presence, and audience presence. *Journal of Personality and Social Psychology, 36*, 324–332.

Carver, C. S., & Scheier, M. F. (1981). *Attention and self-regulation: A control theory approach to human behavior.* New York: Springer.

Chaiken, S. (1980). Heuristic versus systematic information processing and the use of source versus message cues in persuasion. *Journal of Personality and Social Psychology, 39*, 752–766.

Chaiken, S. (1987). The heuristic model of persuasion. In M. P. Zanna, J. M. Olson, & C. P. Herman (Eds.), *Social influence: The Ontario Symposium* (Vol. 5, pp. 3–39). Hillsdale, NJ: Erlbaum.

Chaiken, S., Giner-Sorolla, R., & Chen, S. (1996). Beyond accuracy: Defense and impression motives in heuristic and systematic information processing. In P. M. Gollwitzer & J. A. Bargh

(Eds.), *The psychology of action: Linking cognition and motivation to action* (pp. 553–578). New York: Guilford Press.

Chaiken, S., Liberman, A., & Eagly, A. H. (1989). Heuristic and systematic information processing within and beyond the persuasion context. In J. S. Uleman & J. A. Bargh (Eds.), *Unintended thought* (pp. 212–252). New York: Guilford Press.

Chaiken, S., & Trope, Y. (Eds.). (1999). *Dual-process theories in social psychology*. New York: Guilford Press.

Chapman, L. J. (1967). Illusory correlation in observational report. *Journal of Verbal Learning and Verbal Behavior, 6,* 151–155.

Chartrand, T. L., & Bargh, J. A. (1996). Automatic activation of impression formation goals: Nonconscious goal priming reproduces effects of explicit task instructions. *Journal of Personality and Social Psychology, 71,* 464–478.

Chartrand, T. L., & Bargh, J. A. (1999). The chameleon effect: The perceptionbehavior link and social interaction. *Journal of Personality and Social Psychology, 76,* 893–910.

Chase, W. G., & Simon, H. A. (1973). Perception in chess. *Cognitive Psychology, 4,* 55–81.

Chawla, P., & Krauss, R. M. (1994). Gesture and speech in spontaneous and rehearsed narratives. *Journal of Experimental Social Psychology, 30*(6), 580–601.

Chen, M., & Bargh, J. A. (1997). Nonconscious behavioral confirmation processes: The self-fulfilling consequences of automatic stereotype activation. *Journal of Experimental Social Psychology, 33,* 541–560.

Chen, M., & Bargh, J. A. (1999). Consequences of automatic evaluation: Immediate behavioral predispositions to approach or avoid the stimulus. *Personality and Social Psychology Bulletin, 25,* 215–224.

Chen, S. (2001). The role of theories in mental representation and their use in social perception: A theory-based approach to significant-other representations and transference. In G. B. Moskowitz (Ed.), *Cognitive social psychology: The Princeton Symposium on the Legacy and Future of Social Cognition* (pp. 125–142). Mahwah, NJ: Erlbaum.

Chen, S. (2003). Psychological-state theories about significant others: Implications for the content and structure of significant-other representations. *Personality and Social Psychology Bulletin, 29*(10), 1285–1302.

Chen, S., Shechter, D., & Chaiken, S. (1996). Getting at the truth or getting along: Accuracy versus impressionmotivated heuristic and systematic processing. *Journal of Personality and Social Psychology, 71,* 262–275.

Cheng, P. W., & Novick, L. R. (1990). A probabilistic contrast model of causal induction. *Journal of Personality and Social Psychology, 58,* 545–567.

Cheng, P. W., & Novick, L. R. (1992). Covariation in natural causal induction. *Psychological Review, 99*(2), 365–382.

Choi, I., & Nisbett, R. E. (1998). Situational salience and cultural differences in the correspondence bias and actor–observer bias. *Personality and Social Psychology Bulletin, 24,* 949–960.

Cialdini, R. B., Borden, R. J., Thorne, A., Walker, M. R., Freeman, S., & Sloan, L. R. (1976). Basking in reflected glory: Three (football) field studies. *Journal of Personality and Social Psychology, 34,* 366–375.

Clark, H. H., & Haviland, S. E. (1977). Comprehension and the given-new contract. In R. O. Freedle (Ed.), *Discourse production and comprehension* (Vol. 1, pp. 1–40). Norwood, NJ: Ablex.

Clore, G. L., Schwarz, N., & Conway, M. (1994). Affective causes and consequences of social information processing. In R. S. Wyer, Jr. & T. K. Srull (Eds.), *Handbook of social cognition* (2nd ed.): *Vol. 1.* (pp. 323–417). Hillsdale, NJ: Erlbaum.

Cohen, A. R. (1961). Cognitive tuning as a factor affecting impression formation. *Journal of Personality, 29,* 235–245.

Collins, A. M., & Loftus, E. (1975). A spreading-activation theory of semantic processing. *Psychological Review, 82,* 407–428.

Collins, A. M., & Quillian, M. R. (1969). Retrieval time from semantic memory. *Journal of Verbal Learning and Verbal Behavior, 8*(2), 240–247.

Collins, M. A., & Zebrowitz L. A., (1995). The contributions of appearance to occupational outcomes in civilian and military settings. *Journal of Applied Social Psychology, 25*(2), 129–163.

Cooley, C. H. (1983). *Human nature and the social order.* New Brunswick, NJ: Transaction Books. (Original work published 1902)

Correll, J., Park, B., Judd, C. M., & Wittenbrink, B. (2002). The police officer's dilemma: Using ethnicity to disambiguate potentially threatening individuals. *Journal of Personality and Social Psychology, 83*(6), 1314–1329.

Craik, F. I. M., & Lockhart, R. S. (1972). Levels of processing: A framework for memory research. *Journal of Verbal Learning and Verbal Behavior, 11*, 671–676.

Crano, W. D., & Chen, X. (1998). The leniency contract and persistence of majority and minority influence. *Journal of Personality and Social Psychology, 74*, 1437–1450.

Crocker, J., Hannah, D. B., & Weber, R. (1983). Person memory and causal attributions. *Journal of Personality and Social Psychology, 44*, 55–66.

Crocker, J., & Luhtanen, R. (1990). Collective selfesteem and ingroup bias. *Journal of Personality and Social Psychology, 58*, 60–67.

Crocker, J., Thompson, L. L., McGraw, K. M., & Ingerman, C. (1987). Downward comparison, prejudice, and evaluations of others: Effects of self esteem and threat. *Journal of Personality and Social Psychology, 52*, 907–916.

Crocker, J., Voelkl, K., Testa, M., & Major, B. (1991). Social stigma: The affective consequences of attributional ambiguity. *Journal of Personality and Social Psychology, 60*(2), 218–228.

Crosby, F., Bromley, S., & Saxe, L. (1980). Recent unobtrusive studies of Black and White discrimination and prejudice: A literature review. *Psychological Bulletin, 87*, 546–563.

Darley, J. M., & Fazio, R. H. (1980). Expectancy confirmation processes arising in the social interaction sequence. *American Psychologist, 35*, 867–881.

Darley, J. M., & Gross, P. H. (1983). A hypothesis-confirming bias in labelling effects. *Journal of Personality and Social Psychology, 44*, 20–33.

Darwin, C. (1998). *The expression of the emotions in man and animals.* Oxford: Oxford University Press. (Original work published 1872)

Dasgupta, N., Greenwald, A. G., & Banaji, M. R. (2003). The first ontological challenge to the IAT: Attitude or mere familiarity? *Psychological Inquiry, 14*, 238–243.

Davis, M. H. (1983). *Measuring individual differences in empathy: Evidence for a multidimensional approach. Journal of Personality and Social Psychology, 44*, 113–126.

Davis, M. H., Conklin, L., Smith, A., & Luce, C. (1996). Effect of perspective taking on the cognitive representation of persons: A merging of self and other. *Journal of Personality and Social Psychology, 70*, 713–726.

Deaux, K., & Lewis, L. (1984). Structure of gender stereotypes: Interrelations among components and gender label. *Journal of Personality and Social Psychology, 5*, 991–1004.

Deci, E. L. (1992). On the nature and functions of motivation theories. *Psychological Science, 3*, 167–171.

Deci, E. L., & Ryan, R. M. (1991). A motivational approach to self: Integration in personality. In R. Dienstbier (Ed.), *Nebraska Symposium on Motivation* (Vol. 38, pp. 237–288). Lincoln: University of Nebraska Press.

de Dreu, C. K. W., & de Vries, N. K. (1996). Differential processing and attitude change following majority versus minority arguments. *British Journal of Social Psychology, 35*(1) 77–90.

DePaulo, B. M., & Kashy, D. A. (1998). Everyday lies in close and casual relationships. *Journal of Personality and Social Psychology, 74*(1), 63–79.

DePaulo, B. M., Kashy, D. A., Kirkendol, S. E., Wyer, M. M., & Epstein, J. A. (1996). Lying in everyday life. *Journal of Personality and Social Psychology, 70*(5), 979–995.

DePaulo, B. M., Lanier, K., & Davis, T. (1983). Detecting the deceit of the motivated liar. *Journal of Personality and Social Psychology, 45*, 1096–1103.

DePaulo, B. M., LeMay, C. S., & Epstein, J. A. (1991). Effects of importance of success and expectations for success on effectiveness at deceiving. *Personality and Social Psychology Bulletin, 17*(1), 14–24.

De Soto, C. B., Hamilton, M. M., & Taylor, R. B. (1985). Words, people, and implicit personality theory. *Social Cognition, 3*(4), 369–382.

Deutsch, J. A., & Deutsch, D. (1963). Attention: Some theoretical considerations. *Psychological Review, 70*, 80–90.

Devine, P. G. (1989). Stereotypes and prejudice: Their automatic and controlled components. *Journal of Personality and Social Psychology, 56*, 5–18.

Devine, P. G., & Elliot, A. J. (1995). Are racial stereotypes really fading?: The Princeton Trilogy revisited. *Personality and Social Psychology Bulletin, 21*, 1139–1150.

Devine, P. G., Monteith, M. J., Zuwerink, J. R., & Elliot, A. J. (1991). Prejudice with and without compunction. *Journal of Personality and Social Psychology, 60*, 817–830.

Dewey, J. (1929). *The quest for certainty*. New York: Minton, Balch.

Dijksterhuis, A., & Bargh, J. A. (2001). The perception–behavior expressway: Automatic effects of social perception on social behavior. In M. P. Zanna (Ed.), *Advances in experimental social psychology* (Vol. 33, pp. 1–40), San Diego, CA: Academic Press.

Dijksterhuis, A., Spears, R., Postmes, T., Stapel, D. A., Koomen, W., van Knippenberg, A., & Scheepers, D. (1998). Seeing one thing and doing another: Contrast effects in automatic behavior. *Journal of Personality and Social Psychology, 75*, 862–871.

Dijksterhuis, A., & van Knippenberg, A. (1996). The knife that cuts both ways: Facilitated and inhibited access to traits as a result of stereotype activation. *Journal of Experimental Social Psychology, 32*, 271–288.

Dijksterhuis, A., & van Knippenberg, A. (1998). The relation between perception and behavior, or how to win a game of Trivial Pursuit. *Journal of Personality and Social Psychology, 74*, 865–877.

Dion, K., Berscheid, E., & Walster, E. (1972). What is beautiful is good. *Journal of Personality and Social Psychology, 24*(3), 285–290.

Dion, K., & Earn, B. M. (1975). The phenomenology of being a target of prejudice. *Journal of Personality and Social Psychology, 32*(5), 944–950.

Ditto, P. H., & Lopez, D. F. (1992). Motivated skepticism: Use of differential decision criteria for preferred and nonpreferred conclusions. *Journal of Personality and Social Psychology, 63*, 568–584.

Dovidio, J. F., Evans, N., & Tyler, R. B. (1986). Racial stereotypes: The contents of their cognitive representations. *Journal of Experimental Social Psychology, 22*, 22–37.

Dovidio, J. F., & Gaertner, S. L. (1986). Prejudice, discrimination, and racism: Historical trends and contemporary approaches. In J. F. Dovidio & S. L. Gaertner (Eds.), *Prejudice, discrimination, and racism* (pp. 1–34). Orlando, FL: Academic Press.

Downey, G., & Feldman, S. I. (1996). Implications of rejection sensitivity for intimate relationships. *Journal of Personality and Social Psychology, 70*, 1327–1343.

Downey, G., Freitas, A. L., Michaelis, B., & Khouri, H. (1998). The self-fulfilling prophecy in close relationships: Rejection sensitivity and rejection by romantic partners. *Journal of Personality and Social Psychology, 75*, 545–560.

Duff, K. J., & Newman, L. S. (1997). Individual differences in the spontaneous construal of behavior: Idiocentrism and the automatization of the trait inference process. *Social Cognition, 15*, 217–241.

Duncan, B. L. (1976). Differential social perception and attribution of intergroup violence: Testing the lower limits of stereotyping of Blacks. *Journal of Personality and Social Psychology, 34*, 590–598.

Dunning, D., Leuenberger, A., & Sherman, D. A. (1995). A new look at motivated inference: Are self-serving theories of success a product of motivational forces? *Journal of Personality and Social Psychology, 69*, 58–68.

Duval, S., & Wicklund, R. A. (1972). *A theory of objective self-awareness*. New York: Academic Press.

Dweck, C. S. (1991). Self-theories and goals: Their role in motivation, personality, and development. In R. Dienstbier (Ed.), *Nebraska Symposium on Motivation* (Vol. 38, pp. 199–255). Lincoln: University of Nebraska Press.

Dweck, C. S. (1996). Implicit theories as organizers of goals and behavior. In P. M. Gollwitzer & J. A. Bargh (Eds.), *The psychology of action: Linking cognition and motivation to action* (pp. 69–90). New York: Guilford Press.

Dweck, C. S., & Leggett, E. L. (1988). A social-cognitive approach to motivation and personality. *Psychological Review, 95*, 256–273.

Eagly, A. H., Ashmore, R. D., Makhijani, M. G., & Longo, L. C. (1991). What is beautiful is good, but . . . : A meta-analytic review of research on the physical attractiveness stereotype. *Psychological Bulletin, 110*(1), 109–128.

Eagly, A. H., & Chaiken, S. (1975). An attribution analysis of the effect of communicator characteristics on opinion change: The case of communicator attractiveness. *Journal of Personality and Social Psychology, 32*, 136–144.

Eagly, A. H., & Chaiken, S. (1976). Why would anyone say that?: Causal attributions of statements about the Watergate scandal. *Sociometry, 39*, 236–243.

Eagly, A. H., & Chaiken, S. (1993). *The psychology of attitudes.* Fort Worth, TX: Harcourt Brace Jovanovich.

Eagly, A. H., Wood, W., & Chaiken, S. (1978). Causal inferences about communicators and their effect on opinion change. *Journal of Personality and Social Psychology, 36*, 424–435.

Ekman, P. (1971). Universals and cultural differences in facial expressions of emotion. In J. K. Cole (Ed.), *Nebraska Symposium on Motivation* (Vol. 18, pp. 207–283). Lincoln: University of Nebraska Press.

Ekman, P. (1992). *Telling lies: Clues to deceit in the marketplace, marriage, and politics.* New York: Norton.

Ekman, P. (1998). Afterword. In C. Darwin, *The expression of the emotions in man and animals.* Oxford: Oxford University Press.

Ekman, P., & Friesen, W. V. (1969). *Nonverbal leakage and clues to deception. Psychiatry, 32*, 88–106.

Ekman, P., & Friesen, W. V. (1971). Constants across cultures in the face and emotion. *Journal of Personality and Social Psychology, 17*(2) 124–129.

Ekman, P., & Friesen, W. V. (1974). Detecting deception from the body or face. *Journal of Personality and Social Psychology, 29*(3), 288–298.

Elliott, E. S., & Dweck, C. S. (1988). Goals: An approach to motivation and achievement. *Journal of Personality and Social Psychology, 54*, 5–12.

Epley, N., & Dunning, D. (2000). Feeling "holier than thou": Are self-serving assessments produced by errors in self- or social prediction? *Journal of Personality and Social Psychology, 79*(6), 861–875.

Erb, H.-P., Bohner, G., Schämlzle, K., & Rank, S. (1998). Beyond conflict and discrepancy: Cognitive bias in minority and majority influence. *Personality and Social Psychology Bulletin, 24*, 620–633.

Erdelyi, M. H. (1974). A new look at the New Look: Perceptual defense and vigilance. *Psychological Review, 81*, 1–25.

Erikson, E. H. (1959). *Identity and the life cycle.* New York: Norton.

Fazio, R. H. (1990). A practical guide of the use of response latency in social psychological review. In C. Hendrick & M. S. Clark (Eds.), *Research methods in personality and social psychology* (pp. 74–97). Newbury Park, CA: Sage.

Fazio, R. H., & Dunton, B. C. (1997). Categorization by race: The impact of automatic and controlled components of racial prejudice. *Journal of Experimental Social Psychology, 33*, 451–470.

Fazio, R. H., Jackson, J. R., Dunton, B. C., & Williams, C. J. (1995). Variability in automatic activation as an unobtrusive measure of racial attitudes: A bona fide pipeline? *Journal of Personality and Social Psychology, 69*, 1013–1027.

Fazio, R. H., Sanbonmatsu, D. M., Powell, M. C., & Kardes, F. R. (1986). On the automatic activation of attitudes. *Journal of Personality and Social Psychology, 50*, 229–238.

Fein, S., Hilton, J. L., & Miller, D. T. (1990). Suspicion of ulterior motivation and the correspondence bias. *Journal of Personality and Social Psychology, 58*, 753–764.

Fein, S., & Spencer, S. J. (1997). Prejudice as self-image maintenance: Affirming the self through negative evaluations of others. *Journal of Personality and Social Psychology, 73*, 31–44.

Fenigstein, A., Scheier, M. F., & Buss, A. H. (1975). Public and private self-consciousness: Assessment and theory. *Journal of Consulting and Clinical Psychology, 43*, 522–527.

Festinger, L. (1954). A theory of social comparison processes. *Human Relations, 7*, 117–140.

Festinger, L. (1957). *A theory of cognitive dissonance.* Stanford, CA: Stanford University Press.

Festinger, L., & Carlsmith, J. M. (1959). Cognitive consequences of forced compliance. *Journal of Abnormal and Social Psychology, 58*, 203–210.

Finch, J. F., & Cialdini, R. B. (1989). Another indirect tactic of (self-)image management: Boosting. *Personality and Social Psychology Bulletin, 15*(2), 222–232.

Fishbach, A., Friedman, R. S., & Kruglanski, A. W. (2003). Leading us not unto temptation: Momentary allurements elicit overriding goal activation. *Journal of Personality and Social Psychology, 84*, 296–309.

Fiske, S. T. (1980). Attention and weight in person perception: The impact of negative and extreme behavior. *Journal of Personality and Social Psychology, 38*, 889–906.

Fiske, S. T. (1992). Controlling other people. *American Psychologist, 48*, 621–628.

Fiske, S. T., Bersoff, D. N., Borgida, E., Deaux, K., & Heilman, M. E. (1991). Social science research on trial: Use of sex stereotyping research in *Price Waterhouse v. Hopkins. American Psychologist, 46*, 1049–1060.

Fiske, S. T., & Linville, P. W. (1980). What does the schema concept buy us? *Personality and Social Psychology Bulletin, 6*, 543–557.

Fiske, S. T., & Neuberg, S. L. (1990). A continuum model of impression formation, from category based to individuating processes: Influences of information and motivation on attention and interpretation. In M. P. Zanna (Ed.), *Advances in experimental social psychology* (Vol. 23, pp. 1–74). New York: Academic Press.

Fiske, S. T., & Taylor, S. E. (1984). *Social cognition.* Reading, MA: Addison-Wesley.

Fiske, S. T., & Taylor, S. E. (1991). *Social cognition* (2nd ed.). New York: McGraw-Hill.

Fitzsimons, G. M., Chartrand, T. L., & Fitzsimons, G. J. (2003). *Automatic effects of anthropomorphized objects on behavior: Dog people, cat people, and why we are what we buy.* Manuscript submitted for publication.

Fitzsimons, G. M., & Bargh, J. A. (2003). Thinking of you: Nonconscious pursuit of interpersonal goals associated with relationship partners. *Journal of Personality and Social Psychology, 84*, 148–164.

Flavell, J. H. (1979). Metacognition and cognitive monitoring: A new area of cognitive-developmental inquiry. *American Psychologist, 34*(10), 906–911.

Förster, J., Higgins, E. T., & Idson, L. C. (1998). Approach and avoidance strength during goal attainment: Regulatory focus and the "goal looms larger" effect. *Journal of Personality and Social Psychology, 75*, 1115–1131.

Förster, J., Higgins, E. T., & Strack, F. (2000). When stereotype disconfirmation is a personal threat: How prejudice and prevention focus moderate incongruency effects. *Social Cognition, 18*, 178–197.

Försterling, F. (1989). Models of covariation and attribution: How do they relate to the analogy of analysis of variance? *Journal of Personality and Social Psychology, 57*(4), 615–625.

Försterling, F. (1992). The Kelley model as an analysis of variance analogy: How far can it be taken? *Journal of Experimental Social Psychology, 28*(5), 475–490.

Fox, E. (1995). Negative priming from ignored distractors in visual selection: A review. *Psychonomic Bulletin and Review, 2*(2), 145–173.

Frenkel-Brunswik, E. (1949). Intolerance of ambiguity as an emotional and perceptual personality variable. *Journal of Personality, 18*, 108–143.

Frese, M., & Sabini, J. (1985). *Goal-directed behavior: The concept of action in psychology.* Hillsdale, NJ: Erlbaum.

Freud, S. (1958). The dynamics of transference. In J. Strachey (Ed. & Trans.), *The standard edition of the complete psychological works of Sigmund Freud* (Vol. 12, pp. 97–108). London: Hogarth Press. (Original work published 1912)

Friedrich, F. J., Henik, A., & Tzelgov, J. (1991). Automatic processes in lexical access and spreading activation. *Journal of Experimental Psychology: Human Perception and Performance, 17,* 792–806.

Funder, D. C. (1999). *Personality judgment: A realistic approach to person perception.* New York: Academic Press.

Funder, D. C., & Colvin, C. R. (1988). Friends and strangers: Acquaintanceship, agreement, and the accuracy of personality judgment. *Journal of Personality and Social Psychology, 55,* 149–158.

Gaertner, S. L. (1973). Helping behavior and racial discrimination among liberals and conservatives. *Journal of Personality and Social Psychology, 25*(3) 335–341.

Gaertner, S. L., & Dovidio, J. (1986). The aversive form of racism. In J. Dovidio & S. Gaertner (Eds.), *Prejudice, discrimination, and racism* (pp. 61–89). Orlando, FL: Academic Press.

Gage, N. L., & Cronbach, L. J. (1955). Conceptual and methodological problems in interpersonal perception. *Psychological Review, 62,* 411–422.

Galinsky, A. D., & Ku, G. (2004). The effects of perspectivetaking on prejudice: The moderating role of selfevaluation. *Personality and Social Psychology Bulletin, 30*(5), 594–604.

Galinsky, A. D., & Moskowitz, G. B. (2000b). Perspective taking: Decreasing stereotype expression, stereotype accessibility and in-group favoritism. *Journal of Personality and Social Psychology, 78,* 708–724.

Galinsky, A. D., Moskowitz, G. B., & Skurnik, I. (2000). Counterfactuals as self-generated primes: The effects of prior counterfactual activation on person perception judgments. *Social Cognition, 18*(3), 252–280.

Ganzach, Y., & Schul, Y. (1995). The influence of quantity of information and goal framing on decision. *Acta Psychologica, 89,* 23–36.

Garcia-Marques, L., & Hamilton, D. L. (1996). Resolving the apparent discrepancy between the incongruency effect and the expectancy-based illusory correlation effect: The TRAP model. *Journal of Personality and Social Psychology, 71,* 845–860.

Geen, R. G. (1995). *Human motivation: A social psychological approach.* Pacific Grove, CA: Brooks/Cole.

Geller, V., & Shaver, P. (1976). Cognitive consequences of self-awareness. *Journal of Experimental Social Psychology, 12,* 99–108.

Gelman, S. A., & Markman, E. M. (1986). Categories and induction in young children. *Cognition, 23,* 183–208.

Gibson, J. J. (1979). *The ecological approach to visual perception.* Boston: Houghton Mifflin.

Gilbert, D. T. (1989). Thinking lightly about others: Automatic components of the social inference process. In J. S. Uleman & J. A. Bargh (Eds.), *Unintended thought* (pp. 189–211). New York: Guilford Press.

Gilbert, D. T. (1998). Ordinary personology. In D. T. Gilbert, S. T. Fiske, & G. Lindzey (Eds.), *The handbook of social psychology* (4th ed., Vol. 2, pp. 89–150). Boston: McGraw-Hill.

Gilbert, D. T., & Hixon, J. G. (1991). The trouble of thinking: Activation and application of stereotypic beliefs. *Journal of Personality and Social Psychology, 60,* 509–517.

Gilbert, D. T., Krull, D. S., & Malone, P. S. (1990). Unbelieving the unbelievable: Some problems in the rejection of false information. *Journal of Personality and Social Psychology, 59,* 601–613.

Gilbert, D. T., & Malone, P. S. (1995). The correspondence bias. *Psychological Bulletin, 117,* 21–38.

Gilbert, D. T., Pelham, B. W., & Krull, D. S. (1988). On cognitive business: When person perceivers meet person perceived. *Journal of Personality and Social Psychology, 54,* 733–740.

Gilbert, D. T., Pinel, E. C., Wilson, T. D., Blumberg, S. J., & Wheatley, T. P. (1998). Immune neglect: A source of durability bias in affective forecasting. *Journal of Personality and Social Psychology, 75,* 617–638.

Gill, M. J. (2004). When information does not deter stereotyping: Prescriptive stereotyping can foster bias under conditions that deter descriptive stereotyping. *Journal of Experimental Social Psychology, 40,* 619–632.

Gill, M. J., & Swann, W. B. (2004). On what it means to know someone: A matter of pragmatics. *Journal of Personality and Social Psychology, 86*(3), 405–418.

Gilovich, T. (1991). *How we know what isn't so: The fallibility of human reason in everyday life*. New York: Free Press.

Gilovich, T., Jennings, D. L., & Jennings, S. (1983). Causal focus and estimates of consensus: An examination of the false-consensus effect. *Journal of Personality and Social Psychology, 45*(3), 550–559.

Gilovich, T., Savitsky, K., & Medvec, V. H. (1998). The illusion of transparency: Biased assessments of others' ability to read our emotional states. *Journal of Personality and Social Psychology, 75*, 332–346.

Godfrey, D. K., Jones, E. E., & Lord, C. G. (1986). Self-promotion is not ingratiating. *Journal of Personality and Social Psychology, 50*(1), 106–115.

Goffman, E. (1959). *The presentation of self in everyday life*. Garden City, NY: Doubleday.

Gollwitzer, P. M. (1990). Action phases and mind-sets. In E. T. Higgins & R. M. Sorrentino (Eds.), *Handbook of motivation and cognition: Foundations of social behavior* (Vol. 2, pp. 53–92). New York: Guilford Press.

Gollwitzer, P. M. (1991). *Abwaegen und Planen*. Göttingen, Germany: Hogrefe.

Gollwitzer, P. M. (1993). Goal achievement: The role of intentions. In W. Stroebe & M. Hewstone (Eds.), *European review of social psychology* (Vol. 4, pp. 141–185). Chichester, UK: Wiley.

Gollwitzer, P. M. (1996). The volitional benefits of planning. In P. M. Gollwitzer & J. A. Bargh (Eds.), *The psychology of action: Linking cognition and motivation to action* (pp. 287–312). New York: Guilford Press.

Gollwitzer, P. M. (1999). Implementation intentions: Strong effects of simple plans. *American Psychologist, 54*, 493–503.

Gollwitzer, P. M., Heckhausen, H., & Steller, B. (1990). Deliberative vs. implemental mind-sets: Cognitive tuning toward congruous thoughts and information. *Journal of Personality and Social Psychology, 59*, 1119–1127.

Gollwitzer, P. M., & Moskowitz, G. B. (1996). Goal effects on action and cognition. In E. T. Higgins & A. W. Kruglanski (Eds.), *Social psychology: Handbook of basic principles* (pp. 361–399). New York: Guilford Press.

Gopnik, A., & Meltzoff, A. N. (1997). *Words, thoughts, and theories*. Cambridge, MA: MIT Press.

Gopnik, A., & Wellman, H. M. (1994). The theory theory. In L. A. Hirschfeld & S. A. Gelman (Eds.), *Mapping the mind: Domain specificity in cognition and culture* (pp. 257–293). New York: Cambridge University Press.

Gosling, S. D., Ko, S. J., Mannarelli, T., & Morris, M. E. (2002). A room with a cue: Personality judgments based on offices and bedrooms. *Journal of Personality and Social Psychology, 82*(3), 379–398.

Grant, P. R., & Holmes, J. G. (1981). The integration of implicit personality theory schemas and stereotype images, *Social Psychology Quarterly, 44*(2), 107–115.

Greenwald, A. G., & Banaji, M. R. (1995). Implicit social cognition: Attitudes, self-esteem, and stereotypes. *Psychological Review, 102*, 4–27.

Greenwald, A.G., & Farnham, S. D. (2000). Using the implicit association test to measure self-esteem and self-concept. *Journal of Personality and Social Psychology, 79*(6), 1022–1038.

Greenwald, A. G., McGhee, D. E., & Schwartz, J. L. K. (1998). Measuring individual differences in implicit cognition: The implicit association test. *Journal of Personality and Social Psychology, 74*, 1464–1480.

Grice, H. P. (1975). Logic and conversation: The William James lectures, Harvard University, 1967–68. In P. Cole & J. Morgan (Eds.), *Syntax and semantics: Vol. 3. Speech acts* (pp. 95–113). New York: Academic Press.

Hafer, C. L, (2000). Do innocent victims threaten the belief in a just world? Evidence from a modified Stroop task. *Journal of Personality and Social Psychology, 79*, 165–173.

Hamilton, D. L. (1981). Cognitive representations of persons. In E. T. Higgins, C. P. Herman, & M. P. Zanna (Eds.), *Social cognition: The Ontario Symposium* (Vol. 1, pp. 135–159). Hillsdale, NJ: Erlbaum.

Hamilton, D. L. (1988). Causal attribution viewed from an information processing perspective. In

D. Bar-Tal & A. W. Kruglanski (Eds.), *The social psychology of knowledge* (pp. 359–385). Cambridge, UK: Cambridge University Press.

Hamilton, D. L. (1991, August). *Perceiving persons and groups: A social cognitive perspective.* Paper presented at the 99th Annual Convention of the American Psychological Association, San Francisco.

Hamilton, D. L., & Gifford, R. K. (1976). Illusory correlation in interpersonal perception: A cognitive basis of stereotypic judgments. *Journal of Experimental Social Psychology, 12,* 392–407.

Hamilton, D. L., Katz, L. B., & Leirer, V. O. (1980a). Cognitive representation of personality impressions: Organizational processes in first impression formation. *Journal of Personality and Social Psychology, 39,* 1050–1063.

Hamilton, D. L., Katz, L. B., & Leirer, V. O. (1980b). Organizational processes in impression formation. In R. Hastie, T. M. Ostrom, E. B. Ebbesen, R. S. Wyer, Jr., D. L. Hamilton, & D. E. Carlston (Eds.), *Person memory: The cognitive basis of social perception* (pp. 121–153). Hillsdale, NJ: Erlbaum.

Hamilton, D. L., & Rose, T. L. (1980). Illusory correlation and the maintenance of stereotypic beliefs. *Journal of Personality and Social Psychology, 39,* 832–845.

Hamilton, D. L., & Trolier, T. K. (1986). Stereotypes and stereotyping: An overview of the cognitive approach. In J. F. Dovidio & S. L. Gaertner (Eds.), *Prejudice, discrimination, and racism* (pp. 127–163). Orlando, FL: Academic Press.

Hansen, C. H., & Hansen, R. D. (1988). Finding the face in the crowd: An anger superiority effect. *Journal of Personality and Social Psychology, 54*(6), 917–924.

Hardin, C. D., & Conley, T. D. (2001). A relational approach to cognition: Shared experience and relationship affirmation in social cognition. In G. B. Moskowitz (Ed.), *Cognitive social psychology: The Princeton Symposium on the Legacy and Future of Social Cognition* (pp. 3–17). Mahwah, NJ: Erlbaum.

Hart, H. L. A., & Honoré, A. M. (1961). Causation in the law. In H. Morris (Ed.), *Freedom and responsibility: Readings in philosophy and law.* Stanford, CA: Stanford University Press.

Hasher, L., Goldstein, D., & Toppino, T. (1977). Frequency and the conference of referential validity. *Journal of Verbal Learning and Verbal Behavior, 16,* 107–112.

Hasher, L., & Zacks, R. T. (1979). Automatic and effortful processes in memory. *Journal of Experimental Psychology: General, 108*(3), 356–388.

Hastie, R. (1981). Schematic principles in human memory. In E. T. Higgins, C. P. Herman, & M. P. Zanna (Eds.), *Social cognition: The Ontario Symposium* (Vol. 1, pp. 39–88). Hillsdale, NJ: Erlbaum.

Hastie, R., & Kumar, P. A. (1979). Person memory: Personality traits as organizing principles in memory for behavior. *Journal of Personality and Social Psychology, 37,* 25–38.

Hastie, R., Ostrom, T. M., Ebbesen, E. B., Wyer, R. S., Jr., Hamilton, D. L., & Carlston, D. E. (Eds.). (1980). *Person memory: The cognitive basis of social perception.* Hillsdale, NJ: Erlbaum.

Hastie, R., & Park, B. (1986). The relationship between memory and judgment depends on whether the judgment task is memory-based or on-line. *Psychological Review, 93,* 25–268.

Hastorf, A. H., & Cantril, H. (1954). They saw a game: A case study. *Journal of Abnormal and Social Psychology, 49,* 129–134.

Hastorf, A. H., Schneider, D., & Polefka, J. (1970). *Person Perception.* Reading, MA: Addison-Wesley.

Hayes-Roth, B. (1977). Evolution of cognitive structures and processes. *Psychological Review, 84,* 260–278.

Hebb, D. O. (1949). *The organization of behavior: A neuropsychological theory.* New York: Wiley.

Heckhausen, H. (1991). *Motivation and action.* Heidelberg: Springer-Verlag.

Heider, F. (1944). Social perception and phenomenal causality. *Psychological Review, 51,* 358–374.

Heider, F. (1958). *The psychology of interpersonal relations.* New York: Wiley.

Heider, F., & Simmel, M. (1944). An experimental study of apparent behavior. *American Journal of Psychology, 57,* 243–259.

Helmholtz, H. von. (1925). *Treatise on physiological optics* (3rd ed.) (J. P. C. Southall Ed. & Trans.). Rochester, NY: Optical Society of America. (Original work published 1866)

Herr, P. M. (1986). Consequences of priming: Judgment and behavior. *Journal of Personality and Social Psychology, 51,* 1106–1115.

Herr, P. M., Sherman, S. J., & Fazio, R. H. (1983). On the consequences of priming: Assimilation and contrast effects. *Journal of Experimental Social Psychology, 19,* 323–340.

Hetts, J. J., & Pelham, B. W. (2001). A case for the nonconscious self-concept. In G. B. Moskowitz (Ed.), *Cognitive social psychology: The Princeton Symposium on the Legacy and Future of Social Cognition* (pp. 105–124). Mahwah, NJ: Erlbaum.

Heywood, C. A., Cowey, A., & Newcomb, F. (1994). On the role of parvocellular (P) and magnocellular (M) pathways in cerebral achromatopsia. *Brain, 117*(2), 245–254.

Higgins, E. T. (1987). Self-discrepancy theory: A theory relating self and affect. *Psychological Review, 94,* 319–340.

Higgins, E. T. (1989). Self-discrepancy theory: What patterns of self-beliefs cause people to suffer? In L. Berkowitz (Ed.), *Advances in experimental social psychology* (Vol. 22, pp. 93–136). New York: Academic Press.

Higgins, E. T. (1996). Knowledge activation: Accessibility, applicability, and salience. In E. T. Higgins & A. W. Kruglanski (Eds.), *Social psychology: Handbook of basic principles* (pp. 133–168). New York: Guilford Press.

Higgins, E. T. (1998). The aboutness principle: A pervasive influence on human inference. *Social Cognition, 16,* 173–198.

Higgins, E. T., Bargh, J. A., & Lombardi, W. (1985). Nature of priming effects on categorization. *Journal of Experimental Psychology: Learning, Memory, and Cognition, 11,* 59–69.

Higgins, E. T., & Brendl, C. M. (1995). Accessibility and applicability: Some "activation rules" influencing judgment. *Journal of Experimental Social Psychology, 31,* 218–243.

Higgins, E. T., & Chaires, W. M. (1980). Accessibility of interrelational constructs: Implications for stimulus encoding and creativity. *Journal of Experimental Social Psychology, 16*(4), 348–361.

Higgins, E. T., Herman, C. P., & Zanna, M. P. (1981). *Social cognition: The Ontario Symposium* (Vol. 1). Hillsdale, NJ: Erlbaum.

Higgins, E. T., King, G. A., & Mavin, G. H. (1982). Individual construct accessibility and subjective impressions and recall. *Journal of Personality and Social Psychology, 43,* 35–47.

Higgins, E. T., Rholes, W. S., & Jones, C. R. (1977). Category accessibility and impression formation. *Journal of Experimental Social Psychology, 13,* 141–154.

Higgins, E. T., Roney, C., Crowe, E., & Hymes, C. (1994). Ideal versus ought predilections for approach and avoidance: Distinct self-regulatory systems. *Journal of Personality and Social Psychology, 66,* 276–286.

Hilton, D. J., & Slugoski, B. R. (1986). Knowledge-based causal attribution: The abnormal conditions focus model. *Psychological Review, 93,* 75–88.

Hume. D. (1961). *An enquiry concerning human understanding.* In *The empiricists.* Garden City, NY: Dolphin Books. (Original work published 1748)

Ichheiser, G. (1943). Misinterpretations of personality in everyday life. *Character and Personality, 11,* 145–160.

Ickes, W. (2003). *Everyday mind reading: Understanding what other people think and feel.* Amherst, NY: Prometheus Books.

Izard, C. E. (1971). *The face of emotion.* New York: Appleton-Century-Crofts.

Jacoby, L. L. (1991). A process dissociation framework: Separating automatic from intentional uses of memory. *Journal of Memory and Language, 30,* 513–541.

Jacoby, L. L., & Dallas, M. (1981). On the relationship between autobiographical memory and perceptual learning. *Journal of Experimental Psychology: General, 110,* 306–340.

Jacoby, L. L., Kelley, C., Brown, J., & Jasechko, J. (1989). Becoming famous overnight: Limits on the ability to avoid unconscious influences of the past. *Journal of Personality and Social Psychology, 56*(3), 326–338.

Jacoby, L. L., & Whitehouse, K. (1989). An illusion of memory: False recognition influenced by unconscious perception. *Journal of Experimental Psychology: Learning, Memory, and Cognition, 20*, 304–317.

Jacoby, L. L., Woloshyn, V., & Kelley, C. M. (1989). Becoming famous without being recognized: Unconscious influences of memory provided by dividing attention. *Journal of Experimental Psychology: General, 118*, 115–125.

James, W. (1950). *The principles of psychology* (2 vols.). New York: Dover. (Original work published 1890)

James, W. (1991). *Pragmatism*. Buffalo, NY: Prometheus Books. (Original work published 1907)

Jarvis, W. B. G., & Petty, R. E. (1996). The need to evaluate. *Journal of Personality and Social Psychology, 70*, 172–194.

Johnson, M. K. (1988). Reality monitoring: An experimental phenomenological approach. *Journal of Experimental Psychology, 117*(4), 390–394.

Johnson, M. K., Hashtroudi, S., & Lindsay, D. S. (1993). Source monitoring. *Psychological Bulletin, 114*, 3–28.

Johnson, M. K., & Raye, C. L. (1981). Reality monitoring. *Psychological Review, 88*, 67–85.

Jones, E. E. (1964). *Ingratiation*. New York: Appleton-Century-Crofts.

Jones, E. E. (1979). The rocky road from acts to dispositions. *American Psychologist, 34*, 107–117.

Jones, E. E. (1990). *Interpersonal perception*. New York: Macmillan.

Jones, E. E., & Berglas, S. (1978). Control of attributions about the self through self-handicapping strategies: The appeal of alcohol and the role of underachievement. *Journal of Personality and Social Psychology, 4*, 200–206.

Jones, E. E., & Davis, K. E. (1965). From acts to dispositions: The attribution process in person perception. In L. Berkowitz (Ed.), *Advances in experimental social psychology* (Vol. 2, pp. 219–266). New York: Academic Press.

Jones, E. E., Davis, K. E., & Gergen, K. J. (1961). Role playing variations and their informational value for person perception. *Journal of Abnormal and Social Psychology, 63*, 302–310.

Jones, E. E., & Harris, V. A. (1967). The attribution of attitudes. *Journal of Experimental Social Psychology, 3, 1–24.*

Jones, E. E., & Nisbett, R. E. (1971). *The actor and the observer: Divergent perceptions of the causes of behavior*. Morristown, NJ: General Learning Press.

Jones, E. E., & Thibaut, J. W. (1958). Interaction goals as bases of inference in interpersonal perception. In L. Petrullo & R. Tagiuri (Eds.), *Person perception and interpersonal behavior* (pp. 151–178). Stanford, CA: Stanford University Press.

Jones, J. M. (1986). Racism: A cultural analysis of the problem. In J. F. Dovidio & S. L. Gaertner (Eds.), *Prejudice, discrimination, and racism* (pp. 279–293). Orlando, FL: Academic Press.

Jones, J. M. (1997). *Prejudice and racism*. New York: McGraw-Hill.

Jonides, J. (1995). Working memory and thinking, In E. E. Smith & D. N. Osherson (Eds.), *Thinking: An invitation to cognitive science* (2nd ed., Vol. 3, pp. 215–265). Cambridge, MA: MIT Press.

Kahneman, D. (1973). *Attention and effort*. Englewood Cliffs, NJ: Prentice-Hall.

Kahneman, D. (1995). Varieties of counterfactual thinking. In N. J. Roese & J. M. Olson (Eds.), *What might have been: The social psychology of counterfactual thinking* (pp. 375–396). Hillsdale, NJ: Erlbaum.

Kahneman, D., Fredrickson, B. L., Schreiber, C. A., & Redelmeier, D. A. (1993). When more pain is preferred to less: Adding a better end. *Psychological Science, 4*(6), 401–405.

Kahneman, D., & Miller, D. (1986). Norm theory: Comparing reality to its alternatives. *Psychological Review, 93*, 136–153.

Kahneman, D., & Snell, J. (1992). Predicting a changing taste: Do people know what they will like? *Journal of Behavioral Decision Making, 5*, 187–200.

Kahneman, D., & Tversky, A. (1973). On the psychology of prediction. *Psychological Review, 80*, 237–251.

Kahneman, D., & Tversky, A. (1982). The simulation heuristic. In D. Kahneman, P. Slovic, & A. Tversky (Eds.), *Judgment under uncertainty: Heuristics and biases* (pp. 201–208). New York: Cambridge University Press.

Kahneman, D., & Tversky, A. (1984). Choices, values, and frames. *American Psychologist, 39*(4), 341–350.

Kanouse, D. E. (1971). *Language, labeling, and attribution.* Morristown,NJ: General Learning Press.

Kanouse, D. E., & Hanson, L. R. J. (1972). Negativity in evaluations. In E. E. Jones, D. E. Kanouse, H. H. Kelley, R. E. Nisbett, S. Valins, & B. Weiner (Eds.), *Attribution: Perceiving the causes of behavior* (pp. 47–62). Morristown, NJ: General Learning Press.

Kant, I. (1990). *Critique of pure reason* (J. M. D. Meidlejohn, Trans.). Buffalo, NY: Prometheus Books. (Original work published 1781)

Karpinski, A., & Hilton, J. L. (2001). Attitudes and the Implicit Association Test. *Journal of Personality and Social Psychology, 81,* 774–788.

Kassin, S. M., & Kiechel, K. L. (1996). The social psychology of false confessions: Compliance, internalization, and confabulation. *Psychological Science, 7*(3), 125–128.

Kassin, S. M., & Sukel, H. (1997). Coerced confessions and the jury: An experimental test of the "harmless error" rule. *Law and Human Behavior, 21*(1), 27–46.

Katz, D., & Braly, K. W. (1933). Racial stereotypes of 100 college students. *Journal of Abnormal and Social Psychology, 28,* 280–290.

Kawakami, K., Dovidio, J., Moll, J., Hermsen, S., & Russin, A. (2000). Just say no (to stereotyping): Effects of training in the negation of stereotype associations on stereotype activation. *Journal of Personality and Social Psychology, 78,* 871–888.

Kawashima, R., Sugiura, M., Kato, T., Nakamura, A., Hatano, K., Ito, K., et al. (1999). The human amygdala plays an important role in gaze monitoring: A PET study. *Brain, 122*(4), 779–783.

Kelley, H. H. (1967). Attribution theory in social psychology. In D. Levine (Ed.), *Nebraska Symposium on Motivation* (Vol. 15, pp. 192–238). Lincoln: University of Nebraska Press.

Kelley, H. H. (1972a). Attribution in social interaction. In E. E. Jones, D. E. Kanouse, H. H. Kelley, R. E. Nisbett, S. Valins, & B. Weiner (Eds.), *Attribution: Perceiving the causes of behavior* (pp. 1–26). Morristown, NJ: General Learning Press.

Kelley, H. H. (1972b). Causal schemata and the attribution process. In E. E. Jones, D. E. Kanouse, H. H. Kelley, R. E. Nisbett, S. Valins, & B. Weiner (Eds.), *Attribution: Perceiving the causes of behavior* (pp. 151–174). Morristown, NJ: General Learning Press.

Kelley, H. H. (1973). Processes of causal attribution. *American Psychologist, 28,* 107–128.

Kelley, H. H., & Michela, J. L. (1980). Attribution theory and research. *Annual Review of Psychology, 31,* 457–501.

Kelly, G. (1955). *A theory of personality: The psychology of personal constructs.* New York: Norton.

Kelly, W. L. (1971). Analysis of covariance for certain symbolic functions. *International Journal of Symbology, 2,* 26–39.

Kelman, H. C. (1961). Processes of opinion change. *Public Opinion Quarterly, 25,* 57–78.

Keltner, D. (1997). Signs of appeasement: Evidence for the distinct displays of embarrassment, amusement, and shame. In P. Ekman & E. L. Rosenberg (Eds.), *What the face reveals: Basic and applied studies of spontaneous expression using the Facial Action Coding System (FACS)* (pp. 133–160). London: Oxford University Press.

Kenny, D. A. (1994). *Interpersonal perception: A social relations analysis.* New York: Guilford Press.

Kenny, D. A., Horner, C., Kashy, D. A., & Chu, L. (1992). Consensus at zero acquaintance: Replication, behavioral cues, and stability. *Journal of Personality and Social Psychology, 62*(1), 88–97.

Kenny, D. A., Kiefer, S. C., Smith, J. A., Ceplenski, P., & Culo, J. (1996). Circumscribed accuracy among well-acquainted individuals. *Journal of Experimental Social Psychology, 32,* 1–12.

Kenrick, D. T., Maner, J. K., Butner, J., Li, N. P., Becker, D. V., & Schaller, M. (2002). Dynamic evolutionary psychology: Mapping the domains of the new interactionist paradigm. *Personality and Social Psychology Review, 6,* 347–356.

Keysar, B., Barr, D. J., Balin, J. A., & Paek, T. (1998). Definite reference and mutual knowledge: Process models of common ground in comprehension. *Journal of Memory and Language, 39,* 1–20.

Khouri, R. (2003, April 4). The war Americans don't see. *New York Times.*

Kihlstrom, J. F., & Klein, S. B. (1994). The self as a knowledge structure. In R. S. Wyer, Jr. & T. K. Srull (Eds.), *Handbook of social cognition* (2nd ed.): *Vol. 2. Applications* (pp. 153–208). Hillsdale, NJ: Erlbaum.

King, M. L., Jr. (1963, April 16). *Letter from a Birmingham jail* [Pamphlet]. Birmingham, AL: American Friends Service Committee.

Kitayama, S., & Karasawa, M. (1997). Implicit self-esteem in Japan: Name letters and birthday numbers. *Personality and Social Psychology Bulletin, 23*, 736–742.

Klayman, J., & Ha, Y. W. (1987). Confirmation, disconfirmation, and information in hypothesis-testing. *Psychological Review, 94*, 211–228.

Kleck, R. E., & Strenta, A. (1980). Perceptions of the impact of negatively valued physical characteristics on social interaction. *Journal of Personality and Social Psychology, 39*(5), 861–873.

Klein, S. B., Loftus, J., Trafton, J. G., & Fuhrman, R. W. (1992). Use of exemplars and abstractions in trait judgments: A model of trait knowledge about the self and others. *Journal of Personality and Social Psychology, 63*, 739–753.

Kohlberg, L. (1976). Moral stages and moralization: The cognitive-developmental approach. In T. Lickona (Ed.), *Moral development and behavior* (pp. 31–53). New York: Holt, Rinehart & Winston.

Köhler, W. (1930). *Gestalt psychology*. London: Bell.

Koole, S. L., Dijksterhuis, A., & van Knippenberg, A. (2001). What's in a name: Implicit self-esteem and the automatic self. *Journal of Personality and Social Psychology, 80*(4), 669–685.

Krauss, R. M., Chen, Y., & Chawla, P. (1996). Nonverbal behavior and nonverbal communication: What do conversational hand gestures tell us? In M. P. Zanna (Ed.), *Advances in experimental social psychology* (Vol. 28, pp. 389–450). San Diego, CA: Academic Press.

Kruglanski, A. W. (1980). Lay epistemologic process and contents: Another look at attribution theory. *Psychological Review, 87*, 70–87.

Kruglanski, A. W. (1990). Motivations for judging and knowing: Implications for causal attribution. In E. T. Higgins & R. M. Sorrentino (Eds.), *Handbook of motivation and cognition: Foundations of social behavior* (Vol. 2, pp. 333–368). New York: Guilford Press.

Kruglanski, A. W., & Freund, T. (1983). The freezing and unfreezing of lay inferences: Effects on impressional primacy, ethnic stereotyping, and numerical anchoring. *Journal of Experimental Social Psychology, 19*, 448–468.

Kruglanski, A. W., & Mackie, D. M. (1990). Majority and minority influence: A judgmental process analysis. In W. Stroebe & M. Hewstone (Eds.), *European review of social psychology* (Vol. 1, pp. 229–261). Chichester, UK: Wiley.

Krull, D. S. (1993). Does the grist change the mill? The effect of the perceiver's inferential goal on the process of social inference. *Personality and Social Psychology Bulletin, 19*, 340–348.

Krull, D. S., & Dill, J. C. (1996). On thinking first and responding fast: Flexibility in social inference processes. *Personality and Social Psychology Bulletin, 22*, 949–959.

Krull, D. S., Loy, M. H., Lin, J., Wang, C., Chen, S., & Zhao, X. (1999). The fundamental fundamental attribution error: Correspondence bias in individualist and collectivist cultures. *Personality and Social Psychology Bulletin, 25*(10), 208–1219.

Kuhl, J., & Beckmann, J. (1985). *Action control: From cognition to behavior*. New York: Springer-Verlag.

Külpe, O. (1904). *Versuche ber abstraktion. Berlin International Congress of Experimental Psychology*, 56–68.

Kunda, Z. (1987). Motivated inference: Self-serving generation and evaluation of causal theories. *Journal of Personality and Social Psychology, 53*(4), 636–647.

Kunda, Z., & Oleson, K. C. (1995). Maintaining stereotypes in the face of disconfirmation: Constructing grounds for subtyping deviants. *Journal of Personality and Social Psychology, 68*, 565–579.

Kunda, Z., Sinclair, L., & Griffin, D. (1997). Equal ratings but separate meanings: Stereotypes and the construal of traits. *Journal of Personality and Social Psychology, 72*(4), 720–734.

Kunda, Z., & Thagard, P. (1996). Forming impressions from stereotypes, trait, and behaviors: A parallel constraint satisfaction theory. *Psychological Review, 103*, 284–308.

La France, M., & Ickes, W. (1981). Posture mirroring and interactional involvement: Sex and sex typing effects. *Journal of Nonverbal Behavior, 5*(3), 139–154.

Lambert, A. J., Cronen, S., Chasteen, A. L., & Lickel, B. (1996). Private vs. public expressions of racial prejudice. *Journal of Experimental Social Psychology, 32*(5), 437–459.

Lambert, W. E., & Klineberg, O. (1967). *Children's views of foreign peoples*. New York: Appleton-Century-Crofts.

Langer, E. J. (1975). The illusion of control. *Journal of Personality and Social Psychology, 32*, 311–328.

Langer, E. J. (1978). Rethinking the role of thought in social interaction. In J. H. Harvey, W. I. Ickes, & R. F. Kidd (Eds.), *New directions in attribution research* (Vol. 2, pp. 35–58). Hillsdale, NJ: Erlbaum.

Langer, E. J., Blank, A., & Chanowitz, B. (1978). The mindlessness of ostensibly thoughtful action: The role of "placebic" information in interpersonal interaction. *Journal of Personality and Social Psychology, 3*(6), 635–642.

Langer, E. J., & Rodin, J. (1976). The effects of choice and enhanced personal responsibility for the aged: A field experiment in an institutional setting. *Journal of Personality and Social Psychology, 34*(2), 191–198.

Langton, S. R. H., Watt, R. J., & Bruce, V. (2000). Do the eyes have it? Cues to the direction of social attention. *Trends in Cognitive Sciences, 4*, 50–59.

Latane, B., & Darley, J. M. (1968, July). When will people help in a crisis? *Psychology Today*, pp. 54–57, 70–71.

Latane, B., & Darley, J. M. (1970). *The unresponsive bystander: Why doesn't he help?* New York: Appleton-Century-Crofts.

LeDoux, J. E. (1995). Emotion: Clues from the brain. *Annual Review of Psychology, 46*, 209–235.

Lefcourt, H. M. (1976). Locus of control and the response to aversive events. *Ontario Psychologist, 8*(5), 41–49.

Lepore, L., & Brown, R. (1997). Category and stereotype activation: Is prejudice inevitable? *Journal of Personality and Social Psychology, 72*, 275–287.

Lerner, M. J. (1965). The effect of responsibility and choice on a partner's attractiveness following failure. *Journal of Personality, 33*, 178–187.

Lerner, M. J. (1980). *The belief in a just world: A fundamental delusion*. New York: Plenum Press.

Lerner, M. J., & Miller, D. T. (1978). Just world research and the attribution process: Looking back and ahead. *Psychological Bulletin, 85*(5), 1030–1051.

Lewin, K. (1935). *A dynamic theory of personality: Selected papers* (D. K. Adams & K. E. Zener, Trans.). New York: McGraw-Hill.

Lewin, K. (1936). *Principles of topological psychology*. New York: McGrawHill.

Leyens, J., & Fiske, S. T. (1994). Impression formation: From recitals to Symphonie Fantastique. In P. G. Devine, D. L., Hamilton, & T. M. Ostrom (Eds.), *Social cognition: Impact on social psychology* (pp. 39–75). San Diego, CA: Academic Press.

Li, P. (2004). *Two types of cognitive resources in stereotype activation*. Unpublished doctoral dissertation, Lehigh University.

Li, P., & Moskowitz, G. B. (2004a). *The fate of activated concepts: Free-floating versus engaged fluency*. Manuscript submitted for publication.

Li, P., & Moskowitz, G. B. (2004b). *Imitative mindsets, covert mimicry, and perspective taking in person perception*. Manuscript submitted for publication.

Liberman, A. (2001). Exploring the boundaries of rationality: A functional perspective on dual-process models in social psychology. In G. B. Moskowitz (Ed.), *Cognitive social psychology: The Princeton Symposium on the Legacy and Future of Social Cognition* (pp. 291–305). Mahwah, NJ: Erlbaum.

Liberman, N., & Förster, J. (2000). Expression after suppression: A motivational explanation of postsuppressional rebound. *Journal of Personality and Social Psychology, 79*, 190–203.

Libet, B. (1985). Unconscious cerebral initiative and the role of conscious will in voluntary action. *Behavioral and Brain Sciences 8*(4), 529–566.

Lingle, J. H., Altom, M. W., & Medin, D. L. (1984). Of cabbages and kings: Assessing the extendibility of natural object concepts models to social things. In R. S. Wyer, Jr. & T. K. Srull (Eds.), *Handbook of social cognition* (Vol. 1, pp. 71–118). Hillsdale, NJ: Erlbaum.

Linville, P. W. (1998). The heterogeneity of homogeneity. In J. M. Darley & J. Cooper (Eds.), *Attribution and social interaction: The legacy of Edward E. Jones* (pp. 423–487). Washington, DC: American Psychological Association.

Linville, P. W., & Jones, E. E. (1980). Polarized appraisals of outgroup members. *Journal of Personality and Social Psychology, 38*, 689–703.

Linville, P. W., Salovey, P., & Fischer, G. W. (1986). Stereotyping and perceived distributions of social characteristics: An application to ingroup–outgroup perception. In J. F. Dovidio & S. L. Gaertner (Eds.), *Prejudice, discrimination, and racism* (pp. 165–208). Orlando, FL: Academic Press.

Lippmann, W. (1922). *Public opinion.* New York: Harcourt, Brace.

Livingston, R. W., & Brewer, M. B. (2002). What are we really priming?: Cue-based versus category-based processing of facial stimuli. *Journal of Personality and Social Psychology, 82*(1), 5–18.

Locke, E. A., & Latham, G. P. (1991). Self-regulation through goal setting. *Organizational Behavior and Human Decision Processes, 50*(2), 212–247.

Locke, J. (1961). An essay concerning human understanding. In *The empiricists.* Garden City, NY: Dolphin Books. (Original work published 1690)

Locksley, A., Borgida, E., Brekke, N., & Hepburn, C. (1980). Sex stereotypes and social judgment. *Journal of Personality and Social Psychology, 39*, 821–831.

Locksley, A., Hepburn, C., & Ortiz, V. (1982). Social stereotypes and judgments of individuals: An instance of the base-rate fallacy. *Journal of Experimental Social Psychology, 18*, 23–42.

Logan, G. D. (1979). On the use of a concurrent memory load to measure attention and automaticity. *Journal of Experimental Psychology: Human Perception and Performance, 5*, 189–207.

Logan, G. D. (1989). Automaticity and cognitive control. In J. S. Uleman & J. A. Bargh (Eds.), *Unintended thought* (pp. 52–74). New York: Guilford Press.

Lombardi, W. J., Higgins, E. T., & Bargh, J. A. (1987). The role of consciousness in priming effects on categorization. *Personality and Social Psychology Bulletin, 13*, 411–429.

Lord, C. G., Ross, L., & Lepper, M. R. (1979). Biased assimilation and attitude polarization: The effects of prior theories on subsequently considered evidence. *Journal of Personality and Social Psychology, 37*, 2098–2109.

Lorenz, K. (1971). *Studies in animal and human behavior: II* (R. Martin, Trans.). Cambridge, MA: Harvard University Press.

Lorge, I. (1936). Attitude stability in older adults. *Psychological Bulletin, 33*, 759

Lupfer, M. B., Clark, L. F., & Hutcherson, H. W. (1990). Impact of context on spontaneous trait and situational attributes. *Journal of Personality and Social Psychology 58*(2), 239–249.

Maass, A., Milesi, A., Zabbini, S., & Stahlberg, D. (1995). Linguistic intergroup bias: Differential expectancies or in-group protection? *Journal of Personality and Social Psychology, 68*, 116–126.

Macrae, C. N., Bodenhausen, G. V., & Milne, A. B. (1995). The dissection of selection in person perception: Inhibitory processes in social stereotyping. *Journal of Personality and Social Psychology, 69*, 397–407.

Macrae, C. N., Bodenhausen, G. V., Milne, A. B., & Jetten, J. (1994). Out of mind but back in sight: Stereotypes on the rebound. *Journal of Personality and Social Psychology, 67*, 808–817.

Macrae, C. N., Bodenhausen, G., Milne, A., Thorn, T., & Castelli, L. (1997). On the activation of social stereotypes: The moderating role of processing objectives. *Journal of Experimental Social Psychology, 33*, 471–489.

Macrae, C. N., Hewstone, M., & Griffiths, R. J. (1993). Processing load and memory for stereotype-based information. *European Journal of Social Psychology, 23*, 77–87.

Macrae, C. N., Hood, B. M., Milne, A. B., Rowe, A. C., & Mason, M. F. (2002). Are you looking at me?: Eye gaze and person perception. *Psychological Science, 13*, 460–464.

Macrae, C. N., & MacLeod, M. D. (1999). On recollections lost: When practice makes imperfect. *Journal of Personality and Social Psychology, 77*, 463–473.

Macrae, C. N., Milne, A. B., & Bodenhausen, G. V. (1994). Stereotypes as energy-saving devices: A peek inside the cognitive toolbox. *Journal of Personality and Social Psychology, 66*, 37–47.

Maheswaran, D., & Chaiken, S. (1991). Promoting systematic processing in low motivation settings: The effect of incongruent infromation on processing and judgment. *Journal of Personality and Social Psychology, 61*, 13–25.

Major, B., & Crocker, J. (1993). Social stigma: The consequences of attributional ambiguity. In D. M. Mackie & D. L. Hamilton (Eds.), *Affect, cognition, and stereotyping: Interactive processes in group perception* (pp. 345–370). San Diego, CA: Academic Press.

Malle, B. F. (1999). How people explain behavior: A new theoretical framework. *Personality and Social Psychology Review, 3*(1), 23–48.

Malt, B. C., Sloman, S. A., Gennari, S., Shi, M., & Wang, Y. (1999). Knowing versus naming: Similarity and the linguistic categorization of artifacts. *Journal of Memory and Language, 40*(2), 230–262.

Malt, B. C., & Smith, E. E. (1984). Correlated properties in natural categories. *Journal of Verbal Learning and Verbal Behavior, 23*(2), 250–269.

Mandler, G. (1980). Recognizing: The judgment of previous occurrence. *Psychological Review, 87*(3), 252–271.

Manis, M., Nelson, T. E., & Shedler, J. (1988). Stereotypes and social judgment: Extremity, assimilation, and contrast. *Journal of Personality and Social Psychology, 55*, 28–36.

Markman, A. B., & Ross, B. H. (2003). Category use and category learning. *Psychological Bulletin, 129*, 592–613.

Markus, H. R. (1977). Self-schemata and processing information about the self. *Journal of Personality and Social Psychology, 35*, 63–78.

Markus, H. R., & Kitayama, S. (1991). Culture and the self: Implications for cognition, emotion, and motivation. *Psychological Review, 98*, 224–253.

Martin, L. L. (1986). Set/reset: Use and disuse of concepts in impression formation. *Journal of Personality and Social Psychology, 51*, 493–504.

Martin, L. L., Seta, J. J., & Crelia, R. A. (1990). Assimilation and contrast as a function of people's willingness and ability to expend effort in forming an impression. *Journal of Personality and Social Psychology, 59*, 27–37.

Martin, L. L., & Tesser, A. (1996). Some ruminative thoughts. In R. S. Wyer (Ed.), *Advances in social cognition* (Vol. 9, pp. 1–48). Hillsdale, NJ: Erlbaum.

Maslow, A. H. (1943). The authoritarian character structure. *Journal of Social Psychology, 18*, 401–411.

Mather, M., Johnson, M. K., & De Leonardis, D. M. (1999). Stereotype reliance in source monitoring: Age differences and neuropsychological test correlates. *Cognitive Neuropsychology, 16*, 437–458.

Mayseless, O., & Kruglanski, A. W. (1987). Accuracy estimates in the social comparison of abilities. *Journal of Experimental Social Psychology, 23*, 217–229.

McArthur, L. Z. (1972). The how and what of why: Some determinants and consequences of causal attribution. *Journal of Personality and Social Psychology, 22*, 171–193.

McArthur, L. Z. (1981). What grabs you?: The role of attention in impression formation and causal attribution. In E. T. Higgins, C. P. Herman, & M. P. Zanna (Eds.), *Social cognition: The Ontario Symposium* (Vol. 1, pp. 201–246). Hillsdale, NJ: Erlbaum.

McArthur, L. Z., & Apatow, K. (1983–1984). Impressions of baby-faced adults. *Social Cognition, 2*(4), 315–342.

McArthur, L. Z., & Baron, R. (1983). Toward an ecological theory of social perception. *Psychological Review, 90*, 215–238.

McArthur, L. Z., & Ginsberg, E. (1981). Causal attribution to salient stimuli: An investigation of visual fixation mediators. *Personality and Social Psychology Bulletin, 7*(4), 547–553.

McArthur, L. Z., & Post, D. L. (1977). Figural emphasis and person perception. *Journal of Experimental Social Psychology, 13*, 520–535.

McClure, J., & Hilton, D. (1997). For you can't always get what you want: When preconditions are better explanations than goals. *British Journal of Social Psychology, 36*(2), 223–240.

McConahay, J. B., & Hough, J. C. (1976). Symbolic racism. *Journal of Social Issues, 32*, 23–45.

McConnell, A. R., Sherman, S. J., & Hamilton, D. L. (1994). Illusory correlation in the perception of groups: An extension of the distinctiveness-based account. *Journal of Personality and Social Psychology, 67*, 414–429.

McGinnies, E. (1949). Emotionality and perceptual defense. *Psychological Review, 56*, 244–251.

McGuire, C. (1964). Research in the process approach to the construction and analysis of medical examinations. *The 20th Yearbook of the National Council on Measurement in Education*, 7–16.

Mead, M. (1935). *Sex and temperament in three primitive societies*. New York: Morrow.

Mead, G. H. (1956). *The social psychology of George Herbert Mead* (A. Strauss, Ed.). Chicago: University of Chicago Press.

Meckler, L. (2000, September 13). *Bush dismisses "rat" allegation*. Available online at www.excite.com

Medin, D. L. (1989). Concepts and conceptual structure. *American Psychologist, 44*, 1469–1481.

Medin, D. L., Goldstone, R. L., & Gentner, D. (1993). Respects for similarity. *Psychological Review, 100*, 254–278.

Medvec, V. H., Madey, S. F., & Gilovich, T. (1995). When less is more: Counterfactual thinking and satisfaction among Olympic medalists. *Journal of Personality and Social Psychology, 69*, 603–610.

Mehrabian, A., & Wiener, M. (1967). Decoding of inconsistent communications. *Journal of Personality and Social Psychology, 6*(1), 109–114.

Meltzoff, A. N., & Moore, M. K. (1977). Imitation of facial and manual gestures by human neonates. *Science, 198*, 75–78.

Merton, R. K. (1948). The bearing of empirical research upon the development of social theory. *American Sociological Review, 13*, 505–515.

Meyer, D. E., & Schvandeveldt, R. W. (1971). Facilitation in recognizing pairs of words: Evidence of a dependence between retrieval operations. *Journal of Experimental Psychology, 90*, 227–234.

Milgram, S. (1963). Behavioral study of obedience. *Journal of Abnormal and Social Psychology, 67*, 371–378.

Miller, D. T. (1976). Ego involvement and attributions for success and failure. *Journal of Personality and Social Psychology, 34*, 901–906.

Miller, D. T., Downs, J. S., & Prentice, D. A. (1998). Minimal conditions for the creation of a unit relationship: The social bond between birthdaymates. *European Journal of Social Psychology, 28*(3), 475–481.

Miller, D. T., & Norman, S. A., & Wright, E. (1978). Distortion in person perception as a consequence of the need for effective control. *Journal of Personality and Social Psychology, 36*(6), 598–607.

Miller, D. T., & Prentice, D. A. (1999). Some consequences of a belief in group essence: The category divide hypothesis. In D. A. Prentice & D. T. Miller (Eds.), *Cultural divides: Understanding and overcoming group conflict* (pp. 213–238). New York: Russell Sage Foundation.

Miller, G. A., Galanter, E., & Pribram, K. H. (1960). *Plans and the structure of behavior*. New York: Holt, Rinehart & Winston.

Miller, J. G. (1984). Culture and the development of everyday social explanation. *Journal of Personality and Social Psychology, 46*, 961–978.

Minsky, M. (1975). A framework for representing knowledge. In P. H. Winston (Ed.), *The psychology of computer vision* (pp. 211–277). New York: McGraw-Hill.

Mischel, W. (1968). *Personality and assessment*. New York: Wiley.

Mischel, W. (1973). Toward a cognitive-social reconceptualization of personality. *Psychological Review, 80*, 252–283.

Mischel, W., & Peake, P. K. (1982). Beyond déjà vu in the search for cross-situational consistency. *Psychological Review, 89*, 730–755.

Mischel, W., & Shoda, Y. (1995). A cognitive affective system theory of personality: Reconceptualizing situations, dispositions, dynamics, and invariance in personality structure. *Psychological Review, 102*, 246–268.

Mitchell, J. P., Heatherton, T. F., & Macrae, C. N. (2002). Distinct neural systems subserve person and object knowledge. *Proceedings of the National Academy of Sciences USA, 99*, 15238–15243.

Mitchell, J. P., Macrae, C. N., & Gilchrest, I. D. (2002). Working memory and the suppression of reflexive saccades. *Journal of Cognitive Neuroscience, 14*, 95–103.

Mogg, K., & Bradley, B. P. (1999). Orienting of attention to threatening facial expressions presented under conditions of restricted awareness. *Cognition and Emotion, 13*(6), 713–740.

Mogg, K., Bradley, B. P., & Williams, R. (1995). Attentional bias in anxiety and depression: The role of awareness. *British Journal of Clinical Psychology, 34*(1), 17–36.

Mollon, P. (1989). Anxiety, supervision and a space for thinking: Some narcissistic perils for clinical psychologists in learning psychotherapy. *British Journal of Medical Psychology, 62*(2), 113–122.

Monin, B., & Miller, D. T. (2001). Moral credentials and the expression of prejudice. *Journal of Personality and Social Psychology, 81*(1), 33–43.

Monteith, M. J. (1993). Self-regulation of prejudiced responses: Implications for progress in prejudice reduction efforts. *Journal of Personality and Social Psychology, 65*, 469–485.

Monteith, M. J., Ashburn-Nardo, L., Voils, C. I., & Czopp, A. M. (2002). Putting the brakes on prejudice: On the development and operation of cues for control. *Journal of Personality and Social Psychology, 83*, 1029–1050.

Monteith, M. J., Sherman, J. W., & Devine, P. G. (1998). Suppression as a stereotype control strategy. *Personality and Social Psychology Review, 2*, 63–82.

Monteith, M. J., & Voils, C. I. (2001). Exerting control over prejudiced responses. In G. B. Moskowitz (Ed.), *Cognitive social psychology: The Princeton Symposium on the Legacy and Future of Social Cognition* (pp. 375–388). Mahwah, NJ: Erlbaum.

Morf, C. C., & Rhodewalt, F. (1993). Narcissism and self-evaluation maintenance: Explorations in object relations. *Personality and Social Psychology Bulletin, 19*, 668–676.

Morf, C. C., & Rhodewalt, F. (2001). Unraveling the pardoxes of narcissim: A dynamic self-regulatory processing model. *Psychological Inquiry, 12*, 177–196.

Morris, M. W., Ames, D. R., & Knowles, E. D. (2001). What we theorize when we theorize that we theorize: Examining the "implicit theory" construct from a cross-disciplinary perspective. In G. B. Moskowitz (Ed.), *Cognitive social psychology: The Princeton Symposium on the Legacy and Future of Social Cognition* (pp. 143–162). Mahwah, NJ: Erlbaum.

Morris, M. W., Knowles, E. D., Chiu, C., & Hong, Y. (1998). *Culture and responsibility: Judgments of others who obey and disobey authority.* Unpublished manuscript, Stanford Graduate School of Business.

Morris, M. W., & Peng, K. (1994). Culture and cause: American and Chinese attributions for social and physical events. *Journal of Personality and Social Psychology, 67*, 949–971.

Moscovici, S. (1976). *Social influence and social change.* New York: Academic Press.

Moscovici, S. (1980). Toward a theory of conversion behavior. In L. Berkowitz (Ed.), *Advances in experimental social psychology* (Vol. 13, pp. 209–239). New York: Academic Press.

Moscovici, S. (1985a). Innovation and minority influence. In S. Moscovici, G. Mugny, & E. Van Avermaet (Eds.), *Perspectives on minority influence* (pp. 9–51). Cambridge, UK: Cambridge University Press.

Moscovici, S. (1985b). Social influence and conformity. In G. Lindzey & E. Aronson (Eds.), *Handbook of social psychology* (3rd ed., Vol. 2, pp. 347–412). New York: Random House.

Moscovici, S., Lage, S., & Naffrechoux, M. (1969). Influence of a consistent minority on the responses of a majority in a color perception task. *Sociometry, 32*, 365–380.

Moskowitz, G. B. (1993a). Individual differences in social categorization: The effects of personal need for structure on spontaneous trait inferences. *Journal of Personality and Social Psychology,* *65,* 132–142.

Moskowitz, G. B. (1993b). Person organization with a memory set: Are spontaneous trait inferences personality characterizations or behavior labels? *European Journal of Personality, 7,* 195–208.

Moskowitz, G. B. (1996). The mediational effects of attributions and information processing in minority social influence. *British Journal of Social Psychology, 35,* 47–66.

Moskowitz, G. B. (2001). Preconscious control and compensatory cognition. In G. B. Moskowitz (Ed.), *Cognitive social psychology: The Princeton Symposium on the Legacy and Future of Social Cognition* (pp. 333–358). Mahwah, NJ: Erlbaum.

Moskowitz, G. B. (2002). Preconscious effects of temporary goals on attention. *Journal of Experimental Social Psychology, 38,* 397–404.

Moskowitz, G. B., & Chaiken, S. (2001). Mediators of minority social influence: Cognitive processing mechanisms revealed through a persuasion paradigm. In N. de Vries & C. de Dreu (Eds.), *Group innovation: Fundamental and applied perspectives* (pp. 60–90). Oxford: Blackwell.

Moskowitz, G. B., Gollwitzer, P. M., Wasel, W., & Schaal, B. (1999). Preconscious control of stereotype activation through chronic egalitarian goals. *Journal of Personality and Social Psychology, 77,* 167–184.

Moskowitz, G. B., Li, P., & Kirk, E. (2004). The implicit volition model: The invisible goal-tender and the preconscious regulation of temporarily adopted goals. In M. Zanna (Ed.), *Advances in experimental social psychology* (Vol. 36, pp. 317–413). San Diego, CA: Academic Press.

Moskowitz, G. B., & Roman, R. J. (1992). Spontaneous trait inferences as self generated primes: Implications for conscious social judgment. *Journal of Personality and Social Psychology, 62,* 728–738.

Moskowitz, G. B., Salomon, A. R., & Taylor, C. M. (2000). Implicit control of stereotype activation through the preconscious operation of egalitarian goals. *Social Cognition, 18,* 151–177.

Moskowitz, G. B., & Skurnik, I. W. (1999). Contrast effects as determined by the type of prime: Trait versus exemplar primes initiate processing strategies that differ in how accessible constructs are used. *Journal of Personality and Social Psychology, 76,* 911–927.

Moskowitz, G. B., & Uleman, J. S. (1987). *The facilitation and inhibition of spontaneous trait inferences at encoding.* Poster presented at the 95th Annual Convention of the American Psychological Association, New York.

Mugny, G. (1975). Negotiations, image of the other and the process of minority influence. *European Journal of Social Psychology, 5,* 209–229.

Murphy, G. L., & Medin, D. L. (1985). The role of theories in conceptual coherence. *Psychological Review, 92,* 289–316.

Murphy, S. T., & Zajonc, R. B. (1993). Affect, cognition, and awareness: Affective priming with optimal and suboptimal stimulus exposures. *Journal of Personality and Social Psychology, 64,* 723–739.

Neely, J. (1977). Semantic priming and retrieval from lexical memory: Roles of inhibitionless spreading activation and limitedcapacity attention. *Journal of Experimental Psychology: General, 106*(3), 226–254.

Neill, W. T., Valdes, L. A., & Terry, K. M. (1995). Selective attention and the inhibitory control of cognition. In F. N. Dempster & C. J. Brainerd (Eds.), *Interference and inhibition in cognition* (pp. 207–261). San Diego, CA: Academic Press.

Nemeth, C. J., Mayseless, O., Sherman, J., & Brown, Y. (1990). Exposure to dissent and recall of information. *Journal of Personality and Social Psychology, 58,* 429–437.

Neuberg, S. L. (1989). The goal of forming accurate impressions during social interactions: Attenuating impact of negative expectancies. *Journal of Personality and Social Psychology, 56,* 374–386.

Neuberg, S. L., & Fiske, S. T. (1987). Motivation influences on impression formation: Outcome dependency, accuracy-driven attention, and individuating processes. *Journal of Personality and Social Psychology, 53,* 431–444.

Neuberg, S. L., Judice, T. N., & West, S. G. (1997). What the need for closure scale measures and what it does not: Toward differentiating among related epistemic motives. *Journal of Personality and Social Psychology, 72,* 1396–1412.

Neuberg, S. L., & Newsom, J. T. (1993). Individual differences in chronic motivation to simplify: Personal need for structure and social-cognitive processing. *Journal of Personality and Social Psychology, 65,* 113–131.

Newman, L. S. (1993). How individualists interpret behavior: Idiocentrism and spontaneous trait inference. *Social Cognition, 11,* 243–269.

Newman, L. S. (2001). A cornerstone for the science of interpersonal behavior?: Person perception and person memory, past, present, and future. In G. B. Moskowitz (Ed.), *Cognitive social psychology: The Princeton Symposium on the Legacy and Future of Social Cognition* (pp. 191–210). Mahwah, NJ: Erlbaum.

Newman, L. S., & Uleman, J. S. (1990). Assimilation and contrast effects in spontaneous trait inferences. *Personality and Social Psychology Bulletin, 16,* 224–240.

Niedenthal, P. M., Halberstadt, J. B., & Setterlund, M. B. (1997). Being happy and seeing "happy": Emotional state facilitates visual encoding. *Cognition and Emotion, 11,* 403–432.

Nisbett, R. E., & Ross, L. (1980). *Human inference.* Englewood Cliffs, NJ: Prentice-Hall.

Nisbett, R. E., & Wilson, T. D. (1977). Telling more than we can know: Verbal reports on mental processes. *Psychological Review, 84,* 231–259.

Nolen-Hoeksema, S., Girgus, J. S., & Seligman, M. E. P. (1992). Predictors and consequences of childhood depressive symptoms. *Journal of Abnormal Psychology, 101,* 405–422.

Norem, J. K., & Cantor, N. (1986). Defensive pessimism: "Harnessing" anxiety as motivation. *Journal of Personality and Social Psychology, 55,* 1208–1217.

Norenzayan, A., Choi, I., & Nisbett, R. (1999). Eastern and Western perceptions of causality for social behavior: Lay theories about personalities and situations. In D. A. Prentice & D. T. Miller (Eds.), *Cultural divides: Understanding and overcoming group conflict* (pp. 239–242). New York: Russell Sage Foundation.

Nosofsky, R. M., Palmeri, T. J., & McKinley, S. C. (1994). Rule-plus-exception model of classification learning. *Psychological Review, 101,* 53–79.

Nuttin, J. M. (1985). Narcissism beyond Gestalt and awareness: The name letter effect. *European Journal of Social Psychology, 15,* 353–361.

Öhman, A. (1993). Fear and anxiety as emotional phenomena: Clinical phenomenology, evolutionary perspectives, and information processing mechanisms. In M. Lewis & J. M. Haviland (Eds.), *Handbook of emotions.* New York: Guilford Press.

Olson, J. M., Roese, N. J., & Zanna, M. P. (1996). Expectancies. In E. T. Higgins & A. W. Kruglanski (Eds.), *Social psychology: Handbook of basic principles* (pp. 211–238). New York: Guilford Press.

Operario, D., & Fiske, S. T. (2001). Ethnic identity moderates perceptions of prejudice: Judgments of personal versus group discrimination and subtle versus blatant bias. *Personality and Social Psychology Bulletin, 27,* 550–561.

Osgood, E. E., & Tannenbaum, P. H. (1955). The principle of congruity in the prediction of attitude change. *Psychological Review, 62,* 42–55.

Ostrom, T. M., Pryor, J. B., & Simpson, D. D. (1981). The organization of social information. In E. T. Higgins, C. P. Herman, & M. P. Zanna (Eds.), *Social cognition: The Ontario Symposium* (Vol. 1, pp. 1–38). Hillsdale, NJ: Erlbaum.

O'Sullivan, M., Ekman, P., Friesen, W. V., & Scherer, K. R. (1985). What you say and how you say it: The contribution of speech content and voice quality to judgments of others. *Journal of Personality and Social Psychology, 48*(1), 54–62.

Otten, S., & Moskowitz, G. B. (2000). Evidence for implicit evaluative ingroup bias: Affect-biased spontaneous trait inference in a minimal group paradigm. *Journal of Experimental Social Psychology, 36,* 77–89.

Park, B. (1989). Trait attributes as on-line organizers in person impressions. In J. N. Bassili (Ed.), *On-line cognition in person perception* (pp. 39–60). Hillsdale, NJ: Erlbaum.

Parkin, A. (1979). Specifying levels of processing. *Quarterly Journal of Experimental Psychology, 31,* 175–195.

Peirce, C. (1877). The fixation of belief. *Popular Science Monthly.*

Pelham, B. W., Mirenberg, M. C., & Jones, J. T. (2002). Why Susie sells seashells by the seashore: Implicit egotism and major life decisions. *Journal of Personality and Social Psychology, 82*(4), 469–487.

Pérez, J. A., Falomir, J. M., & Mugny, G. (1995). Internalization of conflict and attitude change. *European Journal of Social Psychology, 25,* 117–124.

Pettigrew, T. F. (1979). The ultimate attribution error: Extending Allport's cognitive analysis of prejudice. *Personality and Social Psychology Bulletin, 55,* 461–476.

Pettigrew, T. F. (1997). Generalized intergroup contact effects on prejudice. *Personality and Social Psychology Bulletin, 23,* 173–185.

Petty, R. E., & Cacioppo, J. T. (1986). The elaboration likelihood model of persuasion. In L. Berkowitz (Ed.), *Advances in experimental social psychology* (Vol. 19, pp. 123–205). New York: Academic Press.

Petty, R. E., Cacioppo, J. T., & Schumann, D. (1983). Central and peripheral routes to advertising effectiveness: The moderating role of involvement. *Journal of Consumer Research, 10,* 135–146.

Piaget, J. (1932). *The moral judgment of the child.* London: Kegan Paul.

Piaget, J. (1970). *Structuralism* (C. Maschler, Ed. & Trans.). New York: Basic Books.

Pinker, S. (1997). *How the mind works.* New York: Norton.

Pittman, T. S., & D'Agostino, P. R. (1989). Motivation and Cognition: Control deprivation and the nature of subsequent information processing. *Journal of Experimental Social Psychology, 25,* 465–480.

Pittman, T. S., & Heller, J. F. (1987). Social motivation. *Annual Review of Psychology, 38,* 461–489.

Pittman, T. S., & Pittman, N. L. (1980). Deprivation of control and the attribution process. *Journal of Personality and Social Psychology, 39,* 377–389.

Plant, E. A., & Devine, P. G. (1998). Internal and external motivation to respond without prejudice. *Journal of Personality and Social Psychology, 75,* 811–832.

Posner, M. I., & Snyder, C. R. R. (1975). Attention and cognitive control. In R. L. Solso (Ed.), *Information processing and cognition: The Loyola Symposium* (pp. 55–85). Hillsdale, NJ: Erlbaum.

Postman, L., Bruner, J. S., & McGinnies, E. (1948). Personal factors as selective factors in perception. *Journal of Abnormal and Social Psychology, 43,* 142–154.

Pratto, F., & John, O. P. (1991). Automatic vigilance: The attention-grabbing power of negative social information. *Journal of Personality and Social Psychology, 61,* 380–391.

Pratto, F., Sidanius, J., Stallworth, L. M., & Malle, B. F. (1994). Social dominance orientation: A personality varivale predicting social and political attitudes. *Journal of Personality and Social Psychology, 67,* 741–763.

Prentice, D. A. (1987). Psychological correspondences of attitudes, possessions, and values. *Journal of Personality and Social Psychology, 53,* 993–1003.

Prentice, D. A. (1990). Familiarity and differences in self- and other-representations. *Journal of Personality and Social Psychology, 59,* 369–383.

Pronin, E., Lin, D. Y., & Ross, L. (2002). The bias blind spot: Perceptions of bias in self versus others. *Personality and Social Psychology Bulletin, 28,* 369–381.

Quattrone, G. A. (1982). Overattribution and unit formation: When behavior engulfs the person. *Journal of Personality and Social Psychology, 42,* 593–607.

Read, S. J., & Miller, L. C. (1989). Interpersonalism: Toward a goal-based theory of persons in relationships. In L. Pervin (Ed.), *Goal concepts in personality and social psychology* (pp. 413–472). Hillsdale, NJ: Erlbaum.

Redelmeier, D. A., & Kahneman, D. (1996). Patients' memories of painful medical treatments: Real-time and retrospective evaluations of two minimally invasive procedures. *Pain, 66*(1), 3–8.

Redelmeier, D. A., & Shafir, E. (1995). Medical decision making in situations that offer multiple alternatives. *Journal of the American Medical Association, 273*(4), 302–305.

Reeder, G. D., & Brewer, M. B. (1979). A schematic model of dispositional attribution in interpersonal perception. *Psychological Review, 86*, 61–79.

Regan, B. C., Julliot, C., Simmen, B., Vienot, F., Charles-Dominique, P., & Mollon, J. D. (1998). Frugivory and colour vision in Alouatta seniculus, a trichromatic platyrrhine monkey. *Vision Research, 38*, 3321–3327.

Regan, D. T., & Totten, J. (1975). Empathy and attribution: Turning observers into actors. *Journal of Personality and Social Psychology, 32*, 850–856.

Rhee, E., Uleman, J. S., Lee, H. K., & Roman, R. J. (1995). Spontaneous self-descriptions and ethnic identities in individualistic and collectivistic cultures. *Journal of Personality and Social Psychology, 69*, 142–152.

Richardson, D. R., Hammock, G. S., Smith, S. M., Gardner, W., & Signon, S. (1994). Empathy as a cognitive inhibitor of interpersonal aggression. *Aggressive Behavior, 20*(4), 275–289.

Rips, L. J., & Collins, A. (1993). Categories and resemblance. *Journal of Experimental Psychology, 122*, 468–486.

Robins, R. W., & John, O. P. (1997). Effects of visual perspective and narcissism on self-perception: Is seeing believing? *Psychological Science, 8*(1), 37–42.

Robinson, R. J., Keltner, D., Ward, A., & Ross, L. (1995). Actual versus assumed differences in construal: "Naive realism" in intergroup perception and conflict. *Journal of Personality and Social Psychology, 68*, 404–417.

Rogers, T. B., Kuiper, N. A., & Kirker, W. S. (1977). Self-reference and the encoding of personal information. *Journal of Personality and Social Psychology, 35*, 677–688.

Rokeach, M. (1973). *The nature of human prejudice.* New York: Free Press.

Rosch, E. (1973). Natural categories. *Cognitive Psychology, 4*, 329–350.

Rosch, E. (1975). Cognitive representations of semantic categories. *Journal of Experimental Psychology, 104*, 192–233.

Rosch, E., & Mervis, C. (1975). Family resemblances: Studies in the internal structure of categories. *Cognitive Psychology, 7*, 573–605.

Rosen, S., & Tesser, A. (1970). On reluctance to communicate undesirable information: The MUM effect. *Sociometry, 33*, 253–263.

Rosenberg, S., & Sedlak, A. (1972). Structural representations of implicit personality theory. In L. Berkowitz (Ed.), *Advances in experimental social psychology* (Vol. 6, pp. 235–297). New York: Academic Press.

Rosenthal, R., & Jacobson, L. (1968). *Pygmalion in the classroom: Teacher expectation and pupils' intellectual development.* New York: Holt, Rinehart & Winston.

Roskos-Ewoldsen, D. R., & Fazio, R. H. (1992). On the orienting value of attitudes: Attitude accessibility as a determinant of an object's attraction of visual attention. *Journal of Personality and Social Psychology, 63*, 198–211.

Ross, L. (1977). The intuitive psychologist and his shortcomings: Distortions in the attribution process. In L. Berkowitz (Ed.), *Advances in experimental social psychology* (Vol. 10, pp. 174–221). New York: Academic Press.

Ross, L., Amabile, T. M., & Steinmetz, J. L. (1977). Social roles, social control, and biases in social-perception processes. *Journal of Personality and Social Psychology, 35*, 484–494.

Ross, L., Greene, D., & House, P. (1977). The false consensus effect: An egocentric bias in social perception and attribution processes. *Journal of Experimental Social Psychology, 13*(3), 279–301.

Ross, L., Lepper, M. R., & Hubbard, M. (1975). Perseverance in self-perception and social perception: Biased attributional processes in the debriefing paradigm. *Journal of Personality and Social Psychology, 32*, 880–892.

Ross, L., & Nisbett, R. E. (1991). *The person and the situation: Perspectives of social psychology.* New York: McGraw-Hill.

Rothbart, M., Evans, M., & Fulero, S. (1979). Recall for confirming events: Memory processes and the maintenance of social stereotypes. *Journal of Experimental Social Psychology, 15,* 343–355.

Rothbart, M., Fulero, S., Jensen, C., Howard, J., & Birrell, B. (1978). From individual to group impressions: Availability heuristics in stereotype formation. *Journal of Experimental Social Psychology, 14,* 237–255.

Rothbart, M., Sriram, N., & Davis-Stitt, C. (1996). The retrieval of typical and atypical category members. *Journal of Experimental Social Psychology, 32,* 1–29.

Rotter, J. B. (1966). Generalized expectancies for internal versus external control of reinforcement. *Psychological Monographs, 80*(1, Whole No. 609).

Rudman, L. A., Greenwald, A. G., Mellott, D. S., & Schwartz, J. L. K. (1999). Measuring the automatic components of prejudice: Flexibility and generality of the implicit association test. *Social Cognition, 17,* 437–465.

Ruggiero, K. M., & Taylor, D. M. (1995). Coping with discrimination: How disadvantaged group members perceive the discrimination that confronts them. *Journal of Personality and Social Psychology, 68,* 826–838.

Ryle, G. (1949). *The concept of mind.* London: Hutchinson.

Sachs, S. (2003, April 4). Arab media portray war as killing field. *New York Times.*

Sanderson, C. A., & Cantor, N. (1995). Social dating goals in late adolescence: Implications for safer sexual activity. *Journal of Personality and Social Psychology, 68*(6), 1121–1134.

Savitsky, K., & Gilovich, T. (1998, February). *Speech anxiety and the illusion of transparency.* Paper presented at the meeting of the Eastern Psychological Association, Boston.

Schank, R. C. (1982). *Dynamic memory: A theory of reminding and learning in computers and people.* New York: Cambridge University Press.

Schank, R. C., & Abelson, R. P. (1977). *Scripts, plans, goals, and understanding: An inquiry into human knowledge structures.* Hillsdale, NJ: Erlbaum.

Schkade, D. A., & Kahneman, D. (1997). Does living in California make people happy?: A focusing illusion in judgments of life satisfaction. *Psychological Science, 9*(5), 340–346.

Schlenker, B. R. (1980). *Impression management: The self-concept, social identity, and interpersonal relations.* Monterey, CA: Brooks/Cole.

Schlenker, B. R., & Leary, M. R. (1982). Social anxiety and self-presentation: A conceptual model. *Psychological Bulletin, 92*(3), 641–669.

Schlenker, B. R., & Leary, M. R. (1985). Social anxiety and communication about the self. *Journal of Language and Social Psychology, 4,* 171–192.

Schlenker, B. R., Phillips, S. T., Boniecki, K. A., & Schlenker, D. R. (1995). Championship pressures: Choking or triumphing in one's own territory? *Journal of Personality and Social Psychology, 68*(4), 632–643.

Schneider, D. J. (1973). Implicit personality theory: A review. *Psychological Bulletin, 79,* 294–309.

Schneider, D. J., & Blankmeyer, B. L. (1983). Prototype salience and implicit personality theories. *Journal of Personality and Social Psychology, 44*(4), 712–722.

Schneider, D. J., Hastorf, A. H., & Ellsworth, P. C. (1979). *Person perception* (2nd ed.). Reading, MA: Addison-Wesley.

Schneider, W., & Shiffrin, R. M. (1977). Controlled and automatic human information processing: I. Detection, search, and attention. *Psychological Review, 84,* 1–66.

Schuman, H., & Presser, S. (1981). *Questions and answers: Experiments on question form, wording, and context in attitude surveys.* New York: Academic Press.

Schwarz, N. (1999). Self reports: How the questions shape the answers. *American Psychologist, 54,* 93–105.

Schwarz, N., Bless, H., Strack, F., Klumpp, G., Rittenauer Schatka, H., & Simons, A. (1991). Ease of retrieval as information: Another look at the availability heuristic. *Journal of Personality and Social Psychology, 61,* 195–202.

Schwarz, N., & Clore, G. L. (1983). Mood, misattribution, and judgments of well-being: Informative and directive functions of affective states. *Journal of Personality and Social Psychology, 45,* 513–523.

Schwarz, N., & Clore, G. L. (1988). How do I feel about it?: Informative functions of affective states. In K. Fiedler & J. Forgas (Eds.), *Affect, cognition, and social behavior* (pp. 44–62). Toronto: Hogrefe.

Schwarz, N., Knäuper, B., Hippler, H., Noelle-Neumann, E., & Clark, F. (1991). Rating scales: Numeric values may change the meaning of scale labels. *Public Opinion Quarterly, 55*(4), 570–582.

Schwarz, N., Strack, F., & Mai, H. (1991). Assimilation and contrast effects in part–whole question sequences: A conversational logic analysis. *Public Opinion Quarterly, 55*(1), 3–23.

Schwarz, N., Strack, F., Müller, G., & Chassein, B. (1988). The range of response alternatives may determine the meaning of the question: Further evidence on informative functions of response alternatives, *Social Cognition, 6*(2), 107–117.

Sedikides, C. (1990). Effects of fortuitously activated constructs versus activated communication goals on person impressions. *Journal of Personality and Social Psychology, 58*, 397–408.

Sedikides, C. (1993). Assessment, enhancement, and verification determinants of the self-evaluation process. *Journal of Personality and Social Psychology, 65*, 317–338.

Sedikides, C., & Anderson, C. A. (1994). Causal perceptions of intertrait relations: The glue that holds person types together. *Personality and Social Psychology Bulletin, 20*, 294–302.

Sedikides, C., & Strube, M. J. (1997). Self-evaluation: To thine own self be good, to thine own self be sure, to thine own self be true, and to thine own self be better. In M. P. Zanna (Ed.), *Advances in experimental social psychology* (Vol. 29, pp. 209–227). San Diego, CA: Academic Press.

Seligman, C., Finegan, J. E., Hazlewood, J. D., & Wilkinson, M. (1985). Manipulating attributions for profit: A field test of the effects of attributions on behavior. *Social Cognition, 3*(3), 313–321.

Seligman, M. E. P. (1975). *Helplessness: On depression, development, and death*. San Francisco: Freeman.

Seligman, M. E. P. (1991). *Learned optimism*. New York: Knopf.

Shafir, E. (1993). Choosing versus rejecting: Why some options are both better and worse than others. *Memory and Cognition, 21*, 546–556.

Shah, J. (2003). Automatic for the people: How representations of significant others implicitly affect goal pursuit. *Journal of Personality and Social Psychology, 84*, 661–681.

Shah, J., Higgins, T., & Friedman, R. S. (1998). Performance incentives and means: How regulatory focus influences goal attainment. *Journal of Personality and Social Psychology, 74*, 285–293.

Shakespeare, W. (1974). Hamlet. In G. B. Evans (Ed.), *The Riverside Shakespeare* (pp. 1135–1197). Boston: Houghton Mifflin. (Original work published 1602)

Sherif, M. (1935). A study of some social factors in perception. *Archives of Psychology, 27* (187), 1–60.

Sherif, M. (1936). *The psychology of social norms*. New York: Harper.

Sherif, M. (1966). *The psychology of social norms*. Oxford: Harper Torchbooks.

Sherif, M., & Hovland, C. I. (1961). *Social judgment: Assimilation and contrast effects in communication and attitude change*. New Haven, CT: Yale University Press.

Sherman, J. W. (2001). The dynamic relationship between stereotype efficiency and mental representation. In G. B. Moskowitz (Ed.), *Cognitive social psychology: The Princeton Symposium on the Legacy and Future of Social Cognition* (pp. 177–190). Mahwah, NJ: Erlbaum.

Sherman, J. W. (1996). Development and mental representation of stereotypes. *Journal of Personality and Social Psychology, 70*, 1126–1141.

Sherman, J. W., & Bessenoff, G. R. (1999). Stereotypes as source monitoring cues: On the interaction bewteen episodic and semantic memory. *Psychological Science, 10*, 100–110.

Sherman, J. W., & Frost, L. A. (2000). On the encoding of stereotyperelevant information under cognitive load. *Personality and Social Psychology Bulletin, 26*, 26–34.

Sherman, J. W., & Klein, S. B. (1994). Development and representation of personality impressions. *Journal of Personality and Social Psychology, 67*, 972–983.

Sherman, J. W., Klein, S. B., Laskey, A., & Wyer, N. A. (1998). Intergroup bias in group judgment processes: The role of behavioral memories. *Journal of Experimental Social Psychology, 34*, 51–65.

Sherman, J. W., Lee, A. Y., Bessenoff, G. R., & Frost, L. A. (1998). Stereotype efficiency reconsidered: Encoding flexibility under cognitive load. *Journal of Personality and Social Psychology, 75*, 589–606

Sherman, S. J., & Fazio, R. H. (1983). Parallels between attitudes and traits as predictors of behavior. *Journal of Personality, 51*(3), 308–345.

Shiffrin, R. M. (1988). Attention. In R. C. Atkinson, R. T. Herrnstein, G. Lindzey, & R. D. Luce (Eds.), *Stevens' handbook of experimental psychology* (2nd ed., Vol. 2, pp. 739–811). New York: Wiley.

Shiffrin, R. M., & Dumais, S. T. (1981). The development of automatism. In J. R. Anderson (Ed.), *Cognitive skills and their acquisition* (pp. 111–140). Hillsdale, NJ: Erlbaum.

Shiffrin, R. M., & Schneider, W. (1977). Controlled and automatic human information processing: II. Perceptual learning, automatic attending, and a general theory. *Psychological Review, 84*, 127–190.

Shuell, T. J. (1977). Clustering and organization in free recall. *Psychological Bulletin, 72*, 353–374.

Shweder, R. A., & Bourne, E. J. (1982). Does the concept of the person vary cross culturally. In A. J. Marsella & G. M. White (Eds.), *Cultural conceptions of mental health and therapy* (pp. 97–137). New York: Kluwer Academic.

Sicoly, F., & Ross, M. (1977). Facilitation of ego-biased attributions by means of self-serving observer feedback. *Journal of Personality and Social Psychology, 35*(10), 734–741.

Sidanius, J., & Pratto, F. (1999). *Social dominance: An intergroup theory of social hierarchy and oppression.* New York: Cambridge University Press.

Simon, L., Greenberg, J., & Brehm, J. (1995). Trivialization: The forgotten mode of dissonance reduction. *Journal of Personality and Social Psychology, 68*(2), 247–260.

Simpson, D. D. (1979). *Four empirical investigations of organization of person information in memory.* Unpublished doctoral dissertation, Ohio State University.

Simpson, J. A., Blackstone, T., & Ickes, W. (1995). When the head protects the heart: Empathic accuracy in dating relationships. *Journal of Personality and Social Psychology, 69*, 629–641.

Skowronski, J. J., & Carlston, D. E. (1989). Negativity and extremity biases in impression formation: A review of explanations. *Psychological Bulletin, 105*, 131–142.

Skurnik, I., Moskowitz, G. B., & Johnson, M. (2004). *Biases in remembering true and false information: Illusions of truth and falseness.* Manuscript submitted for publication.

Sloman, S. A., & Ahn, W. (1999). Feature centrality: Naming versus imagining. *Memory and Cognition, 27*(3), 526–537.

Smeesters, D., Warlop, L., Van Avermaet, E., Corneille, O., & Yzerbyt, V. (2003). Do not prime hawks with doves: The interplay of construct activation and consistency of social value orientation on cooperative behavior. *Journal of Personality and Social Psychology, 84*(5), 972–987.

Smith, E. E., Shoben, E. J., & Rips, L. J. (1974). Structure and process in semantic memory: A featural model for semantic decisions. *Psychological Review, 81*(3), 214–241.

Smith, E. R., Fazio, R. H., & Cejka, M. A. (1996). Accessible attitudes influence categorization of multiply categorizable objects. *Journal of Personality and Social Psychology, 71*(5), 888–898.

Smith, E. R., & Medin, D. L. (1981). *Categories and concepts.* Cambridge, MA: Harvard University Press.

Smith, E. R., & Zarate, M. A. (1992). Exemplar-based model of social judgment. *Psychological Review, 99*, 3–21.

Snowden, R. J. (2002). Visual attention to color: Parvocellular guidance of attentional resources? *Psychological Science, 13*, 180–184.

Snyder, M. L., & Frankel, A. (1976). Observer bias: A stringent test of behavior engulfing the field. *Journal of Personality and Social Psychology, 34*, 857–864.

Snyder, M. L., & Swann, W. B. (1978). Hypotheses testing processes in social interaction. *Journal of Personality and Social Psychology, 36*, 1202–1212.

Snyder, M. L., Tanke, E. D., & Berscheid, E. (1977). Social perception and interpersonal behavior: On the selffulfilling nature of social stereotypes. *Journal of Personality and Social Psychology, 35,* 656–666.

Snyder, M. L., & Uranowitz, S. W. (1978). Reconstructing the past: Some cognitive consequences of person perception. *Journal of Personality and Social Psychology, 36,* 941–950.

Sorrentino, R. M., & Higgins, E. T. (Eds.). (1986). *Handbook of motivation and cognition: Foundations of social behavior* (Vol. 1). New York: Guilford Press.

Sorrentino, R. M., & Short, J. C. (1986). Uncertainty orientation, motivation, and cognition. In R. M. Sorrentino & E. T. Higgins (Eds.), *Handbook of motivation and cognition: Foundations of social behavior* (Vol. 1, pp. 379–403). New York: Guilford Press.

Spencer, S. J., Fein, S., Wolfe, C. T., Fong, C., & Dunn, M. A. (1998). Automatic activation of stereotypes: The role of self-image threat. *Personality and Social Psychology Bulletin, 24,* 1139–1152.

Spencer, S. J., Steele, C. M., & Quinn, D. (1999). Stereotype threat and women's math performance. *Journal of Experimental and Social Psychology, 35,* 4–28.

Spielman, L. A., & Bargh, J. A. (1990). Does the depressive self-schema really exist? In C. D. McCann & N. S. Endler (Eds.), *Depression: New directions in theory, research, and practice* (pp. 111–126). Toronto: Wall & Emerson.

Srull, T. K. (1981). Person memory: Some tests of associative storage and retrieval models. *Journal of Experimental Psychology: Human Learning and Memory, 7,* 440–463.

Srull, T. K. (1983). Organizational and retrieval processes in person memory: An examination of processing objectives, presentation format, and the possible role of self-generated retrieval cues. *Journal of Personality and Social Psychology, 44,* 1157–1170.

Srull, T. K., & Brand, J. F. (1983). Memory for information about persons: The effect of encoding operations on subsequent retrieval. *Journal of Verbal Learning and Verbal Behavior, 22,* 219–230.

Srull, T. K., & Wyer, R. S., Jr. (1979). The role of category accessibility in the interpretation of information about persons: Some determinants and implications. *Journal of Personality and Social Psychology, 37,* 1660–1672.

Srull, T. K., & Wyer, R. S., Jr. (1980). Category accessibility and social perception: Some implications for the study of person memory and interpersonal judgment. *Journal of Personality and Social Psychology, 38,* 841–856.

Srull, T. K., & Wyer, R. S., Jr. (1989). Person memory and judgment. *Psychological Review, 96,* 58–83.

Stangor, C., & Duan, C. (1991). Effects of multiple task demands upon memory for information about social groups. *Journal of Experimental Social Psychology, 27,* 357–378.

Stangor, C., Lynch, L., Duan, C., & Glas, B. (1992). Categorization of individuals on the basis of multiple social features. *Journal of Personality and Social Psychology, 62*(2), 207–218.

Stangor, C., & Ruble, D. N. (1989). Strength of expectancies and memory for social information: What we remember depends on how much we know. *Journal of Experimental Social Psychology, 25,* 18–35.

Stapel, D. A., & Koomen, W. (1997). Using primed exemplars during impression formation: Interpretation or comparison? *European Journal of Social Psychology, 27,* 357–367.

Stapel, D. A., & Koomen, W. (1998). When stereotype activation results in (counter)stereotypical judgments: Priming stereotype-relevant traits and exemplars. *Journal of Experimental Social Psychology, 34,* 136–163.

Stapel, D. A., & Koomen, W. (2001). Let's not forget the past when we go to the future: On our knowledge of knowledge accessibility. In G. B. Moskowitz (Ed.), *Cognitive social psychology: The Princeton Symposium on the Legacy and Future of Social Cognition* (pp. 229–246). Mahwah, NJ: Erlbaum.

Stapel, D. A., Koomen, W., & van der Pligt, J. (1996). The referents of trait inferences: The impact of trait concepts versus actor–trait links on subsequent judgments. *Journal of Personality and Social Psychology, 70,* 437–450.

Stapel, D. A., Koomen, W., & van der Pligt, J. (1997). Categories of category accessibility: The impact of trait concept versus exemplar priming on person judgments. *Journal of Experimental Social Psychology, 33*, 47–76.

Stapel, D. A., & Tesser, A. (2001). Self-activation increases social comparison. *Journal of Personality and Social Psychology, 81*(4), 742–750.

Steele, C. M. (1988). The psychology of self-affirmation: Sustaining the integrity of the self. In L. Berkowitz (Ed.), *Advances in experimental social psychology* (Vol. 21, pp. 261–302). New York: Academic Press.

Steele, C. M. (1997). A threat in the air: How stereotypes shape intellectual identity and performance. *American Psychologist, 52*, 613–629.

Steele, C. M., & Aronson, J. (1995). Stereotype threat and the intellectual test performance of African Americans. *Journal of Personality and Social Psychology, 69*, 797–811.

Steele, C. M., & Lui, T. J. (1983). Dissonance processes as self-affirmation. *Journal of Personality and Social Psychology, 45*, 5–19.

Steinbeck, J. (1962). *Travels with Charley.* New York: Viking Press.

Stevens, L., & Jones, E. E. (1976). Defensive attribution and the Kelley cube. *Journal of Personality and Social Psychology, 34*, 809–820.

Steward, J. M., & Cole, B. L. (1989). The effect of object size on the performance of colour ordering and discrimination task. In B. Drum & G. Verriest (Eds.), *Colour vision deficiencies IX: Proceedings of the 9th Symposium of the International Research Group on Colour Vision Deficiencies* (pp. 79–88). Dordrecht, Netherlands: Kluwer.

Stone, J. (2001). Behavioral discrepancies and the role of construal processes in cognitive dissonance. In G. B. Moskowitz (Ed.), *Cognitive social psychology: The Princeton Symposium on the Legacy and Future of Social Cognition* (pp. 41–58). Mahwah, NJ: Erlbaum.

Stone, J., Aronson, E., Crain, A. L., Winslow, M. P., & Fried, C. B. (1994). Inducing hypocrisy as a means of encouraging young adults to use condoms. *Personality and Social Psychology Bulletin, 20*(1), 116–128.

Stone, J., Lynch, C. I., Sjomeling, M., & Darley, J. M. (1999). Stereotype threat effects on Black and White athletic performance. *Journal of Personality and Social Psychology, 77*(6), 1213–1227.

Stone, J., Wiegand, A. W., Cooper, J., & Aronson, E. (1997). When exemplification fails: Hypocrisy and the motive for self-integrity. *Journal of Personality and Social Psychology, 72*(1), 54–65.

Storms, M. D. (1973). Videotape in the attribution process: Reversing actors' and observers' points of view. *Journal of Personality and Social Psychology, 27*, 165–175.

Strack, F., Schwarz, N., Bless, H., Kübler, A., & Wänke, M. (1993). Awareness of the influence as a determinant of assimilation versus contrast. *European Journal of Social Psychology, 23*, 53–62.

Strack, F., Schwarz, N., & Wänke, M. (1991). Semantic and pragmatic aspects of context effects in social and psychological research. *Social Cognition, 9*(1), 111–125.

Strahan, E. J., Spencer, S. J., & Zanna, M. P. (2002). Subliminal priming and persuasion: Striking while the iron is hot. *Journal of Experimental Social Psychology, 38*, 556–568.

Stroessner, S. J., & Plaks, J. E. (2001). Illusory correlation and stereotype formation: Tracing the arc of research over a quarter century. In G. B. Moskowitz (Ed.), *Cognitive social psychology: The Princeton Symposium on the Legacy and Future of Social Cognition* (pp. 247–260). Mahwah, NJ: Erlbaum.

Stroop, J. R. (1935). Studies of interference in serial verbal reactions. *Journal of Experimental Psychology, 18*, 643–662.

Sutton, R. M., & McClure, J. (2001). Covariational influences on goal-based explanation: An integrative model. *Journal of Personality and Social Psychology, 80*, 222–236.

Swann, W. B., Jr. (1984). Quest for accuracy in person perception: A matter of pragmatics. *Psychological Review, 91*, 457–477.

Swann, W. B., Jr. (1990). To be adored or to be known?: The interplay of self-enhancement and self-verification. In E. T. Higgins & R. Sorrentino (Eds.), *Handbook of motivation and cognition: Foundations of social behavior* (Vol. 2, pp. 527–561). New York: Guilford Press.

Swann, W. B., Jr., Bosson, J. K., & Pelham, B. W. (2002). Different partners, different selves: Strategic verification of circumscribed identities, *Personality and Social Psychology Bulletin, 28*(9), 1215–1228.

Swann, W. B., Jr., Pelham, B. W., & Krull, D. S. (1989). Agreeable fancy or disagreeable truth?: Reconciling self-enhancement and self-verification. *Journal of Personality and Social Psychology, 57,* 782–791.

Swim, J., Borgida, E., Maruyama, G., & Myers, D. G. (1989). Joan McKay versus John McKay: Do gender stereotypes bias evaluations? *Psychological Bulletin, 105*(3), 409–429.

Tagiuri, R. (1958). Introduction. In R. Tagiuri & L. Petrullo (Eds.), *Person perception and interpersonal behavior* (pp. ix–xvii). Stanford, CA: Stanford University Press.

Tajfel, H. (1969). Cognitive aspects of prejudice. *Journal of Social Issues, 25,* 79–97.

Tajfel, H., Billig, M. G., Bundy, R. P., & Flament, C. (1971). Social categorization and intergroup behavior. *European Journal of Social Psychology, 1,* 149–178.

Tajfel, H., & Turner, J. C. (1979). An integrative theory of intergroup conflict. In W. G. Austin & S. Worchel (Eds.), *The social psychology of intergroup relations* (pp. 33–47). Monterey, CA: Brooks/Cole.

Tajfel, H., & Turner, J. C. (1986). An integrative theory of intergroup relations. In S. Worchel & W. G. Austin (Eds.), *Psychology of intergroup relations* (2nd ed., pp. 7–24). Chicago: Nelson-Hall.

Tajfel, H., & Wilkes, A. L. (1963). Classification and quantitative judgment. *British Journal of Psychology, 54,* 101–114.

Taylor, D. M., & Jaggi, V. (1974). Ethnocentrism and causal attribution in a South Indian context. *Journal of Cross-Cultural Psychology, 5,* 162–171.

Taylor, D. M., & Moghaddam, F. M. (1987). *Theories of intergroup relations: International social psychological perspectives.* New York: Praeger.

Taylor, D. M., Wright, S. C., & Porter, L. E. (1994). Dimensions of perceived discrimination: The personal/group discrimination discrepancy. In M. P. Zanna & J. M. Olson (Eds.), *The psychology of prejudice: The Ontario Symposium* (Vol. 7, pp. 233–255). Hillsdale, NJ: Erlbaum.

Taylor, S. E. (1981). The interface of cognitive and social psychology. In J. H. Harvey (Ed.), *Cognition, social behavior, and the environment* (pp. 189–212). Hillsdale, NJ: Erlbaum.

Taylor, S. E., & Brown J. D. (1988). Illusion and well being: A social psychological perspective in mental health. *Psychological Bulletin, 103,* 193–210.

Taylor, S. E., & Crocker, J. (1981). Schematic bases of social information processing. In E. T. Higgins, P. Herman, & M. Zanna (Eds.), *Social cognition: The Ontario Symposium* (Vol. 1, pp. 89–134). Hillsdale, NJ: Erlbaum.

Taylor, S. E., Crocker, J., Fiske, S. T., Sprinzen, M., & Winkler, J. D. (1979). The generalizability of salience effects. *Journal of Personality and Social Psychology, 31,* 357–368.

Taylor, S. E., & Fiske, S. T. (1975). Point-of-view and perceptions of causality. *Journal of Personality and Social Psychology, 32,* 439–445.

Taylor, S. E., & Fiske, S. T. (1978). Salience, attention, and attribution: Top of the head phenomena. In L. Berkowitz (Ed.), *Advances in experimental social psychology* (Vol. 11, pp. 249–288). New York: Academic Press.

Taylor, S. E., Fiske, S. T., Etcoff, N., & Ruderman, A. (1978). The categorical and contextual bases of person memory and stereotyping. *Journal of Personality and Social Psychology, 36,* 778–793.

Taylor, S. E., Lichtman, R. R., & Wood, J. V. (1984). Attributions, beliefs about control, and adjustment to breast cancer. *Journal of Personality and Social Psychology, 46* (3), 489–502.

Tesser, A. (1988). Toward a self-evaluation maintenance model of social behavior. In L. Berkowitz (Ed.), *Advances in experimental social psychology* (Vol. 21, pp. 181–227). New York: Academic Press.

Tesser, A., & Martin, L. (1996). The psychology of evaluation. In E. T. Higgins & A. W. Kruglanski (Eds.), *Social psychology: Handbook of basic principles* (pp. 400–432). New York: Guilford Press.

Tetlock, P. E. (1983). Accountablity and complexity of thought. *Journal of Personality and Social Psychology, 45,* 74–83.

Tetlock, P. E. (1985). Accountability: The neglected social context of judgment and choice. *Research in Organizational Behavior, 7,* 297–332.

Tetlock, P. E. (1992). The impact of accountability on judgment and choice: Toward a social contingency model. In M. P. Zanna (Ed.), *Advances in experimental social psychology* (Vol. 25, pp. 331–376). San Diego, CA: Academic Press.

Tetlock, P. E., & Kim, J. I. (1987). Accountability and judgment processes in a personality prediction task. *Journal of Personality and Social Psychology, 52,* 700–709.

Thompson, E. P., Roman, R. J., Moskowitz, G. B., Chaiken, S., & Bargh, J. A. (1994). Accuracy motivation attenuates covert priming effects: The systematic reprocessing of social information. *Journal of Personality and Social Psychology, 66,* 259–288.

Thompson, M. M., Naccarato, M. E., & Parker, K. C. H. (1989). *Assessing cognitive needs: The development of the Personal Need for Structure and the Personal Fear of Invalidity Scales.* Paper presented at the annual meeting of the Canadian Psychological Association, Halifax, Nova Scotia, Canada.

Thompson, M. M., Naccarato, M. E., Moskowitz, G. B., & Parker, K. J. (2001). The personal need for structure and personal fear of invalidity measures: Historical perspectives, current applications, and future directions. In G. B. Moskowitz (Ed.), *Cognitive social psychology: The Princeton Symposium on the Legacy and Future of Social Cognition* (pp. 19–40) Mahwah, NJ: Erlbaum.

Thompson, M. M., Zanna, M. P., & Griffin, D. W. (1995). Let's not be indifferent about (attitudinal) ambivalence. In R. E. Petty & J. A. Krosnick (Eds.), *Attitude strength: Antecedents and consequences* (pp. 361–386). Hillsdale, NJ: Erlbaum.

Tipper, S. P. (1985). The negative priming effect: Inhibitory priming by ignored objects. *Quarterly Journal of Experimental Psychology, 37,* 571–590.

Todorov, A., & Uleman, J. S. (2002). Spontaneous trait inferences are bound to actors' faces: Evidence from a false recognition paradigm. *Journal of Personality and Social Psychology, 83,* 1051–1065.

Tolman, E. C. (1925). Purpose and cognition: The determinants of animal learning. *Psychological Review, 32,* 285–297.

Treisman, A., & Geffen, G. (1967). Selective attention: Perception or response? *Quarterly Journal of Experimental Psychology, 19,* 1–17.

Triandis, H. C. (1989). The self and social behavior in differing cultural contexts. *Psychological Review, 96,* 506–520.

Triandis, H. C. (1990). Cross-cultural studies of individualism and collectivism. In J. Berman (Ed.), *Nebraska Symposium on Motivation* (pp. 41–133). Lincoln: University of Nebraska Press.

Triandis, H. C., Bontempo, R., Villareal, M. J., Asai, M., & Lucca, M. (1988). Individualism and collectivism: Cross-cultural perspectives on self-ingroup relationships. *Journal of Personality and Social Psychology, 54*(2), 323–338.

Trope, Y. (1986a). Identification and inferential processes in dispositional attribution. *Psychological Review, 93,* 239–257.

Trope, Y. (1986b). Self-enhancement and self-assessment in achievement behavior. In R. M. Sorrentino & E. T. Higgins (Eds.), *Handbook of motivation and cognition: Foundations of social behavior* (Vol. 1, pp. 350–378). New York: Guilford Press.

Trope, Y., & Alfieri, T. (1997). Effortfulness and flexibility of dispositional judgment processes. *Journal of Personality and Social Psychology, 73,* 662–674.

Trope, Y., & Bassok, M. (1982). Confirmatory and diagnosing strategies in social information gathering. *Journal of Personality and Social Psychology, 43,* 22–34.

Trope, Y., & Liberman, A. (1993). The use of trait conceptions to identify other people's behavior and to draw inferences about their personalities. *Personality and Social Psychology Bulletin, 19,* 553–562.

Trope, Y., & Neter, E. (1994). Reconciling competing motives in self-evaluation: The role of self-control in feedback seeking. *Journal of Personality and Social Psychology, 66,* 646–657.

Trope, Y., & Pesach-Gaunt, R. (1999). A dual-process model of overconfident attributional inferences. In S. Chaiken & Y. Trope (Eds.), *Dual-process theories in social psychology* (pp. 161–178). New York: Guilford Press.

Trope, Y., & Pomerantz, E. M. (1998). Resolving conflicts among self-evaluative motives: Positive experiences as a resource for overcoming defensiveness. *Motivation and Emotion, 22,* 53–72.

Trost, M. R., Maass, A., & Kenrick, D. T. (1992). Minority influence: Personal relevance biases cognitive processes and reverses private acceptance. *Journal of Experimental Social Psychology, 28,* 234–254.

Tulving, E. (1972). Episodic and semantic memory. In E. Tulving & W. Donaldson (Eds.), *Organization of memory.* New York: Academic Press.

Tulving, E., & Pearlstone, Z. (1966). Availability versus accessibility of information in memory for words. *Journal of Verbal Learning and Verbal Behavior, 5,* 381–391.

Tulving, E., & Thomson, D. M. (1973). Encoding specificity and retrieval processes in episodic memory. *Psychological Review, 80,* 352–373.

Tversky, A., & Kahneman, D. (1973). Availability: A heuristic for judging frequency and probability. *Cognitive Psychology, 5,* 207–232.

Tversky, A., & Kahneman, D. (1974). Judgment under uncertainty: Heuristics and biases. *Science, 185,* 1124–1131.

Tversky, A., & Kahneman, D. (1981). The framing of decisions and the psychology of choice. *Science, 211,* 453–458.

Tversky, A., & Kahneman, D. (1982). Judgments of and by representativeness. In D. Kahneman, P. Slovic, A. Tversky (Eds.), *Judgment under uncertainty: Heuristics and biases* (pp. 84–98). Canbridge, UK: Cambridge University Press.

Tyler, T., Degoey, P., & Smith, H. (1996). Understanding why the justice of group procedures matters: A test of the psychological dynamics of the groupvalue model. *Journal of Personality and Social Psychology, 70*(5), 913–930.

Uleman, J. S., Hon, A., Roman, R. J., & Moskowitz, G. B. (1996). On-line evidence for spontaneous trait inferences at encoding. *Personality and Social Psychology Bulletin, 22*(4), 377–394.

Uleman, J. S., & Moskowitz, G. B. (1994). Unintended effects of goals on unintended inferences. *Journal of Personality and Social Psychology, 66,* 490–501.

Uleman, J. S., Newman, L. S., & Moskowitz, G. B. (1996). People as flexible interpreters: Evidence and issues from spontaneous trait inference. In M. Zanna (Ed.), *Advances in experimental social psychology* (Vol. 28, pp. 211–280). San Diego, CA: Academic Press.

Uleman, J. S., Newman, L., & Winter, L. (1992). Can traits be inferred automatically?: Spontaneous inferences require cognitive capacity at encoding. *Consciousness and Cognition, 1,* 77–90.

Uleman, J. S., Winborne, W. C., Winter, L., & Shechter, D. (1986). Personality differences in spontaneous personality inferences at encoding. *Journal of Personality and Social Psychology, 51,* 396–403.

Vallacher, R. R., & Wegner, D. M. (1985). *A theory of action identification.* Hillsdale, NJ: Erlbaum.

Vallacher, R. R., & Wegner, D. M. (1987). What do people think they're doing?: Action identification and human behavior. *Psychological Review, 94,* 3–15.

Vallacher, R. R., Wegner, D. M., & Samoza, M. P. (1989). That's easy for you to say: Action identification and speech fluency. *Journal of Personality and Social Psychology, 56*(2), 199–208.

Vallone, R. P., Ross, L., & Lepper, M. R. (1985). The hostile media phenomenon: Biased perception and perceptions of media bias in coverage of the Beirut massacre. *Journal of Personality and Social Psychology, 49,* 577–585.

Van Lange, P. A. M., & Semin-Goossens, A. (1998). The boundaries of reciprocal cooperation. *European Journal of Social Psychology, 28*(5), 847–854.

Varey, C. A., & Kahneman, D. (1992). Experiences extended across time: Evaluation of moments and episodes. *Journal of Behavioral Decision Making, 5*(3), 169–185.

Vonk, R. (1999). Effects of outcome dependency on correspondence bias. *Personality and Social Psychology Bulletin, 25*(3), 382–389.

Vonk, R. (2002). Self-serving interpretations of flattery: Why ingratiation works. *Journal of Personality and Social Psychology, 82*(4), 515–526.

Vorauer, J. D. (2001). The other side of the story: Transparency estimation in social interaction. In G. B. Moskowitz (Ed.), *Cognitive social psychology: The Princeton Symposium on the Legacy and Future of Social Cognition* (pp. 261–276). Mahwah, NJ: Erlbaum.

Vorauer, J. D., & Claude, S. (1998). Perceived versus actual transparency of goals in negotiation. *Personality and Social Psychology Bulletin, 24*, 371–385.

Vorauer, J. D., & Ross, M. (1999). Self-awareness and transparency overestimation: Failing to suppress one's self. *Journal of Experimental Social Psychology, 35*, 415–440.

Walster, E., Berscheid, E., & Walster, G. W. (1973). New directions in equity research. *Journal of Personality and Social Psychology, 25*, 151–176

Warren, R. E. (1972). Stimulus encoding and memory. *Journal of Experimental Psychology, 94*, 90–100.

Webster, D. M., & Kruglanski, A. W. (1994). Individual differences in need for cognitive closure. *Journal of Personality and Social Psychology, 67*(6), 1049–1062.

Webster's new world dictionary (2nd college ed.). (1986). New York: Prentice Hall Press.

Wegener, D. T., Dunn, M., & Tokusato, D. (2001). The flexible correction model: Phenomenology and the use of naive theories in avoiding or removing bias. In G. B. Moskowitz (Ed.), *Cognitive social psychology: The Princeton Symposium on the Legacy and Future of Social Cognition* (pp. 277–291). Mahwah, NJ: Erlbaum.

Wegener, D. T., & Petty, R. E. (1995). Flexible correction processes in social judgment: The role of naive theories in corrections for perceived bias. *Journal of Personality and Social Psychology, 68*, 36–51.

Wegener, D. T., Petty, R. E., & Dunn, M. (1998). The metacognition of bias correction: Naive theories of bias and the flexible correction model. In V. Yzerbyt, G. Lories, & B. Dardenne (Eds.), *Metacognition: Cognitive and social dimensions* (pp. 202–227). London: Sage.

Wegner, D. M. (1992). You can't always think what you want: Problems in the suppression of unwanted thoughts. In M. Zanna (Ed.), *Advances in experimental social psychology* (Vol. 25, pp. 193–225). San Diego, CA: Academic Press.

Wegner, D. M. (1994). Ironic processes of mental control. *Psychological Review, 101*, 34–52.

Wegner, D. M., Ansfield, M., & Pilloff, D. (1998). The putt and the pendulum: Ironic effects of the mental control of action. *Psychological Science, 9*(3), 196–199.

Wegner, D. M., & Bargh, J. A. (1998). Control and automaticity in social life. In D. T. Gilbert, S. T. Fiske, & G. Lindzey (Eds.), *The handbook of social psychology* (4th ed., Vol. 1, pp. 446–496). Boston: McGraw-Hill.

Wegner, D. M., & Erber, R. (1992). The hyperaccessibility of suppressed thoughts. *Journal of Personality and Social Psychology, 63*, 903–912.

Wegner, D. M., Schneider, D. J., Carter, S., III, & White, L. (1987). Paradoxical effects of thought suppression. *Journal of Personality and Social Psychology, 58*, 409–418.

Wegner, D. M., & Vallacher, R. R. (1977). *Implicit psychology: An introduction to social cognition.* London: Oxford University Press.

Weiner, B. (1985a). An attributional theory of achievement motivation and emotion. *Psychological Review, 92*, 548–573.

Weiner, B. (1985b). "Spontaneous" causal thinking. *Psychological Bulletin, 97*, 74–84.

Weinstein, N. D. (1980). Unrealistic optimism about future life events. *Journal of Personality and Social Psychology, 39*, 806–820.

Wellman, H. M. (1990). *The child's theory of mind.* Cambridge, MA: MIT Press.

Wellman, H. M., & Bartsch, K. (1990). Three-year-olds understand belief: A reply to Perner. *Cognition, 33*(3), 321–326.

Wells, G. L., & Gavanski, I. (1989). Mental simulation of causality. *Journal of Personality and Social Psychology, 56*, 161–169.

Wheeler, S. C., Jarvis, W. B. G., & Petty, R. E. (2001). Think unto others: The self-destructive impact of negative racial stereotypes. *Journal of Experimental Social Psychology, 37*(2), 173–180.

White, R. W. (1959). Motivation reconsidered: The concept of competence. *Psychological Review, 66,* 296–333.

Whittlesea, B. W. A., & Williams, L. D. (2000). The source of feelings of familiarity: The discrepancy–attribution hypothesis. *Journal of Experimental Psychology: Learning, Memory, and Cognition, 26*(3), 547–565.

Whittlesea, B. W. A., & Williams, L. D. (2001). The discrepancy-attribution hypothesis: I. The heuristic basis of feelings and familiarity. *Journal of Experimental Psychology: Learning, Memory, and Cognition, 27,* 3–13.

Whorf, B. L. (1956). *Language, thought, and reality: Selected writings.* Cambridge, MA: Technology Press of Massachusetts Institute of Technology.

Wicklund, R. A., & Gollwitzer, P. M. (1982). *Symbolic self-completion.* Hillsdale, NJ: Erlbaum.

Wigboldus, D. H. J., Dijksterhuis, A., & Van Knippenberg, A. (2003). When stereotypes get in the way: Stereotypes obstruct stereotype-inconsistent trait inferences. *Journal of Personality and Social Psychology, 84*(3), 470–484.

Wigboldus, D. H. J., Semin, G. R., & Spears, R. (2000). How do we communicate stereotypes?: Linguistic bases and inferential consequences. *Journal of Personality and Social Psychology, 78*(1), 5–18.

Wilson, T. D., & Brekke, N. (1994). Mental contamination and mental correction: Unwanted influences on judgments and evaluations. *Psychological Bulletin, 116,* 117–142.

Wimmer, H., & Perner, J. (1983). Beliefs about beliefs: Representation and constraining function of wrong beliefs in young children's understanding of deception. *Cognition, 13,* 103–128.

Winter, L., & Uleman, J. S. (1984). When are social judgments made?: Evidence for the spontaneousness of trait inferences. *Journal of Personality and Social Psychology, 47,* 237–252.

Wittenbrink, B., Gist, P. L., & Hilton, J. L. (1997). Structural properties of stereotypic knowledge and their influences on the construal of social situations. *Journal of Personality and Social Psychology, 72,* 526–543.

Wittenbrink, B., Judd, C. M., & Park, B. (1997). Evidence for racial prejudice at the implicit level and its relationship with questionnaire measures. *Journal of Personality and Social Psychology, 72,* 262–274.

Wood, W., & Eagly, A. H. (1981). Stages in the analysis of persuasive messages: The role of causal attributions and message comprehension. *Journal of Personality and Social Psychology, 40,* 246–259.

Wood, W., Pool, G. J., Leck, K., & Purvis, D. (1996). Self definition, defensive processing, and influence: The normative impact of majority and minority groups. *Journal of Personality and Social Psychology, 71,* 1181–1193.

Word, C. O., Zanna, M. P., & Cooper, J. (1974). The nonverbal mediation of self-fulfilling prophecies in interracial interaction. *Journal of Experimental Social Psychology, 10,* 109–120.

Wortman, C. B. (1975). Some determinants of perceived control. *Journal of Personality and Social Psychology, 31,* 282–294.

Wortman, C. B., & Silver, R. (1989). The myths of coping with loss. *Journal of Consulting and Clinical Psychology, 57*(3), 349–357.

Wright, E. F., & Wells, G. L. (1988). Is the attitude-attribution paradigm suitable for investigating the dispositional bias? *Personality and Social Psychology Bulletin, 14,* 183–190.

Wright, S. C., Taylor, D. M., & Moghaddam, F. M. (1990). Responding to membership in a disadvantaged group: From acceptance to collective protest. *Journal of Personality and Social Psychology, 58,* 994–1003.

Wundt, W. (1862). *Beiträge zur Theorie der Sinneswahrnehmung.* Leipzig, Germany: C.F. Wintersche Verlagshandlung.

Wyer, R. S., Jr., & Gordon, S. E. (1984). The cognitive representation of social information. In R. S. Wyer, Jr. & T. K. Srull (Eds.), *Handbook of social cognition* (Vol. 2, pp. 73–150). Hillsdale, NJ: Erlbaum.

Wyer, R. S., Jr., & Srull, T. K. (1989). *Memory and cognition in its social context.* Hillsdale, NJ: Erlbaum.

Yzerbyt, V. R., Corneille, O., Dumont, M., & Hahn, K. (2001). The dispositional inference strikes back: Situational focus and dispositional suppression in causal attribution. *Journal of Personality and Social Psychology, 81*(3), 365–376.

Yzerbyt, V. R., Rogier, A., & Fiske, S. T. (1998). Group entitativity and social attribution: On translating situational constraints into stereotypes. *Personality and Social Psychology Bulletin, 24*(10), 1089–1103.

Yzerbyt, V. R., Schadron, G., Leyens, J., & Rocher, S. (1994). Social judgeability: The impact of meta-informational cues on the use of stereotypes. *Journal of Personality and Social Psychology, 66*, 48–55.

Zadny, J. G., & Gerard, H. B. (1974). Attributed intentions and informational selectivity. *Journal of Experimental Social, 10*(1), 34–52.

Zajonc, R. B. (1960). The process of cognitive tuning in communication. *Journal of Abnormal and Social Psychology, 61*, 159–167.

Zajonc, R. B. (1980). Feeling and thinking: Preferences need no inferences. *American Psychologist, 35*, 151–175.

Zanna, M. P., & Cooper, J. (1974). Dissonance and the pill: An attribution approach to studying the arousal properties of dissonance. *Journal of Personality and Social Psychology, 29*, 703–709.

Zebrowitz, L. A. (1997). *Reading faces: Window to the soul?* Boulder, CO: Westview Press.

Zebrowitz, L. A., Andreoletti, C., Collins, M. A., Lee, S. Y., & Blumenthal, J. (1998). Bright, bad, babyfaced boys: Appearance stereotypes do not always yield selffulfilling prophecy effects. *Journal of Personality and Social Psychology, 75*, 1300–1320.

Zeigarnik, B. (1927). Das Behalten erledigter und unerledigter Handlungen [The retention of completed and uncompleted actions]. *Psychologische Forschung, 9*, 1–85.

Zimbardo, P. (1971, October 25). *The psychological power and pathology of imprisonment* (p. 3). Statement prepared for the U. S. House of Representatives Committee on the Judiciary, Subcommittee No. 3: Hearings on Prison Reform, San Francisco.

Zirkel, S. (1992). Developing independence in a life transition: Investing the self in the concerns of the day. *Journal of Personality and Social Psychology, 62*, 506–521.

Author Index

Subject Index

Page numbers followed by an *f* indicate figure; *t* indicate table